CANCER & NATURAL MEDICINE

A Textbook of Basic Science and Clinical Research

NOTICE

Medical knowledge is constantly expanding. As new experimental and clinical experiences are gained, modifications to treatment and research protocols are required. The author and publisher of this book have consulted sources believed to be reliable in their effort to provide information that is complete and true to the body of knowledge available at the time of publication. However, due to the possibility of human error or changes in medical knowledge, neither the author, publisher, nor any other party involved with the publication or preparation of this book warrants that the information contained in this book is fully accurate or complete, and these parties are not responsible for any omissions, errors, or the results obtained from the use of this information. Readers are advised to confirm the information contained in this book with appropriate written sources and experts in the field. This book is not intended as a clinical guide, but rather as a resource for inspiring further medical research.

CANCER & NATURAL MEDICINE

A Textbook of Basic Science and Clinical Research

John Boik

Oregon Medical Press

CANCER & NATURAL MEDICINE: A Textbook of Basic Science and Clinical Research

Oregon Medical Press
315 10th Avenue North
Princeton, Minnesota 55371 USA
Phone and fax: (763) 389-0768.
www.ompress.com
sales@ompress.com

Quantity discounts and single orders are available from the publisher.

Cover design: Jody Turner-Cheung

Publisher's Cataloging in Publication (Prepared by Quality Books Inc.)

Boik, John.
    Cancer & natural medicine : a textbook of basic science and
clinical research / John Boik.
    p. cm.
    Includes biographical references and index.
    LCCN: 95-69639
    ISBN 0-9648280-0-6

    1. Cancer--Alternative treatment. 2. Alternative medicine.
I. Title.

RC271.A62B65 1996   616.99'406
                               QBI96-20101

TABLE OF CONTENTS

PREFACE

Why this book and why this author? Two and a half years ago I developed a strong interest in the effects of natural medicine on cancer patients as an outgrowth of my general clinical work. The few books available on the subject did not satisfy my hunger for knowledge and I soon realized that the comprehensive text I was hoping to find simply did not exist. After some preliminary searches on the National Library of Medicine online data base (Medline), I believed I had hit the jackpot. It didn't take long to collect a few dozen studies that suggested certain natural agents may have some efficacy in cancer treatment. Armed with this information, I began to write an article on the subject. As I was writing, a few more questions arose and I continued my literature searches. New information begot more questions and, before I knew it, the article turned into a booklet, and the booklet into a book. Now 1,200 studies later, I believe I am ready to present to my peers the book I was hoping to find—a comprehensive review of the basic principles of cancer and natural medicine. I stress the word "basic" because, from the standpoint of conventional oncology, the discussions contained in this book on the mechanisms of cancer initiation and progression can only be considered entry level.

It is my hope that this book provides practitioners not trained in oncology with enough background information to understand the principles by which natural anticancer agents may work. Likewise, it is my hope that the book provides practitioners trained in oncology with enough background information to assess the potential for, and the contraindications of natural agents that their patients may be receiving. Above all, it is my hope that this book inspires further research into the use of natural agents in cancer treatment.

A number of items are discussed below that will help the reader to understand the structure and content of this book.

- First, this book contains at least one obvious bias. Although the subject of cancer and natural medicine can be approached from numerous angles, the approach used in this book reflects my training and interest in Traditional Chinese Medicine (TCM), in particular, TCM herbal medicine. To assist those readers who are not familiar with TCM, Chapter 10 provides an overview of its basic theories, especially as they relate to cancer.
- This book is roughly divided into four parts. Part I (Chapters 1-8) provides a discussion of biomedical mechanisms by which cancer is initiated and progresses. Natural agents that may affect these mechanisms are discussed where appropriate. Part II (Chapters 9-10) discusses the treatment of cancer in conventional medicine and in TCM. Part III (Chapters 11-16) discusses the effects of individual agents on cancer. These agents include herbs, dietary components, vitamins, acupuncture, and others. Lastly, Part IV (Chapter 17) summarizes the actions of natural agents previously introduced and discusses their potential clinical use.
- When reviewing studies an attempt was made to identify the exact Latin binomial for each botanical agent discussed. However, the nomenclature used in many studies was vague and exact identification was not always possible. Some studies referred to herbs only by their Mandarin or pharmaceutical names. Usage of these names is inexact since these names can, in some cases, refer to multiple plants (usually multiple species, but in some cases multiple genus). In these cases, the binomial for the most commonly used plant source was estimated and reported.
- The studies on natural agents reported in this book are by no means exhaustive. The primary source of information used to obtain these studies was the National Library of Medicine data base. This data base contains journal citations from around the world, including a number of Chinese journals. Although it is perhaps the largest medical database available, a number of pertinent international studies may not be entered into its files. It is possible, therefore, that some prominent studies on the subject are not included in this book.
- Within the text, individual herbs are discussed according to their biomedical actions. Although it is not clear from this style of presentation, I believe that optimum results will be achieved when herbs and other agents are used within the context of formulas, as is common practice in TCM. In TCM, single agents are rarely prescribed. Rather, the practitioner chooses combinations of agents that are compatible with the patient's overall condition (from a conventional as well as TCM perspective). Agents are also chosen to be compatible, if not synergistic, with one another.
- The fields of oncology and natural medicine are constantly expanding. Tomorrow I will surely find new information that I would like to have included in this book. Therefore, if there is sufficient interest from the community, I plan to publish a periodic newsletter discussing new data. Topics may include new research, clinical applications, research grants, research protocols, toxicity data, and theoretical

insights. Please contact me at the address provided on page *iv* if you would like to be on the mailing list or are interested in receiving the newsletter. I also welcome comments on and corrections to the material presented in this book.

Lastly, I would like to thank the many people who made this book possible. Thanks to Matthew Suffness, Ph.D., John Prudden M.D., Charles Simone, M.D., Subhuti Dharmananda, Ph.D., James Duke, Ph.D., Peter Kaufman, Ph.D., Michael Gould, Ph.D., John Mark Christensen, Ph.D., Stanley Jacob, M.D., Steve Austin, N.D., William Stetler-Stevenson, M.D., Ph.D., Elizabeth Goldblatt, Ph.D., Natalie Arndt, R.N., LAc., Nicholas Gonzalez, M.D., Tom Moore, Dean P. Jones, Ph.D., and Paul Okunieff, M.D., for answering my questions and/or providing review on pertinent sections.

Thanks to Adriane Fugh-Berman M.D. and Rick Marinelli, N.D., LAc., for their review of early drafts of the manuscript.

Thanks to my revolving typing staff: Sara Jernigan, Catalina Paulting, Caroline Weitzer, Karen Hensley, Kevin O'Neil, and especially, Lisa Keppinger, who was saddled with the brunt of the work.

Thanks to Zhong You Ping for her assistance with Chinese translations.

Thanks to the staff at the libraries of Oregon Health Sciences University, Oregon College of Oriental Medicine, Portland State University, National College of Naturopathic Medicine, and American College of Traditional Chinese Medicine.

Thanks to my editor, Julie Zinkus, for long hours of work.

Thanks to Jody Turner-Cheung for designing the cover.

Lastly, a very special thanks to Walter Urba, M.D., Ph.D. for providing detailed comments on the content and tone of much of the book, and for his patience with a novice.

This book is dedicated to my parents, who never lost faith, even in the darkest moments.

CANCER & NATURAL MEDICINE

A Textbook of Basic Science and Clinical Research

I
INTRODUCTION

1.1 CANCER INCIDENCE AND MORTALITY

Humans have been afflicted with cancer since antiquity. Several ancient civilizations described cancer in their writings and pictures, and bone cancers have been diagnosed in Egyptian mummies. Western medicine began its scientific inquiry into the causes of cancer in 1775, when an English doctor, Sir Percival Pott, observed that chimney sweeps developed an unusually high rate of testicular cancer. He suggested that this was due to an agent in the chimney soot.

Today, cancer is one of the leading causes of death in the United States. As shown in Figure 1.1, cancer accounted for 24% of all deaths in the United States in 1991. In 1992 alone, an estimated 1,130,000 new cases of cancer were diagnosed, and 520,000 cancer-related deaths occurred.[1]

In response to high mortality rates, the U.S. Congress declared a "war on cancer" in the early 1970s, and mandated the ongoing collection of data on cancer incidence and mortality. This resulted in the establishment of the Surveillance, Epidemiology, and End Results (SEER) program administered by the National Cancer Institute (NCI). Using SEER data, NCI developed, and continues to update, statistics on a broad range of cancer-related issues. Based on the latest data, 42% of all males and 39% of all females are expected to develop cancer at some point during their lifetimes. The probability that males will develop various specific cancers is shown in Figure 1.2. Figure 1.3 shows the probability for specific cancers in females.

As can be seen from the figures, cancer is the cause of significant morbidity, and a high percentage of Americans will have to face this disease at some point in their lives. In fact, the overall incidence of cancer is 44% greater today than it was 40 years ago and overall mortality is 3% greater.

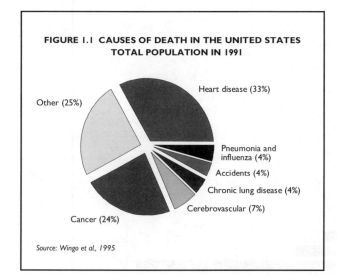

FIGURE 1.1 CAUSES OF DEATH IN THE UNITED STATES TOTAL POPULATION IN 1991

Heart disease (33%)

Other (25%)

Pneumonia and influenza (4%)

Accidents (4%)

Chronic lung disease (4%)

Cerebrovascular (7%)

Cancer (24%)

Source: Wingo et al, 1995

1.2 THE USE OF COMPLEMENTARY MEDICINE BY CANCER PATIENTS

Each year in the United States over one million patients are newly diagnosed with cancer. Approximately half of these patients receive surgery, radiotherapy,

---

[1] The source for incidence and mortality data for this chapter is the U.S. National Cancer Institute (Miller et al., 1992), unless otherwise specified. Incidence and mortality data are for the white population, unless otherwise specified, and are age-adjusted to the 1970 U.S. standard population.

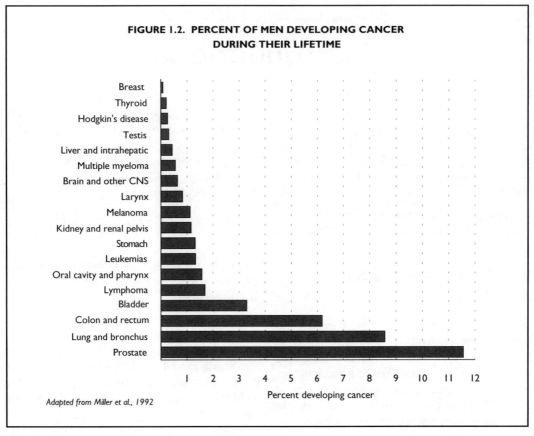

FIGURE 1.2. PERCENT OF MEN DEVELOPING CANCER
DURING THEIR LIFETIME

Adapted from Miller et al., 1992

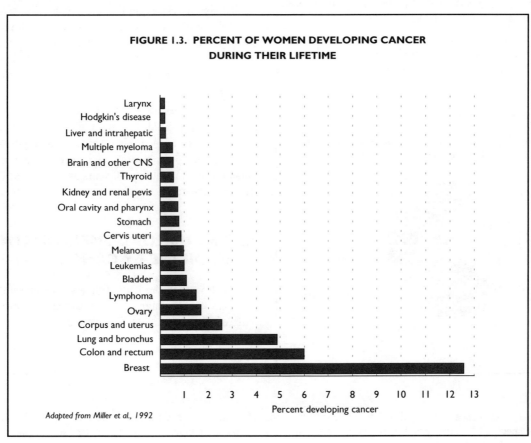

FIGURE 1.3. PERCENT OF WOMEN DEVELOPING CANCER
DURING THEIR LIFETIME

Adapted from Miller et al., 1992

and/or chemotherapy and are cured of their disease.[2] The other half of the population is not so fortunate; even with these therapies they will die within five years. Treatment itself may cause further morbidity. Intensive treatment with radiotherapy or chemotherapy is commonly associated with a range of adverse side effects from nausea to bone marrow failure. Those patients who receive intensive treatment may experience a decline in quality of life. Because of these and other reasons, a significant minority of cancer patients seek out alternatives to conventional care.

A recent survey conducted by the American Cancer Society estimated that 9% of cancer patients use complementary therapies (Kennedy, 1993). Other investigators have placed the figure at 10 to 60% (Hauser, 1993). In a recent study conducted at New York Hospital, approximately 30% of the breast cancer patients interviewed reported that they had consulted nonconventional therapists, and nearly 25% were receiving some form of nonconventional therapy, such as shark cartilage, mushrooms, Chinese herbs, and/or vitamin injections (OAM, 1994). Various other studies have estimated that 10 to 50% of cancer patients use some form of complementary medicine (McGinnis, 1991).[3] The United States Congress has estimated that two billion dollars is spent annually on complementary cancer treatments (Guzley, 1992). A conservative estimate that 10% of cancer patients seek complementary care would imply that every year more than 100,000 cancer patients in the United States are either treated by practitioners of complementary medicine or self-prescribe complementary therapies.

The use of complementary therapies by cancer patients is not limited to the United States. In a survey of 415 cancer patients in two London hospitals, 16% reported that they had used complementary therapies (Downer et al., 1994). According to a survey conducted at the Women's and Children's Hospital in South Australia, approximately 46% of the children with cancer had used at least one complementary therapy, generally in addition to conventional treatment. Less than 50% of the parents discussed the therapy with their doctors (Sawyer et al., 1994). In a survey of 949 oncology outpatients from several hospitals in Holland, 9% were currently using complementary therapy in addition to conventional treatment, and an additional 6% had used complementary therapy in the past, but had since stopped (Van der Zouwe et al., 1994). Up to 25% of the patients with lymphatic cancers admitted to the Center of Oncology in Krakow, Poland had received complementary therapies (Pawlicki et al., 1991). In a German study of 160 cancer outpatients, 53% had used complementary therapy at some time (Morant et al., 1991).

The term "complementary therapies" is not well defined. For the purposes of this book, it will be defined as the medicinal use of naturally occurring substances ("natural agents") that are not licensed as drugs by the U.S. Food and Drug Administration. The term also includes the medicinal use of physical, spiritual, mental, or emotional therapies that are not generally reimbursed by U.S. insurance companies. Note that natural agents, by the above definition, include naturally occurring substances that are currently under investigation by conventional researchers, but have not yet been licensed for use.

1.3 THE CLINICAL EFFICACY OF COMPLEMENTARY MEDICINE IN TREATING CANCER

The widespread use of complementary medicine in treating patients with cancer raises a number of questions. One of these is certainly, Are these patients receiving any clinical benefit? This question is difficult to answer since relatively few clinical trials have been conducted. In one study, 156 pairs of patients with documented extensive malignant disease and a predicted survival time of less than one year were treated either at a prominent complementary cancer clinic in San Diego, California, or treated by conventional medicine. The complementary treatment consisted of an immune-enhancing vaccine, vegetarian diets, and coffee enemas. Some of these patients also received conventional treatment, primarily chemotherapy. Both groups exhibited a mean survival period of 15 months (Cassileth et al., 1991). Of course this trial does not reflect possible outcomes for patients treated with other complementary therapies. Nor does it reflect possible outcomes of patients in early stage disease treated with these complementary therapies.

As will be discussed later in this book, clinical studies conducted in China tend to be more positive, and a number of them suggest that combining herbal medicine with conventional treatment may moderately increase survival time. They also suggest that the combined treatment may improve the quality of life of patients (by reducing nausea and vomiting, improving appetite, and so on). Some of the more successful trials reported that survival time doubled. However, most of the Chinese

---

[2] The five-year relative survival rate is often used as a rough estimate of the cure rate. However, it likely overestimates the cure rate for reasons explained in Chapter 9. The current five-year survival rate for all cancer sites in the U.S. white population is 53% (Miller et al., 1992).

[3] The majority of patients who receive complementary therapy continue to receive conventional care. Approximately 5% of cancer patients abandon conventional therapy to pursue complementary therapy (McGinnis, 1991).

studies on herbal treatments were poorly designed, and it is therefore difficult to interpret the meaning of their results.

In general, the studies contained in this book do not prove or disprove that complementary therapies work. The primary reason for this is that there are a multitude of complementary therapies, and each may be used singularly or in combination to assist the cancer patient. Each treatment protocol must be judged on its own merits on well-defined patient groups. To date, very little clinical research has been conducted on the majority of complementary therapies, and it is simply too early to make many judgments. Since so little is known about the anticancer effects of complementary therapies, their use should, in general, be focused toward research.

1.4 RESEARCH ON COMPLEMENTARY MEDICINE

As already stated, the clinical efficacies of natural anticancer agents are largely unknown. Although some agents are currently being investigated in clinical trials (for example, Phase I (toxicity) trials are in progress in England on limonene, the primary constituent of orange oil), research on the majority of natural agents is in the preclinical phase, or is not being actively pursued.

A large number of studies are frequently necessary before the effects of an agent are accepted as proven. This is especially true if the quality of the studies is questionable or the results are conflicting. Considering the low funding priority that many natural agents receive, it may be a very long time before definitive statements can be made regarding their effectiveness. Practitioners of conventional and complementary medicine can help to reduce these delays by increasing their involvement in research.

Funding for research is difficult to obtain. Professional researchers compete heavily to obtain private and federal funding. For example, approximately 75% of all grant proposals received by the National Cancer Institute are considered to be of high quality and worthy of funding, yet limited resources allow funding for only about 9 to 20% (Urba, 1994, personal communication).[4] Such fierce competition severely limits funding, particularly for studies on controversial agents or agents of limited interest. In the industrial sector, funding is also limited for agents that do not lead to patentable products. For these reasons, the U.S. Congress recently established the Office of Alternative Medicine (OAM) within the National Institutes of Health, and charged it with the mission of facilitating research on complementary medicine. Unfortunately, the OAM itself is poorly funded, and the research grants it awards are generally less then $30,000 per project. This is enough, however, to conduct small projects. There are a number of research designs that may be conducted with even less money. Some designs, such as case studies, can sometimes be financed by patient fees. Research designs will be discussed further in Chapter 17.

1.5 SUMMARY

Cancer accounts for 24% of all deaths in the United States, and approximately 40% of the population will be diagnosed with cancer at some point in their lifetime. Of those who are diagnosed with cancer, a significant minority are using complementary therapies in conjunction with conventional treatment. Complementary therapies vary widely in their makeup, and their efficacy is largely unknown. Further research is needed, and in this regard practitioners can play an important role.

---

[4] Walter Urba, Ph.D., M.D. is Medical Director of the Cancer Program, Providence Portland Medical Center, Portland, Oregon; and past Director of the Clinical Services Program, Frederick Cancer Research and Development Center, National Cancer Institute.

2
INITIATION, PROLIFERATION, AND CELL DEATH

Cancer is a disease marked by uncontrolled, virulent growth of poorly differentiated cells. To gain insight into the nature of cancer, it is useful first to review the processes occurring in individual cancer cells. Three important processes are cell initiation, cell proliferation, and cell death.

2.1 CELL INITIATION

2.1.1 Cancer Initiation and DNA Damage

The transformation of a normal cell into a neoplastic cell occurs in response to one or more initiating factors. These factors may originate externally or internally to the cell. The primary external factors include chemical carcinogens, viruses, and ionizing radiation. The common link between these three is their ability to inflict damage on cellular deoxyribonucleic acid (DNA). DNA carries the genetic information in each cell. Damage to the DNA, if not repaired, may eventually result in the formation of a neoplastic (literally, *newly formed*) cell. Externally-induced DNA damage is commonly mediated by free radicals (see Box 2.1).

The primary internal initiating factor is random damage to DNA during cell division. As cells divide and their DNA replicates, random errors may occur that alter the genetic code.

To prevent internally- or externally-induced DNA damage from producing mutations, cells contain an ever-vigilant DNA repair system.[1] If the repair system malfunctions, as is the case in some inherited disorders, the risk of developing cancer increases. Even when fully functional, the repair system is not perfect, and a small probability exists that damaged DNA will escape repair during any one cell division. This is, in fact, a desirable fault, since slight changes in the DNA are required for evolution and adaptation to proceed.

Evidence to support the theory that DNA is the essential target of all carcinogens includes the following (reviewed by Tannock and Hill, 1992:2):

- Individuals who are unable to repair damaged DNA due to an inherited defect have higher cancer rates.

- Chromosomal changes in certain types of cancer are well-defined. For example, in chronic myelogenous leukemia, the abnormal Philadelphia chromosome is created through a translocation of two normal chromosomes.

- Some genes (oncogenes) can transform normal cells into cancer cells. Some of these genes have been identified in cancer-causing viruses. In the early 1900s, investigators discovered that cancer could be transferred between animals by injecting healthy laboratory animals with cell-free extracts from cancer-bearing animals, thereby implicating a viral cause. Although viruses do not appear to initiate the majority of human cancers, a few viruses that cause cancer in humans have been identified.

- Some genes (tumor suppressor genes), when inactive lead to the development of cancer.

Table 2.1 contains a partial list of oncogenes and tumor suppressor genes. More than 30 oncogenes and 10 tumor suppressor genes have been discovered to date (Greenwald, et al., 1995).

2.1.2 Viruses

Proto-oncogenes are genes that, upon overexpression, become oncogenes. In normal cells, proto-oncogenes may be expressed in a regulated fashion and

---

[1] A number of natural agents may stimulate DNA repair. For example, extracts of *Panax ginseng (ren shen)* can inhibit cancer formation in hamster lung cells exposed to alkylating chemotherapy agents or a number of other carcinogenic chemicals. This inhibition is due, in part, to enhanced DNA repair (Rhee et al., 1991).

BOX 2.1. FREE RADICALS

Free radical-induced damage to DNA, protein, and lipids has been implicated as a major contributor to aging and also degenerative diseases such as cancer, cardiovascular disease, immune dysfunction, brain dysfunction, and cataracts (Ames et al., 1993). Free radicals can be produced by external factors, such as radiation and cigarette smoke, as well as internal factors such as products of aerobic cellular respiration, immune cell activity, inflammation, and other processes. In humans, up to 5% of the oxygen taken in is converted to free radicals (Reiter et al., 1995).

Free radicals are molecules that contain an odd number of electrons. As such they have a strong tendency to react with the electrons of other molecules. When a free radical contacts electrons of a stable molecule, the radical gains or loses electrons to achieve stability. However, this process disturbs the electron balance of the stable molecule, thereby creating a new free radical. In this manner free radicals initiate a chain reaction of destruction.

During cellular respiration, mitochondria consume oxygen (O_2) and produce water (H_2O). Byproducts of this process include the free radical superoxide ($O_2 \cdot$). (The odd electron is represented by a dot in the chemical formula.) Through the actions of the enzyme superoxide dismutase (which is zinc-and copper-dependent), superoxide is converted to hydrogen peroxide (H_2O_2). Hydrogen peroxide is converted to water through the actions of catalase and glutathione peroxidase (a selenium-dependent enzyme). Although hydrogen peroxide is not a free radical, it can be toxic at high concentrations. It can also be reduced to the hydroxyl radical ($OH \cdot$) in the presence of superoxide. The hydroxyl radical is the most toxic of the oxygen-based free radicals. Yet another important free radical is the peroxyl radical ($ROO \cdot$), which mediates lipid peroxidation, thereby damaging cell membranes.

The body maintains a variety of antioxidants as a multilevel defense against free radical damage. These include the enzymes mentioned above (superoxide dismutase, catalase, and glutathione peroxidase); nonessential antioxidants, such as glutathione, proteins, and uric acid; and essential radical scavengers such as vitamins C, A, E, and beta-carotene (Gey, 1993). For example, macrophages and neutrophils are types of immune cell that destroy foreign microbes by producing a respiratory burst of hydrogen peroxide and free radicals. To prevent self-inflicted damage, macrophages contain high amounts of vitamin C.

Antioxidant defenses are not perfect and DNA is damaged regularly. Ames et al. (1993) estimate that there are 10,000 oxidative hits to DNA per cell per day in humans. The vast majority of these lesions are repaired by cellular enzymes. Those that are not repaired may progress toward neoplasia. Due to the continual bombardment of DNA and other tissues by free radicals, the body must obtain ample antioxidant supplies through the diet. These include vitamins, flavonoids, and other compounds found in fresh fruits and vegetables. Epidemiological studies consistently report that populations who consume inadequate amounts of these foods are at a higher risk for heart disease, cancer, and other degenerative diseases.

Recent studies on breast cancer patients suggest that oxidative stress is associated with malignant disease (Hietanen et al., 1994). The nature of this association is not yet clear, but perhaps malignant disease, in and of itself, may actually increase oxidative stress.

TABLE 2.1. SELECTED KNOWN OR SUSPECTED ONCOGENES AND TUMOR SUPPRESSOR GENES

ONCOGENE	CANCER TYPE	SUPPRESSOR GENE	CANCER TYPE
erbb2	breast	*apc*	colon
fos	lung	*dcc*	colon
jun	lung	*p53*	numerous
hras *	pancreatic	*rb1*	retinoblastoma
kras *	colon		
nras *	lung and others		
myc	breast, colon, small-cell lung		

* These belong to a large group of *ras* oncogenes.
Source: Greenwald et al., 1995

they appear to play a role in normal cell function (reviewed by Tannock and Hill, 1992:62). In animals, ribonucleic acid (RNA) viruses can induce overexpression of proto-oncogenes, and cause cancer.[2] However, in humans it appears that only a small number of viruses are capable of overexpressing proto-oncogenes.

2.1.3 Radiation

Radiation initiates neoplasia by creating free radicals that damage the DNA. Under certain conditions, radiation causes water to ionize, resulting in the formation of hydroxyl (OH·) and hydrogen (H·) radicals. These radicals can cause different levels of damage, depending on the number of radicals produced. Low-level radiation may produce moderate damage, which allows the mutated cells to continue to proliferate and develop into a cancer. High-level radiation may produce severe damage, completely stopping proliferation (mitosis).[3] The radiation used in cancer treatment is designed to produce a sufficient amount of DNA damage to completely inhibit the proliferation of targeted tumor cells.

2.1.4 Chemical Carcinogens

Neoplasia due to chemical carcinogens is thought to involve a two-stage process of initiation and promotion as shown in Figure 2.1. In the initiation stage, a carcinogenic agent contacts a normal cell and alters the DNA.

This stage is reversible because the body maintains several processes that can repair damaged DNA. Initiation becomes irreversible when the damaged cell passes through one cycle of division, which makes the DNA lesion a permanent component of the gene code in the daughter cell.

Some chemicals categorized as carcinogens are not actually carcinogenic themselves, but their metabolites are.[4] In an effort to facilitate urinary excretion of foreign fat-soluble compounds, the body converts them to water-soluble compounds. During this process, the body may convert a variety of noncarcinogenic compounds into carcinogenic ones. Carcinogen metabolism occurs in a number of different tissues, although the greatest quantity occurs in the liver.

When initiation is complete, the preneoplastic cell may remain indistinguishable from normal cells until a promoting agent stimulates it into neoplasia. In the promotion stage, a noncarcinogenic promoting agent contacts the initiated cell and produces a series of cellular changes that eventually result in formation of a neoplastic cell. Whereas the initiation stage tends to be rapid, the promotion stage tends to be prolonged. Tumor-promoting agents include the active component of croton oil 12-O-tetradecanoylphorbol-13-acetate (TPA), phenobarbital, saccharin, and 2,3,7,8-tetrachlorodi-benzo-p dioxin (TCDD). The promotion stage is reversible up until final formation of the neoplastic cell.

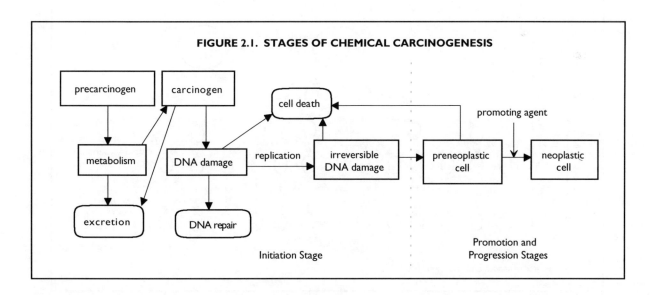

FIGURE 2.1. STAGES OF CHEMICAL CARCINOGENESIS

---

[2] RNA is a nucleic acid that controls protein synthesis in cells. Viruses are minute, simple organisms that live within and are parasitic to cells. They are composed of a single strand of either RNA or DNA and a covering of protein.

[3] Mitosis is the process of cell division whereby DNA is copied from the parent cell and instilled in the daughter cell. Cells of human tissue proliferate by mitosis.

[4] For example, polycyclic aromatic hydrocarbons do not act directly to induce neoplasia; however the phenols, quinones, and other compounds produced during their metabolism do induce neoplasia (reviewed by Tannock and Hill, 1992:107-8).

2.2 CELL GROWTH

2.2.1 Cell Proliferation

Once a cell becomes neoplastic, its continued replication may result in the formation of a solid tumor.[5] In general, the size of a solid tumor increases because the neoplastic cells within the tumor live long enough for the cell proliferation rate to overcome the cell death rate. This is in contrast to the common belief that tumor size increases primarily because the cells proliferate rapidly. Although a few cancers do exhibit rapid cell proliferation rates, the cells of the majority of adult cancers proliferate relatively slowly.

Cancers are thought to arise from the proliferation of a single precursor cell called a *stem cell*. As the initial transformed cell divides and its clones proliferate, individual cells mutate, thereby producing variants of the original transformed cell. This heterogeneity allows tumors to adapt more easily to adverse conditions. This is one way that tumors can become resistant to cytotoxic chemotherapy drugs. Internal mutation also allows tumors to develop ever-increasing malignant properties, and explains why tumors obtained from different sites in the same patient may exhibit different properties.[6]

2.2.2 Cell Differentiation

Stem Cells

Stem cells are capable of both self-renewal (self-replacement) and clonal expansion and, therefore, appear immortal (see Figure 2.2). In non-neoplastic conditions, stem cells act as a source of new cells during tissue repair. Under neoplastic conditions, the proliferation of stem cells is unchecked. Furthermore, their daughter cells do not fully *differentiate*, or acquire the functions of more mature cells. If they did differentiate, their ability to proliferate would be reduced. For example, fully differentiated bone cells are not able to proliferate. Tumors contain a limited number of stem cells from which they propagate, and these are the targets of cytotoxic chemotherapy and radiotherapy.

Stem cells are present in high numbers in tissues that constantly renew their population such as the bone marrow and intestinal lining. Bone marrow cells have a turnover rate of approximately five days, as opposed to several years for some vascular cells. Due to their rapid proliferation, these cells are at greater risk of transformation induced by chance mutation.

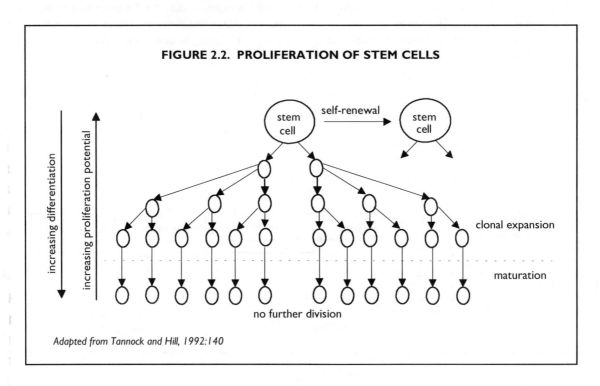

FIGURE 2.2. PROLIFERATION OF STEM CELLS

Adapted from Tannock and Hill, 1992:140

---

[5] In the case of hematological neoplasms, such as leukemia and lymphoma, a solid tumor does not develop since the neoplastic cells are suspended within the blood or in the lymph glands.

[6] Tumor heterogeneity within an individual is also an impediment to successful immunotherapy. Immunotherapy is most effective if all tumors cells are genetically identical, since this allows the immune system to recognize tumor cells with the least amount of difficulty.

BOX 2.2. HISTOLOGICAL ORIGINS OF CANCER CELLS

Malignant tumors can be described according to their tissue of origin. Histiogenic classification schemes recognize the following five tumor types:

Tumors arising from epithelial tissue: These tumors include all carcinomas, such as squamous cell carcinoma, transitional cell carcinoma, adenocarcinoma, and basal cell carcinoma.

Tumors arising from mesenchymal tissue: Mesenchymal tissues include muscles, skeleton, blood vessels, lymph vessels, and reticular tissue. Tumors arising from these tissues include all sarcomas, such as osteosarcoma, myosarcoma, and fibrosarcoma.

Tumors arising from lymphatic reticular tissue: Tumors arising from this subset of mesenchymal tissue include Hodgkin's disease, lymphatic leukemia, and myeloid leukemia.

Tumors arising from nerve tissue: These tumors include glioblastoma multiforme, neuroblastoma, meningioma, and pheochromocytoma.

Tumors arising from other tissues: These tumors include malignant hydatidiform mole and malignant teratoma.

Other tissues contain fewer stem cells and have slower replacement rates. In these tissues, cancer is more likely to be initiated from external irritants that increase tissue repair (for example, by cigarette smoke in lung tissue), or by DNA damage due to external factors (such as chemical carcinogens), rather than by chance mutation.

Generally, the majority of cells in a tumor partially differentiate. However, a sufficient number of cells fully differentiate, such that, on inspection, a pathologist can determine the tissue of origin. For example, a limited number of cells from a bone cancer may differentiate into mature and identifiable bone cells.

Tumor cells can be described by a variety of classifiers. As described in Box 2.2, tumors can be classified according to their tissue of origin. They can also be described by their level of differentiation. Tumor *grade* indicates the degree of differentiation in the tumor as a whole. Tumors that are poorly differentiated generally grow faster and are assigned a higher grade. The opposite is true for tumors that are well differentiated. If tumor cells do not differentiate, the tumor is called *anaplastic* (literally, not formed).

Natural Agents that Induce Differentiation

The progression of some malignancies is thought to be due to a block in differentiation. Agents that induce differentiation may be useful in treating these malignancies (Breitman, 1987). A number of natural agents demonstrate the ability to induce differentiation in human leukemia (T-cell, B-cell, and promyelocytic), melanoma, colon carcinoma, bladder carcinoma, brain cancer (glioblastoma multiforme), as well as in a variety of mouse cell lines (Marks and Rifkind, 1991). When these cells are exposed to differentiating agents, they can develop into normal cells and lose their ability to proliferate. Natural agents that induce differentiation are listed in Table 2.2. Due to the amount of information available regarding dimethyl sulfoxide (DMSO), it is discussed separately in the text following the table.

TABLE 2.2. NATURAL AGENTS THAT INDUCE DIFFERENTIATION IN VITRO		
AGENT	**EFFECT**	**REFERENCE**
Berberine	Berberine is an alkaloid found in *Coptis chinensis (huang lian)* and a number of other herbs. Berberine induced differentiation of human embryonal carcinoma cells in as little as 24 hours at the relatively high, but nontoxic, concentration of 100 µg/ml (298 µM). Treatment with retinoic acid also induced cells to differentiate, but induction took at least several days to develop. Results indicated that the process was associated with down-regulation of a *ras* proto-oncogene (c-Ki-ras2).	Chang et al., 1990; Chang 1991
Bromelain, trypsin, and chymotrypsin	Bromelain is a proteolytic enzyme derived from pineapple stems, and trypsin and chymotrypsin are proteolytic enzymes produced by the pancreas. These enzymes induced differentiation in human leukemia cells.	See Section 15.3.
Bufo bufo gargarizans (chan su)	Bufalin, a component found in the skin of the toad *Bufo bufo gargarizans*, induces differentiation in four human leukemia cell lines. Crude extracts of the skin have been used clinically in patients with acute leukemia, apparently with some success.	Zhang et al, 1991; see Section 11.5.5.
(Table continues)		

TABLE 2.2 *(continued)*		
AGENT	**EFFECT**	**REFERENCE**
Butyric acid	Butyric acid is a compound formed in the colon by the action of intestinal bacteria on fiber. Although it has the capacity to induce differentiation and may play a role in limiting the development of colon cancers, it quickly biodegrades in vivo and, therefore, is not a good candidate for a systemic therapeutic agent.	Reviewed by Marks and Rifkind, 1991
Cytokines	Cytokines are endogenous chemicals that regulate cellular growth and function, including the growth and function of immune cells. Cytokines such as granulocyte colony stimulating factor (CSF), granulocyte-macrophage-CSF, macrophage-CSF, and interferon, induce differentiation in a variety of neoplastic cell lines.	Reviewed by Marks and Rifkind, 1991
Daidzein	Daidzein is an isoflavone found in legumes such as *Pueraria lobata* (*ge gen*) and in soy products. Daidzein induced differentiation in B16 melanoma and HL-60 human leukemia cells.	Jing and Han, 1992; Jing et al., 1993; Han, 1994
Docosahexaenoic acid (DHA)	Docosahexaenoic acid (DHA), a component of fish oil, markedly accelerates retinoic acid-induced differentiation in human leukemic (HL-60) cells. The effect appears to be due to the ability of DHA to alter plasma membrane fluidity. Although it was not tested in this study, eicosapentaenoic acid (EPA), a primary component of fish oil, could be expected to produce similar effects, since it alters membrane fluidity in a similar manner. Increased membrane fluidity is associated with greater freedom of molecular motion, greater drug transport, increased metabolism, and a greater capacity for division. Excessive membrane fluidity can cause cell death.	Burrns et al., 1989
Eugenia caryophyllata, (ding xiang) and *Arctium lappa (niu bang zi)*	In studies of over 200 extracts of crude drugs, extracts of *E. caryophyllata* and *A. lappa* were found to exhibit potent abilities to induce differentiation of mouse myeloid leukemia (M1) cells. In the studies on arctium, lignan fractions were the most active and initiated differentiation at concentrations as low as 5 µM. However, these fractions were not effective in inducing differentiation in human promyelocytic leukemia (HL-60) cells.	Umehara et al., 1992, 1993
Ganoderma lucidum (ling zhi)	The polysaccharide fraction of *Ganoderma lucidum (ling zhi)* has been shown to act as an immune stimulant. When human immune cells (monocytes/macrophages) were incubated with ganoderma, they produced a medium that induced differentiation in human monocytic leukemia (U937) cells.	Lieu et al., 1992
Perillyl alcohol	The monoterpene perillyl alcohol is a potent inducer of differentiation in mouse neuroblastoma cells. This may explain, in part, the antitumor effects of perillyl alcohol and the related monoterpene limonene.	Shi and Gould, 1995
Retinoic acid	Retinoic acid (RA) is the acid form of vitamin A.* RA is one of the most potent inducers of differentiation. However, relatively high concentrations of RA are required to induce differentiation, and the use of RA as a differentiating agent is severely hampered by its toxic effects. One strategy to overcome the toxicity problem may be to combine RA with a synergistic agent, such as DMSO. Although investigators have been studying less toxic derivatives of RA, few have proven better than the naturally occurring 13-cis-retinoic acid or all-trans retinoic acids. All-trans retinoic acid has recently been recommended for approval for treating patients with acute myelogenous leukemia.	Breitman and He, 1990; reviewed by Linder, 1991:494
Vitamin D_3	The active metabolite of vitamin D_3, 1,25-dihydroxyvitamin D_3 (1,25-diOHD$_3$), induces differentiation in a variety of cell lines. However, like retinoic acid, it can be toxic at high levels. Retinoic acid appears to up-regulate vitamin D_3 receptors and, in this manner, the two compounds may act synergistically. 1,25-diOHD$_3$ also induces differentiation in myelocytes (precursors of leukocytes in the bone marrow), affects lymphocyte function, and induces differentiation in epidermal cells. In a study of 136 breast cancer patients, those with 1,25-diOHD$_3$ receptor-positive tumors exhibited a significantly longer disease-free survival than those with receptor-negative tumors. Administration of synthetic analogs of 1,25-diOHD$_3$ to rats bearing breast cancer resulted in significant inhibition of tumor progression. In a study of 620 healthy volunteers, risk of developing colon cancer during the next 8 years decreased threefold in subjects with moderate 1,25-diOHD$_3$ serum levels (>20 ng/ml).	Marks and Rifkind, 1991; Scott and Harris, 1994; Reichel and Norman, 1989; Colston et al., 1989; Garland et al., 1989; Reichel et al., 1989
* The other two forms of vitamin A are alcohol (retinol) and aldehyde (retinal).		

TABLE 2.3. CELL LINES THAT DIFFERENTIATE IN RESPONSE TO DMSO IN VITRO	
CELL LINE	**REFERENCE**
Human promyelocytic leukemia (HL-60)	Bradford and Autieri, 1991; Yung et al., 1994; Ahmed and Weidemann, 1994
Human hepatoma (PLC/PRF/5) and human hepatoblastoma (Hep G2)	Saito et al., 1992; Kuprina et al., 1993; Vesey et al., 1991
Human ovarian carcinoma (AMOC-2)	Yabushita and Sartorelli, 1993; Grunt et al., 1992
Human rhabdomyosarcoma (A-673, RD, and A-204)	Prados et al., 1993
Cultured human T lymphoma	Lonnbro and Wadso, 1991
Human neuroblastoma (SH-SY5Y)	Koman et al., 1993
Six human glioma cell lines	Geder et al., 1989
Human melanoma (MM96E)	Takahashi et al., 1992

As shown in Table 2.2, certain cytokines, and immunostimulants such as bromelain and *Ganoderma lucidum (ling zhi)*, all induce differentiation. Quite likely, immunostimulants induce differentiation by increasing the production of cytokines (Suffness and Pezzuto, 1991).

DMSO

Dimethyl sulfoxide (DMSO) induces differentiation in a wide range of human neoplastic cell lines in vitro (see Table 2.3).[7] High concentrations (1 to 2% v/v) of DMSO are required. Plasma concentrations of this magnitude can be expected to produce severe adverse effects in humans, including hepatotoxicity (Toren and Rechavi, 1993). However, the concentration of DMSO required to induce differentiation in vivo may be lower than that required in vitro due to the presence of retinoic acid in the plasma. Trans-retinoic acid and DMSO act synergistically in inducing differentiation of human HL-60 leukemia cells. In the presence of normal plasma levels of retinoic acid (30 nM), the concentration of DMSO required to induce differentiation in vitro is reduced by as much as 400% (Breitman and He, 1990).

The process by which DMSO and other compounds induce differentiation is unknown, although numerous theories have been postulated. Most of these theories involve the effects of DMSO on the plasma membrane of individual tumor cells. Some of these theories are listed below:

- The effects of DMSO may be modulated by various extracellular cations. DMSO is a powerful solvent capable of transporting cations through the plasma membrane. This alteration of the intracellular ionic composition can alter the membrane surface potential (the electrical charge across the membrane).

One study reported a linear correlation between a shift in the surface potential and induction of differentiation in some cell lines (Arcangeli et al., 1993).

- DMSO can cause a rapid reduction in the binding of growth factors (granulocyte-macrophage colony-stimulating factor and insulin) to cell surface receptors (Schwartz et al., 1993). This suggests that DMSO may induce differentiation by disrupting the structure and/or organization of the cell surface receptors that govern growth and differentiation.

- DMSO can cause a reduction in cell surface protein *p185*, a protein involved in regulating differentiation. This suggests that DMSO may induce differentiation by altering the location of *p185* and inhibiting *p185*-mediated signal transduction pathways (Matin and Hung, 1993).

- DMSO can cause a down-regulation of *myc* and *T* oncogenes (Grunt et al., 1992; Witte et al., 1992). This suggests that DMSO may induce differentiation by down-regulating oncogenes involved in suppressing differentiation.

The Clinical Relevance of Experimentally Derived Concentration Data

In Table 2.2 and elsewhere in this book, references are made to the concentration at which an agent is effective in vitro. The ability of an agent to produce a biologic effect depends on its concentration at the target site. To reduce the amount of experimentation on humans, researchers commonly use in-vitro and animal data to determine approximate concentrations needed to produce a desired effect in humans. The clinical relevance of this data is discussed in Box 2.3.

---

[7] Although not a natural agent by the definition given in Chapter 1, DMSO is discussed in this book due to a continued interest in the compound by practitioners of complementary medicine, and its widespread use by the public.

BOX 2.3. IN-VITRO CONCENTRATIONS AND THEIR CLINICAL RELEVANCE

The concentration of a compound in a solution is often described by its *molarity*. The molarity (M) is equal to the number of gram molecular weights (moles) in one liter of solution. For example, the flavonoid quercetin has a molecular weight of 302 grams/mole. Therefore, a concentration of 1 μg/ml of quercetin is equal to 3.3 μM (micromoles). The advantage of referring to a concentration by its molarity is that the molarity takes into account the variability in molecular weights between compounds.

In general, compounds that are effective at low concentrations in vitro are also effective at low concentrations in vivo. In the U.S. National Cancer Institute plant screening program, a pure compound has generally been considered to have in-vitro cytotoxic activity if the concentration that causes a 50% cell kill (in KB carcinoma cells) is less than about 4 μg/ml (less than 20 μg/ml for crude extracts). (The NCI screening program is discussed in more detail in Chapter 11.) For our purposes this value can be used as a rough reference point for assessing the activity of natural agents in a number of other in-vitro assays. Many of the compounds discussed in this book are of low molecular weight (approximately 300 grams/mole), and the molarity corresponding to 4 μg/ml is approximately 13 μM. Agents that are active at concentrations markedly greater than this value, depending on the assay involved, may be considered relatively weak. For example, berberine (molecular weight 336), at 100 μg/ml (298 μM), induces differentiation of human embryonal carcinoma cells in vitro (see Table 2.2). This suggests that relatively high concentrations of berberine are required to produce differentiation in this line. The method given here to interpret concentration data provides only a rough approximation and is not appropriate for all assays.

2.2.3 Tumor Growth

Tumor growth is roughly exponential, and as such, the amount of time it takes a tumor to double in size is approximately constant. Therefore, an increase in diameter from 0.5 to 1.0 centimeters requires the same amount of time as an increase from 5 to 10 centimeters. The larger the tumor, the faster the volume growth. Average doubling times for human tumors are typically in the range of one to three months (reviewed by Tannock and Hill, 1992:155). Doubling would occur in less then 20 days if not for the large percentage of nonproliferating cells within a tumor (partially differentiated cells, immune cells such as macrophages, and other cells) and for the high rate of cell death within a tumor (up to 90% of the rate of cell production).

The cell population within a tumor must reach an enormous number before modern diagnostic equipment can detect the tumor mass. Detection of a tumor becomes possible when the tumor cell population reaches a minimum of approximately 10^9 cells (a weight of approximately one gram).[8] A successful chemotherapy or radiotherapy treatment results in a remission, meaning that the tumor is no longer detectable. In a number of cancers, cell kill can be sufficiently complete to effectively cure the patient. However, in the majority of adult cancers, chemotherapy and radiotherapy are not capable of producing this degree of cell kill, and multiple logs of viable cells often remain.

By the time a tumor can be detected clinically, its cell populations has doubled approximately 30 times since initial transformation. Just 10 more doublings are required before the tumor weighs one kilogram, a size that is often incompatible with life. Therefore, most of a cancer's life span occurs before the cancer is clinically detectable.

Although the doubling time is roughly constant, growth rate does slow as the tumor gets larger. This is likely due to a deficiency of nutrition and oxygen in larger tumors. As tumors grow, some of the cells become distanced from the tumor's internal blood supply. Solid tumors often contain tissue nodules made up of dead cells near the center and active cells near the periphery.[9] Not surprisingly, the rate of cell proliferation decreases rapidly as the distance from the blood supply increases. Tumors in the initial stages of growth also exhibit reduced growth rates. In small tumors (<1 mm³) an internal blood supply *(angiogenesis)* is not yet developed and nutrition is limited. In addition, small tumors may exhibit reduced growth rates due to the effects of the immune system (which is most effective against small tumors).[10]

---

[8] Tumors are easily detected by imaging equipment when they contain approximately 10^{10} cells, and weigh approximately 10 grams.

[9] A second factor in nodule formation is the deposition of a fibrin stroma around clumps of tumor cells during tumor growth.

[10] Chemotherapy is also more successful against small tumors, in part, due to the limited blood circulation within large tumors.

2.3 CELL DEATH

2.3.1 Apoptosis vs. Necrosis

Cell death has long been thought to occur only through necrosis, a process in which death is caused by an adverse environment. In the last decade, researchers have clarified a second cause of cell death: *apoptosis.* This type of cell death is programmed into the cell at birth and triggers its death at old age or under other conditions where cell death benefits the host.

There are many differences between the two types of cell death. Unlike necrosis, apoptosis affects scattered, individual cells, does not produce inflammation, and therefore, does not damage adjacent cells. Apoptosis represents an orderly method of removing old, damaged, or otherwise unwanted cells.

Apoptosis has been noted in numerous mammal, insect, plant, and amphibian species. In humans, apoptosis has been identified in a wide variety of processes, including the shedding of cells from the intestinal lining, atrophy of the prostate after castration, regression of the lactating breast after weaning, elimination of mature immune cells, and cell turnover during wound healing.

Both necrosis and apoptosis play a role in limiting tumor growth. Necrosis may occur, for example, in cells distanced from the blood supply or as a result of immune activity or cytotoxic chemotherapy. Until recently, the single goal in conventional anticancer therapy was to produce tumor cell necrosis. This has now been expanded to include the induction of differentiation as discussed previously, and the induction of apoptosis, as discussed below.

2.3.2 Apoptosis and Cancer

Defects in apoptosis may play a role in both the initiation and proliferation of cancer cells. One possible cause of cancer is the failure of apoptosis to remove cells whose DNA has been damaged (Schwartzman and Cid-

lowski, 1993; Carson and Riberio, 1993). This may allow the cell to survive long enough to progress from the initiation stage, where DNA damage is reversible, to the promotion and proliferation stages, where the damage is permanent (see Figure 2.1). Some newly transformed cells can self-inhibit the genes that induce apoptosis, thereby lengthening their life span. Although apoptosis occurs at a lower rate in tumor cells than in normal cells, it does play a significant role in limiting net tumor growth.

In laboratory experiments on cancer cells, a number of common cytotoxic anticancer drugs induce necrosis at high doses and apoptosis at low doses. This suggests that cells with mild damage may "commit suicide" rather than live to produce mutations (Schwartzman and Cidlowski, 1993; Desoize and Sen, 1992; Meyn et al., 1994). Additional research is necessary to determine if low doses of cytotoxic drugs may be useful in inducing apoptosis in vivo. If this is true, it may open new possibilities for therapy with natural agents that exhibit mild cytotoxic activity.

2.3.3 Natural Agents that Stimulate Apoptosis

Since apoptosis is a rather recent discovery, few studies on the effects of natural substances on apoptosis have been conducted. However, several studies do report that naturally occurring compounds induce apoptosis in cancer cells in vitro. These studies are summarized in Table 2.4.

2.4 SUMMARY

Neoplastic cells are initiated, proliferate, and expire by certain mechanisms that have been partially defined. Each of these mechanisms is a potential target for anticancer therapy.

Initiation involves changes in the cellular DNA, which can be caused by viruses, chemicals, or radiation.

TABLE 2.4. NATURAL AGENTS THAT INDUCE APOPTOSIS IN CANCER CELLS IN VITRO		
AGENT	**EFFECT**	**REFERENCE**
Butyric acid (in the form of its sodium salt, sodium butyrate)	Sodium butyrate induces apoptosis in colon cancer cells. Recall from Table 2.2 that butyric acid is formed in the colon by the action of intestinal bacteria on fiber. This may explain, in part, the apparent protective effect of dietary fiber against colon cancer.	Hague et al., 1993
Caffeine	Caffeine can stimulate apoptosis and enhance the cytotoxicity of radiotherapy and some alkylating chemotherapy agents.* However, caffeine prevents apoptosis when used with some nonalkylating agents.	Traganos et al., 1993; Shinomiya et al., 1994
(Table continues)		

	TABLE 2.4. *(continued)*	
AGENT	**EFFECT**	**REFERENCE**
DMSO	DMSO induced apoptosis in mouse erythroleukemia cells transfected with a mutant *p53* gene. The normal *p53* protein, a product of the *p53* gene (see Table 2.1), is a tumor suppressor protein that has been identified as a key regulator of apoptosis in normal and malignant hematopoietic cells. It also regulates other processes of the cell cycle. Mutant *p53* genes do not perform their functions of inducing apoptosis and controlling cell cycle and have been identified within a wide variety of neoplasms.	Ryan and Clarke, 1994; Finnegan et al., 1994
Genistein	Genistein is an isoflavone found in legumes. It induces apoptosis at 30 μg/ml in some cell lines.	See Section 14.6.
Quercetin	Quercetin is a flavonoid that induces apoptosis in human leukemia (K563 and MOLT-4) and Burkitt's lymphoma (Raji) cells.	Wei et al., 1994
Retinoic acid	Retinoic acid induces transglutaminases, which are enzymes that catalyze the cross-linking of proteins. This reaction is important in a number of biochemical processes, such as blood clotting and macrophage function. It is also important in apoptosis.	Reviewed by Linder, 1991:154
Viscum album (mistletoe)	Induced apoptosis in human lymphocytes, and was cytotoxic. The authors suggest that viscum extracts may inhibit cancer cells by both mechanisms.	Bussing et al., 1996
Vitamin D$_3$	1,25-Dihydroxyvitamin D$_3$ induced apoptosis in human colon cancer HT 29 cells.	Vandewalle et al., 1995
Xiao Chai Hu Tang (formula),** and its components *Bupleurum chinensis (chai hu)* and *Scutellaria baicalensis (huang qin)*	Water-soluble components of the formula inhibited proliferation of human hepatocellular carcinoma (KIM-1) and cholangiocarcinoma (KMC-1) cells in vitro. The crude extract inhibited proliferation by 50% at the relatively high concentration of 236 to 353 μg/ml. The crude extract did not suppress normal human peripheral blood lymphocytes or normal rat hepatocytes, suggesting that the extract may exhibit specific effects against neoplastic cells. The extract appeared to induce both apoptosis and necrosis, depending on the phase of the cell cycle during exposure. Studies on the individual components revealed that the saponin saikosaponin-a (from *B. chinensis*) induced apoptotic cell death in human hepatoma (HuH-7) cells in vitro at concentrations of 50 μg/ml. The flavonoid baicalein (from *S. baicalensis*) nearly completely inhibited cell growth at 50 μg/ml. The flavonoid baicalin (also from *S. baicalensis*) inhibited human hepatoma cell growth by 50% at a concentration of 20 μg/ml. Baicalein and saikosaponin-a produced this effect at 50 μg/ml.	Yano et al., 1994; Okita et al., 1993; Motoo and Sawabu, 1994

* Alkylating chemotherapy agents include carboplatin, busulfan, cyclophosphamide, and numerous others. Alkylating agents are listed in Table 9.1.
** The ingredients of herbal formulas discussed in this book are provided in Appendix B.

Free radical scavengers can be used to protect cells from oxidative damage and subsequent initiation.

Proliferation is controlled by stem cells and is an exponential process. The descendants of stem cells can either partially or fully differentiate. The more they differentiate, the less they proliferate. A number of natural agents have been identified that induce differentiation and thereby limit proliferation.

Cell death can occur through necrosis or apoptosis. Natural agents that induce apoptosis have been identified. A large number of natural agents are cytotoxic and induce necrosis. These will be discussed further in Chapter 11.

3
ANGIOGENESIS

3.1 THE MECHANICS OF ANGIOGENESIS

Although it has been known for over 100 years that tumors contain an abnormally dense blood vessel network, it was not until the 1960s that investigators realized that tumors induce their own blood supply. And it was not until the 1970s that investigators realized the growth of solid tumors is, in fact, dependent upon angiogenesis.[1] In a landmark study, Folkman and Hochberg (1972) reported that tumors implanted in the eyes of rabbits grew only to a size of approximately 1 mm^3 before developing their own blood supply. Tumor growth was linear prior to vascularization, but exponential after vascularization. Angiogenesis facilitates growth by supplying the tumor with oxygen and nutrients. Angiogenesis also provides tumor cells with a ready access to the blood circulation, which assists metastasis.

Angiogenesis is not limited to malignant tumors. It is also present in benign tumors (such as highly neovascularized adrenal adenomas), various non-neoplastic diseases, and some normal processes. Non-neoplastic diseases that involve aberrant angiogenesis include: rheumatoid arthritis, hemangiomas, angiofibromas, psoriasis, atherosclerosis, and eye diseases such as diabetic retinopathy and neurovascular glaucoma (Folkman and Klagsbrun, 1987). Angiogenesis also occurs in healthy adults and is evident during wound healing, ovulation, menstruation, and pregnancy.

Angiogenesis is a complex process in which existing mature vessels generate sprouts that develop into complete new vessels. Studies have shown that during tumor angiogenesis, vascular cells grow at abnormally rapid rates. Normal endothelial cells divide approximately once every 7 years, but in experimental tumors endothelial cells may divide once every 7 to 10 days (Scott and Harris, 1994). Angiogenesis involves at least three events (Denekamp, 1993):

1) The basement membrane surrounding a mature capillary dissolves, and a bud grows out of the capillary. (The basement membrane is a layer of specialized connective tissue that attaches the extracellular matrix (ECM), the extracellular "glue," to the epithelial cells of capillaries (see Figure 3.1)).

2) A hollow sprout grows from the bud and migrates toward the angiogenic stimulus (often toward a hypoxic environment).

3) The sprout eventually joins its end with another sprout to form a new capillary vessel.

Further budding from the newly formed capillary follows as the process repeats itself. Angiogenesis is a relatively rapid process, as epithelial buds can form within 48 hours of exposure to an angiogenic factor (Folkman, 1976).

In spite of active angiogenesis, the blood supply in a solid tumor is relatively limited compared to that of normal tissue. Tumor angiogenesis results in chaotic vessel growth, and the new vessels are surrounded by poorly developed basement membranes. Because of this, the

---

[1] Nonsolid tumors, such as leukemias and lymphomas, do not depend upon angiogenesis for obtaining nutrients and oxygen.

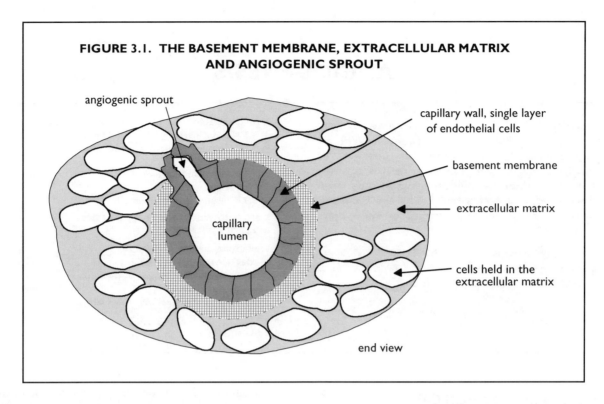

FIGURE 3.1. THE BASEMENT MEMBRANE, EXTRACELLULAR MATRIX AND ANGIOGENIC SPROUT

angiogenic sprout

capillary wall, single layer of endothelial cells

basement membrane

extracellular matrix

capillary lumen

cells held in the extracellular matrix

end view

vessels tend to be thin-walled and leaky. Some sprouts may not fuse with one another and become dead-end sacs. These factors, in conjunction with a lack of tumor lymph vessels, lead to the creation of pressure gradients within tumors. Pressure gradients, in turn, compress the vessels and restrict or occlude blood flow. This appears to be a primary cause of the hypoxia-induced central necrosis found in many large tumors. Hypoxic necrosis occurs in tumor cells that are farther than 150 to 200 μm from a capillary (the diffusion distance of oxygen) (Folkman and Klagsburn, 1987). The increased interstitial pressure also limits the uptake of chemotherapy drugs (and natural anticancer agents) into the tumor. Similarly, it limits the ability of immune cells, or factors that stimulate immune cells, to reach intratumor targets (Jain, 1990).[2]

Capillary density in tumor tissue (a measure of active angiogenesis) may independently predict metastatic disease in women with breast cancer (Weidner et al., 1991). Measuring the capillary density may help to determine if a patient's tumor is in a preangiogenic or angiogenic phase. During this phase, tumor growth and metastasis are usually limited. Tumor growth in the angiogenic phase is exponential and frequently metastatic.

Antiangiogenesis as a cancer therapy was first proposed in 1971. Investigators have since identified numerous factors that either increase or inhibit angiogenesis, and these factors and their effects are being widely studied.

3.2 ANGIOGENIC FACTORS

Numerous angiogenic compounds have been discovered. Some of these are listed in Table 3.1. Angiogenic compounds are commonly found throughout the body and stimulate angiogenesis only under specific, but poorly understood, circumstances. They also vary in the ways they induce angiogenesis, and may act independently or in concert with one another. They may, for example, directly stimulate the growth of endothelial cells, attract macrophages to the site (which then secrete angiogenic factors), or release intracellular stores of angiogenic factors (Folkman and Klagsbrun, 1987).

As mentioned previously, angiogenesis occurs during wound healing, as well as in neoplasia. The repair of wounds involves blood coagulation, inflammation, and the formation of new connective tissue. Each of these processes produces factors that stimulate angiogenesis. Not surprisingly, the factors that stimulate angiogenesis in non-neoplastic circumstances appear to be the same agents that stimulate angiogenesis under neoplastic conditions. In this respect, cancer can be thought of as a wound that will not heal (Nagy et al., 1989). A look at

---

[2] Natural agents that reduce blood viscosity theoretically should facilitate the perfusion of immune factors or other anticancer agents into solid tumors. Agents that decrease fibrinogen levels may have this effect (Jain, 1988). Fibrinolytic agents are discussed in more detail later in this chapter.

TABLE 3.1. PARTIAL LISTING OF ANGIOGENIC FACTORS

ANGIOGENIC CYTOKINES*	NONCYTOKINE ANGIOGENIC FACTORS
Interleukin-1 (IL-1) (secreted by immune cells)	Copper
Interleukin-8 (IL-8) (secreted by immune cells)	Fibrin degradation products
Basic fibroblast growth factor (bFGF)	Eicosanoids such as prostaglandin E_1 and E_2 and Leukotriene B_4
Transforming growth factor-alpha (TGF-α) (secreted by immune cells)	Lactic acid**
Transforming growth factor-beta (TGF-β) (secreted by immune cells)	Kinins
Platelet-derived endothelial cell growth factor (PD-EGF)	Heparin
Vascular permeability factor (VPF)***	Insulin
Platelet activating factor (PAF) (secreted by immune cells)	Nicotinamide
Tumor necrosis factor-alpha (TNF-α, or cachectin) (secreted by immune cells)	Thrombin

* Cytokines are protein factors produced by cells that regulate local cellular growth and function.
** Lactic acid is produced in the hypoxic environment within tumors and may stimulate macrophages to secrete angiogenic factors.
*** VPF, vascular endothelial growth factor (VEGF), and folliculostellate-derived growth factor (FSdGF) have nearly identical amino acid sequences and may be the same factor. These factors bind heparin.
Sources: Folkman, 1993a, or as otherwise specified in the text

the angiogenic factors listed in Table 3.1 reveals that the majority are active during wound healing. These include basic fibroblast growth factor, transforming growth factor, platelet-derived endothelial growth factor, vascular permeability factor, tumor necrosis factor, platelet activating factor, interleukin 1, interleukin-8, fibrin, thrombin, eicosanoids, heparin, and kinins. To better understand the role of some of these agents in angiogenesis, a review of their role in wound healing (in particular, their role in coagulation, inflammation, and connective tissue repair) is presented below. That tumor angiogenesis is stimulated by the same mechanisms that are active in normal wound healing suggests that natural agents that affect wound healing (for example, certain anti-inflammatory and fibrinolytic agents) may inhibit angiogenesis.

3.2.1 Blood Coagulation

In response to vessel injury, platelets at the site of injury initiate immediate clot formation, or *primary hemostasis*. Primary hemostasis occurs in three steps: 1) platelet adhesion to the injured vessel; 2) secretion of various factors from the activated platelets; and 3) platelet aggregation (see Figure 3.2).

Platelet adhesion is initiated when platelets contact the exposed connective tissue of injured tissues (in particular, exposed collagen). Collagen fibrils from the vessel bind with collagen receptors on the platelets.

Adhesion is stabilized by the presence of the adhesive protein von Willebrand factor. Adhesion stimulates platelets to secrete a variety of factors, including fibrinogen and additional von Willebrand factor. The secreted fibrinogen facilitates aggregation (or platelet stickiness) by linking platelets together, and the secreted von Willebrand factor further secures the platelet plug on the vessel wall. Activated platelets also secrete thromboxane A_2, a prostaglandin that further stimulates platelet aggregation. Platelet aggregation is also stimulated by the secretion of platelet activating factor (PAF) by activated immune cells.

Activated platelets also secrete a number of other compounds, including the following: platelet-derived growth factor, which stimulates fibroblasts to produce new connective tissue; fibronectin, an adhesive protein that acts as a track for the placement of new connective tissue; and heparinase, an enzyme that degrades heparin.

Whereas primary hemostasis occurs within seconds of injury, *secondary hemostasis* occurs within minutes. Secondary hemostasis is the process by which a fibrin clot forms to secure and eventually replace the platelet plug. Secondary hemostasis develops along two pathways: the *extrinsic pathway*, which the cells of the vascular lining induce; and the *intrinsic pathway*, induced by plasma factors contacting exposed collagen. The steps in secondary hemostasis are illustrated in Figure 3.3.

In the extrinsic pathway, damaged vascular cells secrete a protein (thromboplastin) that reacts with a

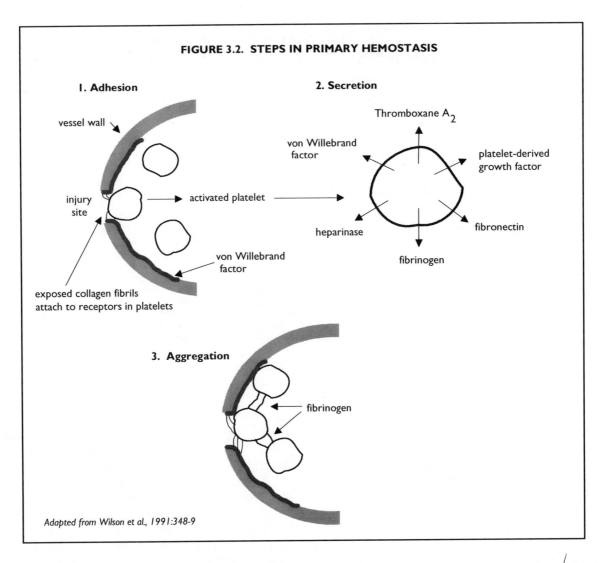

FIGURE 3.2. STEPS IN PRIMARY HEMOSTASIS

I. Adhesion

vessel wall

injury site

activated platelet

von Willebrand factor

exposed collagen fibrils attach to receptors in platelets

2. Secretion

Thromboxane A$_2$

von Willebrand factor

platelet-derived growth factor

heparinase

fibronectin

fibrinogen

3. Aggregation

fibrinogen

Adapted from Wilson et al., 1991:348-9

plasma coagulation factor and calcium to initiate fibrin production. In the intrinsic pathway, fibrin production is initiated when plasma factors (high molecular weight kininogen, factor XII, and prekallikrein) contact collagen. In both cases, a series of steps follows in which thrombin activates fibrinogen and fibrin is produced.

The proteolytic enzyme plasmin breaks down fibrin (fibrinolysis), which balances fibrin formation. Plasmin is produced from plasminogen in the presence of plasminogen activator. Although fibrin production and fibrinolysis occur simultaneously, fibrin production prevails in the early stages of secondary hemostasis. In the later stages, as new connective tissue forms to replace the fibrin clot, fibrinolysis prevails.

3.2.2 Inflammation

Inflammation is a normal consequence of immune reaction. Phagocytic immune cells (neutrophils,

monocyte-macrophages, eosinophils, and basophils) form the core of the inflammatory response. Since the immune system is discussed in detail in Chapter 8, only a brief description of immunity relevant to inflammation is presented here.

During the first stage in inflammation, vasodilation occurs and vascular permeability increases. Both are induced, in large part, by the release of histamine from ruptured or activated mast cells, circulating basophils, and platelets (see Figure 3.4).[3] Mast cells also release serotonin, another compound that induces vasodilation. Increased vascular permeability leads to local edema, during which phagocytes and humoral factors are released into the extravascular space. Some of these humoral factors, such as fibrinogen, assist in clot formation. Others are compounds that assist the migration of phagocytes into the affected site. Humoral factors include the following:

---

[3] Mast cells are basophils that reside in connective tissue.

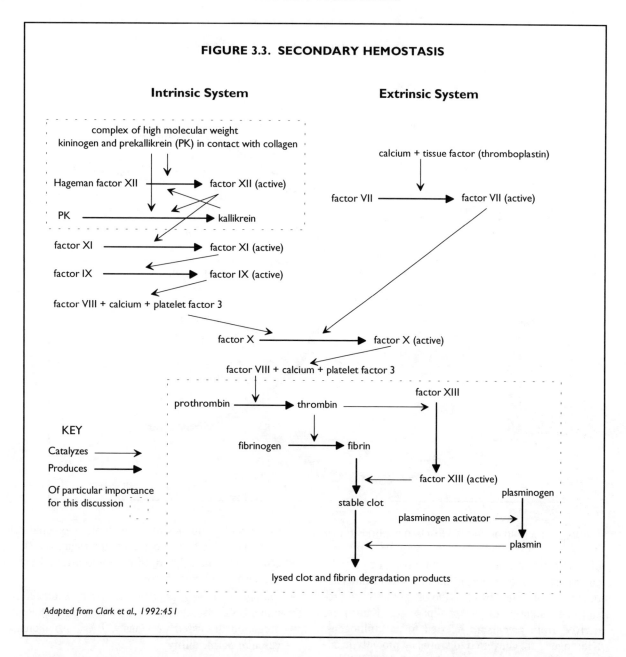

FIGURE 3.3. SECONDARY HEMOSTASIS

Intrinsic System Extrinsic System

complex of high molecular weight
kininogen and prekallikrein (PK) in contact with collagen

Hageman factor XII → factor XII (active)

PK → kallikrein

factor XI → factor XI (active)

factor IX → factor IX (active)

factor VIII + calcium + platelet factor 3

calcium + tissue factor (thromboplastin)

factor VII → factor VII (active)

factor X → factor X (active)

factor VIII + calcium + platelet factor 3

KEY

Catalyzes →

Produces ➔

Of particular importance
for this discussion

prothrombin → thrombin → factor XIII

fibrinogen → fibrin

factor XIII (active)

stable clot

plasminogen

plasminogen activator →

plasmin

lysed clot and fibrin degradation products

Adapted from Clark et al., 1992:451

- Proteins of the *complement system* consist of a series of plasma proteins that attach themselves to antigen-antibody complexes. One of the effects of the complement system is to stimulate mast cells to release histamine and heparin. Histamine release causes further edema. Heparin release assists angiogenesis, as will be described shortly.

- *Eicosanoids* are products of arachidonic acid metabolism. They will be discussed in detail in Chapter 6, with only a brief introduction here. Arachidonic acid is a fatty acid present in the plasma membrane of immune cells and other cells. Arachidonic acid is removed from the plasma membrane by the enzyme phospholipase A_2. Other enzymes catalyze the conversion of free arachidonic acid into a variety of hormone-like compounds called eicosanoids, which can be further classified as prostaglandins and leukotrienes. The production of prostaglandins and leukotrienes is initiated by heparin, kinins (described below), and other inflammatory stimuli. Some prostaglandins, such as prostaglandin E_2 (PGE_2), promote edema and inflammation by increasing vascular permeability. Leukotrienes, for example leukotriene B_4 (LTB_4), have a similar inflammatory effect. PGE_2 also suppresses the activity of immune cells, probably as a negative feedback mechanism to prevent excessive immune response (and resultant tissue damage). Solid tumors are known to produce large amounts of PGE_2.

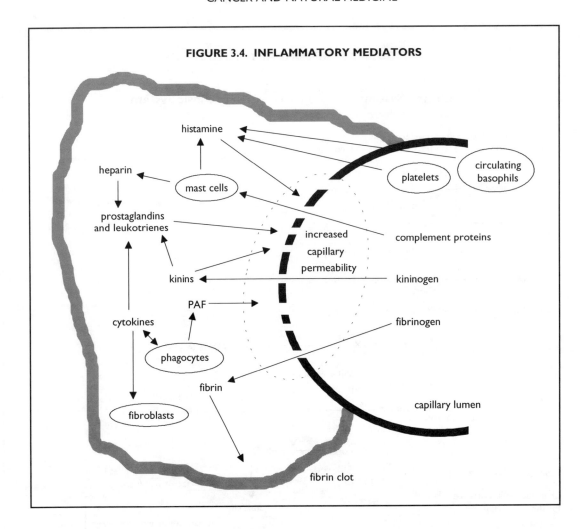

FIGURE 3.4. INFLAMMATORY MEDIATORS

- *Kinins* are a group of highly bioactive peptides found in a variety of body tissues. They produce a number of physiological changes, including increases in vascular permeability. Some of the actions of kinins appear to be mediated by eicosanoids, possibly as a result of stimulation of phospholipase A_2. Kinins are derived from precursors referred to as kininogens. Kininogens are converted to kinins by proteolytic enzymes, the most important of which is kallikrein. The precursor to kallikrein is prekallikrein. As illustrated in Figure 3.3, kallikrein is activated when the serum components kininogen, Hageman factor, and prekallikrein contact exposed collagen.

- *Cytokines* are protein factors produced by cells that regulate local cellular growth and function, including the growth and function of immune cells. They will be discussed in detail with the immune system in Chapter 8. The cytokine interleukin-1 (IL-1) stimulates the proliferation and activity of various immune cells, and stimulates the release of PGE_2. It also stimulates fibroblasts to produce connective tissue, and stimulates the growth of endothelial cells (angiogenesis). The cytokine interleukin-8 (IL-8) causes immune cells to migrate into affected tissues and also stimulates angiogenesis.

- *Platelet activating factor* is secreted by activated immune cells. In addition to its effects on platelet aggregation discussed previously, PAF also increases vascular permeability.

3.2.3 Tissue Repair

After a fibrin clot forms around an injured area and foreign material is removed, the clot is slowly dissolved by plasmin and replaced by connective tissue. Connective tissue is produced by cells called fibroblasts, which are stimulated by basic fibroblast growth factor (bFGF) and other agents. Lastly, angiogenesis supplies the new connective tissue with blood vessels.

The preceding section mentioned that the release of heparin from mast cells facilitates angiogenesis.[4] Heparin is a polysaccharide that performs a number of

---

[4] Contrary to other reports, Jakobson and Hahnenberger (1991) reported that heparin, by itself, inhibited angiogenesis in the CAM assay.

functions. One of its primary functions is to inhibit co-agulation.[5] Heparin binds with basic fibroblast growth factor, which protects bFGF from degradation by proteo-lytic enzymes released during tissue damage. This facili-tates angiogenesis, since bFGF is strongly angiogenic (Folkman, 1993a). One way that bFGF may stimulate angiogenesis is by stimulating the fibroblast cells to pro-duce more connective tissue, since new blood vessels re-quire connective tissue for support. Current research suggests that prior to tissue injury, bFGF is stored in the extracellular matrix, safely bound to heparan sulfate. Tissue injury stimulates secretion of heparin and the en-zymes collagenase and heparinase, which, in turn, may liberate the bound bFGF, thereby allowing angiogenesis to begin (Folkman, 1993a).[6] Heparin also binds and pro-tects a number of other angiogenic factors, such as endo-thelial cell growth factor (Folkman and Klagsbrun, 1987).

In contrast to the above discussions, some heparin complexes actually inhibit angiogenesis. Heparin-cortisone complexes inhibit angiogenesis, apparently by dissolving or limiting the development of the basement membranes of new capillaries (Folkman, 1993a). The exact method by which this is accomplished is unknown. One possibility is that heparin-cortisone complexes may interfere with the synthesis of collagen, a component of the basement membrane. Testing certain proline ana-logs, which interfere with collagen synthesis, in conjunc-tion with cortisone and heparin resulted in 100% inhibi-tion in angiogenic assays using chick embryos (the cho-rioallantoic membrane or CAM assay).[7] The antiangio-genic effects of these compounds appeared to be due to their ability to inhibit collagen synthesis (Ingber and Folkman, 1988). Similarly, beta-aminoproprionitrile, a compound that prevents collagen cross-linking, also in-hibited angiogenesis in the CAM assay. These findings suggest that preventing collagen synthesis can inhibit an-giogenesis. Nicosia et al. (1991) supported this theory by reporting that vitamin C, which is necessary for collagen synthesis, enhanced angiogenesis in CAM assays by stimulating the production and deposition of collagen.[8]

3.3 ANGIOGENIC FACTORS AND NEOPLASIA

Having finished our review of coagulation, inflam-mation, and tissue repair, we can now discuss individual angiogenic factors.

3.3.1 Basic Fibroblast Growth Factor

Basic fibroblast growth factor is a potent angiogenic factor. It has been identified in the urine of patients with malignancies, and its presence has been correlated with survival of patients with breast cancer (Scott and Harris, 1994). As mentioned previously, heparin can both pro-tect and liberate bFGF.[9] Mast cells accumulate at tumor sites prior to angiogenesis, and, the release of heparin by mast cells may be a primary initiator of tumor angiogene-sis (Folkman and Klagsbrun, 1987).

Other sources of bFGF include tumor cells them-selves and tumor-stimulated endothelial cells. This has been documented in a variety of tumors, including basal cell carcinoma, squamous cell carcinoma, hemangioma, colon carcinoma, neuroblastoma, and adrenal carcinoma. Some other tumors, such as Kaposi's sarcoma, ovarian carcinoma, and hemangiosarcoma, do not appear to pro-duce bFGF. However, even these may produce bFGF-like compounds, as demonstrated for Kaposi's sarcoma (Folk-man, 1993a). Therefore, it appears that bFGF or bFGF-like peptides may be produced within a wide variety of human tumors.

There are few, if any, studies on the direct effects of natural agents on bFGF secretion. Therefore, the indirect manipulation of bFGF by agents that inhibit mast cell granulation may offer the most logical strategy at this time. Agents that inhibit mast cell granulation could re-duce vascular permeability (by inhibiting histamine re-lease), and inhibit the heparin-induced liberation and protection of bFGF (by inhibiting heparin release). Nu-merous natural agents inhibit mast cell granulation. Some of these are listed in Table 3.2. Many of these agents occur in traditional formulas that are used to treat asthma and allergies—diseases that are mediated by his-tamine release.

A few natural agents either contain heparin or stimulate bFGF secretion, and should be used with

---

[5] Heparin inhibits the conversion of prothrombin to thrombin and prevents the liberation of thromboplastin from platelets.

[6] Proteins such as protamine and platelet factor IV may inhibit angiogenesis by competing with bFGF for binding sites on heparin.

[7] The amino acid proline is a major component of connective tissue.

[8] The clinical effect of vitamin C supplementation on tumor angiogenesis has not been determined. However, administering high doses of vitamin C to cancer patients did not appear to shorten patient lifespans in clinical trials. Vitamin C is discussed in more detail in Chapter 13.

[9] Liberation of bFGF also occurs during tumor invasion, in which tumor-induced collagenases or other proteolytic enzymes degrade the ECM and release heparin from mast cells. Mast cells contain heparin and histamine in intracellular granules.

TABLE 3.2 NATURAL AGENTS THAT INHIBIT MAST CELL GRANULATION

AGENT	EFFECT	REFERENCE
Acanthopanax sp. (*wu jia pi, ci wu jia*)	Phenolic glycoside fractions of this herb strongly inhibited histamine release from rat mast cells in vitro in a concentration-dependent manner. The most active fraction was 6800 times stronger than disodium cromoglycate, a successful flavonoid-like antiallergy drug.	Umeyama et al., 1992
Aloe vera gel	Inhibited the release of histamine from mast cells in vitro.	Reviewed by Klein et al., 1988
Centipeda minima (*shi hu sui*)	Flavonoid and sesquiterpene compounds obtained from both aqueous and alcohol extracts inhibited histamine release from mast cells in vitro, and demonstrated antiallergic effects in mice in the passive cutaneous anaphylaxis (PCA) test after oral administration.* Extracts from centipeda were more potent than extracts from *Citrus sp., Magnolia sp., Scutellaria sp.,* and *Glycyrrhiza sp.* in inhibiting histamine release from mast cells.	Wu et al., 1991; Sankawa and Chun, 1985
Ganoderma lucidum (*ling zhi*)	Inhibited histamine release from rat mast cells in vitro.	Kohda et al., 1985
Ginkgo biloba extract	Water-soluble components given orally exhibited antiallergic effects in the PCA test in mice. Given intraperitoneally, they inhibited histamine release from mast cells in rats. They were also effective in treating cyclic edema in young women.	Zhang et al., 1990a; Lagrue et al., 1986
Glycyrrhiza sp. (*gan cao*)	Glycyrrhetinic acid markedly inhibited the release of histamine from rat mast cells in vitro.	Imanishi et al, 1989
Hesperidin	The flavonoid hesperidin inhibited histamine release from rat mast cells in vitro and exhibited antiallergic effects in the PCA test in rats.	Matsuda et al., 1991
Magnolia salicifolia (*xin yi hua*)	Inhibited histamine release from rat mast cells in vitro and exhibited antiallergic effects in the PCA test in rats.	Tsuruga et al., 1991
Peucedanum praeruptorum (*qian hu*)	Coumarins inhibited histamine release from rat mast cells in vitro.	Suzuki et al., 1985
Picrorrhiza kurroa (*hu huang lian*)	Oral doses inhibited allergic reaction to antigen challenge in guinea pigs. It was more effective than disodium cromoglycate. Extracts stabilized mast cells in vivo.	Mahajani and Kulkarni, 1977; Panday and Das, 1988
Proanthocyanidins	These flavonoid-like compounds reduce histamine levels in aortic endothelium tissue in vitro.	Masquelier, 1980
Quercetin	The flavonoid quercetin inhibited histamine release from rat mast cells in vitro.	Johri et al., 1985; see Section 14.4.1
Saiboku To (formula)	Inhibited histamine release from mouse and guinea pig mast cells in vitro and exhibited antiallergic effects in the PCA test in rats.	Toda et al., 1988; Nishiyori et al., 1985
Scutellaria baicalensis (*huang qin*)	Flavonoids inhibited histamine release from guinea pig mast cells in vitro and exhibited antiallergic effects in the PCA test in guinea pigs and mice.	Reviewed by Chang and But, 1987:1022-3
Tanacetum parthenium (feverfew)	Inhibited histamine release from rat mast cells in vitro.	Hayes and Foreman et al., 1987

* In this test, an antigen is injected under the skin, and the allergy reaction is recorded after administration of the antiallergy agent.

caution. Leech (*Hirudo nipponia, shui zhi*), for example, contains heparin. However, the clinical effects of heparin administration on angiogenesis are uncertain. In a trial of 603 patients with postsurgical colorectal cancer, subcutaneous heparin injections actually increased five-year survival rates (Kingston et al., 1993). This effect may be due to inhibition of metastasis secondary to a reduction in platelet aggregation, as will be discussed in Chapter 5, or it may be due to increased fibrinolysis, as will be discussed in Section 3.3.4.

A second herb that should be used with caution is *Artemisia princeps (ai ye)*. Hot water extracts induced the production of bFGF and stimulated the proliferation of endothelial cells in vitro (Kaji et al., 1990a, 1990b).

TABLE 3.3. NATURAL AGENTS THAT INHIBIT THE PRODUCTION OF PAF IN VITRO

AGENT	REFERENCE
Bupleurum chinense (chai hu) and *Glycyrrhiza uralensis (gan cao)* from the formula *Saiboku To* *	Nakamura et al., 1993
Docosahexaenoic acid (DHA) (found in fish oil)	Shikano et al., 1993
Ginkgo biloba extract	Etienne et al., 1986**; Baranes et al., 1986; Sanchez-Crespo et al., 1985
Piper kadsura (hai feng tang) and *P. wallichii (shi nan teng)*	Ma et al., 1993a, 1993b; Chen et al., 1993; Han et al., 1989; Shen et al., 1985***; Li et al., 1989
Prehispanolone, isolated from *Leonurus heterophyllus* (*yi mu cao*)	Lee et al., 1991

   * *Scutellaria baicalensis (huang qin),* which is also in this formula, had no effect.
   ** Orally effective in rat studies.
   *** Kadsurenone, the active ingredient, was effective in reducing PAF-induced increases in cutaneous vascular permeability in guinea pigs at an oral dose of 25 to 50 mg/kg.

3.3.2 Platelet Activating Factor

Platelet activating factor (PAF), a molecule produced by immune cells, stimulates platelet aggregation. In addition, PAF increases vascular permeability, produces bronchospasms, and is, therefore, an important mediator in inflammation, allergic reactions, and asthma. Platelet activating factor may affect carcinogenesis by acting as a tumor promoting agent, and may affect tumor growth by inducing angiogenesis.[10]

Animal studies using the sponge-implant method have shown that platelet activating factor increases angiogenesis (Andrade et al., 1992).[11] Cells of some tumors, such as Kaposi's sarcoma, can be stimulated to produce PAF in vitro (Sciacca et al., 1994), and elevated PAF levels have been observed in patients with certain cancers (Marathe et al., 1991). For example, plasma PAF levels may be markedly higher in patients with breast cancer compared to those with benign tumors or healthy subjects (Nigam et al., 1989; Pitton et al., 1989). In these studies, PAF was also elevated in the cancer tissue itself.

A few studies have shown that a small number of natural agents inhibit the production of PAF in vitro. These agents may have potential for inhibiting PAF-induced angiogenesis in vivo. Further studies are needed to determine the clinical efficacy of this approach. Natural agents that inhibit the production of PAF by immune cells are listed in Table 3.3. It is not surprising that some of these agents are used traditionally to inhibit inflammation. For example, *Piper kadsura* is used in Chinese medicine to treat the pain of arthritis, and *Leonurus heterophyllus* is used to treat premenstrual abdominal pain. The traditional Japanese formula *Saiboku To* is used to treat asthma, which may be due in part to its anti-PAF activity.[12]

3.3.3 Kinins

Kinins are a group of highly bioactive peptides found in the pancreas (Greek: *kallikreas*) and a variety of other body tissues. They lower blood pressure and increase heart rate by causing vasodilatation, and produce edema by causing increased vascular permeability. In addition, they induce contraction of various smooth muscles (such as in the lungs), and stimulate nerve endings and produce pain (Goodman and Gilman, 1985:656). The two primary groups of kinins, kallidin and bradykinin, are derived from precursors referred to as kininogens. As discussed previously, kininogens are converted to kinins by proteolytic enzymes, the most important of which is kallikrein. The precursor of kallikrein is prekallikrein. Both prekallikrein and kallikrein play active roles in blood coagulation (see Figure 3.3). Some of the actions of kinins appear to be mediated by eicosanoids, possibly as a result of kinin stimulation of phospholipase A_2, the enzyme that liberates arachidonic acid from plasma membranes for eicosanoid production.

Kinins appear to play a role in angiogenesis and other aspects of cancer. Substance P, a type of kinin and

---

[10] The effects of PAF on tumor promotion are likely related to its ability to stimulate inflammation (Bennett et al., 1993). Numerous tumor promoting agents possess the ability to stimulate inflammation.

[11] In this assay, a sponge is implanted under the skin of animals, and test compounds are added to determine if they can stimulate the growth of new blood vessels into the sponge.

[12] Its antiasthmatic effects are also thought to be due to the steroid-sparing effects of *Magnolia officinalis (hou po)* (Homma et al., 1993), and its antihistamine effects (mentioned in Table 3.2).

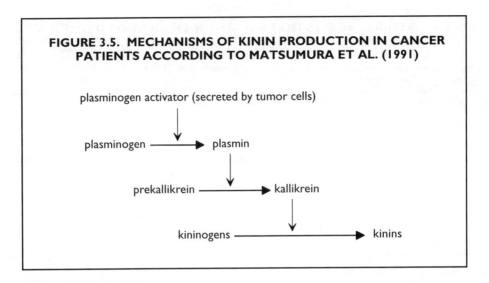

FIGURE 3.5. MECHANISMS OF KININ PRODUCTION IN CANCER PATIENTS ACCORDING TO MATSUMURA ET AL. (1991)

a major mediator of neurogenic inflammation, causes intense angiogenesis in the rat sponge-implant model (Fan et al., 1993), induces angiogenesis in the rabbit cornea model, and increases proliferation of human endothelial cells in vitro (Ziche et al., 1990). Bradykinin also enhances angiogenesis in the rat sponge-implant model (Hu and Fan, 1993).

Kinins are elevated in the plasma of patients with some forms of cancer, in part, due to factors secreted from tumor cells. Both prekallikrein and kininogen levels were significantly lower in the plasma of 28 patients with advanced cancer as compared to controls (Matsumura et al., 1991). Prekallikrein levels were low, apparently due to conversion to kallikrein, and kininogen levels were low due to conversion to kinins (see Figure 3.5). In-vitro testing indicated that plasminogen activates prekallikrein. Plasminogen is a precursor to plasmin, and is activated by plasminogen activator. In view of these results, the authors of this study suggest that the production of plasmin by tumor-secreted plasminogen activator initiates kinin generation in patients with advanced cancer. Tumor cells may produce plasmin to facilitate tumor invasion, since plasmin degrades the extracellular matrix. Other investigators have also reported abnormally low levels of prekallikrein and kininogen in the serum of cancer patients (Roeise et al., 1990; Deutsch et al., 1983). The production of kinins may result in edema and increased angiogenesis. In addition, the production of kallikrein may lead to coagulation disorders. Figure 3.3 showed that increased levels of kallikrein catalyze the start of the intrinsic coagulation system. This may account in part for the increased incidence of coagulation disorders seen in patients with advanced cancer.

Natural agents that inhibit kinin production or degrade kinins may inhibit kinin-induced angiogenesis. These agents include the proteolytic enzyme bromelain (derived from pineapple stems) and the gel of *Aloe vera*. The kinin-degrading and fibrinolytic effects of bromelain are discussed in Section 15.3.3 along with the many other activities of bromelain. *Aloe vera* gel deactivates bradykinin and inhibits the formation of histamine in vitro (reviewed by Klein and Penneys, 1988). Glycoproteins isolated from other aloe species, such as *A. arborescens* and *A. saponaria,* also degrade bradykinin in vitro (Yagi et al., 1982, 1987). Aloe gel has also demonstrated antiangiogenic activity in vivo in the inflamed synovial pouch model in mice.[13] In this model, local application of *Aloe vera* reduced angiogenesis by 50%, reduced the number of mast cells in the pouch by 50%, and increased the number of fibroblasts (Davis et al., 1992).

3.3.4 Fibrin and Thrombin

Recent research suggests that fibrin and thrombin may play roles in tumor-induced angiogenesis.[14] Fibrinogen (the precursor of fibrin) and thrombin reach the extracellular space through capillaries made hyperpermeable during inflammation. Tissues surrounding solid tumors are commonly inflamed, and as illustrated in Figure 3.3, thrombin activates fibrin, which then encases the inflamed area. In neoplasia, the primary agent that causes hyperpermeability is likely to be vascular permeability factor (VPF), which tumor cells secrete.[15] VPF is a

---

[13] In this model, air is injected under the skin of animals to create a synovial-like pouch, into which an inflammatory agent is injected.

[14] Thrombin stimulates angiogenesis in the CAM assay apart from its involvement in fibrin formation (Tsopanoglou et al., 1993).

[15] Vascular permeability factor is very similar, if not identical to vascular endothelial growth factor (VEGF). It is believed to be a primary angiogenic factor (Scott and Harris, 1994). Using a monoclonal antibody specific to VEGF, three *(continued next page)*

protein that is 50,000 times more active than histamine in enhancing vascular permeability (Nagy et al., 1989).

Fibrin deposition occurs within minutes of the entry of fibrinogen and other clotting factors into the extracellular space. At the same time that fibrin is forming, the fibrinolytic system is stimulated and substantial destruction of fibrinogen and fibrin occurs. Up to 90% of fibrinogen may be degraded immediately. In spite of this, fibrin production prevails and sufficient fibrin accumulates to produce a provisional fibrin stroma surrounding the tumor (Brown et al., 1989; Beranek, 1989; Nagy et al., 1989). In fact, the formation of this fibrin stroma may be the most important precondition for angiogenesis. Studies show that the removal of fibrin through fibrinolysis terminates angiogenesis (Liu, 1992).

The ongoing maintenance of this stroma facilitates the growth of the tumor in at least two ways:

1) The fibrin stroma provides a structure that physically supports the tumor (Nagy et al., 1989). In early stages of tumor growth, the fibrin stroma encases individual tumor cells or clumps of tumor cells.[16] These clumps remain discrete units as the tumor grows, and eventually macrophages, fibroblasts, and new blood vessels invade the older stroma transforming it into mature connective tissue. The newer stroma, deposited on the periphery of the tumor, retains its fibrin composition. In total, the stroma in some tumors can comprise up to 90% of a tumor's mass. By increasing fibrinolysis, the stroma that supports tumor growth may be destroyed, and the periphery of the tumor may be exposed to greater immune attack.

2) Certain products of fibrin degradation (produced during fibrinolysis) are factors that stimulate angiogenesis (Thompson et al., 1992, 1991, 1990a, 1990b; Liu, 1992; Liu et al., 1990; Dvorak et al., 1987).

The stimulation of angiogenesis by fibrin degradation products appears to play a significant role in normal wound healing. Once a fibrin stroma forms and inflammation recedes, three processes are initiated: 1) Plasmin begins to degrade the fibrin clot; 2) macrophages and fibrocytes infiltrate the stroma; and 3) angiogenesis proceeds. Eventually, connective tissue replaces the stroma. Once fibrinolysis is complete, angiogenesis stops. However, in the case of a tumor, inflammation continues, as do fibrin production and degradation. Therefore, angiogenesis is continuous in tumors.[17] This process may be related to the development of coagulation disorders in cancer patients, as discussed in Box 3.1.

The natural process of wound healing is vital to survival of the species and, quite likely, is guarded by redundancy to assure its ability to function. It is not surprising

---

BOX 3.1. COAGULATION DISORDERS IN CANCER PATIENTS

Numerous authors have reported reduced fibrinolysis in humans with neoplastic disease (Mitter and Zielinski, 1991; Bu et al., 1990; Honn et al., 1982). The most important coagulation disease in cancer patients is disseminated intravascular coagulation (DIC), which can be acute or chronic (reviewed by Calabresi and Schein, 1993:192-5).

Chronic DIC is a complex disease marked by diffuse coagulation and thrombus formation, caused by the systemic introduction of procoagulant materials into the blood. These procoagulant materials may include fibrinogen, thrombin, and other compounds. In contrast, acute DIC is a disease marked by excessive bleeding. This also involves intravascular activation of clotting pathways (although not necessarily thrombus formation) leading to a depletion of coagulation factors.

The reasons for the increased incidence of coagulation disorders in cancer patients is not clear. As discussed, fibrinogen and other procoagulant products may leave the vasculature near a tumor. In addition, plasma fibrinogen levels may be increased secondary to increased synthesis in the liver—an event that may occur in 50 to 80% of patients. In patients with leukemia (particularly acute promyelocytic leukemia), DIC is thought to be a result of the release of granules in leukemic cells which contain promoters of coagulation.

(continued) human tumors lines transplanted into mice were markedly inhibited (up to 96% decrease in tumor weight) by administration of the antibody (Kim et al., 1993). The density of vessels at the tumor sites was decreased, suggesting that VEGF is an angiogenic factor.

[16] In addition to solid tumors, fibrin deposits have also been observed in lymphomas (Nagy et al., 1989).

[17] Other differences also exit. For example, the conversion of fibrinogen to fibrin in normal wounds is in large part mediated by clotting factors discharged by platelets. In tumors, the neoplastic cells secrete the clotting factors thromboplastin and prothrombin (see Figure 3.3) (Nagy et al., 1989).

then, that so many factors appear to stimulate angiogenesis. This complexity is an obstacle to efforts to undermine this process, and a simple solution is not likely. The rate-limiting step in this process appears to be increased vascular permeability, rather than the availability of coagulation factors (Nagy et al., 1989). Therefore, inhibiting increased permeability should receive primary attention.

So far this chapter has identified a number of agents that increase vascular permeability, act as angiogenic factors, and/or assist angiogenic factors. These include VPF, histamine, heparin, PAF, kinins, thrombin, and fibrin. Since the natural angiogenic process appears to be guarded by redundancy, it would seem likely that a therapy that targets all of these factors, with special emphasis on normalizing vascular permeability, may have the greatest chance of success. To my knowledge, the clinical efficacy of this combined approach has not been tested. To some degree, parts of this approach have been used in Traditional Chinese Medicine, where one of the

traditional herbal strategies for treating cancer is "invigoration" of the blood circulation using fibrinolytic and other agents. However, the effects of this traditional strategy on angiogenesis has not been determined. Obviously, the degree to which fibrinolysis can be stimulated may be limited. Patients with cancer often are recovering from surgeries or have tumors that bleed. Excessive fibrinolysis in these patients could be catastrophic.

Natural agents that inhibit the production of histamine, heparin, PAF, and kinins were discussed previously. Natural agents that inhibit fibrin production or stimulate fibrinolysis are listed in Table 3.4. Also listed in Table 3.4 are previously unmentioned agents that inhibit increases in vascular permeability. Agents that may inhibit thrombus formation by inhibiting platelet aggregation are not discussed further here, since platelet aggregation is not a critical factor in tumor-induced fibrin production. Agents that increase plasmin production are discussed further in Chapter 4.

TABLE 3.4. NATURAL AGENTS THAT INHIBIT FIBRIN PRODUCTION, STIMULATE FIBRINOLYSIS, OR INHIBIT INCREASED VASCULAR PERMEABILITY		
AGENT	**MECHANISM**	**REFERENCE**
AGENTS THAT INHIBIT FIBRIN PRODUCTION OR STIMULATE FIBRINOLYSIS		
Allium sativum (garlic, *da suan*)	Daily ingestion of garlic by humans increased fibrinolysis during the first four weeks. Levels dropped to baseline by the 12th week.	Ernst, 1981; Arora et al., 1981; reviewed by Chang and But, 1986:90
Agkistrodon acutus (bai hua she), Pheretima aspergillum (di long), Hirudo nipponia (shui zhi), Scolopendra subspinipes mutilans (wu gong), and Buthus martensi (quan xie)	In a study on 112 extracts prepared from 37 different animal species, water extracts of these species demonstrated marked fibrinolytic activity in vitro.	Wang et al., 1989
Artemisia argyi (ai ye) *	Inhibits both thrombin and plasmin, and prolongs prothrombin time in vitro. Prothrombin time is a measure of bleeding time.	Niwa et al., 1985
Atractylodes macrocephala (bai zhu)	Intragastric administration to rats for one to four weeks significantly prolonged prothrombin time. Oral administration to humans had the same effect. Levels returned to normal after 10 days.	Reviewed by Chang and But, 1986:374
Brinase, a proteolytic enzyme from *Aspergillus oryzae*	Induces fibrinolytic activity in animals and humans after intravenous administration. Degrades fibrinogen in human plasma in vitro, but does not activate plasmin.	Vanhove et al., 1979; Roschlau and Fisher, 1966; FitzGerald et al., 1979
Bromelain	Stimulates plasmin production and has direct fibrinolytic activity.	See Section 15.3.3
Brown alge, *Laminaria sp. (kun bu), Sargassum sp. (hai zao)*	High molecular weight polysaccharides inactivate thrombin and also act by mechanisms similar to heparin.	Grauffel et al., 1989
Bu Yang Huan Wu Tang (formula)	Inhibits conversion of fibrinogen to fibrin by thrombin in vitro. The formula contains *Paeonia lactiflora* (see below) and increases blood circulation. It is used in cases of stroke.	Li XL et al., 1989
Capsicum annuum (cayenne pepper)	Stimulates fibrinolytic activity after oral administration in humans.	Visudhiphan et al., 1982
(Table continues)		

TABLE 3.4. *(continued)*		
AGENT	**MECHANISM**	**REFERENCE**
AGENTS THAT INHIBIT FIBRIN PRODUCTION OR STIMULATE FIBRINOLYSIS *(continued)*		
Carthamus tinctorius (hong hua)	Alcohol extracts inhibit prothrombin and thrombin activity, and prolong prothrombin time in vitro. Widely used in China to treat patients with coronary heart disease.	Reviewed by Chang and But, 1986:535
Curcuma longa (jiang huang)	Enhances fibrinolytic activity and inhibits platelet aggregation in vitro. Also possesses anti-inflammatory activity in vivo. Used in China to treat patients with angina pectoris.	Reviewed by Chang and But, 1987:936-8
Paeonia lactiflora (chi shao and *bai shao)*	Stimulates fibrinolysis by increasing plasmin production in vitro, and inhibits fibrin production by inhibiting thrombin in vitro.	Wang and Ma, 1990
Salvia miltiorrhiza (dan shen)	Stimulated plasminogen activator to produce plasmin in vitro. Also stimulated the conversion of fibrinogen to fibrin in vitro. Used widely in China to treat patients with coronary heart disease and has demonstrated some success in treating DIC.	Reviewed by Chang and But, 1986:258-62
AGENTS THAT INHIBIT INCREASED VASCULAR PERMEABILITY		
Aesculus hippocastanum (horse chestnut)	Used orally in humans to treat hemorrhoids and edema. Scavenges free radicals and may inhibit enzymatic breakdown of the basement membrane. Improves venous tone. Inhibits increased capillary permeability induced by a variety of agents (including bradykinin) in human and animal veins in vitro. Its ability to increase the tension of isolated human veins may be due to increased $PGF_{2-alpha}$ production and is inhibited by cyclooxygenase inhibitors. Given orally or intravenously, it inhibited experimentally-induced brain edema in animals and inhibited experimentally-induced paw edema and increased capillary permeability in rats. Given intravenously it reduced lymph flow in rats, apparently by reducing the size of capillary small pores (quercetin increased lymph flow). The active agent appears to be the saponin escin.	Reviewed by Murray and Pizzorno, 1991:538; Bisler et al., 1986; Guillaume and Padioleau, 1994; Longiave et al., 1978; Czernicki, 1977; Arnold and Przerwa, 1976; Ogura et al., 1975; Vogel et al., 1970; Vogel and Stroecker, 1966
Angelica sinensis (dang gui)	Inhibits increased vascular permeability induced by a variety of agents in vitro.	Hu et al., 1991
Bupleurum chinense (chai hu)	Inhibits increased vascular permeability induced by histamine and ascetic acid.	Reviewed by Chang and But, 1987:968
Corydalis turtschaninovii (yan hu suo)	Inhibits increased vascular permeability induced by acetic acid in mice.	Kubo et al., 1994
Ligustrum lucidum (nu zhen zi)	Inhibits increased vascular permeability induced by acetic acid in mice.	Dai et al., 1989
Omega-3 fatty acids such as EPA and DHA from fish oil	Favors production of PGE_3 over PGE_2. PGE_3 is less inflammatory than PGE_2.	See Section 12.1
Proanthocyanidins	High affinity for vascular tissue. Inhibits enzymatic breakdown of basement membrane. Improves integrity of vascular wall. Inhibits increased vascular permeability induced by a variety of agents in vitro and in vivo. Inhibits formation of postoperative edema in humans. Increases capillary resistance in animal studies and in hypertensive and diabetic patients.	Reviewed by Murray and Pizzorno, 1991:538; reviewed by Schwitters and Masquelier, 1993:52; Baruch, 1984; Lagrua et al., 1981; Robert et al., 1990; Cahn and Borzeix, 1983
Ruscus aculeatus (butcher's broom)	History of use in treating hemorrhoids and varicose veins. Vasoconstrictive. Inhibits increased vascular permeability induced by a variety of agents in vitro. Effective orally in humans. The active ingredients appear to be ruscogenins.	Reviewed by Murray and Pizzorno, 1991:538; Bouskela et al., 1993; Rudofsky, 1989

* Although *Artemisia argyi* inhibits fibrin production, the related species *A. princeps* (also called *ai ye*) has been shown to induce bFGF production. Since bFGF is a very potent angiogenic factor, artemisia species should be used with caution.

TABLE 3.5. NATURAL AGENTS THAT DECREASE TISSUE COPPER LEVELS OR INHIBIT FIBRONECTIN SYNTHESIS		
AGENT	**EFFECT**	**REFERENCE**
Cysteine	At high intravenous doses complexes with copper and may reduce excess copper levels.	Reviewed by Braverman and Pfeiffer, 1987:115; Hjortso et al., 1990
Epimedium sagittatum (yin yang huo)	Inhibited the deposition of fibrin and fibronectin on the glomerular capillary wall in rats with experimentally induced chronic renal failure.	Cheng et al., 1994
Salvia miltiorrhiza (dan shen)	An isolated component of the herb inhibited proline uptake by fibroblasts, and inhibited fibronectin and collagen synthesis by cultured fibroblasts.*	Liu et al., 1992b
* In contrast, in rats with experimentally induced acute liver failure, *Salvia miltiorrhiza (dan shen)* and *Paeonia lactiflora (bai shao and chi shao)* increased plasma fibronectin levels (Qi, 1991).		

3.3.5 Copper

Copper complexes have been shown to increase angiogenesis, and angiogenesis fails to occur in copper-deficient rabbits. Copper sulfate induces angiogenesis in the rabbit cornea model (Parke et al., 1988). Heparin-copper complexes also induce angiogenesis in the rabbit cornea model, and may play a prominent role in tumor-induced angiogenesis in humans (Folkman and Klagsbrun, 1987). Apparently, copper stimulates angiogenesis and endothelial cell migration through enhancing fibronectin synthesis (Hannan and McAuslan, 1982). Fibronectin is an adhesive glycoprotein found in the basement membrane. During the early stage of angiogenesis specialized endothelial cells produce fibronectin. These specialized cells are the first to migrate in response to an angiogenic signal and deposit a trail of fibronectin in their wake. The fibronectin acts as a track on which the other endothelial cells can follow (McAuslan and Gole, 1980).

Copper-chelating drugs, such as penicillamine-D, also inhibit angiogenesis, which adds further support for the angiogenic role of copper (Folkman, 1993a).[18] Penicillamine-D is used to treat arthritis, and may inhibit angiogenesis in arthritic joints.[19] Further evidence comes from studies that correlate increased tumor copper levels with increased angiogenic and metastatic ability of mouse mammary adenocarcinomas (Fuchs and DeLustig, 1989).

Not all tumors are affected by copper levels, however. An in-vivo study on chondrosarcoma implants in rat muscles showed that copper-deficient diets did not affect tumor angiogenesis (Schuschke et al., 1992). The authors suggest that the ability of copper to mediate angiogenesis may be a function of the tumor type, the host tissue, or specific conditions of copper depletion.[20] One group of tumors that may be especially sensitive to copper depletion is brain tumors. Cerebral neoplasms sequester copper, and penicillamine treatment inhibits the growth and vascularity of brain tumors in rabbits (Brem et al., 1990). Penicillamine treatment failed to affect the same tumor when implanted into the thigh muscle.

Agents that decrease tissue copper levels, or inhibit fibronectin synthesis may be useful in preventing copper-dependent angiogenesis. Natural agents that may have this affect are listed in Table 3.5.

3.3.6 Insulin and Nicotinamide

Insulin stimulated angiogenesis in the inflamed synovial pouch model in rats (Kimura, 1987). Diabetic mice exhibited reduced angiogenic action. Angiogenesis induced by insulin preceded collagen fiber formation, and may be an early step in angiogenesis. As will be discussed in Chapter 7, insulin is also a growth factor that stimulates proliferation of tumor cells. Since insulin production greatly increases in response to dietary sugars, it may be prudent for patients with cancer to avoid refined sugars or other agents that unnecessarily increase insulin production. However, a correlation between high sugar intake and increased angiogenesis has not yet been demonstrated clinically.

Nicotinamide has been identified as an angiogenic factor in animal tumors, and commercial nicotinamide

---

[18] Razoxane, an antimetastatic drug structurally related to the metal chelator EDTA, inhibits tumor invasion, presumably by complexing copper and/or other metals (Karakiulakis et al., 1989). Penicillamine-copper complexes may inhibit angiogenesis by producing hydrogen peroxide, which inhibits endothelial cell proliferation (Matsubara et al., 1989).

[19] In contrast, copper has also been successful with some arthritic patients. Quite likely this may be due to the fact that copper is necessary for the production of connective tissue (reviewed by Murray and Pizzorno, 1991:451).

[20] The rats used in this study were on a copper-deficient diet for only seven days prior to implant.

induced neovascularization in the CAM assay (Kull et al., 1987; Collins et al., 1989). Nicotinamide (niacinamide) is a form of niacin (nicotinic acid, or vitamin B_3). The body synthesizes it from the amino acid tryptophan, and it is also available as a vitamin supplement. The effects of nicotinamide supplementation on angiogenesis in humans has yet to be demonstrated. Nicotinamide also decreases blood flow resistance in tumors, and subsequently, lowers the intratumor vascular pressure (Lee et al., 1992). The method by which nicotinamide produces this effect is not understood. Since high vascular pressure limits the uptake of drugs by a tumor, it may be possible, under certain conditions, to use nicotinamide to increase the efficacy of anticancer drugs.

3.4 NATURAL AGENTS THAT INHIBIT ANGIOGENESIS

A number of natural agents exhibit antiangiogenic properties. Some of these are listed in Table 3. 6. Antiangiogenic agents that also exhibit antioxidant activity are discussed below.

Gold thiomalate has been shown to inhibit angiogenesis and block the release of angiogenic factors by macrophages. Gold thiomalate is used to treat arthritis and appears to prevent angiogenesis in arthritic joint spaces. The antiangiogenic activity of gold thiomalate may be due more to the thiol it contains than the effects of gold itself. Thiol compounds, such as those found in glutathione and *Allium sp.*, markedly inhibited the production of angiogenic factors by macrophages, whereas gold compounds that did not contain thiol were not inhibitory (Koch et al., 1991).

Preparations of *Allium sativum* (garlic, *da suan*) have been tested clinically in China as anticancer agents. In a study on 57 patients with various advanced carcinomas, administration of garlic produced marked improvement in 13% and some improvement in 50% (reviewed by Chang and But, 1986:90). The results of this study are hard to interpret from the data presented due to the lack of controls and unreported design specifications (such as the criteria for judging improvement). Theoretically, garlic may inhibit cancer by a variety of mechanisms, including reduced angiogenesis, reduced platelet aggregation, and increased fibrinolysis. Thioallyl compounds found in garlic inhibit umbilical endothelial cell proliferation in vitro (Lee et al., 1994).

The antiangiogenic effect of thiol compounds may be due to their ability to inhibit free radical production by macrophages (Koch et al., 1992). Other free radical scavengers, such as urea and catalase, also inhibited angiogenesis in vitro. The effect was due in part to a reduction of tumor necrosis factor production by macrophages (recall that TNF is an angiogenic factor). However, additional cytokines or other factors were also responsible.

TABLE 3.6. ANTIANGIOGENIC SUBSTANCES		
SUBSTANCE	**COMMENT**	**REFERENCE**
Cartilage extract, including collagenase inhibitors	Discussed in detail in Section 15.2	Reviewed by Folkman, 1993a
Genistein	Discussed in detail in Section 14.6	
Gold thiomalate	Discussed in text	
Hydrocortisone and heparin complexes	Dissolves or limits the development of the basement membranes of new capillaries	Reviewed by Folkman, 1993a
Interferon-alpha (IFN-α)	A cytokine secreted by immune cells	Reviewed by Folkman, 1993a, 1993b
Magnolia liliflora (xin yi hua)	The lignan magnosalin inhibited angiogenesis in the inflamed synovial pouch model in mice and inhibited the proliferation of rat endothelial cells in vitro. The compound was active at 10 μg/ml, but was less effective in inhibiting angiogenesis than hydrocortisone.	Kimura et al, 1990, 1991, 1992
Penicillamine-D	Penicillamine-D is a copper chelator	Reviewed by Folkman, 1993a
Platelet factor IV	Binds heparin	Reviewed by Folkman, 1993a
Protamine	Binds heparin	Reviewed by Folkman, 1993a
(Table continues)		

	TABLE 3.6. *(continued)*	
SUBSTANCE	**COMMENT**	**REFERENCE**
SCM-chitin	SCM-chitin is a modified derivative of chitin. Chitin is a polysaccharide found in insect exoskeletons such as cicada molting *(Cryptotympana atrata, chan tui)*. It is composed of N-acetyl-glucosamine (NAG) residues, and inhibits collagenase and heparinase. It is not clear if NAG itself possesses antiangiogenic properties. NAG is available commercially and has been used to treat osteoarthritis.	Reviewed by Folkman, 1993a
Thiol compounds, such as glutathione and *Allium sp.*	Discussed in text	
Viscum album (mistletoe)	Aqueous extracts inhibited angiogenesis in vivo, and were cytotoxic.	Yoon et al., 1995
Vitamin A	Vitamin A analogs inhibit the growth of endothelial cells in vitro and inhibit angiogenesis in the CAM assay. This may be due, in part, to the ability of vitamin A to inhibit collagen synthesis.	Braunhunt and Palomares, 1991; Paige et al., 1991; Oikawa et al., 1989; Ingber and Folkman, 1988
Vitamin D_3 metabolites	Vitamin D_3 may up-regulate vitamin A receptors, and therefore potentiate vitamin A's antiangiogenic effects. The combination of 1,25-dihydroxyvitamin D_3—the active metabolite of vitamin D_3 in humans—and various retinol analogs synergistically inhibited tumor-induced angiogenesis in mice. Vitamin D_3 may also exhibit antiangiogenic activity apart from its association with vitamin A. Although vitamin D_3 itself was not active in the CAM assay, 1,25-dihydroxyvitamin D_3 was active. Effective concentrations were at the nanogram level and were comparable to the effective concentrations of retinoic acid. The mechanism by which 1,25-dihydroxyvitamin D_3 inhibits angiogenesis is unknown.	Scott and Harris, 1994; Majewski et al., 1993; Oikawa et al., 1990b

BOX 3.2. HYPOXIA AND ANGIOGENESIS

Low oxygen levels (hypoxia) play a significant role in limiting the proliferation of neoplastic cells in solid tumors. Hypoxic conditions are created, in large part, by the chaotic and faulty development of the neovasculature during tumor angiogenesis. If sufficiently extreme, hypoxia causes cell death. This accounts for the common observation of central necrosis within solid tumors. Hypoxia may also stimulate angiogenesis. Macrophages cultured under hypoxic environments secrete abundant amounts of an angiogenesis factor, but secrete little angiogenesis factor under normal oxygen conditions. Under high oxygen conditions, no angiogenesis factor is produced (Knighton et al., 1983). Since macrophages comprise 10 to 30% of the cells in a solid tumor, and solid tumors commonly contain hypoxic areas, hypoxia-stimulated macrophages may produce substantial quantities of angiogenesis factor. That hypoxic conditions stimulate angiogenesis is not surprising. As discussed in the text, tumor-induced angiogenesis and wound-induced angiogenesis share many of the same mechanisms. In normal wound healing, hypoxic tissues are most in need of angiogenesis and the body likely contains redundant mechanisms to ensure that angiogenesis in these locations is successful.

The success of radiotherapy treatment also depends on the degree of oxygen saturation in tumor cells. In general, cells within hypoxic areas respond poorly to radiotherapy. Agents that increase tumor blood flow, and therefore oxygen, have been investigated as adjuvants in radiotherapy.

One possibility is that free radical scavengers induce the release of angiogenic inhibitors.

Macrophages may be stimulated to produce more angiogenesis factor in low oxygen conditions, such as that found in solid tumors. This is discussed in more detail in Box 3.2. Note that the oxygen distribution within tumors is not uniform. It can vary according to a number of factors, one of which may be age. For example, the hypoxic fraction in EMT6 tumors in aging mice was 41%, whereas the hypoxic fraction in tumors from young mice was 19% (Rockwell et al., 1991).

3.5 NEOVASCULATURE AS AN ANTICANCER TARGET

3.5.1 Antiangiogenesis vs. Antivascular Therapies

Antivascular therapies are distinct from antiangiogenic therapies (Denekamp, 1993). Antiangiogenic therapies target the inhibition of endothelial cell proliferation. In contrast, antivascular therapies target the microvasculature itself. Antivascular therapies attempt to induce a blockade, collapse, stasis, hemorrhage, or thrombosis of the capillaries in order to disrupt the supply of blood to the tumor. Denekamp argues that antiangiogenesis therapies stop new blood vessel growth, but do not lead to tumor regression, as the existing vascular network continues to supply the tumor. Antivascular therapies, on the other hand, reduce the existing blood supply and, therefore, theoretically should lead to tumor regression. Antivascular therapies employ one or more of the following mechanisms:

- Destruction of endothelial cells, which may account, in part, for the antitumor action of some common chemotherapy agents. Most cytotoxic chemotherapy drugs target the fastest growing cells and, therefore, may target endothelial cells, which divide rapidly during angiogenesis.
- Blocking the capillaries by destroying endothelial cells, increasing platelet aggregation, and/or increasing coagulation.
- Causing hemorrhage within the capillaries by damaging fragile vessel walls.
- Causing the collapse of capillaries by decreasing local blood flow.

3.5.2 Natural Agents that Have Antivascular Activity

Of the antivascular mechanisms listed above, the destruction of endothelial cells and vascular blockage may best lend themselves to manipulation by natural agents. A large number of natural agents are toxic to tumor cells (and normal cells), and more than a few of these may be toxic to endothelial cells. Neovasculature as an anticancer target is a new and little-studied concept. Not surprisingly, few, if any, studies have specifically investigated the toxic effects of natural agents on endothelial cells. Additional research is needed to identify those agents that may be useful in antivascular therapies.

Agents that induce tumor necrosis, such as the cytokine tumor necrosis factor, may block the vasculature by clogging the capillaries with debris. For example, polysaccharide fractions (acemannan) isolated from *Aloe vera*

increased the survival of sarcoma-bearing mice. The tumors in animals treated with acemannan exhibited vascular congestion, edema, leukocyte infiltration, central necrosis with hemorrhage, and peripheral fibrosis (Peng et al., 1991). The authors suggest that acemannan may induce these effects by stimulating macrophages to produce the cytokines interleukin-1 and tumor necrosis factor.

The synthetic flavonoid, flavone acetic acid (FAA) also stimulates macrophages to produce tumor necrosis factor, which leads to vascular blockage by necrotic debris. Administering a single dose of FAA to tumor-bearing mice significantly reduced tumor burdens due to a dramatic reduction of blood flow within the tumors (Mahadevan and Hart, 1991). The effect was both specific to tumor vasculature and depended on the presence of an existing tumor vasculature, since administering FAA to mice with sponge-implant-induced granulomas did not affect blood flow within the granulomas. Many other investigators have reported similar dramatic antitumor effects of FAA in a wide variety of mouse models. FAA may not be unique in this property, since other flavonoids appear to produce similar effects. For example, the flavonoid quercetin blocks tumor blood flow in mice (Teicher et al., 1991). Unfortunately, human tumors respond poorly to FAA treatment (Bibby and Double, 1993), presumably due to differences in immune response.

Other agents that cause vascular blockage may be used, but some may have adverse effects. For example, papain, a proteolytic enzyme found in papaya, can increase platelet aggregation and may facilitate the formation of a thrombus within the capillaries. However, increasing platelet aggregation may also increase metastasis and cause other adverse effects, such as stroke and myocardial infarction in patients with vascular disease.

3.6 SUMMARY

Solid tumors must induce angiogenesis to grow larger than a few cubic millimeters in size. Multiple factors contribute to inducing angiogenesis, and many of these are also active during normal wound healing. Some of the more important factors include basic fibroblast growth factor, vascular permeability factor, platelet activating factor, kinins, and fibrin. Certain natural agents may inhibit the production of these factors and break the cycle that allows tumors to act as a nonhealing wound. In addition, some natural agents may inhibit angiogenesis by other means, such as by scavenging free radicals. Lastly, therapy can target the neovasculature, rather than angiogenesis, to destroy the existing blood supply of tumors.

4

INVASION

Invasion is the infiltration of tumor cells into adjacent tissues and, along with metastasis, is one of the distinguishing features of malignancy. Tumor-induced proteolytic enzymes play a central role in invasion, as they provide the means by which tumors digest the extracellular matrix. Protease inhibitors and nutritional factors likewise play central roles in invasion, as they prevent excessive proteolytic activity and stabilize connective tissue.

4.1 CONNECTIVE TISSUE, PROTEASES, AND THE EXTRACELLULAR MATRIX

Cells in the body are held together and supported by connective tissue. Connective tissue is the most abundant tissue in the body. It includes tendons, bones, cartilage, vascular tissue, adipose tissue, and reticular tissue (the tissue that forms the stroma of organs and binds together smooth muscle cells). Connective tissue is normally vascular (except cartilage) and contains few cells. It is primarily composed of macromolecules assembled into what is called the extracellular matrix (ECM). These macromolecules include at least 13 different types of collagen, the fibrous protein elastin, a variety of mucopolysaccharides (also known as glycosaminoglycans) including hyaluronic acid, and additional components that have not been well defined. Connective tissue provides a natural barrier to tumor invasion, which is why proteases that dissolve connective tissue play an important role in neoplasia.

Proteases break apart the amino acid chains that comprise protein structures, and are active in a wide variety of biological processes. They are produced both inside the digestive tract, where they digest food proteins, and outside the digestive tract, where they play important roles in numerous homeostatic mechanisms. Normal wound healing provides two examples: macrophages secrete proteolytic enzymes that dissolve damaged tissue (Knighton et al., 1983), and the proteolytic enzyme plasmin dissolves fibrin clots.

Since the exact nature of many endogenous proteases are unknown, they are often described in relationship to well-defined proteases such as the following: trypsin and chymotrypsin (produced in the pancreas to aid in protein digestion), papain (produced from unripe papaya fruits), ficin (produced from the sap of fig trees), and bromelain (produced from the stems of pineapple plants). For example, human skin contains a variety of proteases that resemble chymotrypsin and trypsin. As a second example, the endogenous protease cathepsin B resembles papain (Fischer and Slaga, 1985:223).

Categories of proteolytic enzymes important in cancer include the following:

* *Metalloproteinases,* which contain a metal ion in their structure. A number of important collagenases are metalloproteinases. Calf and shark cartilage, which may possess anticancer activity, appear to contain inhibitors of metalloproteinases.

* *Serine proteases,* which degrade proteins that contain the amino acid serine. Serine proteases include trypsin and plasmin.

* *Cysteine proteases,* which include cathepsin B and bromelain, degrade proteins that contain the amino acid cysteine. Cysteine is an amino acid that, in the form of cystine, acts as a "solder" to maintain a durable structure in various tissues.

4.2 PROTEASES AND PROTEASE INHIBITORS IN NEOPLASIA

The effects of proteases on carcinogenesis were first reported in 1970, when researchers found that protease inhibitors could reduce the tumor-promoting effect of croton oil on mouse skin (Troll et al., 1970). Since that time, numerous investigators have reported that proteases and their inhibitors play a role in tumor promotion and

TABLE 4.1. NATURAL AGENTS THAT INHIBIT COLLAGENASE ACTIVITY

AGENT	REFERENCE	FURTHER DISCUSSION
Anthocyanins from red-blue fruits and other plants	Monboisse et al., 1983; reviewed by Pizzorno and Murray, 1987; Rao et al., 1983	Section 14.4.4
Calf and shark cartilage	Lee and Langer, 1983	Section 15.2
(+)-Catechin (found in green tea and other plants)	Makimura et al., 1993; Osawa et al., 1991; Beretz and Cazenave, 1988	Section 14.4.4
Eicosapentaenoic acid (EPA) (found in certain fish oils)	Reich et al., 1989	Section 12.3
Proanthocyanidins (found in grape seeds, pine bark, and other plants)	Corbe et al., 1988; Schwitters and Masquelier, 1993:43	Section 14.4.4

tumor invasion, although the exact role that they play is still uncertain.

The endogenous proteases plasminogen activator, plasmin, collagenase, cathepsin B, and elastinase all appear to be involved in invasion. For example, in one study 20 patients with breast cancer showed an increase of cathepsins in malignant breast tissue as compared to adjacent nonmalignant tissue (Gabrijelcic et al., 1992). Similarly, a number of protease inhibitors, such as urinary trypsin inhibitors, have been shown to inhibit invasion in vitro.

Proteases appear to mediate at least four processes that influence neoplasia:

- *Inflammation:* The inflammatory response associated with tumor-promoting agents involves the release of histamine, free radicals, eicosanoids (prostaglandins and leukotrienes), and proteases such as collagenases, elastinase, and cathepsins.[1] It appears that each individual product of inflammation affects the release of others. For example, trypsin, chymotrypsin, pronase, and papain reportedly cause macrophages to produce two to six times more free radicals in response to the tumor-promoting agent croton oil (Fischer and Slaga, 1985:219). Similarly, various proteases increase PGE_2 synthesis, and a variety of protease inhibitors inhibit PGE_2 synthesis.
- *Cell proliferation:* Proteases have been shown to regulate cell proliferation. Trypsin, pronase and ficin stimulate DNA synthesis, and trypsin stimulates mitosis in chick embryo cells. Transformed cells may exhibit greater proteolytic activity than normal cells, and the cell surface activity that some proteases induce may increase proliferation rates (reviewed by Belman and Garte, 1985).

- *Invasion and metastasis:* Invasion requires a delicate balance between substrate-specific proteolytic activity and proteolytic inhibition (Stetler-Stevenson, 1994, personal communication).[2] When protease activity is insufficient or protease inhibition is excessive, tumors cannot digest the ECM and are unable to invade. Similarly, when protease activity is excessive or protease inhibition is insufficient, tumors essentially dissolve the ECM into a "soup" and, without the structure provided by the ECM, again, are unable to invade. Proteases also play a role in metastasis by facilitating invasion into the basement membrane of capillaries, thereby allowing tumor cells access to the blood circulation.
- *Angiogenesis:* The migration of endothelial cells during angiogenesis could be considered a form of regulated invasion, and agents that inhibit invasion may also inhibit angiogenesis (Alessandro and Kohn, 1995). For example, calf cartilage contains a protein that is both a protease inhibitor and is antiangiogenic (Langer et al., 1976).

The proteases collagenase, plasmin, and elastinase are prominently involved in invasion and agents that inhibit these enzymes are discussed below.

4.2.1 Inhibitors of Collagenases and Other Metalloproteinases

Collagenases are a family of enzymes that digest collagen, the fibrous protein found in connective tissue. Collagen is derived from the German words *kolla* (glue), and *gennan* (to produce), reflecting its role in "gluing" cells together. Approximately 30% of the body's total protein store is contained in collagen. Each of the

---

[1] Free radicals by themselves may stimulate invasion. Oxygen radicals have been shown to increase the invasive potential of mouse hepatoma cells, probably by altering their plasma membranes (Shinkai et al., 1986). Phagocytes are recruited to tumor sites in large numbers, and are known to produce oxygen radicals. Therefore, phagocytes may play a role in stimulating the invasive potential of neoplastic cells.

[2] William Stetler-Stevenson, M.D., Ph.D. is Chief of the Extracellular Matrix Pathology Section at the U.S. National Cancer Institute.

different types of collagenases degrade a specific type of collagen. The basement membrane contains type IV collagen, and therefore, type IV collagenase is a particularly important enzyme in tumor invasion. Since type IV collagenase is a metalloproteinase, it may be affected by metalloproteinase inhibitors, such as found in shark and bovine cartilage. These and other natural agents that inhibit collagenase activity are listed in Table 4.1.

A number of other natural agents may stimulate the production of endogenous metalloproteinase inhibitors. Both retinol and retinoic acid increase the production of metalloproteinase inhibitors by capillary cells in vitro (Braunhut and Moses, 1994). The solvent DMSO causes a reversible decrease in the production of the metalloproteinase stromelysin by transformed rat fibroblasts (Popowicz et al., 1993). In two fibrosarcoma cell lines that express high levels of stromelysin, DMSO caused a decrease in stromelysin production and a decrease in invasive propensity (Popowicz et al., 1993).

4.2.2 Inhibitors of Plasmin

Plasmin is a serine protease capable of degrading a number of protein substrates, including fibrin, the structural component of blood clots. The agents responsible for fibrinolysis are plasmin and its precursor, plasmino-gen. Plasminogen is activated by plasminogen activator (see Figure 4.1).

In addition to degrading fibrin, plasmin is also capable of degrading components of the extracellular matrix and is one of the proteolytic enzymes active in tumor invasion (Fazioli and Blasi, 1994). For example, plasmin may be involved in the invasion of the ECM by human ovarian cancers (Kobayashi et al., 1994a, 1994b). Serum levels of plasminogen tend to be elevated in cancer patients in comparison to healthy controls (Kliachkin et al., 1985). For example, an increase in plasminogen activator appears to be a late event in the progression of human melanoma (De Vries et al., 1994).

Two forms of plasminogen activator are involved in invasion and metastasis. These are urokinase-type plasminogen activator (uPA), and tissue-type plasminogen activator (tPA).[3] Studies have shown that uPA plays a central role in the invasion of breast cancer (Janicke et al., 1994). It also enhances the invasion of mouse prostate cancer into both skeletal and nonskeletal tissue (Achbarou et al., 1994) and plays a key role in the invasiveness of brain tumors (Caccamo et al., 1994; Landau et al., 1994). In some cases, it is responsible for tumor-induced dissolution of the basement membrane, which allows the tumor access to the vasculature for metastasis (Sugimura et al., 1994).

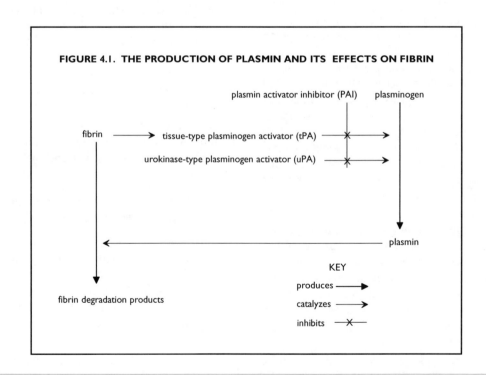

FIGURE 4.1. THE PRODUCTION OF PLASMIN AND ITS EFFECTS ON FIBRIN

---

[3] Urokinase-type plasminogen activator derives its name from human urine, the source from which it was originally isolated. Tissue-type plasminogen activator stimulates the production of plasmin in response to fibrin, whereas urokinase-type plasminogen activator stimulates the production of plasmin regardless of the presence of fibrin. tPA is the principal mediator of fibrinolysis.

TABLE 4.2 NATURAL AGENTS THAT AFFECT PLASMINOGEN ACTIVATOR		
AGENT	**EFFECT**	**REFERENCE**
Allium sativum (garlic, *da suan*)	Administration of garlic powder to healthy subjects for 1 to 14 days increased tPA and fibrinolytic activity	Legnani et al., 1993
(+)-Catechin	Binds tPA in vitro and renders it inactive	Bracke et al., 1991, 1988a, 1988b 1986, 1985, 1984; Mareel and De Mets, 1989
Panax ginseng (ren shen)	A ginsenoside isolated from panax increased the secretion of plasminogen activator from cultured human endothelial cells. This effect was observed with and without stimulation of the cells by thrombin.	Ushio, 1992
Salvia miltiorrhiza (dan shen)	Stimulated plasminogen activator to produce plasmin in vitro	Reviewed by Chang and But, 1986:258-62.
Typha angustifolia (pu huang)	Stimulated endothelial cells to produce tPA in vitro	Zhao et al., 1990

Tumor cells are known to produce both uPA and tPA and their inhibitors, and invasion appears to depend on the relative balance between them. All elements of the plasmin activation-inhibition system may be overexpressed in human breast cancers (Jankun et al., 1993). In the serum of patients with renal carcinoma, uPA and tPA were elevated and levels of both decreased after surgery (Bashar et al., 1994). Levels of plasminogen activator inhibitor (PAI-1) were higher in those with metastasis compared to those without metastasis. High levels of uPA and PAI-1 were also associated with poor outcome of breast cancer patients (Bouchet et al., 1994), and poor outcome of patients with adenocarcinoma of the lung and bladder cancer (Pedersen et al., 1994; Hasui et al., 1993). High tPA activity may be responsible, in part, for the high incidence of chronic disseminated intravascular coagulation (DIC) observed in patients with leukemia (Wada et al., 1993).

Natural agents that inhibit or stimulate plasminogen activator are listed in Table 4.2.[4] As suggested above, agents that stimulate the production of plasminogen activator may facilitate invasion. However, this is probably not sufficient in and of itself to increase invasion. It is likely that a number of other proteolytic enzymes, including metalloproteinases and cathepsins, must act in unison with plasmin to degrade the basement membrane (Tannock and Hill, 1992:183; Thorgeirsson et al., 1985). Quite likely, these enzymes must also act in unison to degrade the ECM in general. However, it is not known if plasmin production is the rate-limiting step in invasion.

As discussed in Chapter 3, it may be advantageous to stimulate fibrinolysis to inhibit angiogenesis. However, stimulating plasmin production may also facilitate invasion. If true, it may still be possible to stimulate fibrinolysis with certain agents, such as brinase, which do not activate the plasminogen-plasmin system.

4.2.3 Inhibitors of Elastinase

As mentioned previously, elastin is a component of the ECM, and elastinase is involved in invasion. The degradation of elastin by elastinase is inhibited by proanthocyanidins and (+)-catechin, both in vitro and in rabbits (Tixier et al., 1984).

4.2.4 Inhibitors of Other Proteases

Exogenous protease inhibitors are present in a number of seed foods and apparently evolved as a survival mechanism to prevent digestion of the seed in the stomach of animals. Soybeans are a particularly rich source of protease inhibitors and will be discussed further in Section 14.5.

Protease inhibitors are also found within the body. For example, inhibitors of trypsin and chymotrypsin can be elevated in the blood and urine of cancer patients (Belman and Garte, 1985). Urinary trypsin inhibitor (purified from human urine) inhibits plasmin and reduces the invasion of human ovarian cancer in vitro (Kobayashi et al., 1994a, 1994b).

4.3 NATURAL AGENTS THAT FACILITATE COLLAGEN PRODUCTION

A number of natural agents facilitate collagen production or collagen cross-linking and, theoretically, may

---

[4] In relation to cancer, the production of plasminogen activator by tumor cells is of more concern than the production of plasminogen activator by normal cells. The actions of the agents listed in Table 4.2 are not specific for tumor cells.

TABLE 4.3. AGENTS THAT FACILITATE COLLAGEN PRODUCTION OR CROSS-LINKING

AGENT	EFFECT	REFERENCE
Anthocyanins	Anthocyanins, the flavonoids found in red-blue fruits such as *Vaccinium myrtillus* (bilberry) and *Crataegus oxyacantha (shan zha)* reportedly protect collagen from degradation by inducing cross-linking of collagen fibers, by promoting collagen synthesis, and by preventing enzymatic cleavage of collagen. Other red-blue fruits, such as blackberries, cherries, blueberries, and red grapes might also produce these effects.	Reviewed by Pizzorno and Murray, 1987; Rao et al., 1983
(+)-Catechin	This flavonoid, found in green tea and other plants, promotes the cross-linking of collagen.	Beretz and Cazenave, 1988
Glucosamine	Glucosamine is a component of proteoglycans, and stimulates its synthesis. Proteoglycans are essential components of connective tissue. Glucosamine may effectively treat osteoarthritis, in part by stimulating collagen production in damaged joints. In a trial of 1208 patients with osteoarthritis, administration of 1.5 grams of glucosamine sulfate daily resulted in improvements in 95% of cases. Glucosamine is commercially available as glucosamine sulfate or N-acetyl glucosamine.	Vaz, 1982; Tapadinhas et al., 1982
Proanthocyanidins	Proanthocyanidins were more effective than catechin, tannin, and other flavonoids in protecting collagen strips from shrinkage due to hot water.	Schwitters and Masquelier, 1993:40-3
Proline, glycine, and arginine	The amino acids proline, glycine, and arginine may stimulate the healing of surgical wounds and burns. These agents supply the raw material necessary for collagen synthesis.	Reviewed by Braverman and Pfeiffer, 1987:243
Silicon and copper	Silicon facilitates the synthesis of collagen, and may facilitate collagen cross-linking. Copper is also required for collagen cross-linking.	Reviewed by Linder, 1991:231, 247
Vitamin C	Vitamin C is necessary for maintenance of the extracellular matrix. Low levels of vitamin C produce scurvy, a disease characterized by destruction of the ECM, vascular disorganization, and undifferentiated cellular proliferation—symptoms similar to those produced during tumor growth and invasion. Vitamin C stimulates collagen synthesis in human fibroblast cells in vitro, and enhances angiogenesis in CAM assays.	Chan et al., 1990; Heino et al., 1989; Grinnell et al., 1989; McDevitt et al., 1988; Nicosia et al, 1991

inhibit invasion.[5] However, as discussed in Section 3.2.3, agents that stimulate collagen production may also facilitate angiogenesis. Additional research is needed to determine the end effect of these agents on invasion and angiogenesis. Natural agents that facilitate collagen production are listed in Table 4.3.

4.4 SUMMARY

Invasion is one of the distinguishing features of malignancy and is mediated, in part, by tumor-derived proteases. Proteases may affect at least four processes that influence neoplasia. These are inflammation, cell proliferation, invasion, and metastasis. Proteases influence invasion by dissolving the ECM. They influence metastasis by dissolving the basement membrane of capillaries, thereby allowing tumor cells access to blood circulation.

Two important proteases are collagenases and plasmin. A number of natural agents inhibit these proteases,

although the clinical effects of administering protease inhibitors to cancer patients has not been determined.

Nutritional factors and agents that stimulate collagen synthesis and cross-linking likewise play central roles in neoplasia. They prevent excessive proteolytic activity and stabilize connective tissue.

---

[5] The cross-linking of collagen fibers provides collagen with strength.

5
METASTASIS

Metastasis is the movement of malignant cells from the primary tumor site to a distant location, where a secondary tumor subsequently develops. Metastatic cells travel through the blood and lymphatic circulation systems. The growth of a tumor at its primary location is generally not a cause of death, except in the case of brain, liver, and lung cancers. Brain cancer is one of the few cancers that rarely metastasize.

5.1 THE MECHANISMS OF METASTASIS

The metastatic process is inherently inefficient. In a study of patients with renal cell carcinoma, tumors released from ten million to one billion cancer cells into the patient's bloodstream per day. In spite of this enormous release, 20% of the patients showed no evidence of new tumor development, even after 30 months (Glaves et al., 1988). In animal tumors, only 0.001% of the tumor cells released develop into metastatic colonies (Honn et al., 1987a, 1987b). The inefficiency of the metastatic process is due largely to the inhospitable environment that greets malignant cells as they migrate through the circulatory systems.

A metastatic colony develops according to the steps listed below and as illustrated in Figure 5.1. Like many aspects of cancer, metastasis is a complicated and poorly understood process, and numerous factors can affect each of these steps. The steps are:

1) Cells detach from the primary tumor and invade the basement membrane of a blood vessel (intravasation) to enter the blood stream.
2) In circulation, the migrating cells must evade the host's immune system and other adverse conditions.
3) The migrating cells adhere to the wall of the blood vessel at the metastatic site (cell arrest).
4) The arrested cells invade through the basement membrane to leave the blood vessel (extravasation).
5) The tumor cells proliferate and the new tumor induces angiogenesis.

Although this discussion primarily refers to metastasis via hematogenous dissemination, metastasis via the lymphatic system can occur through similar processes.

Each of these five steps is discussed individually in the following sections.

5.2 CELL DETACHMENT AND INTRAVASATION

The initial step in metastasis is the detachment of cells from the primary tumor. Once detached, cancer cells contact a blood vessel (usually within the tumor) and secrete or induce the secretion of proteolytic enzymes, which digest the basement membrane. Tumor cells then slip between vascular endothelial cells to enter the vessel lumen (intravasation). Intravasation is facilitated by the poorly developed basement membranes and fragile capillaries produced during neovascularization. An intact basement membrane provides a barrier that inhibits intravasation.

Cell detachment rates tend to increase as a tumor enlarges and as a tumor undergoes central necrosis. Other factors that may stimulate detachment include mechanical stress, increased hydrostatic pressure within tumors, increased activity by various proteolytic enzymes, and decreased expression of adhesion molecules (CAMs) on the cell's surface.

Cell adhesion molecules are complex protein and carbohydrate molecules that occur on the plasma membrane of all cells. In recent years they have been recognized as pivotal mediators of normal and neoplastic cell function. Originally, CAMs were believed to control primarily cell-cell and cell-matrix interactions, such as cellular adhesion. It is now known that they also control signal transduction from the plasma membrane and, as such, inform the cell of membrane interactions with soluble hormones, mechanical forces, and other factors

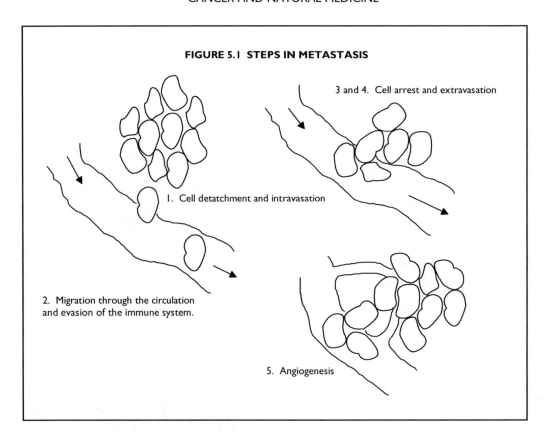

FIGURE 5.1 STEPS IN METASTASIS

3 and 4. Cell arrest and extravasation

1. Cell detatchment and intravasation

2. Migration through the circulation and evasion of the immune system.

5. Angiogenesis

(Schwartz and Ingber, 1994).[1] Through these actions, CAMs regulate organ architecture, cell migration, differentiation, apoptosis, mitosis, platelet aggregation, and the activity of immune cells (Roth, 1994; Agrez and Bates, 1994; Pignatelli and Vessey, 1994; Juliano and Varner, 1993). In fact, loss of differentiation in tumor cells may be a consequence of reduced intercellular adhesion (Birchmeier and Behrens, 1994).

One family of CAMs important in neoplasia are cadherins. For example, E-cadherin appears to inhibit both invasion and metastasis (Jiang et al., 1995), and reduced expression allows cells to more easily detach from their surroundings and invade adjacent tissues. A reduced expression of cadherins has been observed on invasive cells from a variety of human cancers (Isaacs et al., 1994; Furukawa et al., 1994).

Two other families of CAMs important in neoplasia are cell-surface lectins and lectin-binding proteoglycans.[2] Due to recent advances laboratory techniques, research on proteoglycans has flourished. Proteoglycans are proteins attached to a large carbohydrate called a glycosaminoglycan (GAG).[3] Many proteoglycans are constituents of the extracellular matrix, where they provide structural

functions such as forming the elastic pad in cartilage. They also occur intracellularly and on the surface membrane of cells. Recent evidence suggests that they act as CAMs, thereby influencing a wide range of cellular processes (Kjellen and Lindahl, 1991).

Sulfated GAGs have a strong negative charge that allows them to bind to many substances, including a variety of growth factors. For example, a heparan sulfate proteoglycan is responsible for binding fibroblast growth factor and immobilizing it in the extracellular matrix (ECM) as discussed in Section 3.2.3 (Ruoslahti and Yamaguchi, 1991). The varied effects of proteoglycans may be due, in part, to their ability to undergo extensive structural modulation during cellular expression (Hardingham and Fosang, 1992). For example, a number of transformed cells appear to synthesize an under-sulfated heparan sulfate proteoglycan, which appears to impede matrix formation and stability (Robinson et al., 1984; David and Van Den Berghe, 1983). Similar differences in sulfonation were observed in heparan sulfate obtained from normal and cancerous human liver tissue (Nakamura and Kojima, 1981). As another example, cartilage from dogs with experimentally induced osteoarthritis synthesizes chondroitin sulfate with longer carbohydrate

---

[1] Signal transduction may occur via tyrosine phosphorylation (Juliano, 1994; Juliano and Varner, 1993) (see Section 14.6.).

[2] Lectins are proteins with two or more binding sites that can interact with specific sugars, thereby binding cell-surface proteoglycans (or glycolipids) and causing cell adhesion.

[3] GAGs exist in four main forms: heparan sulfate and heparin, chondroitin sulfate and dermatan sulfate, hyaluronic acid, and keratan sulfate. Of these, only hyaluronic acid is not bound to a protein and is not sulfated in its natural form.

chains, which appears to facilitate matrix repair by chondrocytes (Hardingham and Fosang, 1992).

Oral administration of polysaccharides may inhibit neoplasia by directly affecting CAMs. For example, tumor galactoside-binding proteins (gal-lectins) are CAMs believed to facilitate cell adhesion by linking oligosaccharides on the tumor cell surface with galactose residues on adjacent tumor cells. As will be discussed shortly, tumor cell aggregation increases the chances for successful metastasis. The carbohydrate side chains of pH-modified citrus pectin (MCP)[4] contain galactose residues, and orally and intravenously administrated MCP appears to saturate the tumor cell gal-lectins, thereby inhibiting aggregation and metastasis. MCP inhibits metastasis in vitro and in rodents injected with melanoma and human prostate cancer cells (Pienta et al., 1995; Platt and Raz, 1992; Naik et al., 1995; Inohara and Raz, 1994). With oral dosing, optimal effects were observed in rats at approximately 1.3 gram/kg per day (equivalent to approximately 21 grams/day in a 70-kg human). In these studies, growth of the primary tumor was not affected, suggesting that MCP acts only on the metastatic colonies, and then only at the earliest stages of metastasis.

Administration of polysaccharides may also inhibit neoplasia by directly affecting ECM GAGs. For example, a variety of sulfated polysaccharides have been shown to inhibit tumor metastasis, apparently by inhibiting ECM digestion induced by tumor cell-derived heparanases (Coombe et al., 1987; Parish et al., 1987). Specifically, these heparanases appear to degrade the GAG side chains of heparan sulfate proteoglycans in the basement membrane, thereby allowing tumor cell intravasation. Sulfated polysaccharides may inhibit these heparanases by acting as non-cleavable substrates that attach to and block the active site of the enzymes.[5] This effect may not be limited to sulfated polysaccharides. For example, the non-sulfated polysaccharide peptide PSK (isolated from the mushroom *Coriolus versicolor, yun zhi*) also inhibited tumor cell invasion in vitro, apparently by a similar mechanism (Ebina and Murata, 1994). A related compound, polysaccharide peptide PSP (also from *Coriolus versicolor*) has shown antitumor activity in animals and appears to prolong the lifespan of cancer patients (reviewed in Yang and Kwok, 1993). Although much of PSP's activity may be secondary to immunostimulation, it is possible that heparanase inhibition is also occurring.

Sulfated polysaccharides may also inhibit angiogenesis, although through a different mechanism. A sulfated polysaccharide-peptide complex obtained from the bacterial cell wall of the *Arthrobacter sp.* inhibited angiogenesis in the CAM assay, apparently by inhibiting endothelial cell DNA synthesis (Tanaka et al., 1989). It is interesting to speculate that this may be due to a direct effect on endothelial cell CAMs.

Administration of non-polysaccharide agents may also inhibit neoplasia by directly affecting cell surface proteoglycans. For example, proteolytic enzymes such as bromelain may inhibit metastasis by altering proteoglycans on tumor cells. This will be discussed in more detail in Section 15.3.3.

In addition to external influences on CAMs, some natural agents may also affect CAM expression. For example, gamma linolenic acid (GLA) increased the expression of E-cadherin in a range of human tumor lines in vitro. This effect was associated with reduced invasion in vitro (Jiang et al., 1995). In another study, proteins purified from *Ganoderma lucidum (ling zhi)* produce a dramatic rise in the expression of one type of CAM (ICAM-1) (Haak-Frendscho et al., 1993).

Although gene expression clearly affects cell-matrix interactions, the opposite is also true: cell-matrix interactions affect gene expression (Stetler-Stevenson et al., 1993). Therefore, natural agents that protect matrix integrity may reduce invasion, metastasis, loss of differentiation, and possibly other features of malignancy. Agents that protect matrix integrity include protease inhibitors (see Table 4.1) and agents that facilitate collagen production or cross-linking (see Table 4.3).

5.3 MIGRATION THROUGH THE CIRCULATION

The second step in metastasis is the migration of tumor cells through the blood circulation. The vast majority of migrating tumor cells die due to forces present in the circulation, the most important of which may be the immune system. Although there is considerable evidence that the immune system plays a prominent role in inhibiting metastasis, the issue is complex, and no simple correlation between immune status and metastatic spread has been found. The immune cells that appear to be most active in attacking migrating cancer cells are natural killer (NK) cells and macrophages.

Numerous animal experiments support a role for the immune system in limiting metastasis (reviewed by Calabresi and Schein, 1993:69):

---

[4] Pectin is a polysaccharide found in the cell walls of all plant tissues. Lemon and orange rind contain approximately 30% pectin (Budavari et al., 1989:7009).

[5] Macrophages and other immune cells can also degrade the ECM in a similar fashion, causing inflammation. For this reason, some sulfated polysaccharides are likely to possess potent anti-inflammatory activity.

- Metastasis is more frequent in animals with T-lymphocyte deficits.
- When animals are injected with exogenous tumor tissue, metastasis is more frequent if the macrophages present within the tumor tissue are extracted prior to injection.
- Metastasis is more frequent in animals that are treated with immune-suppressing drugs prior to tumor implant.
- Metastasis is less frequent in mice that have high levels of NK cells.

These observations suggest that agents that stimulate the immune system, particularly those that stimulate NK cell activity, may inhibit metastasis. A large number of natural agents may have this effect. See Chapter 8 for a discussion of the immune system.

In addition to the immune system, other forces may destroy migrating tumor cells. These include mechanical stress as the cells move through the small vessels, and toxicity caused by high oxygen levels in the blood (Tannock and Hill, 1992:181).

5.4 CELL ARREST AT A NEW LOCATION

The third step in metastasis is cell arrest. Since intravascular conditions create an inhospitable environment for migrating tumor cells, the cells must exit the vasculature in order to survive. This is initiated by attachment to the capillary wall, or *cell arrest*. Several factors promote cell arrest. These include denuding of the basement membrane, tumor cell aggregation, platelet aggregation, and thrombus formation. Each of these is discussed below.

5.4.1 Denuding of the Basement Membrane

Similar to platelets, tumor cells adhere more efficiently to exposed collagen of a denuded (or damaged) vessel than to normal endothelial cells.[6] Denuded areas provide prime targets for cell arrest. Vessels can become denuded due to trauma or inflammation. Natural agents that counteract these processes may inhibit cell arrest. For example, vitamin C and a host of other antioxidant compounds inhibit inflammation and may, therefore, inhibit denuding and cell arrest. Some antioxidants, such as proanthocyanidins, appear to exhibit specificity for vascular tissue.

Arrest onto endothelial cells can also occur directly through the action of cell adhesion molecules. Vessels of different organs express varying amounts of CAMs, which may account, in part, for the varying rates of metastatic colony formation observed between organs (reviewed by Tannock and Hill, 1992:182-3).[7] Cell arrest is also facilitated by laminin receptors that may occur on the surface of tumor cells. The receptors bind to laminin on basement membranes.

5.4.2 Tumor Cell Aggregation

Tumor cells tend to aggregate with each other while migrating in the blood, thereby forming a larger complex that may lodge in the capillary beds more easily. In experimental studies on mice, the efficiency of metastasis increased with the injection of a large number of tumor cells or with clumps of tumor cells (Hill et al., 1986). Unfortunately, tumor cell aggregation cannot be controlled easily, and manipulation of tumor cell aggregation is not a promising antimetastasis therapy.

5.4.3 Platelet Aggregation and Thrombus Formation

The importance of thrombus formation in facilitating metastatic spread is controversial. Thrombus formation may shield tumor cells from immune attack and protect tumor cells against damage due to mechanical stress. Although thrombi have been observed around arrested cells, they appear to break down within a few hours and, therefore, many investigators believe they play a minor role in metastasis (reviewed by Tannock and Hill, 1992:182).

The importance of platelet aggregation in metastasis is more widely accepted. Two mechanisms by which platelet aggregation may promote metastasis are as follows (Honn et al., 1987a, 1987b):

1) Activated platelets are sticky and may enhance the adhesion of tumor cells to the endothelial lining.
2) Platelet-secreted factors, such as platelet-derived growth factor, may stimulate the growth of tumor cells and contribute to their survival within the blood circulation.

Experimental studies have shown that migrating cells from some cancers induce platelet aggregation by modifying the eicosanoid balance (reviewed by Tannock and Hill, 1992:182). Eicosanoids are discussed in more detail in Chapter 6, but two eicosanoids are briefly introduced here. Platelet aggregation depends on a balance of the eicosanoids prostacyclin (PGI_2) and thromboxane

---

[6] See Figure 3.2 for an illustration of platelets contacting a denuded area of a vessel.

[7] Other reasons for varying colony-formation rates between organs include differences in blood flow and capillary beds.

TABLE 5.1. NATURAL ANTICOAGULANT AGENTS AND THEIR MECHANISMS OF ACTION			
AGENT	**REDUCE TXA$_2$ OR INCREASE PGI$_2$**	**INHIBIT PLATELET AGGREGATION** (unspecified mechanisms)	**FIBRINOLYTIC AND/OR ANTITHROMBOTIC** (unspecified mechanisms)
Agkistrodon acutus (bai hua she)			in vitro
Allium bakeri (xie bai)	in vitro		
Allium sativum (garlic, *da suan*)	in vitro (allitridi)	in humans	in humans
Aloe vera	in vitro		
Andrographis paniculata (chuan xin lian)	in vivo	in vivo, in humans	in vitro, in humans
Angelica dahurica (bai zhi)	in vitro		
Angelica sinensis (dang gui)	in vitro	in humans	
Artemisia argyi (ai ye)			in vitro
Artemisia capillaris (yin chen hao)	in vitro		
Astragalus membranaceus (huang qi)	in vitro	in vitro, in humans	
Atractylodes macrocephala (bai zhu)			in vivo, in humans
Bombyx mori (jiang can)			in vitro
Brinase, a proteolytic enzyme from *Aspergillus oryzae*			in vivo, in humans
Bromelain	in vitro	in vivo, in humans	in vitro, in vivo
Bu Yang Huan Wu Tang (formula)			in vitro
Buthus martensi (quan xie)			in vitro
Capsicum frutescens and *Capsicum annuum* (cayenne pepper)		in vitro	in humans
Carthamus tinctorius (hong hua)			in vitro, in humans
Codonopsis pilosula (dang shen)	in vitro, in humans	in vitro, in humans	
Curcuma longa (jiang huang)			in vitro
Flavonoids (including some anthocyanins and catechins)		in humans	
Genistein (isoflavone)		in vitro	
Ginkgo biloba			in vivo
Glehnia littoralis (bei sha shen)	in vitro		
Gynostemma pentaphyllum (jiao gu lan)	in vivo	in vivo	
Hirudo nipponia (shui zhi)			in vitro
Ligusticum chuanxiong (chuan xiong)	in vivo, in humans	in humans, in vivo	
Paeonia lactiflora (chi shao and *bai shao)*			in vitro
Panax ginseng (ren shen)	in vitro	in humans	
Pheretima aspergillum (di long)			in vitro
Rheum palmatum (da huang)	in vitro, in vivo		
Salvia miltiorrhiza (dan shen)			in vitro, in humans
Scolopendra subspinipes mutilans (wu gong)			in vitro
Scutellaria baicalensis (huang qin)	in vitro		
Tanacetum parthenium (feverfew)		in vitro	in vitro
Typha angustifolia and *Typha latifolia* (*pu huang*)	in vitro	in vitro	in vitro

41

(TXA$_2$). PGI$_2$, which cells of the endothelial lining produce, inhibits platelet aggregation. TXA$_2$, which platelets produce, enhances aggregation. Tumors promote platelet aggregation by stimulating the production of TXA$_2$, and/or by inhibiting the production of PGI$_2$.

In contrast to tumor cell aggregation, platelet aggregation and thrombus formation can readily be manipulated. Three types of drugs inhibit the coagulation-clotting process: 1) anticoagulants, which interfere with the action of clotting factors; 2) fibrinolytic agents, which activate plasmin; and 3) inhibitors of platelet aggregation.

Anticoagulants, such as warfarin and heparin, and platelet-inhibitors, such as aspirin, have been studied as antimetastasis agents. In a study of 431 patients with small cell lung cancer, warfarin treatment prolonged the time to first evidence of disease progression and increased survival time (Zacharski, 1984). However, this effect was not observed in patients with a variety of other cancers. In subsequent studies on patients with breast and colorectal cancer, warfarin treatment did not increase survival time (Daly, 1991; Levine et al., 1994). In a study on cancer-bearing mice, aspirin significantly reduced the number of lung metastases (reviewed by Calabresi and Schein, 1993:71). Aspirin inhibits platelet aggregation by preventing the formation of TXA$_2$. A single dose of aspirin can suppress platelet aggregation for 48 hours and longer. Fibrinolytic agents may also inhibit metastasis. Both streptokinase (a drug used to stimulate plasmin production), and tissue-type plasminogen activator (tPA), inhibited the seeding of metastatic cells in the lungs of animals (Brown et al., 1994).

A large number of natural agents inhibit clotting factors, have fibrinolytic action, or inhibit platelet aggregation and, therefore, may be useful as antimetastasis agents. Agents that stimulate fibrinolysis were discussed in Chapter 3 (Table 3.4) and agents that specifically affect plasminogen activator were discussed in Chapter 4 (Table 4.2). For convenience they are listed again in Table 5.1. Also listed in Table 5.1 are agents that inhibit platelet aggregation or otherwise inhibit clotting. See Appendix D for further information and references. Only one of the agents reviewed specifically inhibited coagulation factors. This was *Cucurbita maxima* (pumpkin seed, *nan gua zi*), which inhibited human Hageman-factor-dependent clotting in vitro (Hojima et al., 1982).

As discussed in Chapter 3, patients with cancer often bleed. In fact, unexpected bleeding can be the initial symptom of some cancers, such as lung, colon, kidney, and uterine cancers. In addition, patients can bleed after surgery. The indiscriminate use of fibrinolytic agents or agents that inhibit platelet aggregation could be disastrous in some patients.

5.5 EXTRAVASATION

The fourth step in metastasis is extravasation, or the movement of the metastatic colony out of the blood vessel. Extravasation is mediated by protease enzymes and other factors in a process similar to intravasation. In both cases, the basement membrane provides an obstacle to the movement of tumor cells through the endothelium. It may be possible to inhibit extravasation (and intravasation) by inhibiting the actions of collagenase or other proteases (see Tables 4.1 and 4.2).

Local trauma may likewise facilitate movement through the vessels. When cancer cells were injected into rabbits with traumatized tissues, metastasis to the trauma site was increased 20-fold over nontraumatized tissues (reviewed by Calabresi and Schein, 1993:69-70). Therefore, it is possible that agents that stabilize the vasculature or basement membrane may inhibit extravasation and metastasis. These include agents that facilitate collagen synthesis or cross-linking (see Table 4.3) and agents that increase capillary resistance (see Table 3.4).

5.6 INDUCTION OF ANGIOGENESIS

The fifth and last step in tumor metastasis is the induction of angiogenesis by the new tumor. Without angiogenesis a tumor is unable to grow larger than a few millimeters in diameter. Once angiogenesis is established, the new tumor can seed itself in a new cycle of metastasis. In fact, tumors generally do not metastasize until angiogenesis is initiated. The leaky vessels produced during angiogenesis allow tumor cells greater access to the circulation. Agents that may inhibit angiogenesis were discussed in Chapter 3.

5.7 SUMMARY

Metastasis is a central feature of neoplasia, and occurs in the majority of solid cancers. The five steps in metastasis are: 1) cell detachment and intravasation; 2) migration through the circulation; 3) cell arrest; 4) extravasation; and 5) angiogenesis. Each of these steps offers targets for anticancer therapy. Cell detachment may be inhibited by affecting the binding, degradation, or expression of cell adhesion molecules, or by protecting ECM integrity. Intravasation and extravasation may be inhibited by protecting vascular integrity and inhibiting protease action. Migration may be inhibited by stimulating the immune system. Cell arrest may be inhibited by inhibiting platelet aggregation. Lastly, angiogenesis may be inhibited by agents discussed in Chapter 3.

6
HUMORAL FACTORS THAT AFFECT NEOPLASIA

The cells in our bodies communicate with each other through a complex set of interactions, some of which are still being discovered. These interactions include chemical signals in the form of autocrine, paracrine, and endocrine factors. *Autocrine factors* are produced by and affect an individual cell. *Paracrine factors* are produced by an individual cell and affect adjacent cells. *Endocrine factors*, or hormones, are produced in specialized cells and travel through the blood to affect target cells at distant locations.

All three types of humoral factors can affect the transformation and proliferation of neoplastic tissue. Factors of particular importance in neoplasia include sex hormones, eicosanoids, and autocrine/pancrine growth factors, which are the subject of this chapter.

6.1 SEX HORMONES

From their origin in the endocrine glands, hormones travel to, and affect, distant target cells. Endocrine glands include the pineal, pituitary, thyroid, parathyroid, adrenals, pancreas, ovaries, testes, thymus, kidney, stomach, small intestine, and placenta. Hormones regulate the body's internal environment, including responses to environmental conditions, growth and development, and reproduction. Hormones can be divided into two categories: water-soluble (for example, insulin), and lipid-soluble (for example, sex hormones). Although all hormones may affect neoplasia in some way, this chapter will focus specifically on sex hormones. The effects of insulin on neoplasia will be discussed in Chapter 7.

Sex hormones are steroidal compounds derived from cholesterol metabolism. The primary male sex hormone is testosterone, and the primary female sex hormones, the estrogens, are estradiol and estrone. Testosterone is mainly produced in the testes, and estrogens are mainly produced in the ovaries. Testosterone and estrogens are also produced in the adrenal glands, although to a lesser extent.

Some tumors may be responsive to, or even depend on, stimulation by sex hormones. A large percentage of cancers that originate from tissues that are responsive to hormones retain some degree of hormone responsiveness, especially in their early stages. These can include breast, endometrial, and prostate tumors.[1] Therefore, treatments for breast and endometrial cancer may include removal of the ovaries or administration of hormones that oppose estrogens. Treatments for prostate cancer may include removal of the testes or administration of hormones that oppose testosterone. In breast cancer, the success of hormonal manipulation correlates with the presence of specific hormone receptors in the tumor cells. Although hormonal manipulation is not a cure, up to 74% of breast cancer patients with estrogen receptor-positive and progesterone receptor-positive tumors respond to hormonal treatment. Up to 30% of patients with endometrial cancer obtain remission, and 80% of patients with prostate cancer obtain improvement in symptoms with hormonal treatment (Tannock and Hill, 1992:224-29).

A variety of common medications can affect estrogen or testosterone levels. For example, oral contraceptives contain estrogen.[2] A variety of natural agents may also affect estrogen or testosterone levels or bioavailability. These agents may:

- affect hormone production
- affect hormone metabolism
- affect the production of the serum protein sex-hormone-binding globulin (SHBG), which binds and reduces the bioavailability of sex hormones
- affect the hormone excretion rate
- compete for, or otherwise affect, hormone binding sites on target tissues

Studies on natural agents that affect these mechanisms are summarized in Table 6.1. In general, patients with breast or endometrial cancer may want to avoid

---

[1] Other cancers, such as ovarian cancer, may contain estrogen receptors, but generally are not responsive to estrogen stimulation.

[2] The effect of oral contraceptives on the development of breast cancer is still uncertain. Some studies indicate that their use increases cancer risk and other studies indicate that their use does not.

agents that increase estrogen bioavailability, especially if their tumors are estrogen receptor-positive. Likewise, patients with prostate cancer may want to avoid agents that increase testosterone bioavailability. Agents that decrease sex hormone bioavailability may be useful for either group.

The effects of natural agents on hormone bioavailability are complex, and the information contained in Table 6.1 may not accurately predict actual results of treatment. This would be particularly true if the data were not obtained from studies on humans. In addition, some data in the table are self-contradicting. The formulas *Dang Gui Shao Yao San, Gui Zhi Fu Ling Wan, Er Chen Tang,* and *Xiao Yao San* are all listed as agents that reduce estrogen bioavailability. However, three of these four formulas contain *Paeonia lactiflora,* which reportedly increases estrogen bioavailability, and two contain *Glycyrrhiza sp.,* which also reportedly increases estrogen bioavailability. This inconsistency does not seem to be explained by other herbs common to the formulas.

TABLE 6.1. NATURAL AGENTS THAT AFFECT HORMONE BIOAVAILABILITY		
AGENT	**EFFECT**	**REFERENCE**
AGENTS THAT REDUCE ESTROGEN BIOAVAILABILITY IN FEMALES		
Camellia sinensis (green tea)	Inhibits the interaction between estrogen and estrogen receptors in estrogen-responsive tumors in vitro.	Komori et al., 1993
Dang Gui Shao Yao San (formula)	Suppresses estradiol secretion by rat ovarian follicles in vitro.	Usuki, 1991
Dietary fat reduction	Decreases estrogen production and increases estrogen metabolism.	See Section 12.2
Fiber	Binds estrogen in human feces and facilitates estrogen elimination.	See Section 12.4.3
Genistein (isoflavone)	Increases the production of sex hormone-binding globulin in vitro.	See Section 14.6
Gui Zhi Fu Ling Wan (formula)	Acts as a weak antiestrogen agent in female rats by inhibiting ovarian DNA synthesis. Reduced plasma estradiol levels by 50% when given orally to female rats. Suppresses estradiol secretion by rat ovarian follicles in vitro.	Sakamoto et al., 1992, 1988; Usuki, 1991
Humulus lupulus (hops)	Prevented estrogen production in female rats that were stimulated with gonadotropins. Gonadotropins are hormones produced by the pituitary gland and placenta that stimulate the male or female sex organs.	Okamoto and Kumai, 1992
Lignans	Although lignans, such as those found in flax seed *(Linum usitatissimum),* possess weak estrogen activity, they may produce weak antiestrogen effects by competing for estrogen receptor sites, especially in premenopausal women.	See Section 14.7
Phytoestrogens	Phytoestrogens, such as those found in soy, compete with estrogen for binding to receptor sites. Phytoestrogens also act as weak estrogens, and appear to produce estrogen effects in postmenopausal women, and antiestrogen effects in premenopausal women.	See Section 14.2
Xiao Yao San and *Er Chen Tang* (formulas)	Markedly decreased saliva estradiol levels in women with proliferative breast disease.	Zhang, 1991
AGENTS THAT INCREASE ESTROGEN BIOAVAILABILITY IN FEMALES		
Foeniculum vulgare (fennel)	Stimulated estrogen production in animals. The active ingredients are thought to be in the essential oils.	Albert-Puleo, 1980
Glycyrrhiza uralensis (gan cao) and *Paeonia lactiflora (bai shao* and *chi shao)*	These herbs stimulate the activity of aromatase, an enzyme that converts testosterone to estrogen. Paeoniflorin (from *P. lactiflora*), and glycyrrhizin and glycyrrhetinic acid (from *G. uralensis*) stimulated aromatase activity in the rat ovary to promote estradiol synthesis. Formulas containing *P. lactiflora* increased estradiol secretion from cultured rat ovarian follicles. A formula consisting of *P. lactiflora* and *G. uralensis* increased DHEA-S, a precursor of estrogen, and increased serum estrogen concentrations in rats whose ovaries were surgically removed. *(column continues)*	Takeuchi et al., 1991, 1989; Ota et al., 1989; Kato and Okamoto, 1992; Takahashi and Kitao, 1994
(Table continues)		

44

TABLE 6.1. (continued)		
AGENT	**EFFECT**	**REFERENCE**
AGENTS THAT INCREASE ESTROGEN BIOAVAILABILITY IN FEMALES (continued)		
Glycyrrhiza uralensis (gan cao) and *Paeonia lactiflora (bai shao* and *chi shao)*	*(continued)* This formula lowered serum testosterone levels in sterilized female rats by stimulating aromatase activity. When the formula was administered to females with polycystic ovarian disease, serum testosterone levels decreased and the ratio of estrogen to testosterone increased. In conventional medicine, inhibitors of aromatase have been used in the treatment of breast cancer.	See previous page
Liu Wei Di Huang Tang (formula)	This formula increased plasma estradiol levels and increased estrogen receptors on leukocytes in menopausal women. In contrast, the formula increased plasma testosterone and lowered plasma estradiol in patients with *kidney yin vacuity,* a disease pattern in Chinese medicine that is common in menopausal women.	Zhang and Zhou, 1991; Zhu et al., 1993
Pimpinella anisum (anise)	Stimulated estrogen production in animals. The active ingredients are thought to be in the essential oils.	Albert-Puleo, 1980
Salvia miltiorrhiza (dan shen)	Increased the level of plasma estradiol in female rats.	Li et al., 1992b
AGENTS THAT DECREASE TESTOSTERONE BIOAVAILABILITY IN MALES		
Cannabis sativa (marijuana)	Smoking the herb reduced plasma testosterone levels or inhibited testosterone receptors in humans and in animals.	Barnett et al., 1983; Fujimoto et al., 1982; Purohit et al., 1980
San Zhuang Wan (formula)	The formula decreased serum testosterone levels in male rats.	Zhang and Pomerantz, 1989
Serenoa repens (saw palmetto)	Used in Western herbology to treat benign prostatic hypertrophy (BPH). In 20 men with BPH, administration of the lipid extract for 30 days did not affect plasma testosterone levels. Rather, serenoa appears to inhibit the metabolism of testosterone (by the enzyme 5 alpha-reductase) to its more potent form, dihydrotestosterone, and appears to block the binding of testosterone to tissues by competing for binding sites. Lipid extracts of serenoa inhibited 5 alpha-reductase activity and effectively blocked testosterone receptor binding in human fibroblasts in vitro. The lipid extract inhibited the binding of testosterone by 42% and dihydro-testosterone by 41% in 11 different tissue specimens. In contrast to these studies, other investigators reported that lipid extract did not exhibit 5 alpha reductase inhibitory activity in vitro.	Casarosa et al., 1988; Sultan et al., 1984; Delos et al., 1994; El-Sheikh et al., 1988; Carilla et al., 1984; Rhodes et al., 1993
Vitex negundo (huang jing zi)	Flavonoids from vitex reduced testosterone production in male dogs.	Bhargava, 1989
AGENTS THAT INCREASE TESTOSTERONE BIOAVAILABILITY IN MALES		
Cinnamomum cassia (rou gui)	Increased serum testosterone in male mice.	Kuang et al., 1989
Ba Wei Di Huang Wan (formula)	The formula increased testosterone production in rat testes in vitro and in vivo. This formula contains *Cinnamomum cassia*.	Usuki, 1988
Panax ginseng (ren shen)	Oral administration increased the plasma testosterone level in adult male rats.	Fahim et al., 1982
Wu Zi Yan Zong (formula)	The formula increased plasma testosterone in older rats, but not in younger ones.	Wang and Zie, 1993

6.2 EICOSANOIDS

Eicosanoids are autocrine and paracrine factors produced from the metabolism of arachidonic acid and other plasma membrane fatty acids. They are produced in nearly every cell in the body.

Eicosanoids are very potent substances. As little as one billionth of a gram can have measurable biological effects. The body produces a variety of eicosanoids, and they affect a wide range of functions, including blood pressure, gastric secretion, platelet aggregation, tension of the intestinal and uterine muscles, inflammation, steroid hormone production, pain sensation, and induction of labor.

6.2.1 Eicosanoid Biosynthesis

Prostaglandins were the first eicosanoids to be recognized. They derive their name from the prostate gland, where they were first thought to be produced. A number of important prostaglandins are derived from arachidonic acid. Arachidonic acid is obtained in the diet primarily through animal products, and along with other fatty acids, is incorporated into the phospholipid bilayer of the plasma membrane of all cells. Through the action of the enzymes phospholipase A_2 and phospholipase C, it is cleaved from the cell membrane to form free arachidonic acid (see Figure 6.1 for a diagram of arachidonic acid metabolism).[3] The enzymes cyclooxygenase and lipoxygenase metabolize free arachidonic acid to form prostaglandins, thromboxane, HETE, and leukotrienes. All products of cyclooxygenase or lipoxygenase activity are termed eicosanoids. Products of cyclooxygenase activity in particular, are termed prostanoids. Eicosanoids are synthesized according to their immediate need and are not stored. Once synthesized, they quickly degrade in the body.

The prostanoids that form from arachidonic acid are given the subscript 2 (for example, PGE_2), and the leukotrienes are given the subscript 4 (i.e., LTA_4). Two dietary fatty acids, other than arachidonic acid, that can produce eicosanoids are linoleic acid, found in most vegetable oils, and eicosapentaenoic acid (EPA), found in fish oil. Linoleic acid is converted to dihomo-gamma-linolenic (DGLA) through the actions of various enzymes, and the prostanoids that form from DGLA are given the subscript 1 (for example, PGE_1), and the leukotrienes are given the subscript 3 (i.e., LTA_3). The prostanoids that form from EPA are given the subscript 3 (for example, PGE_3), and the leukotrienes are given the subscript 5 (for example, LTA_5). The subscript denotes the number of double bonds present between carbon atoms.

The bioactivity of eicosanoids vary depending on the type of eicosanoids formed and the fatty acid that they derive from. For example, PGE_2, derived from arachidonic acid, is highly inflammatory, whereas PGE_3, derived

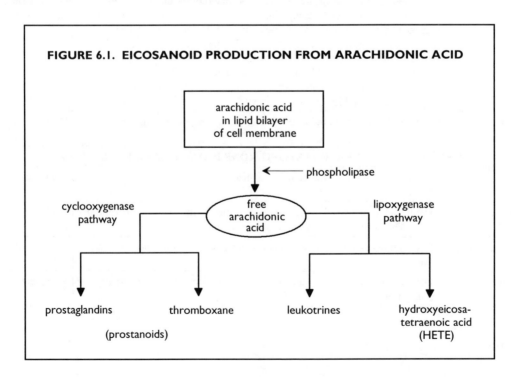

FIGURE 6.1. EICOSANOID PRODUCTION FROM ARACHIDONIC ACID

arachidonic acid in lipid bilayer of cell membrane

← phospholipase

cyclooxygenase pathway

free arachidonic acid

lipoxygenase pathway

prostaglandins   thromboxane

(prostanoids)

leukotrines   hydroxyeicosa-tetraenoic acid (HETE)

---

[3] With regard to inflammation, phospholipase C is mainly involved in eicosanoid production, and phospholipase A_2 is mainly involved in mast cell degranulation and histamine release (Neves et al., 1993).

TABLE 6.2. PHYSIOLOGICAL EFFECTS OF ARACHIDONIC ACID-DERIVED EICOSANOIDS	
EICOSANOID	**PHYSIOLOGICAL EFFECT**
PROSTANOIDS	
PGE_2	Broad physiological effects. Inhibits lipolysis by decreasing the hormone-induced activation of cAMP in fat cells, increases the formation of cAMP in macrophages, stimulates renin secretion, vasodilator, inhibits gastric acid production, inhibits norepinephrine release, inhibits insulin secretion, induces calcium release from bones and bone resorption, induces fever, and increases pain. PGE_2 is the primary proinflammatory prostanoid.
PGD_2	Affects platelet aggregation and brain function.
$PGF_{2\text{-alpha}}$	Vasoconstrictor that affects uterine and ovarian function. Slight proinflammatory action.
PGI_2 (prostacyclin)	Vasodilator that inhibits platelet aggregation, stimulates renin secretion, and inhibits gastric acid production. Moderate proinflammatory action.
TXA_2 (thromboxane)	Enhances platelet aggregation and is a vasoconstrictor. Slight proinflammatory action.
LEUKOTRIENES	
LTA_4	Histamine-like actions (increases vascular permeability and bronchospasms). Markedly more potent than histamine in causing bronchospasms. Most leukotrienes are vasoconstrictors. Leukotrienes contribute to the development of allergic and inflammatory reactions.
LTB_4	
LTC_4	
LTD_4	
LTE_4	
Sources: Wilson et al., 1991:397-401; Vane, 1987	

from EPA, is anti-inflammatory. The physiological effects of some eicosanoids derived from arachidonic acid are listed in Table 6.2.

Prostanoid synthesis can be affected by drugs such as aspirin, ibuprofen, and cortisol. Aspirin and other nonsteroidal anti-inflammatory drugs inhibit the cyclooxygenase pathway, and glucocorticoids, such as cortisol, inhibit the action of phospholipase A_2. In either case, the production of proinflammatory eicosanoids is inhibited.

6.2.2 Eicosanoids and the Immune System

The effects of eicosanoids on the human immune system are not fully understood. Macrophages, T lymphocytes, and natural killer cells are types of immune cells that may play a central role in the body's defense against cancer, and eicosanoids affect these cells in diverse ways. Macrophages readily synthesize both prostanoids and leukotrienes from arachidonic acid, and these eicosanoids, in turn, affect the functioning of the macrophages. PGE_2 inhibits macrophage activity in vitro, whereas leukotrienes, especially LTC_4, stimulate macrophage activity (Bailey and Fletcher-Cieutat, 1987; Droge et al., 1987). Leukotriene C_4 in combination with inhibitors of cyclooxygenase (PGE_2 inhibitors) produced additive effects in stimulating macrophages against mouse tumor cells in vitro (Bonata and Ben-Efraim, 1987).

One mechanism by which PGE_2 may suppress macrophage activity is by increasing adenosine 3',5'-cyclic monophosphate (cAMP) production. Cyclic AMP acts as an intracellular messenger by carrying information from hormone receptors at the surface of the cell to receptors internal to the cell (see Box 6.1). An increase in cAMP could increase the inhibitory action of water-soluble hormones (such as insulin) on immune cells.[4]

PGE_2 also suppresses T-lymphocyte activity in vitro. This may occur through two mechanisms: 1) by increasing cAMP levels, and 2) by inhibiting the production of interleukin-2, a cytokine that stimulates T-lymphocyte activity. Aspirin, an inhibitor of PGE_2 production, has been shown to stimulate T-lymphocyte proliferation.

In contrast to in-vitro inhibitory effects, PGE_2 stimulates lymphocyte proliferation and activity in vivo. When administered to healthy humans, a PGE_2 analog (misoprostol) improved lymphocyte proliferation in response to mitogens and increased tumor necrosis factor production (Waymack et al., 1992). In some cases, the effects of PGE_2 may be bidirectional, depending on the state of the immune system. Natural killer cell activity was inhibited by PGE_2 in normal animals, and stimulated in immunosuppressed animals (Favalli et al., 1987). Further study

---

[4] Lipid-soluble hormones, such as sex hormones, easily penetrate the plasma membrane to reach intracellular targets and do not require cAMP to act as an intermediary.

BOX 6.1. CYCLIC AMP

Adenosine 3',5'-cyclic monophosphate (cAMP) acts as an intracellular switch, regulating cellular growth and differentiation. It does this by mediating the intracellular stimulation of a number of nonsteroid hormones such as corticotropin, epinephrine, glucagon, follicle stimulating hormone, luteinizing hormone, norepinephrine, thyroid stimulating hormone, and vasopressin (Stryer, 1988:987). As such, cAMP is often referred to as a *second messenger* in the action of these hormones. Cyclic AMP affects a wide variety of cellular processes, including stimulation of gastric acid secretion, lipolysis, and inhibition of platelet aggregation. Cyclic AMP is degraded by the enzyme cAMP phosphodiesterase.

A number of in-vitro and in-vivo studies suggest that cAMP inhibits tumor growth. For example, various cAMP derivatives inhibited hormone-responsive mammary tumors in vitro (Yoon Sang et al., 1985). The amino acid arginine appears to act synergistically with cAMP in this respect. In one animal study, the combination of cAMP and arginine reduced tumor size by 85% within two weeks. Analogs of cAMP inhibit human leukemia and colon carcinoma cells in vitro (Yokozaki et al., 1992), and cAMP inhibits Ehrlich ascites tumor cells in vitro (Wang et al., 1982a). Rapidly growing tumor cells exhibited low cAMP levels and slowly growing cells exhibited high levels. Elevated levels of cAMP phosphodiesterase have been observed in human Kaposi's sarcoma tissue (Ambrus et al., 1992). Pan (1992:35) summarized a number of studies on cAMP conducted in China:

- Intracellular levels of cAMP are lower in human tumor cells than in normal cells.
- Patients whose tumors contain lower levels of cAMP exhibit more serious signs of disease.
- When cAMP was added to cultures of neoplastic and normal cells, the neoplastic cells were inhibited by 70 to 80% within 4 days, whereas the normal cells were inhibited by 13%.
- Injection of cAMP into tumor-bearing animals retarded tumor growth.

However, not all research has demonstrated a clear relationship between cAMP levels and neoplastic growth. For example, the inhibitory effect of cAMP on macrophage and T-cell activity was discussed in the text. Other investigators have also reported conflicting results and general conclusions on the effect of cAMP on cancer cells cannot be made at this time (Tannock and Hill, 1992:216).

A number of natural agents have been reported to increase cAMP levels in vitro or in vivo. These include the herbs *Andrographis paniculata (chuan xin lian), Polyporus umbellatus (zhu ling), Salvia miltiorrhiza (dan shen), Ziziphus jujuba (da zao), Cnidium monnieri (she chuang zi), Actinidia chinensis (teng li gen), Aconitum carmichaeli (fu zi)*, and *Cinnamomum cassia (rou gui)*; and the formulas *Li Wei Di Huang Tang, Saiboku To, Yi Qi Jian Pi, You Gui Yin*, and *Kanzo Shashin To*; and caffeine. For the interested reader, studies on these agents are summarized in Appendix E.

---

is necessary to clarify the immunomodulatory effects of PGE$_2$ in vivo.

6.2.3 Eicosanoids and Cancer

Eicosanoids may play a variety of roles in the initiation, promotion, and progression of cancer. Observations of the relationship between eicosanoids and cancer include the following:[5]

- Tumors synthesize eicosanoids through both the cyclooxygenase and lipoxygenase pathways. The lipoxygenase pathway of arachidonic acid is important, if not essential, to tumor promotion.
- A variety of tumor-promoting agents stimulate prostaglandin synthesis. This is as expected, since inflammation is associated with both tumor-promoting agents and prostaglandin production. In animal models, application of various prostaglandins, in conjunction with tumor promoters, can modify the number of tumors produced, with the direction being determined by which prostaglandins are applied.

- Malignant cells synthesize excessive levels of prostaglandins, especially PGE$_2$ and PGF$_{2\text{-alpha}}$, compared to normal cells. Elevated levels of prostaglandins have been detected in the blood and urine of tumor-bearing animals.
- Some investigators have reported that PGE$_2$ inhibits tumor cell replication in vitro. Other investigators have reported that PGE$_2$ and PGF$_{2\text{-alpha}}$ appear to enhance growth of neoplastic tissues in vivo, although this varied with tumor type.
- PGE$_2$ induces cellular differentiation, and prostaglandins may potentiate the differentiating effect of vitamin A. Combining vitamin A with PGE$_1$ or PGE$_2$ lowers the dose of vitamin A required to induce differentiation.
- PGE-induced inflammation may mediate tumor invasion and angiogenesis. The effects of

---

[5] Sources: Fischer and Slaga, 1985:174, 42; Jaffe and Santoro, 1987; Levine, 1987; Breitman, 1987; Powles, 1987; Favalli et al. 1987; Waymack and Chance, 1990.

TABLE 6.3. NATURAL AGENTS THAT AFFECT PGE SYNTHESIS

AGENT	EFFECT	REFERENCE
Aloe vera	Inhibited the metabolism of arachidonic acid in vitro.	Klein et al., 1988
EPA and other dietary fats	Dietary fats are the source of fatty acids for eicosanoid production and greatly influence the type of eicosanoid produced.	See Section 12.1
Ligustrum lucidum (nu zhen zi)	Reduces the level of PGE_2 in experimentally inflamed rat ear tissues.	Dai et al., 1989
Rheum palmatum (da huang)	Blocked the biosynthesis of PGA_2, PGE_2 and PGF_2 in rabbit kidneys. The authors suggest that these effects may be due to an inhibition of cyclooxygenase.	Guo et al., 1989
Salvia miltiorrhiza (dan shen)	A constituent of *S. miltiorrhiza* increased urinary PGE_2 excretion in rats with sodium-induced hypertension. This effect may explain the hypotensive action of this herb.	Yokozawa et al., 1992
Serenoa repens	Inhibited both the cyclooxygenase and lipoxygenase pathways of eicosanoid production. This may account for the herb's reported anti-inflammatory and antiedema activity.	Breu et al., 1992

inflammation on angiogenesis were discussed in Chapter 3.

- Prostaglandins have been shown to facilitate the metastasis of tumors to bone.
- Prostaglandins may affect metastasis by affecting platelet aggregation.
- The effects of prostaglandins on tumor growth may be related to modulation of the immune system. These effects may be positive or negative depending on the experimental conditions (treatment schedule, tumor type, level of immunosuppression, and extent of metastasis).

Due to the complexity of eicosanoid synthesis and the broad range of effects of different eicosanoids, the exact role of each eicosanoid in cancer is far from clear. Research has shown contradictory results in that some prostaglandins can both inhibit and accelerate tumor proliferation, and inhibit and stimulate immune cells (Favalli et al., 1987). Therefore, agents that affect eicosanoid production play an uncertain role in the treatment of cancer. Some of these agents have been discussed previously. Table 5.1 summarized information regarding natural agents that alter prostaglandin synthesis and inhibit platelet aggregation. Table 3.4 summarized information regarding natural agents that prevent increased vascular permeability. Natural agents that affect PGE synthesis in other regards are listed in Table 6.3. Potentially, agents that inhibit PGE_2 synthesis could reduce PGE_2-induced inflammation, inhibit tumor cell proliferation, and stimulate the activity of immune cells. However, as suggested above, more research is needed to determine the accuracy of this assertion.

6.3 GROWTH FACTORS

Growth factors are small soluble proteins that bind to specific receptors on plasma membranes.[6] They include both autocrine and paracrine factors. Growth factors regulate cell maintenance, differentiation, proliferation, and other functions. As discussed in previous chapters, this regulatory function is shared by cell adhesion molecules and matrix components, among other factors. The binding of growth factors on membrane receptors stimulates the receptor to send an intracellular signal. Signal transduction is commonly accomplished through phosphorylation of tyrosine kinases.

Kinases are intracellular enzymes that catalyze the transfer of phosphate from adenosine triphosphate (ATP) to an acceptor. ATP, the energy storehouse of cells, contains three phosphoric acid groups. Tyrosine kinases (named for the amino acid tyrosine they contain) may be stimulated by cAMP, or as is the case with certain hormones, may be stimulated by growth factor binding on a cell membrane receptor. As an example, the receptor binding of a generic growth factor is shown in Figure 6.2. In this case, the phosphate acceptor is the receptor itself (called autophosphorylation) and an intracellular protein substrate. Phosphorylation stimulates an intracellular protein substrate to produce certain activities, such as inducing differentiation. Although all cells contain tyrosine kinases, the quantity or quality of kinases in transformed cells may vary in response to proto-oncogene activation (Bergamaschi et al., 1993). The effects of insulin on membrane receptors are similar to that shown in the figure. In the case of insulin, phosphorylation stimulates the cell to increase glucose uptake, among other actions.

---

[6] Growth factors, or other agents that stimulate a membrane receptor, are called *ligands*.

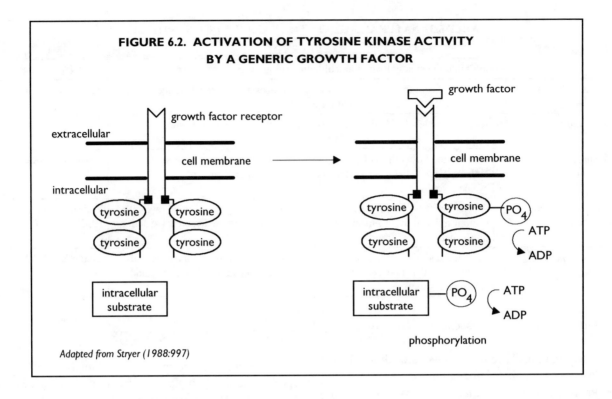

FIGURE 6.2. ACTIVATION OF TYROSINE KINASE ACTIVITY BY A GENERIC GROWTH FACTOR

Adapted from Stryer (1988:997)

TABLE 6.4. GROWTH FACTORS THAT MAY AFFECT NEOPLASIA	
GROWTH FACTOR	**COMMENT**
Bombesin-like peptides	Homologous to bombesin, a peptide found in amphibians. Secreted by some human small-cell lung cancer lines.
Epidermal growth factor (EDF)	The EGF receptor may be overexpressed in human cancers such as brain cancers (glioblastomas), and breast and bladder cancers.
Fibroblast growth factor (FGF)	Expressed by many types of tumor cells. FGFs are heparin-binding growth factors that are involved in angiogenesis. See Section 3.3.1 for more information on FGF in relation to angiogenesis.
Insulin-like growth factors (IGF)	Homologous to insulin. Produced by a variety of malignant cells. IGF receptors occur on a variety of human tumors, including breast cancers. Antiestrogen therapy with tamoxifen may reduce serum levels of IGF. Certain natural agents that exhibit antiestrogen activity, such as quercetin, may also reduce IGF secretion, although this has not been verified.
Cytokines, such as interleukin-2, interferon, and granulocyte-macrophage colony stimulating factor	These growth factors regulate immune cell function and are discussed with the rest of the immune system in Chapter 8. Numerous natural agents induce the production of these growth factors.
Transforming growth factor-alpha (TGF-α)	Alternative ligand for epidermal growth factor receptors. May be involved in angiogenesis.
Transforming growth factor-beta (TGF-β)	Inhibits the proliferation of several cell types, including endothelial cells. Distributed widely in adult tissues, as is its receptors. The production of TGF-β_1 is stimulated by a number of agents such as retinoids, vitamin D, antiestrogens (including tamoxifen), quercetin, and interferons, and may account, in part, for their antitumor effects (see Section 14.4.4).
Source: Tannock and Hill, 1992:148-52	

By affecting the response of cells to external factors, tyrosine kinases play a role in numerous cellular activities, including induction of platelet aggregation, inhibition of apoptosis, stimulation of mitosis, and production of prostaglandins. For example, growth factors such as interleukin-3 and granulocyte-macrophage colony stimulating factor are known to stimulate cell proliferation and inhibit apoptosis. In fact, neoplastic cells may require growth factor-induced tyrosine phosphorylation to maintain their extended life span. Some growth factors that are important in neoplasia are listed in Table 6.4.

Natural agents that inhibit tyrosine kinase activity may inhibit growth factor-induced activities, and, therefore, various aspects of neoplasia. These agents include emodin (Jayasuriya et al., 1992) genistein, and quercetin (Matsukawa et al., 1993).[7] It is likely that numerous natural agents produce their biologic effects in part through modulation of tyrosine kinase or growth factor activity. The effects of natural agents on these activities are just beginning to be discovered.

6.4 SUMMARY

This chapter discussed three important groups of compounds that regulate cellular function and are important in neoplasia. These are sex hormones, eicosanoids, and growth factors. Although a number of natural agents affect the production or action of these compounds, their biologic regulation is complex. In addition, the influence that these compounds exert on human cancers is, in many cases, incompletely defined, and additional investigations are required to identify the most profitable clinical applications.

---

[7] More than one type of tyrosine kinase exists, and quercetin inhibits various tyrosine kinases, as well as other protein kinases. Genistein appears to affect phosphorylation of the cdc2 kinase (Matsukawa et al., 1993).

7

EFFECTS OF pH ON NEOPLASIA

The proliferation rate of tumor cells is greatly affected by the intracellular acid-alkaline balance (pH). Abnormalities in pH have been investigated both as a cause for, and treatment of, cancer.

Intracellular pH may be altered by endogenous agents, such as insulin and certain growth factors, and by exogenous agents such as dietary sugars, hyperthermia and, possibly, the metal cesium.

7.1 THE REGULATION OF pH

The extracellular environment within solid tumors is generally acidic (low pH), and may be particularly acidic in those regions that are most hypoxic (Dobrowsky et al., 1991; Kennedy and Rockwell, 1990).[1] Some human tumors have an extracellular pH as low as 7.09 units (Van der Zee et al., 1989). In contrast, the intracellular pH of tumor cells is generally equal to that of normal cells, which is approximately 7.3 units—slightly less than the pH of arterial blood (7.35 to 7.45 units) (Newell et al., 1993).

At the systemic level, arterial pH is controlled by three mechanisms: respiration, kidney excretion, and buffer systems (i.e., carbonic acid-bicarbonate, phosphate, hemoglobin-oxyhemoglobin, and protein buffer systems). At the cellular level, pH is mediated by a protein contained in the plasma membrane that controls the exchange of sodium ions for hydrogen ions (the sodium-hydrogen exchanger).[2] The energy to drive the sodium-hydrogen exchanger is obtained from the steep inwardly-directed sodium gradient maintained by the sodium-potassium ATPase (adenosine triphosphatase) system (the sodium-potassium pump) (Mahnensmith and Aronson, 1985). The sodium-potassium pump creates a sodium vacuum that, under subnormal pH conditions,

enables the sodium-hydrogen exchanger to push hydrogen ions out of the cell in exchange for sodium ions, thereby raising the intracellular pH (see Figure 7.1).[3] In addition to, or as part of regulating the intracellular pH, the sodium-hydrogen exchanger plays a central role in the regulation of cell proliferation, metabolic response to hormones such as insulin, and regulation of cell volume (Mahnensmith and Aronson, 1985). Through these mechanisms, this system may be intimately involved in the pathophysiology of cancer.

7.2 CELL PROLIFERATION AND pH

Activating the sodium-hydrogen exchanger brings sodium into the cell. Numerous investigators have reported that tumor cells from a variety of human cancers have a higher sodium-to-potassium ratio than nonmalignant tissue.[4] In tissue biopsies obtained from 18 patients with suspected laryngeal cancer, benign tissues exhibited a sodium-to-potassium ratio one-fifth as large as that for malignant tissues. The higher ratios in malignant tissue were primarily due to increased sodium content (Nagy et al., 1987). Similar studies on thyroid and urogenital cancers associated elevated sodium-to-potassium ratios with increasing malignancy (Nagy et al., 1981, 1983; Lukacs et al., 1983). Taken together, these studies suggest that

---

[1] pH is defined as: log (1 ÷ hydrogen ion concentration).

[2] The intracellular pH of cells may also be regulated by Cl^- - HCO_3^- exchange (which lowers pH), lactic acid transport out of the cell (which raises pH), and intracellular buffer systems such as the protein buffer system (Vaughn-Jones, 1988).

[3] Due to the large interior-negative electrical membrane potential, if intracellular pH were in electrochemical equilibrium across the membrane, it would be 6.3 to 6.5 units. However, the intracellular pH of normal cells ranges from 6.8 to 7.3 units. Therefore, energy must be used to drive hydrogen ions out of the cell to raise the pH to its normally observed value.

[4] Jansson (1987, 1990) reported that dietary ratios of sodium-to-potassium are 20 times higher in the Western diet than in the historic diet of humans, and postulates that high dietary Na/K ratios are responsible for an increase in cancer incidence. This hypothesis was also put forth by Max Gerson (1881-1959), a pioneer in nutritional metabolic therapy (Walters, 1993:189-203). However, this theory conflicts with the observation that some Asian populations eat a high-salt diet and do not exhibit increased rates of cancer incidence, except for increased rates of stomach cancer.

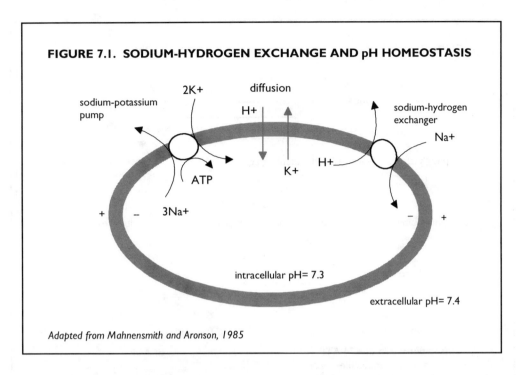

FIGURE 7.1. SODIUM-HYDROGEN EXCHANGE AND pH HOMEOSTASIS

Adapted from Mahnensmith and Aronson, 1985

sodium levels are often elevated in neoplastic tissues. One possible cause is activation of the sodium-hydrogen exchanger.

Activating the sodium-hydrogen exchanger raises the intracellular pH. A number of in-vitro studies have shown that a rise in intracellular pH to hypernormal levels stimulates cell proliferation. Under normal conditions the sodium-hydrogen exchanger maintains intracellular pH at approximately 7.3 units. At this pH, the protein that controls the sodium-hydrogen exchanger has a low affinity for hydrogen ions and is nearly inactive. However, when intracellular pH becomes more acidic, the protein's affinity for hydrogen ions increases, thereby activating the sodium-hydrogen exchanger. The presence of certain growth factors, tumor promoters, and mitogens can abnormally increase the protein's affinity for hydrogen ions. This excessively activates the exchanger which, in turn, abnormally elevates the intracellular pH. This increase in alkalinity appears to be part of the mechanism by which these agents stimulate cell proliferation.

Elevating the pH of the extracellular environment can also raise intracellular pH. A number of studies have associated increased extracellular pH with increased proliferation in a variety of malignant neoplasms (reviewed by Harguindey, 1982). These include experiments on tumor-bearing rabbits, in which alkalizing drinking water with bicarbonate increased the growth of tumors, and acidifying drinking water with acetic acid induced tumor regressions.

A variety of hormones also may increase the intracellular pH (Mahnensmith and Aronson, 1985). Insulin,

glucocorticoids, and thyroid hormone all stimulate the activities of the sodium-potassium pump and sodium-hydrogen exchanger and increase intracellular pH. Glycolysis, or the breakdown of sugar to form energy, is induced by insulin and can be inhibited by preventing a rise in intracellular pH. Lowering extracellular sodium can inhibit an insulin-induced increase in intracellular pH, presumably because reducing the transmembrane sodium gradient reduces the driving force of the sodium-hydrogen exchanger.

Activating the sodium-hydrogen exchanger may explain how malignant tumors produce excessive lactic acid and subsequently acidify their microenvironment (Mahnensmith and Aronson, 1985). Glucose produces lactic acid by the glycolysis pathway, shown in Figure 7.2. Glycolysis is limited, in part, by the availability of adenosine diphosphate (ADP), and ADP is made available by the breakdown of ATP to ADP by ATPase. Insulin, growth factors, tumor promoters, and certain mitogens all stimulate an increase in intracellular pH, and this increase is associated with elevated levels of sodium. Elevated intracellular sodium stimulates the sodium-potassium ATPase pump, thereby providing a source of ADP for glycolysis. In addition, an increase in intracellular pH itself stimulates glycolysis, since the rate-limiting enzyme in glycolysis, phosphofructokinase (PFK), becomes markedly more functional as the pH rises. Under aerobic conditions, increased glycolysis results in increased production of pyruvate, a small amount of which transforms into lactic acid. However, under the hypoxic conditions present in solid tumors, anaerobic glycolysis greatly increases the transformation of

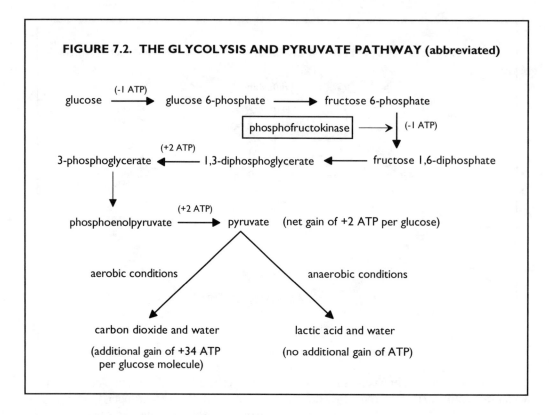

FIGURE 7.2. THE GLYCOLYSIS AND PYRUVATE PATHWAY (abbreviated)

pyruvate into lactic acid. The production of lactic acid stimulates the sodium-hydrogen exchanger to remove excess hydrogen ions which, if carried to excess, further stimulates glycolysis. The production and discharge of lactic acid by tumors acidifies the extracellular pH.

The glycolysis pathway described above is greatly stimulated in tumor cells. Tumor cells consume glucose at a rate three to five times higher than normal cells (Demetrakopoulos and Brennan, 1982) and, therefore, produce inordinate amounts of lactic acid. Numerous studies have demonstrated that oral administration of glucose reduces the extracellular pH in tumors. In one study on patients with cervical cancer, 100 grams of orally administered glucose lowered the extracellular tumor pH from 7.12 to 6.96 units (Leeper et al., 1990). Table 7.1 illustrates the relationship between intracellular pH, glucose, oxygen, and cellular metabolism.

Lactic acid production is undesirable for two reasons. First, it may increase the ability of tumor cells to metastasize. In mouse models, subjecting tumor cells to a low pH environment prior to injection increased the potential for metastatic colonization (Schlappack et al., 1990). Second, lactic acid production may stimulate the production of angiogenic factors by macrophages (Folkman, 1993a). Since lactic acid production increases after oral administration of glucose, it may be prudent for patients with cancer to avoid dietary intake of simple sugars, although this has not been confirmed clinically. In addition, ingestion of dietary sugar leads to

ACTIVITY	INCREASING pH	DECREASING OXYGEN	DECREASING pH	INCREASING OXYGEN	INCREASING GLUCOSE
Glycolysis	increased	increased	inhibited	inhibited	increased
Pyruvate production	increased	increased	inhibited	inhibited	
Sodium-potassium ATPase activity	increased	—	decreased	—	—
Lactic acid production	increased (in aerobic glycolysis)	greatly increased (in anaerobic glycolysis)	inhibited	inhibited	increased

TABLE 7.1. EFFECTS OF INTRACELLULAR pH, OXYGEN, AND GLUCOSE ON CELLULAR METABOLISM

Sources: Harguindey, 1982; Mahnensmith and Aronson, 1985; Hedley, 1989

hyperglycemia, which stimulates the production of insulin, which may further stimulate cell proliferation.

As discussed above, the primary cause of the acidic extracellular pH may be the increased production of lactic acid via anaerobic glycolysis. However, some researchers have demonstrated that mechanisms other than lactic acid production may also reduce the pH. Glycolysis-deficient hamster tumors do not produce lactic acid in vitro and do not contain hypoxic areas in vivo, but they do produce acidic conditions in vivo (Newell et al., 1993). A possible cause is the production of carbonic acid (H_2CO_3) from the carbon dioxide produced during oxidative energy metabolism. The inadequate neovasculature formation and reduced circulation present within tumors may allow sufficient accumulation of carbon dioxide to create carbonic acid.

7.3 LOW pH TREATMENTS

As shown in Table 7.1, high intracellular pH and low oxygen conditions favor increased glycolysis and lactic acid production. These observations suggest that either a reduction in intracellular pH or an increase in oxygen may inhibit the growth of cancer cells. Lowering extracellular pH by hyperthermia or metabolic acidosis may also reduce intracellular pH. Both of these are discussed below.

7.3.1 Hyperthermia

Cellular respiration can occur only within a limited pH range. Tumor cells cannot live in an environment with an extracellular pH below 6.0 to 6.5 units (Dobrowsky et al., 1991). As mentioned above, lactic acid production and other factors reduce the extracellular pH. However, these mechanisms are not sufficient in and of themselves to reduce the extracellular pH to the point of cell death. To decrease the extracellular pH to this range requires the use of external agents. One such agent is heat (Van de Merwe et al., 1990; Dietzel, 1983). Hyperthermia has been used clinically with some success against superficial cancers where localized application is possible, but its use is more limited in the treatment of internal tumors due to its adverse effects on healthy tissues.

Certain flavonoids may potentiate the ability of hyperthermia to destroy tumor cells. The flavonoid quercetin inhibits intracellular synthesis of heat shock proteins, which protect cells against damage from heat (Elia and Santoro, 1994).[5] Heat shock proteins are universally induced in human cells exposed to high temperatures (and other stresses such as radiation and chemicals). Inhibiting the synthesis of these proteins increases the vulnerability of tumor cells to stress damage.[6]

Quercetin can also inhibit lactic acid transport out of human cervical and colon carcinoma cells and Ehrlich ascites tumor cells in vitro (Kim et al., 1984; Graziani et al., 1977; Agullo et al., 1994). By inhibiting lactic acid transport, quercetin may lower intracellular pH. Therefore, under heat stress, quercetin may inhibit proliferation of tumor cells by inhibiting heat shock protein synthesis and by reducing the intracellular pH. In cervical carcinoma cells, quercetin did not induce cytotoxic effects at normal body temperature, but did potentiate hyperthermia-induced cytotoxicity at 41 °C (105.8 °F) (Kim et al., 1984).

7.3.2 Metabolic Acidosis

A reduction in systemic pH may inhibit proliferation of tumor cells by reducing tumor pH. Administering hydrochloric acid tablets and acidic diets to tumor-bearing dogs lowered the blood pH to 7.3 units and almost completely eliminated circulating lactic acid and pyruvate. In addition, systemic acidosis in humans has been cited as a cause of tumor regression (reviewed by Harguindey, 1982). Harguindey suggests that many "spontaneous regressions" in humans may be due to systemic acidosis caused by fever or other mechanisms. For example, fever, and associated acidosis, may be partly responsible for regressions due to administration of Coley's toxins.[7] Lactic acid, pyruvate, and lactic dehydrogenase, an enzyme that degrades lactate, all may be elevated in tumor-bearing animals, and Harguindey suggests that they may be useful in monitoring tumor activity.

Manipulating the systemic acid-base balance in humans is not a viable treatment option due to the narrow

---

[5] Quercetin has been shown to be cytotoxic against a variety of tumor cell lines, and some investigators have suggested that the cytotoxic effects may be due in part to inhibition of the sodium-potassium pump (Agullo et al., 1994).

[6] Heat shock proteins may allow a tumor to develop resistance to chemotherapy drugs and toxins by protecting cells against chemical stresses. Resistance can also develop against immune-mediated toxins, such as tumor necrosis factor. Heat shock proteins may also be involved in inhibiting apoptosis. The ability of quercetin to induce apoptosis in human leukemia and Burkitt's lymphoma cells may be related to its ability to inhibit the synthesis of heat shock proteins (Wei et al., 1994).

[7] There is an inverse relationship between temperature and pH in all biological systems (Harguindey, 1982). Administering Coley's toxins is an unorthodox cancer treatment developed by Dr. William Coley (1862-1936) that employs a vaccine made of bacterial toxins. The vaccine has been thought to activate the immune system in cancer patients, in particular by inducing the production of tumor necrosis factor. The fever induced by Coley's toxins may also cause some degree of metabolic acidosis.

55

limits within which the blood pH must be maintained. Exceeding these limits can be fatal. Normally, pH is maintained between 7.35 and 7.45 units. This leaves little room for manipulation. Approximate critical values are less than 7.2 and greater than 7.6 units. This area deserves further study however, since even a slight decrease in pH may drastically affect tumor cell proliferation. An elevation of only 0.8 units can induce a 40-fold increase in glycolysis and an 18-fold increase in DNA synthesis in chick embryos (Harguindey, 1982), and the opposite effect could be expected with a decrease in pH.

7.4 HIGH pH TREATMENTS

Agents that markedly raise intercellular pH may also be useful as anticancer agents. Although a moderate elevation in intracellular pH stimulates cell proliferation, a large elevation causes necrosis. A small group of investigators have postulated that the element cesium may selectively raise the intracellular pH of tumor cells to the point of cell death.

Cesium belongs to the 1A group of alkali metals in the periodic chart. Other metals in this group include lithium, sodium, and potassium. The metals in this group possess similar biophysical properties, and in some cases, can substitute for each other in biochemical processes. In this respect, cesium most resembles and can substitute for potassium. Lithium most resembles and can substitute for sodium (El-Domeiri et al., 1981). Administration of these metals may alter the ionic composition of the intracellular environment.

Initial studies in 1927 (Ishiwara) on the anticancer effects of metals identified cesium, germanium, selenium, cerium, scandium, and ytterbium as potential antitumor agents. Studies by Burton and Marsh (1931) failed to identify a substantial antitumor effect in mammary adenocarcinoma-bearing mice, and research on cesium chloride ceased soon thereafter.[8] Interest was renewed in the late 1970s by Brewer and Passwater (1976) and Messiha et al. (1979). By this time it was known that tumor cells exhibit a preferential uptake of cesium relative to normal tissue and, for this reason, radioactive cesium had been investigated as a tumor-imaging agent.

Brewer (1984) developed what he called "high pH therapy," in which cesium chloride is administered to cancer patients in dosages of 6 grams per day (approximately 0.6 mEq/kg).[9] High doses of cesium reportedly, within a few days, raise intracellular pH in tumor cells to 8 units, a level incompatible with life. The elevated pH

also may buffer acids the tumor produces and reduce toxemia-induced pain. Doses below 3 grams per day may actually increase tumor growth by mildly elevating pH to a range more conducive to mitosis.

Cesium has been studied in a number of experimental tumor models. Cesium chloride at 3.0 mEq/kg reduced mortality by up to 50% in sarcoma-bearing mice (Messiha, 1984b).[10] Cesium chloride has also reduced tumor growth in sarcoma-bearing mice (El Domeiri et al., 1981), and colon 38-bearing mice (Tufte et al., 1984). Administration of cesium chloride inhibited tumor growth in mice bearing MT296 mammary adenocarcinomas and chemically-induced epithelial carcinomas (Pinsky and Bose, 1984).

Some of these authors suggest that the anticancer effects of cesium may be due to its imperfect substitution with potassium. A deficiency of intracellular potassium results in an increase of intracellular sodium through the actions of the sodium-potassium pump. As discussed in the preceding sections, activation of the sodium-potassium pump can activate the sodium-hydrogen exchanger and raise intracellular pH.

Studies using radioactive cesium in mice demonstrated a preferential uptake of cesium by MT296 tumors, and by tissues of the small intestine and kidneys, as compared to tissues with a naturally high affinity for cesium chloride, such as skeletal muscle (Pinsky and Bose, 1984).

In contrast to the above studies, administration of 3.7 to 8.0 mEq/kg of cesium chloride to Novikoff hepatoma-bearing rats increased mortality in test animals when 1.0 ml of the tumor inoculant was injected.[11] However, mortality decreased when 2.0 ml of the inoculant was injected (Messiha and Stocco, 1984). This protective effect may be due, in part, to the potassium content of the inoculant, since an experiment using potassium, rather than cesium chloride, as the test agent also reduced mortality. Other ratios of cesium chloride and potassium increased mortality, suggesting that the balance between cesium chloride and potassium is critical to optimize the antitumor effect.

Cesium chloride was administered to 50 patients with preterminal neoplastic disease, 47 of whom had generalized metastases (Sartori, 1984). These 47 patients received treatment with surgery, radiotherapy, and/or chemotherapy prior to cesium chloride treatment. Patients received 6 to 9 grams of cesium chloride orally per day, along with a variety of supportive compounds including zinc, selenium, vitamin A, vitamin C, and

---

[8] Dosages used in Burton's experiments were very low at 0.05 mg cesium chloride daily (approximately 0.02 mEq/kg).

[9] One mEq of cesium is equal to 133 mg of cesium.

[10] Based on metabolic mass extrapolation, this represents a human dose of approximately 0.3 mEq/kg.

[11] Based on metabolic mass extrapolation, this represents a human dose of approximately 0.8 to 1.7 mEq/kg.

DMSO. Results indicated that half of the patients with cancers of the breast, colon, prostate, pancreas, and lung survived at least one year (the length of the study). Patients with liver cancer and lymphoma had lower survival rates. Many patients reportedly experienced marked symptomatic improvement. Approximately half of those patients who died did so within the first 14 days of the trial, suggesting that the treatment provided a protective effect only after two weeks of administration. On the other hand, this observation could also suggest that cesium chloride is toxic to some patients and hastens their death. The authors reported that cesium chloride also eliminated pain in all patients within three days of treatment. This would seem unlikely, since even morphine does not relieve pain in every patient.

Cesium chloride is a common off-the-shelf chemical. Known side effects of cesium chloride treatment include nausea and diarrhea, which proper dosing can control to some extent. Cesium is only moderately toxic, producing CNS symptoms, such as initial antidepressant activity followed by suppression of locomotor activity (Pinsky and Bose, 1984). Cesium chloride may stimulate preganglionic cholinergic nerve fibers (those liberating acetylcholine) as evidenced by a transient rise in blood pressure and autonomic changes such as salivation, pi-loerection (hair standing on end), urination, and diarrhea. Based on radioisotope studies, the half-life of cesium in humans is 65 to 84 days. The primary toxicological concerns are CNS and renal involvement (Messiha, 1994, personal communication). In addition, cesium could saturate the potassium pool, leading to potassium deficiency and cardiotoxicity.

7.5 SUMMARY

Both intracellular and extracellular tumor pH may play significant roles in determining proliferation rates of tumor cells. The intracellular pH is controlled by the sodium-hydrogen exchanger, which derives its energy from the sodium-potassium pump. The sodium-hydrogen exchanger may be involved in the stimulation of proliferation caused by a variety of growth factors and hormones. Mild elevations in pH stimulate cell proliferation, and extreme elevations, or reductions, inhibit proliferation. Hyperthermia, hyperglycemia, and metabolic acidosis may all reduce pH to a range that inhibits proliferation. Treatment with cesium chloride may increase pH to a range that inhibits proliferation.

8

THE IMMUNE SYSTEM

The immune system is a complex organization of white blood cells, antibodies, and humoral factors that distinguish and protect the self from the nonself. Many investigators believe that the immune system plays a key role in preventing the progression of new cancers, a concept known as "immune surveillance." It also may limit the progression of established tumors. This chapter discusses the mechanics of immunity and its role in cancer treatment.

8.1 OVERVIEW OF THE IMMUNE SYSTEM

Without an immune system we would quickly fall prey to the plethora of viruses, bacteria, and parasites that live within and around us. In its widest sense, the immune system is a multilayered defense system that includes physical barriers, such as the skin and the lining of the gastrointestinal tract; chemical barriers, such as stomach acid; microbial barriers, such as beneficial intestinal microflora; and the immune system proper (white blood cells, antibodies, and the humoral factors, called cytokines, that affect them).[1] White blood cells (leukocytes) and red blood cells (erythrocytes) are derived from pluripotent stem cells in the bone marrow as shown in Figure 8.1. After their formation, leukocytes migrate through the blood and lymph to congregate in lymphoid tissues (such as the spleen, lymph nodes, and tonsils) and in other tissues, where they reside until activated by antigen or by other means.[2] Figure 8.1 also shows the cytokines that stimulate maturation of blood cells.

The human immune system functions by two separate, but interconnected, branches: humoral immunity and cell-mediated, or cellular, immunity. These are discussed individually below.

8.1.1 Humoral Immunity

Humoral immunity relies primarily upon the production of antibodies by white blood cells known as B lymphocytes.[3] In response to foreign antigens, B lymphocytes divide and differentiate into either plasma cells, which produce antibodies, or memory B cells (see Figure 8.2). Memory B cells remember the antigen that originally stimulated the parent B cell, and facilitate the rapid production of antibodies if the antigen is encountered in the future. Vaccines prevent infection by stimulating the production of memory B cells that recognize specific antigens.

After binding to antigens, antibodies destroy, incapacitate, or eliminate antigens by one or more of five mechanisms:

---

[1] Cytokines are chemicals that regulate cellular growth and function. When they are secreted by lymphocytes (or monocytes) and regulate the growth of other lymphocytes, they are called lymphokines. For example, interleukin-2 is a type of lymphokine.

[2] Antigens are endogenous or exogenous substances that are alien to the self and induce the formation of antigen-specific antibodies. They can be soluble proteins, or structures on foreign or infected cells. Antibodies are soluble proteins produced by B lymphocytes. Antibodies bind to specific antigens.

[3] Humoral immunity (Latin *humor*, fluid) derives its name from its dependence on the blood-borne factors (antibodies) that mediate it. B lymphocytes obtain their name from the bursa of Fabricius, a structure in birds in which B lymphocytes mature. A similar structure in humans has not been identified, but the fetal liver is presumed to serve the same function.

FIGURE 8.1. ORIGIN OF BLOOD CELLS

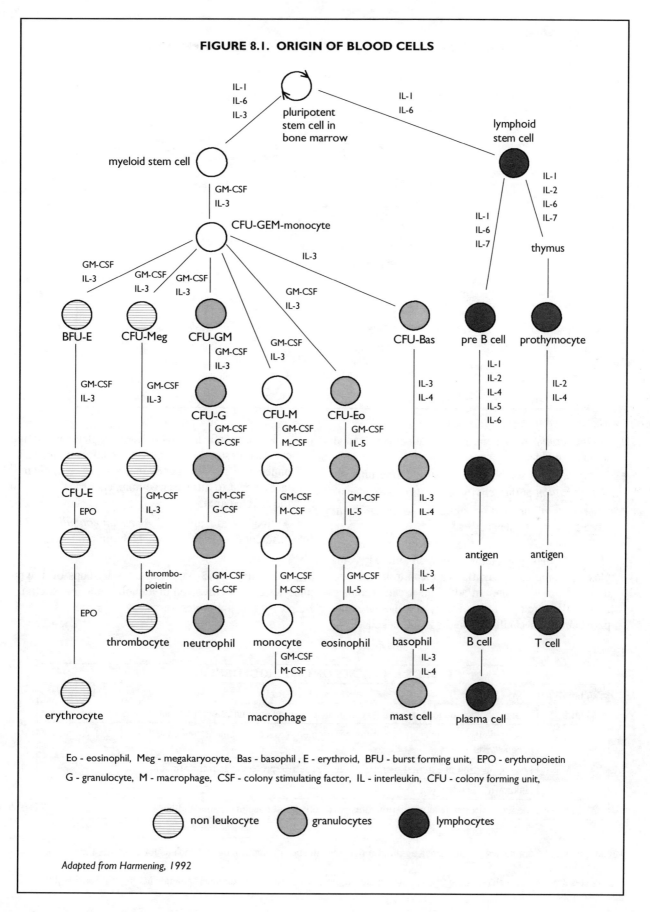

Eo - eosinophil, Meg - megakaryocyte, Bas - basophil , E - erythroid, BFU - burst forming unit, EPO - erythropoietin

G - granulocyte, M - macrophage, CSF - colony stimulating factor, IL - interleukin, CFU - colony forming unit,

non leukocyte   granulocytes   lymphocytes

Adapted from Harmening, 1992

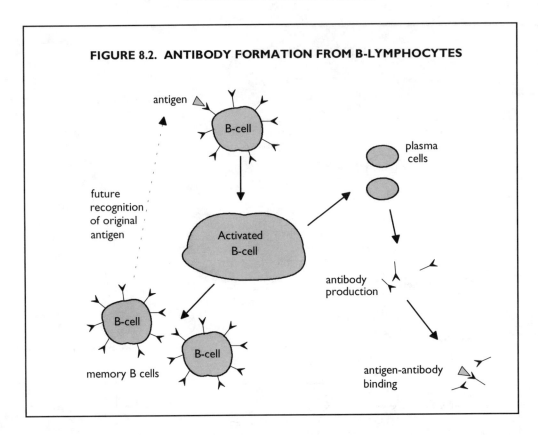

FIGURE 8.2. ANTIBODY FORMATION FROM B-LYMPHOCYTES

- *Agglutination,* or clumping of antibodies around soluble antigens.[4]
- *Precipitation* of soluble antigens from the serum.
- *Neutralization* of the activity or motility of antigens.
- *Opsonization,* or coating antigens to make them more attractive to phagocytes.[5]
- *Complement-fixation,* or the sequential attachment of specific plasma proteins to antigen-antibody complexes. Complement-fixation can lead to neutralization and opsonization. In addition, it can stimulate mast cells to release histamine, which increases the permeability of capillaries and assists leukocytes in

penetrating affected tissues. Complement-fixation can also destroy a foreign cell or microorganism by puncturing its cell membrane, and act as a chemotactic agent to attract large numbers of leukocytes to the affected area.

Antibodies are also called *immunoglobulins.* The five different classes of immunoglobulin are listed in Table 8.1.

In addition to B lymphocytes, subgroups of T lymphocytes are also involved in humoral immune reactions. Helper T lymphocytes assist the switching of B

TABLE 8.1. CLASSES OF IMMUNOGLOBULIN	
CLASS	FUNCTION
IgM	First antibody produced in a primary immune response; stimulates complement system
IgG	Produced after IgM in a primary immune response; fixes complement, and coats bacteria to facilitate phagocytosis
IgA	Local protection in external secretions, such as saliva; protects gastrointestinal system
IgD	Unknown function
IgE	Mediates allergic reactions; stimulates mast cells to produce histamine and heparin

---

[4] Blood typing is accomplished by measuring agglutinin reactions to specific agglutinogens, such as for example, the Rh agglutinogen.

[5] Phagocytes are immune cells that ingest foreign particulates or debris. They include macrophages, neutrophils, eosinophils, and basophils.

lymphocytes into plasma cells, thereby enhancing antibody production.

8.1.2 Cellular Immunity

Cellular immunity is the branch of the immune system most responsible for destruction of infected cells and tumor cells. Unlike humoral immunity, cellular immunity does not depend on an antibody response to antigens. Rather, antigen recognition is carried out directly by immune cells, called T lymphocytes, or antigen recognition is absent, as is the case with macrophages and natural killer cells. T lymphocytes, macrophages, and natural killer cells are discussed individually below.

T Lymphocytes

Although T lymphocytes do recognize antigens, the method of recognition is dramatically different than that of antibodies.[6] Whereas antibodies bind directly to soluble antigens, T lymphocytes only react to antigens when they are "presented" to the T lymphocyte in the context of *histocompatibility antigens* present on the surface of cells. Histocompatibility antigens are normal surface proteins of all nucleated cells, and are unique to each individual. As such, histocompatibility antigens provide a marker by which the immune system can distinguish self from nonself.[7] The expression of histocompatibility antigens responsible for the strongest identification of self (or the strongest rejection of nonself) is controlled by localized groups of genes in the chromosomes called the *major histocompatibility complex* (MHC).[8] Foreign cells can be identified by foreign MHC products (as is the case

with tissue transplants) and altered cells can be identified by foreign antigens complexed with self MHC products (as is the case with infected cells). Due to their dependence on MHC products, T lymphocytes are said to be MHC-restricted. Some tumor cells may not express self MHC products (the antigens may be absent), and failure of the immune system to recognize these cells may allow cancers to progress.

T lymphocytes can be divided into two subpopulations, helper T cells and cytotoxic (killer) T cells, based on their expression of surface proteins and their function. In recent years, molecular biology has developed to the point where distinct configurations of cell surface proteins can be identified. These configurations, called *cluster designations,* allow greater discrimination of different cell types.

Cluster designations for various leukocytes are listed in Table 8.2. Frequently, a leukocyte is referred to by its cluster designations. For example, a mature T lymphocyte may be referred to as a CD3 cell. Some groupings of cluster designations are found only in pathologies. For example, $CD2^+CD7^+$ are found only on leukemic T lymphocytes.

Helper T cells, which express $CD4^+$, derive their name from their ability help an immune response by stimulating B lymphocytes to produce antibodies and by stimulating immune reactions of other lymphocytes. Cytotoxic T cells, which express $CD8^+$, derive their name from their ability to destroy target cells. They can also suppress the immune response of other lymphocytes. However, the correlations between cluster designation and cell function are not absolute. A stronger correlation exists between cluster designation and the ability of

TABLE 8.2. PARTIAL LISTING OF CLUSTER DESIGNATIONS			
CD	**CELL TYPE IDENTIFIED**	**CD**	**CELL TYPE IDENTIFIED**
CD3	Mature T lymphocytes	CD13	Myeloid and monocytic cells
$CD3^+DR^+$	Activated T lymphocytes	CD14	Monocytes
CD4	Helper/inducer T lymphocytes	CD19	B lymphocytes
$CD4^+29^+$	CD4 inducer of activation	$CD5^+19^+$	Chronic B lymphocytic leukemia
$CD4^+45^+$	CD4 inducer of suppression	$CD3^-16^+56^+$	Natural killer cells
CD8	Cytotoxic/suppressor T lymphocytes	CD33	Acute myelogenous leukemia and most monocytes
$CD8^+DR^+$	Activated CD8 T lymphocytes	CD34	Hematopoietic stem cells
$CD8^+57^+$	Activated CD8 T lymphocytes	$CD2^+CD7^+$	Acute T-lymphocyte leukemias

---

[6] T lymphocytes derive their name from the thymus gland. They arise from stem cells in the bone marrow, and migrate to the thymus gland, which programs them to perform their individual functions.

[7] Rejection of organ transplants by the immune system is largely due to recognition of foreign histocompatibility antigens. Autoimmune diseases can develop when self-histocompatibility antigens are not recognized.

[8] In humans, the MHC was identified via studies on leukocyte antigens and is termed the human leukocyte antigen (HLA) complex.

helper and cytotoxic T cells to recognize different classes of MHC products (reviewed by Tannock and Hill, 1992:238-9).

There are two classes of MHC products that are of particular importance here. Class I products are proteins that are expressed on the surface of all cells. Class II products are proteins expressed primarily on some active immune cells.[9]

Grooves on the top of MHC class I molecules bind with a large number of short peptides that have similar structure. When the MHC molecule is being formed within the cell, it samples, and when possible binds to, peptides being produced within the cytoplasm. The MHC molecule-peptide complex is then transported to the surface, and presents the peptide for possible recognition by class I-restricted T cells. Most CD8+ cells recognize class I MHC products, and their bias toward cytotoxic/suppressor function appears to be an indirect consequence of class I-restriction.

In contrast, class II MHC molecules sample and bind to peptides that derive from extracellular proteins that have been taken up by cellular vesicles and degraded. These MHC molecule-peptide complexes are again transported to the cell surface and may be recognized by T cells. Most CD4+ cells recognize class II MHC products, and their bias toward helper function appears to be an indirect consequence of class II-restriction.

Macrophages, B-cells, dendritic cells, and, in some cases, epithelial cells can all express class II MHC products. These cells endocytose soluble antigens and the degradation products of these antigens can be brought back to the cell surface complexed to MHC products. CD4+ (helper) T cells may recognize these complexes and be stimulated to produce cytokines that assist the function of these cells.

In a similar fashion, foreign and altered cells may produce foreign peptides within their cytoplasm, and these peptides can be brought to the cell surface complexed to class II MHC products. CD8+ (cytotoxic/suppressor) T cells may recognize these complexes and be stimulated to destroy these cells by secreting toxic substances, such as tumor necrosis factor. They may also be stimulated to produce certain cytokines, or otherwise transmit signals, that inhibit aspects of the immune system. The mechanisms that lead to T cell-induced immunosuppression are poorly understood. In some cases, suppression may function as a negative feedback mechanism, whereby second or third generation T cells inhibit the function of first generation cells. This may serve to prevent excessive immune activity. Under certain conditions, the immunosuppression induced by T cells can be extensive.

Natural Killer Cells

The second group of cells responsible for cellular immunity are natural killer (NK) cells.[10] NK cells are non-T non-B lymphocytes that bind to a target and secrete cytotoxic molecules. NK cells and monocyte-macrophages provide the host with natural immunity, that is, immunity that does not depend on prior sensitization. The mechanism NK cells use to recognize nonself is poorly understood. They do not recognize antigens and do not depend on MHC product recognition, but may recognize an absence of MHC products.

In contrast to cytotoxic T lymphocytes, NK cells also express a surface receptor for immunoglobulin (FcR). Because of this, they assist in antibody-dependent cellular cytotoxicity (ADCC). Antibody-dependent cellular cytotoxicity refers to recognition of the antibody portion of an antigen-antibody complex (often an IgG complex) by a macrophage or NK cell, which is then triggered to destroy the antigen. The primary role for antibodies in tumor destruction appears to be through ADCC, rather than through humoral immune mechanisms.

NK cells were discovered in the mid-1970s, and constitute up to 15% of the total lymphocyte population in healthy subjects. They are capable of killing a broad range of human solid tumor, leukemic, and virus-infected cells. Depressed NK cell activity and depressed NK cell populations may be associated with the development and progression of cancer, AIDS, chronic fatigue syndrome, psychiatric depression, various immunodeficiency syndromes, and certain autoimmune diseases.

NK cells appear to present the first line of defense against metastatic spread of tumors. In animal experiments, low NK cell populations were associated with greater survival of intravenously injected tumor cells and with increased development of lung metastasis. Correction of the NK cell population restored resistance. In human studies, patients with solid tumors commonly have diminished NK cell activity, but the association between low NK cell activity and metastatic spread is not as strong as in animals.

NK cell activity is correlated with disease status in patients with hematologic malignancies, such as leukemias and lymphomas. In some studies on patients with leukemia, a sudden and maintained decrease in NK cell activity was reported nearly always to precede relapse, even if the patient was in complete remission.

---

[9] In humans, there are three different class I gene loci (HLA-A, HLA-B, and HLA-C), and three different class II products (HLA-DP, HLA-DQ, and HLA-DR). Hence the cluster designations CD8+DR+, CD3+DR+, and so on.

[10] Unless specified, the source for this section is a review by Whiteside and Herberman (1989).

Furthermore, significant decreases in NK cell activity were found only in those patients whose leukemia subsequently relapsed. Measurement of NK cell activity may thus provide a useful tool for monitoring clinical status in patients with leukemia. For similar reasons, measuring NK cell activity may also be useful in patients with large cell lymphoma (the type of lymphoma most associated with immunosuppression), and also in patients with head and neck cancer.

NK cell activity varies between normal individuals, and also between laboratories according to the testing procedures used. In healthy individuals, long-term NK cell activity is relatively constant, although daily levels follow a circadian rhythm, with maximum activity early in the day.[11] Exercise may cause short-term levels to vary. The variation of NK cell activity between individuals is due, in part, to differences in age, sex, and general health factors. Although there is a correlation between the population of NK cells and their activity level, the relationship is not very strong. NK cells vary in their active status, and a population count will not substitute for an activity measurement.

NK cell activity appears to be a well-regulated system, subject to both inhibitory and excitatory controls. In-vitro studies show that the cytokines interferon and interleukin-2 stimulate activity, while prostaglandins and other soluble factors inhibit activity. Prostaglandins PGE_1, PGE_2, PGA_1, and PGA_2 all may inhibit NK cell activity (Herberman and Santoni, 1982), as may suppressor T cells. The exact regulation of NK cell activity in vivo has yet to be determined.

Monocyte-Macrophages

The last group of cells responsible for cellular immunity are monocyte-macrophages. Like lymphocytes, monocytes reside in lymphoid tissues and migrate to the site of invasion when needed. Once stimulated, they are called macrophages. Like NK cells, macrophages do not recognize antigens. In addition, they do not recognize MHC products. Their activation mechanisms are poorly understood, but may involve receptors for certain carbohydrates, complement, and immunoglobulin. As such, they mediate antibody-dependent cellular cytotoxicity. Bacterial products, such as lipopolysaccharides (LPS), are among the most potent activators. They can also be activated by contact with tumor cells. Macrophages destroy foreign substances by phagocytosis or by secretion of certain cytokines, such as tumor necrosis factor (TNF), proteases, hydrogen peroxide, or lysosomal enzymes.

Macrophages may play a primary role in anticancer immunity. Supportive evidence includes the following (Holleb et al., 1991):

- Macrophages accumulate in considerable numbers within a variety of tumors.
- Macrophages lyse or inhibit the growth of a wide variety of transformed cells in vitro.
- Treatments that suppress the function of macrophages have been associated with increased tumor incidence and increased metastasis.
- Injection of activated macrophages into tumor-bearing animals inhibits metastatic spread of some tumor cell lines.
- Some carcinogens depress the reticuloendothelial system (the system of cells, including macrophages, which have the power to phagocytose).
- Stimulation of macrophage activity has been associated with decreased tumor growth or decreased tumor incidence in animals.

8.1.3 Granulocytes

In addition to the lymphocytes and macrophages discussed in the preceding sections, there is another group of leukocytes called granulocytes. Granulocytes consist of neutrophils, eosinophils, and basophils. Like macrophages, neutrophils are phagocytic in nature. They ingest foreign objects and are the most active leukocyte in response to bacteria. They also ingest dead matter. Eosinophils aid in the destruction of parasites and are present in high numbers during allergic reactions. Basophils play a key role in allergic responses in that they form into mast cells, which can secrete histamine, serotonin, and heparin.

8.2 IMMUNITY AND CANCER

8.2.1 Immune Surveillance

The immune system appears to play a critical role in preventing tumor development by searching out and destroying newly transformed cells. This concept, known as immune surveillance, was first proposed by Ehrlich in 1909, and is supported by the following observations that associate immune depression with increased cancer risk (Penn, 1991):

- Children with immunodeficiency diseases have increased rates of lymphoma, leukemia, and Hodgkin's disease.

---

[11] Although chronobiologic immune therapy has received little attention, theoretically, morning administration of immunostimulants may produce optimal stimulation of NK cell activity. Morning administration may also be optimal for agents that stimulate hemopoietic cells.

- High rates of Kaposi's sarcoma and lymphoma are seen in patients with immunosuppression caused by the human immunodeficiency virus (HIV).

- In organ-transplant patients who receive immuno-suppressive drugs, the incidence of malignancies increases threefold. Commonly, these malignancies include cancers of the skin, lips, vulva, anus, liver, and lymphoma and Kaposi's sarcoma.

- Cancer risk increases with the duration of immuno-suppressive treatment. In a study of heart transplant patients, cancer incidence increased 3-fold after one year of immunosuppressive treatment, and 26-fold after five years. In some patients, regression of Kaposi's sarcoma and lymphoma was observed after cessation of the immunosuppressive therapy.

- Patients with autoimmune diseases treated with im-munosuppressive therapy show increased incidence of acute leukemia, lymphoma, liver cancer, bladder cancer, and skin cancer.

- Secondary tumors are common in cancer patients who receive immunosuppressive chemotherapy treatment. These may include acute leukemias, lymphoma, and bladder cancers. However, in many cases this may be more related to chemotherapy-induced DNA damage than to immunosuppression.

Immunosuppressed patients appear to have a dispro-portionately high incidence of certain malignancies, such as Kaposi's sarcoma, lymphoma, and acute leukemia. Relatively few of the more common malignancies, such as breast and lung cancer, are seen. The preferential de-velopment of these tumors over other types may be due to the longer latency period (15 to 20 years or more) of many common tumors. Immunosuppressed patients may simply die of faster-developing tumors, or infections, be-fore other slow-growing tumors develop.

An alternate explanation for this disproportion is that cancers commonly associated with immunosup-pressed states may be virally induced. In this theory, rather than failing to destroy the tumor cells, the immune system fails to destroy viruses that cause cancers. A number of human viruses are suspected or known to cause cancer. These include:

- Epstein-Barr virus (EBV), which is associated with nasopharyngeal cancer.

- Human T-cell leukemia virus type I (HTLV-I), which causes adult T-cell leukemia.

- Hepatitis B virus (HBV), which is associated with hepatoma.

- Human papilloma virus (HPV), which probably causes cervical cancer.

- A new herpes virus, which is associated with Ka-posi's sarcoma.

The short induction time of Kaposi's sarcoma and lymphoma in immunosuppressed patients may reflect a viral origin. In organ transplant patients, Kaposi's sar-coma appears, on average, within 20 months, and lym-phoma appears, on average, within 34 months.

In addition to the immune system's postulated role in preventing cancer, the immune system may also influ-ence the course of the disease once it has developed. This "antitumor immunity" may be responsible for a number of unusual observations, such as spontaneous re-gressions, cures after incomplete removal of primary le-sions, sudden development of metastasis years after suc-cessful treatment, and regression of metastasis after local treatment of the primary tumor.

Antitumor immunity may involve both the humoral and cellular branches of the immune system. Antibodies against the patient's own (autologous) tumor have been identified in the sera of some patients with soft-tissue sarcoma, malignant melanoma, ovarian carcinoma, and lung cancer. Cellular cytotoxicity to autologous tumors has also been demonstrated in patients with melanoma (reviewed by Calabresi and Schein, 1993:325-6). The degree to which the immune system is capable of destroy-ing established cancers has not been established. In gen-eral, the immune system may be more effective against small tumors. The success of the immune system is also hampered by the ability of tumors to evade immunologic reactions.

8.2.2 Immunologic Suppression by Tumors

The immune system must recognize a tumor cell as foreign before it can destroy it. The ability of the im-mune system to recognize a foreign substance is called the *antigenicity* of the substance. However, recognition of a foreign body does not necessarily ensure that an im-mune reaction will take place. The ability of a foreign substance to evoke an immunologic reaction in a host is called its *immunogenicity*. Most human tumor cells ap-pear to be strongly antigenic but only weakly immuno-genic. Therefore, rejection of the tumor by the host is difficult. Recent investigations have shown that a few cancers, such as melanoma, are more strongly immuno-genic, but even these escape destruction by the immune system.

Immune evasion occurs through one or more of the following mechanisms (reviewed by Holland et al., 1993:187; reviewed by Calabresi and Schein, 1993:331):

- *Repression of antigen expression:* Tumor cells may down-regulate the expression of genes that control the production of tumor rejection antigens. Due to the heterogeneity of cells within a tumor, antigenic

TABLE 8.3. IMMUNOSUPPRESSION FROM VARIOUS CANCERS	
IMMUNOLOGICAL DEFECT	**CANCER**
B lymphocyte	Chronic lymphocytic leukemia
	Multiple myeloma
	Ovarian carcinoma
T lymphocyte	Hodgkin's disease
	Disseminated carcinomas
	Kaposi's sarcoma/AIDS
Monocyte	Carcinomas and sarcomas
	Hodgkin's disease
Granulocyte	Acute lymphoblastic leukemia
	Acute myeloid leukemia
	Chronic myelogenous leukemia
	Multiple myeloma
Source: Holland et al., 1993:188	

TABLE 8.4. MYELOSUPPRESSIVE EFFECTS OF COMMON CHEMOTHERAPY AGENTS	
IMMUNOLOGICAL EFFECT	**AGENT**
Strongly myelosuppressive	Cyclophosphamide, nitrosoureas (e.g. BCNU)
	6-Mercaptopurine, azathioprine
	5-Fluorouracil, cytosine arabinoside
	Methotrexate
	Vinblastine
	Daunorubicin, doxorubicin
	Glucocorticoids
Weakly myelosuppressive	Bleomycin, mithramycin, vincristine
	Busulfan, dacarbazine (DTIC)
Note: Some agents, such as doxorubicin, may be immuno-stimulating at certain schedules. *Modified from Calabresi and Schein, 1993:342*	

expression may vary between subpopulations. Under attack by the immune system, nonantigenic subpopulations may exhibit increased survival and, therefore, may become the dominant cell type. This is called *clonal selection.* Tumor cells can also fail to express MHC products, which are required to present tumor antigens to T lymphocytes.

- *Antigenic modulation:* Antigenic modulation occurs when the tumor cell loses its surface antigens upon exposure to specific antibodies. The antigen-free cell thus escapes immune recognition.

- *Production of blocking factors:* Cancer patients are frequently immunosuppressed, and this suppression can sometimes be corrected by removing the bulk of the tumor. One mechanism for this suppression is thought to be the excessive shedding of soluble antigens into the blood by tumors. The shed antigens can combine with antibodies to form antigen-antibody complexes, thereby competitively inhibiting binding to tumor antigens.

- *Production of prostaglandins:* Macrophages are present in high numbers within tumors and may cause immunosuppression by producing prostaglandins such as PGE_2.

- *Production of cytokines:* Tumor cells may produce a variety of cytokines, such as transforming growth factor-beta and interleukin-10, that may suppress immune reactions.

Patients with advanced cancers of any type frequently exhibit nonspecific defects in both humoral and cellular immunity. Table 8.3 lists immunological defects associated with various cancers. In general, immunocompetence is reduced by poor nutritional status and high tumor burdens. Immunosuppression may be due to the mechanisms discussed above, or may be due to indirect effects of the cancer, such as cachexia or nutritional impairment secondary to gastrointestinal obstruction.[12]

Chemotherapy, radiotherapy, or surgery may also cause myelosuppression and/or immunosuppression. Myelosuppression refers specifically to a reduction of the white blood cell count and is usually associated with increased bacterial infections. Immunosuppression, on the other hand, normally refers to an inhibition of lymphocyte and possibly monocyte function, and is associated with increased viral infections and infections by other opportunistic pathogens. Surgery may produce a transient depression of NK cells and T- and B-lymphocyte levels; both usually recover within one month. Chemotherapy may produce both myelosuppression and immunosuppression. However, immunosuppression is usually more transient and less profound. Table 8.4 lists the degree of myelosuppression by common cytotoxic chemotherapy drugs.

8.2.3 Tumor-associated Antigens

Investigators have been searching for tumor-specific antigens (TSAs) to use as targets for immune manipulation. TSAs have been known for quite some time in mouse tumors, but only recently have they been identified

---

[12] Cachexia is a syndrome of tissue-wasting that is common in patients with certain cancers. It is associated with abnormalities in fat, protein, and carbohydrate metabolism.

TABLE 8.5. COMMON TUMOR MARKERS

TYPE	MARKER	CANCER
Tumor-associated antigens	CA-125 antigen (CA-125)	Ovarian
	CA-19-9 monoclonal antibody (CA19-9)	Colon, stomach, pancreatic
	Prostate-specific antigen (PSA)	Prostate
Hormones	Human chorionic gonadotropin (HCG)	Tumors of the placenta
Enzymes	Acid phosphatase	Prostate
	Neuron specific enolase (NSE)	Tumors of the central nervous system
	Galactosyl transferase II	Colon, pancreatic, and other gastrointestinal tumors
Immunoglobulins	Various immunoglobulins	Myeloma
Oncofetal antigens	Alpha-fetoprotein (AFP)	Hepatoma (also for diagnosis/screening), testicular
	Carcinoembryonic antigen (CEA)	Colon, breast, lung, pancreas, stomach, ovarian
Other	Polyamines	Leukemia, lymphoma, solid tumors
	Beta$_2$-microglobulin	Lymphoma, myeloma

Sources: Calabresi and Schein, 1993:163-70; Tannock and Hill, 1992:197

in human tumors. Tumor-associated antigens (TAAs) are antigens that are preferentially expressed on tumor cells, but may also be expressed on normal cells. TAAs exist on human cancer cells, and a number of TAAs, such as CA-125 antigen, are used as tumor markers in monitoring the treatment of various cancers. Some common tumor markers are listed in Table 8.5.

8.3 CANCER IMMUNOTHERAPY

The majority of human cancers exhibit low immunogenicity, probably due to one or more of the immune-evading mechanisms described previously. However, this does not mean that immunotherapy is necessarily ineffective against them. Past clinical failures with immunotherapy may be due to suboptimal methods of use (Hanna et al., 1991). Tumor antigens may stimulate potent responses when the appropriate adjuvants are administered. In experiments with the weakly immunogenic L-10 hepatocarcinoma in guinea pigs, a therapeutic immune response could be induced by administration of any one of several adjuvants (Hanna et al., 1991). However, even with appropriate adjuvants, it is expected that immunotherapy in humans will be most effective in patients with a relatively healthy immune system and a low tumor burden, i.e., an early stage of malignancy. Immunotherapy can be divided into two categories: active and passive. Each of these is discussed separately below.

8.3.1 Active Immunotherapy

Active immunotherapy refers to methods that directly stimulate an immune response by the host. In cancer therapy, this is often accomplished through immunization with nonviable tumor cells, or by injection of antigens that are not tumor-specific, such as microbial agents. Active immunotherapy has resulted in transient regression of some human tumors such as carcinoma of the kidney, melanoma, and ovarian cancer (reviewed by Tannock and Hill, 1992:245 and Calabresi and Schein, 1993:334). However, its clinical role may be limited, since prior to therapy, the patient's immune system has had ample time to recognize and react to tumor antigens. Tumor-induced immunosuppression (such as by blocking agents) must be removed or reduced for active immunization to be successful. The use of various active immunotherapy agents has had limited success in treating patients with osteosarcoma, leukemia, lymphoma, melanoma, and lung, renal cell, bladder, ovarian, colon, and breast cancer (Hoover and Hanna, 1991; Hersh and Taylor, 1991). Renal cell carcinoma and melanoma appeared to exhibit the greatest immunogenicity and may respond better to active immunotherapy than other cancers.

8.3.2 Passive Immunotherapy

Passive immunotherapy refers to administration of agents that passively increase immune activity, rather than directly stimulating an immune response in the host. Passive immunotherapy includes the administration of serum or immune cells from immunized animals, administration of monoclonal antibodies, and administration of cloned immune cells and cytokines.

Injection of heterologous serum or immune cells has not been successful. Reasons for the lack of success include the minor role of antibodies in tumor rejection, the lack of tumor specificity of injected antibodies, and the foreign nature of the serum or cells, which itself elicits a rejection reaction. Injection of monoclonal antibodies has also met with limited success for similar reasons, and because of the heterogeneity of antigen expression on tumor cells (Tannock and Hill, 1992:245-52).

Passive immunotherapy with cloned immune cells and cytokines may be more successful. Two types of clones have been investigated: tumor-infiltrating lymphocytes (TIL) and lymphokine-activated killer (LAK) cells. TIL therapy involves the removal of T lymphocytes from a tumor, and their expansion and administration. TIL therapy has had some success against melanoma. LAK cell therapy involves the removal of nontumor lymphocytes, and their expansion, activation, and administration. LAK cells act similar to, but are more active than, NK cells.

The expansion of TIL and LAK cells in culture is made possible by the administration of interleukin-2 (IL-2). High concentrations of IL-2 are also used to activate LAK cells. Interleukin-2, along with interferons, colony stimulating factors, tumor necrosis factor, and other interleukins belong to a group of humoral factors known as biological response modifiers (BRMs) (see Table 8.6).[13] A number of BRMs have been studied as individual agents in clinical trials. Additional discussion of LAK cells, IL-2, interferons, colony stimulating factors and IL-3 is provided below.

IL-2 and LAK Cells

A summary of multiple trials using IL-2 alone or in combination with LAK cells is presented in Table 8.7. The average total response rate for the studies shown in the table is 23%, and the majority of these responses were partial. (Actual average response rates may be lower, since trials with a zero response rate were not included in Table 8.7.) The limited clinical gains occurred in spite of the fact that immune function, such as measured by NK cell activity, was stimulated in the majority of patients (Koretz et al., 1991; Weiss et al., 1992). This suggests that new approaches to immunotherapy are needed, and that it may be necessary to combine immunotherapy with other anticancer therapies to obtain optimal clinical results.

Although IL-2 is a naturally occurring substance in the body, its use at high concentrations produces serious, sometimes life-threatening, adverse effects (see Table 8.6). These effects are apparently due, in part, to increases in capillary permeability. However, newer approaches, employing lower doses of IL-2 given intravenously or subcutaneously, may circumvent some of these problems.

Interferons

Interferons (IFNs) have been the most extensively studied cytokines in cancer treatment. Three types of interferon have been identified: IFN-alpha, produced by leukocytes; IFN-beta, produced by fibroblasts; and IFN-gamma, produced by T lymphocytes.

As a group, interferons affect a wide array of immunological functions. They mediate antiviral and antimicrobial activity, stimulate or inhibit leukocyte proliferation, suppress oncogenes, enhance tumor-associated antigen expression, suppress angiogenesis, and augment the activity of NK cells, T lymphocytes, and macrophages. Interferons and tumor necrosis factor increase the catabolism of body fat stores, possibly to release energy reserves from fat cells for the immune system to use. As such, they play a role in the development of cachexia.

IFN-alpha is effective against a number of lymphoreticular neoplasms, such as hairy cell leukemia (85% response), chronic myelogenous leukemia (75% response), and nodular lymphoma (45% response) (reviewed by Holland et al., 1993:190). Injections are usually administered daily for prolonged periods. IFN-alpha is ineffective against chronic lymphocytic leukemia and multiple myeloma, but in multiple myeloma, administration of IFN-alpha may prolong the duration of a chemotherapy-induced remission. Solid tumors respond less favorably to IFN-alpha therapy. Responses have been observed in Kaposi's sarcoma (33%), glioblastoma (40%), mid-gut carcinoids (20%), melanoma (15%), and renal cell carcinoma (15%). Intralesional and regional therapies, as opposed to systemic therapy, have been used with some success against basal cell (75% response), bladder (40% response), and ovarian carcinomas (45% response).

Although life-threatening complications are rare from IFN administration, quality of life is commonly impaired due to fever, chills, headache, fatigue, anorexia, nausea, and other side effects. Some of these side effects may be due to increased secretion of tumor necrosis factor by stimulated macrophages.

Colony Stimulating Factors and IL-3

The hemopoietic growth factors granulocyte macrophage-colony stimulating factor (GM-CSF), granulocyte-colony stimulating factor (G-CSF), and IL-3 demonstrate significant clinical potential in stimulating

---

[13] Additional BRMs exist besides those listed in Table 8.6 but will not be discussed further here. These include IL-10 through IL-15, erythropoietin, and thrombopoietin.

TABLE 8.6. PROPERTIES OF SOME BIOLOGIC RESPONSE MODIFIERS

CYTOKINES	ORIGIN	INDUCING STIMULI	ACTIONS
Interleukin-1 (IL-1)	○ Monocytes ○ NK cells ○ B cells ○ T cells ○ Endothelial cells	○ Microorganisms ○ Antigens ○ Inflammatory agents ○ Plant lectins ○ Lymphokines ○ Certain chemicals	○ Stimulates lymphokine release from activated T cells, differentiation of activated B cells (with IL-6), NK cell activity, and proliferation of activated B cells (with IL-5). ○ Stimulates growth of fibroblasts, synovial cells, and endothelial cells. ○ Stimulates release of PGE$_2$ and collagenase. ○ Contributes to cachexia. ○ Stimulates stem cells to respond to other growth factors. ○ In large doses, rIL-1 may inhibit gonadotrophins. *
Interleukin-2 (IL-2)	○ Helper T cells that express IL-2 receptors	○ T-lymphocyte activation by IL-1 and/or antigen	○ Stimulates T-lymphocyte proliferation, production of IFN and TNF by T cells, proliferation of B cells (with IL-4), proliferation of chronic lymphocytic leukemia B cells, differentiation of B cells, and eosinophil proliferation. ○ Expands and activates cytotoxic T cells, and activates NK cells. ○ Expands and activates lymphokine-activated killer (LAK) cells. ○ Toxic effects of rIL-2 may include fever, weight loss, hypotension, rash, eosinophilia, fluid retention, pulmonary infiltrates, and transient alterations of renal, hepatic, and CNS function.
Interleukin-3 (IL-3)	○ Activated helper T cells	○ T-lymphocyte activation by IL-1 and/or antigen	○ Stimulates proliferation of stem cells in bone marrow and production and release of histamine from mast cells. ○ Also called multi-CSF because it is able to stimulate multiple cell lines.
Interleukin-4 (IL-4)	○ Activated helper T cells	○ Lymphocyte interactions ○ T-lymphocyte activation by antigen, IL-1, or endotoxin	○ Stimulates antibody synthesis by B cells and B-lymphocyte proliferation. ○ Stimulates mast cells. ○ Induces IL-2-mediated cytotoxic T cells. ○ Growth factor for T cells.
Interleukin-5 (IL-5)	○ Activated helper T cells	○ T-lymphocyte activation by antigen, IL-1, or endotoxin	○ Stimulates synthesis of antibodies by B cells. ○ Stimulates eosinophil differentiation and induces IL-2-mediated cytotoxic T cells.
Interleukin-6 (IL-6)	○ Activated helper T cells ○ Macrophages ○ Fibroblasts ○ Endothelial cells ○ Carcinoma cells ○ Sarcoma cells	○ IL-1-stimulated B cells ○ Antigens ○ Endotoxin	○ Stimulates induction of IL-2, induction of IL-2 receptor expression on T cells, and IL-3-induced colony formation by stem cells. ○ Acts on CNS to cause fever. ○ Inhibits growth of myeloid leukemia. ○ Causes production of acute phase reactants. ○ Exerts thrombopoietic effects.
Interleukin-7 (IL-7)	○ Thymus cells		○ Stimulates proliferation of thymocytes and lymphoid precursors.
Interleukin-8 (IL-8)	○ Monocytes ○ T cells		○ Accumulates neutrophils and/or lymphocytes in tissues.

(Table continues)

TABLE 8.6. *(continued)*

CYTOKINES	ORIGIN	INDUCING STIMULI	ACTIONS
Tumor necrosis factor-alpha (TNF-alpha) or cachectin	○ Macrophages ○ T cells ○ Thymocytes ○ Endothelial cells ○ NK cells	○ Bacterial endotoxin ○ Inflammatory agents ○ IL-1 ○ IFN	○ Kills tumor cells, stimulates fever, sequesters iron, alters glucose metabolism in muscle, and enhances inflammatory responses. ○ Synergistic with IL-1 and IFN. ○ Accelerates lipolysis and contributes to fat catabolism and cachexia. ○ rTNF may cause fever, chills, anorexia, neutropenia, and CNS toxicity.
Interferon-alpha (IFN-alpha)	○ Leukocytes	○ Viral stimulation of neutrophils ○ Endotoxin	○ Antiviral and antiproliferative. ○ Affects T cells, NK cells, and macrophages. ○ rIFN may cause influenza-like symptoms (fever, myalgia, anorexia), neutropenia, and CNS toxicity.
Interferon-beta (IFN-beta)	○ Fibroblasts	○ Cytokines	○ Antiviral and antiproliferative. ○ Affects T cells, NK cells, and macrophages.
Interferon-gamma (IFN-gamma)	○ Activated helper T cells	○ T cell activation by IL-1 or antigen	○ Antiviral and antiproliferative. ○ Stimulates NK cell activity and antitumor activity by macrophages. ○ rIFN-gamma may cause fever, myalgia, anorexia, and fatigue.
Granulocyte-macrophage colony stimulating factor (GM-CSF)	○ Activated helper T cells ○ Fibroblasts ○ Endothelial cells ○ Macrophages	○ T cell activation by IL-1 or antigen ○ Cytokine stimulation by other cell types	○ Stimulates stem cells of macrophages, granulocytes, and eosinophils. ○ Matures granulocytes and monocytes. ○ Stimulates monocyte production of TNF, IL-1, and hydrogen peroxide. ○ Chemotactic for macrophages and eosinophils. ○ Stimulates histamine release. ○ Stimulates maturation of dendritic cells, which present antigens to T cells. ○ Increases leukocyte count in humans following chemotherapy treatment. ○ rGM-CSF may cause bone pain and slight fever.
Granulocyte colony-stimulating factor (G-CSF)	○ Macrophages ○ Fibroblasts ○ Epithelial cells	○ Cell activation by IL-1 or mitogen	○ Stimulates colony formation by neutrophilic precursors. ○ Increases leukocyte count in humans following chemotherapy treatment. ○ rG-CSF may cause bone pain, mild fever, and fatigue.
Macrophage colony stimulating factor (M-CSF)	○ Monocytes ○ Fibroblasts ○ Epithelial cells ○ Carcinoma cells	○ Cell activation by IL-1 or mitogen	○ Stimulates colony formation by macrophage precursors.

* Recombinant cytokines are those that are mass produced by cloning their genes in bacteria. They are designated by the letter r (e.g., rTNF). If of human origin, they may be designated by the letters rh (e.g., rhTNF).

Sources: Linder, 1991:532-35; Tannock and Hill, 1992:248; Holland et al., 1993:179-188

TABLE 8.7. RESULTS OF IL-2 AND LAK CELL THERAPY

CANCER	THERAPY		NUMBER OF PATIENTS	COMPLETE RESPONSE (%)	COMPLETE AND PARTIAL RESPONSE (%)
Melanoma	IL-2*	Trial 1	6	0	50
		Trial 2	31	0	3
		Trial 3	42	0	24
		Trial 4	26	0	12
		Trial 5	12	0	17
	IL-2 plus LAK**		48	8	21
Renal cell carcinoma	IL-2*	Trial 1	17	0	18
		Trial 2	54	7	22
		Trial 3	44	2	11
		***Trial 4	94	5	17
	IL-2 plus LAK**		72	11	35
Colorectal cancer	IL-2 plus LAK**		30	3	17
Lymphoma	IL-2*		9	0	33
	IL-2 plus LAK**		7	14	57
Total Patients and Average Response			492	4	23

* Other trials for this cancer reported zero response rates. *Sources: review by Lotze and Rosenberg, 1991; Koretz et al., 1991.*
** Results of multiple trials. Trials for other cancers reported zero response rates. *Sources: review by Rosenberg, 1991.*
*** *Source: Weiss et al., 1992*

the recovery of bone marrow after cytotoxic chemother-chemotherapy treatment. These growth factors increase the proliferation of leukocytes from the stem cells located in the bone marrow, thereby reversing immunosuppression. Although they also produce a cytotoxic effect against certain tumor cells in vitro, it is not known if such actions will occur in human patients (reviewed by Metcalf and Morstyn, 1991).

8.4 NATURAL AGENTS THAT STIMULATE THE IMMUNE SYSTEM

8.4.1 Herbal Agents

A large number of herbal agents have an effect on the immune system (see Table 8.8). The mechanisms by which these agents exert their immunostimulant effects are not well understood, but often include the production of cytokines.

There are additional, nonherbal natural agents that stimulate the immune system. For example, the effects of melatonin, thymostimulin, and other agents are discussed in the text below.

A number of agents listed in Table 8.8 contain high molecular weight polysaccharides. These agents include *Acanthopanax sp., Astragalus membranaceus (huang qi), Echinacea purpurea, Ganoderma lucidum (ling zhi), Lycium barbarum (gou qi zi), Pseudostellaria heterophylla (tai zi shen)* and others. Studies suggest that the immunostimulating activity of polysaccharides increases in direct proportion to their molecular weight. Polysaccharides from some of these plants have been isolated and are available in pill form in Japan, China, and the United States.

TABLE 8.8. HERBAL AGENTS THAT STIMULATE THE IMMUNE SYSTEM

AGENT	EFFECT	REFERENCE
Acanthopanax sp. (*wu jia pi, ci wu jia*)	Polysaccharides stimulated macrophage phagocytosis, T-cell and B-cell activity, and IL-1 and interferon production in vitro. The *Acanthopanax sp.* is related to the *Panax sp.* (i.e., *P. ginseng, ren shen*). Outside of China, the accepted name of *Acanthopanax senticosus* is *Eleutherococcus senticosus*.	Wagner, 1985
(Table continues)		

TABLE 8.8. *(continued)*		
AGENT	**EFFECT**	**REFERENCE**
Achyranthes bidentata (*niu xi*)	Polysaccharides induced the production of IL-1 and TNF-alpha in mouse macrophages in vitro.	Xiang and Li, 1993
Altheae officinalis (marsh mallow)	Polysaccharide-rich mucilages stimulated macrophage phagocytosis, T-cell and B-cell activity, and IL-1 and interferon production in vitro.	Wagner, 1985
Angelica sinensis (*dang gui*)	Increased the production of IL-2 in mouse spleen mononuclear cells in vitro. This action was blocked by the addition of PGE_2. The herb increased TNF cytotoxicity in mice.	Weng et al., 1987; Haranaka et al., 1985a, 1985b
Aristolochia debilis (*mu xiang or tian xian teng, or ma dou ling*)	Aristolochic acid stimulated macrophage phagocytosis, T-cell and B-cell activity, and IL-1 and interferon production in vitro. Aristolochic acid is mutagenic and carcinogenic in animals.	Wagner, 1985; Farnsworth, 1993; Mengs and Klein, 1988
Astragalus membranaceus (*huang qi*)	Fractions of the herb caused a 10-fold increase in the cytotoxic effects of rIL-2 in vitro. Since the success of using rIL-2 has been hampered by its severe toxicity, cotreatment with astragalus may be useful in allowing IL-2 to be used at lower, less toxic, doses. Extracts of astragalus injected into mice immunosuppressed by cyclophosphamide, radiotherapy, or aging, enhanced the antibody response to antigens and was associated with an increase of helper T-lymphocyte activity in normal and immunosuppressed mice. Fractions of astragalus injected intravenously into cyclophosphamide-treated rats completely reversed immunosuppression caused by cyclophosphamide. This was evidenced by an increased rejection of xenogeneic grafts. Extracts induced IFN production in mouse cells in vitro. Administration for 3 to 4 months to patients with coxsackie B viral myocarditis and depressed NK cell activity increased NK cell activity by a factor of 4, and improved clinical outcomes. Astragalan, a component of the herb, enhanced the production of TNF by human peripheral blood mononuclear cells ex vivo. Polysaccharides stimulated macrophage phagocytosis, T-lymphocyte and B-lymphocyte activity, and IL-1 and interferon production in vitro.	Wang et al., 1992b; Chu et al., 1988a, 1988b, 1990; Zhao and Mancini, 1990; Hou et al., 1981; Yang et al., 1990; Zhao and Kong, 1993; Wagner, 1985
Astragalus membranaceus (*huang qi*) and *Ligustrum lucidum* (*nu zhen zi*)	Aqueous extracts were added to cultures of mononuclear cells obtained from 19 cancer patients and 15 healthy donors. In one experiment, T-cell function, as measured by graft-versus-host reaction, was restored in cells from 9 out of 10 cancer patients. In a second experiment, T-cell function was restored in cells from 9 of 13 cancer patients. The degree of the immune restoration appeared to be complete, as reactions of test cells equaled the levels found in cells from healthy donors.	Sun et al., 1983
Astragalus membranaceus (*huang qi*), *Ligustrum lucidum* (*nu zhen zi*) and *Eclipta prostrata* (*han lian cao*)	Increased lymphocyte activation, serum IgG levels, and the weights of the thymus and spleen in mice. The formula also inhibited cyclophosphamide-induced immunosuppression.	He et al., 1992
Astragalus membranaceus (*huang qi*) and *Panax ginseng* (*ren shen*)	Markedly enhanced the cytotoxic action of LAK cells.	Zhao, 1993
Astragalus membranaceus (*huang qi*) and *Sheng Mai San* (formula)	Markedly enhanced the cytotoxic action of LAK cells.	Zhao, 1993
Atractylodes macrocephala (*bai zhu*)	Stimulated phagocyte activity in mice. Increased leukocyte count in humans with leukocytosis.	Reviewed by Chang and But, 1986:376
Bupleurum chinense (*chai hu*)	Increased TNF cytotoxicity in mice.	Haranaka et al., 1985a, 1985b
(Table continues)		

71

AGENT	EFFECT	REFERENCE
	TABLE 8.8. *(continued)*	
Cinnamomum cassia (rou gui)	Increased TNF cytotoxicity in mice.	Haranaka et al., 1985a, 1985b
Codonopsis pilosula (dang shen)	In a study of 76 cancer patients undergoing radiotherapy, the herb did not affect the leukocyte count, but increased the delayed hypersensitivity reaction and lymphocyte response to mitogens. Plasma IgM was slightly increased in the treatment group and was significantly decreased in controls. Markedly stimulated the phagocytic activity of peritoneal macrophages in mice.	Zeng et al., 1992; Chang and But, 1987:975
Cordyceps sinensis (dong chong xia cao)	The ethanol extract stimulated NK cell activity both in vitro and in mice, and inhibited cyclophosphamide-induced reductions of NK cell activity in mice. The extract increased human NK cell activity of peripheral blood cells ex vivo. The ethanol extract stimulated the proliferation and phagocytosis of mouse macrophages, reduced PGE_2-induced inhibition of IL-2 in mouse splenocytes, and prolonged survival in tumor-bearing mice. The herb increased NK activity in peripheral blood cells obtained from leukemia patients. Water extracts enhanced the proliferation of spleen lymphocytes in rats, and increased the production of IL-2 from spleen cells.	Xu et al., 1992; Liu et al., 1992a; Cheng, 1992
Cuscuta australis (tu si zi)	Alcohol extracts normalized macrophage phagocytosis and lymphocyte proliferation in mice with second degree burns.	Xiao et al., 1990
Echinacea purpurea	Polysaccharides stimulated macrophage phagocytosis, T-lymphocyte and B-lymphocyte activity, and IL-1 and interferon production in vitro.	Wagner, 1985
Er Xiang Tang (formula)	Stimulated the production of GM-CSF in mice with bone marrow suppression.	Lin et al., 1990
Eupatorium perfoliatum (boneset)	Polysaccharides stimulated macrophage phagocytosis, T-lymphocyte and B-lymphocyte activity, and IL-1 and interferon production in vitro.	Wagner, 1985
Eupatorium cannabinum (hemp agrimony)	Polysaccharides stimulated macrophage phagocytosis, T-lymphocyte and B-lymphocyte activity, and IL-1 and interferon production in vitro.	Wagner, 1985
Formula #3	In a study on 40 patients undergoing radiotherapy, the formula increased leukocyte count, whereas the leukocyte count dropped significantly in the control group. The leukocyte count in radiated mice was significantly greater in those receiving the formula as opposed to controls.	Zhang et al., 1990b
Fu Zheng Jie Du Tang (formula)	Enhanced the production of TNF by peritoneal macrophages in EMT6 tumor-bearing mice treated with cyclophosphamide.	Wei, 1990
Ganoderma lucidum (ling zhi)	Oral administration (300 mg/kg) increased the production of IL-2 in mice. Administration of a purified fraction increased the number of peripheral blood lymphocytes in humans. This effect was thought to be due to stimulation of T lymphocytes and increased production of IL-2 and IFN-gamma.	Zhang et al., 1993; Haak-Frendscho et al., 1993
Gynostemma pentaphyllum (jiao gu lan)	Contains dammarane-type saponins, which have adaptagenic effects. (Nonspecific antistress, homeostasis-enhancing effects have been called adaptagens by various investigators.) Dammarane-type saponins may act through modulation of the hormonal system via the hypothalamus-pituitary-adrenal axis. The total saponins prevented inhibition of immunity, elevated NK cell activity, and maintained the weight of the immune organs in cyclophosphamide-treated mice. The saponins also enhanced T- and B-lymphocyte proliferation in the spleens of normal and cyclophosphamide-treated mice. In healthy mice, the extract showed a bidirectional action, normalizing immune indices when higher or lower than median levels. The saponins protect phagocytes and endothelial cells from oxidative stress.	Shibata, 1985; Zhang et al., 1990d; Li et al., 1993
	(Table continues)	

72

TABLE 8.8. *(continued)*		
AGENT	**EFFECT**	**REFERENCE**
Hochu Ekki To (formula)	Augmented the production of TNF, IL-1, and PGE_2 by macrophages, and had a synergistic effect with IFN-gamma in stimulating the production of TNF and increasing macrophage cytotoxicity.	Kataoka et al., 1989
Isatis tinctoria (indigo, *qing dai*)	Elevated the leukocyte count in rats after radiation. Dosages up to 6 g/kg did not produce toxic reactions.	Liu and He, 1991
Jian Pi Jin Dan (formula)	Increased phagocytosis by peritoneal macrophages in mice with cyclophosphamide-induced immunosuppression. The formula also increased the proliferation of spleen T cells and B cells, the production of IL-1 by macrophages, and the production of IL-2 by T cells in both healthy and immunosuppressed mice.	Fan, 1993
Kang Shuai Sen Fang (formula)	Increased the immune response of mouse spleen cells to mitogenic substances, including lipopolysaccharides. Enhanced cytotoxic T-cell activity and stimulated the production of IL-2.	Gong et al., 1991
Kang Fu Xin (formula)	Intraperitoneal injection increased the phagocytosis-induced respiratory burst (chemiluminescence) of mouse peritoneal cells. Chemiluminescence was stimulated in a dose-dependent fashion. Oral administration to normal and immunosuppressed tumor-bearing mice had similar effects. Macrophages from mice injected with the formula were more cytostatic for P815 tumor cells than those from controls.	Liu et al., 1989
Ligusticum chuanxiong (*chuan xiong*)	Increased TNF cytotoxicity in mice.	Haranaka et al., 1985a, 1985b
Lycium barbarum (*gou qi zi*)	Polysaccharides increased the ability of IL-2 to stimulate the proliferation of lymphocytes in mouse splenocyte cultures.	Geng et al., 1989
Panax pseudoginseng (*san qi*)	Contains dammarane-type saponins that are adaptagenic (see *Gynostemma pentaphyllum*).	Shibata, 1985
Panax quinquefolium (American ginseng, *xi yang shen*)	Contains dammarane-type saponins that are adaptagenic (see *Gynostemma pentaphyllum*).	Shibata, 1985
Panax ginseng (*ren shen*)	Contains dammarane-type saponins that are adaptagenic (see *Gynostemma pentaphyllum*). The physiological effects of ginseng saponins include sedation, antifatigue action, stimulation of RNA and protein biosynthesis in the liver and kidneys, stimulation of carbohydrate and lipid metabolism, increase of adrenal cAMP, stimulation of macrophage phagocytosis, promotion of antibody and complement production, and restoration of sexual behavior in stressed animals. Saponins increased the NK cell activity of mouse spleen cells by 40% in vitro. IL-2 and interferon production were each increased approximately 100%. In healthy mice, NK activity was increased as much as 600%.	Shibata, 1985; Hiai, 1985; Wang et al., 1985; Yang and Yu, 1988
Paris formosana (*quan shen*)	Glycosides stimulated the proliferative response of lymphocytes in mice to mitogens, and augmented the production of GM-CSF in vitro. Saponins stimulated NK cell activity, markedly stimulated interferon production, and inhibited the growth of mouse hepatoma cells in mice.	Chiang et al., 1992; Shibata, 1985
Picrorrhiza kurroa (*hu huang lian*)	Orally administered ethanol extracts stimulated T-cells, B-cells, and phagocytes, and increased graft rejection in animals.	Atal et al., 1986, reviewed by Bone, 1995
Plantago sp. (i.e., psyllium seed)	Polysaccharide-rich mucilages stimulated macrophage phagocytosis, T-cell and B-cell activity, and IL-1 and interferon production.	Wagner, 1985
Polygonatum odoratum (*yu zhu*)	Alcohol extracts normalized macrophage phagocytosis and lymphocyte proliferation in mice with second-degree burns.	Xiao et al., 1990
(Table continues)		

	TABLE 8.8. *(continued)*	
AGENT	**EFFECT**	**REFERENCE**
Pseudostellaria heterophylla (tai zi shen)	A water-soluble extract stimulated the production of mouse spleen lymphocytes and TNF in vitro. The extract exhibited potent antitumor activities against Ehrlich ascites tumor in mice. This effect was not seen in vitro, and thus may be due to immune stimulation. Polysaccharides from the plant stimulated the production of GM-CSF in vitro.	Wong et al., 1992, 1994
Ren Shen Yang Rong Tang (formula)	Protected mice injected with the bacteria *Listeria monocytogenes* from lethal infections. The formula stimulated macrophage production via production of IL-1, IL-6, and GM-CSF. The formula significantly stimulated GM-CSF, but not G-CSF, in cultures of human peripheral blood mononuclear cells.	Yonekura et al., 1992; Okamura et al., 1991
Ren Shen Tang (formula)	Oral and intraperitoneal administration enhanced the function of the reticuloendothelial system in mice and increased the relative weights of the thymus, spleen, and liver.	Ito and Shimura, 1985a, 1985b
Rheum palmatum (da huang)	Oral administration increased delayed hypersensitivity reactions to bovine serum albumin, and increased the proliferation response of spleen cells to mitogens in mice.	Ma, 1991
Shen Cao Fu Zheng Kangai (formula)	Inhibited cyclophosphamide-induced immunosuppression in mice. After 3 days of treatment, the leukocyte count was reduced by 60% in the treatment group, and 79% in the control group. No acute toxicity was observed.	Zhao, 1992
Shi Quan Da Bu Tang (formula)	Oral and intraperitoneal administration enhanced the function of the reticuloendothelial system in mice, and increased the relative weights of the thymus, spleen, and liver.	Ito and Shimura, 1985a, 1985b
Symphitum sp. (i.e., comfrey)	Polysaccharide-rich mucilages stimulated macrophage phagocytosis, T-cell and B-cell activity, and IL-1 and interferon production in vitro	Wagner, 1985
Xiao Chai Hu Tang (formula)	Numerous investigators have reported that the formula stimulates the production of colony stimulating factors and interleukins. Oral, intraperitoneal, and intravenous administration induced a dose-dependent induction of CSF in mice. In bone marrow culture, the growth stimulating effects were characteristic of standard GM-CSF. The formula dose-dependently increased the production of G-CSF in peripheral blood mononuclear cell cultures obtained from healthy subjects. Other herbal formulas were less effective at increasing G-CSF. It induced the production of IFN-alpha and beta in mice. This effect was also seen in vitro in mouse spleen cells. Repeated intraperitoneal treatment resulted in a decline in interferon induction. However, repeated oral administration resulted in continuous induction. Intraperitoneal administration of the formula and the constituent herbs *Glycyrrhiza uralensis*, *Scutellaria baicalensis*, *Bupleurum chinense*, and *Pinellia ternata* all induced IFN and IL-6 production in mice. These herbs stimulated the production of IFN by B cells in mouse spleen cell cultures. All herbs except *Scutellaria baicalensis* showed mitogenic activity in spleen cell cultures. Oral administration of the formula increased phagocytosis and diminished PGE_2 production in mice. Results suggest that the formula enhances the immune response through eliminating PGE_2-induced inhibition of lymphocytes, and through presenting antigens more efficiently. The formula reduced the severe shock pattern caused by administration of rhTNF to mice. In addition, the formula enhanced the antitumor activity of rhTNF. Oral and intraperitoneal administration enhanced the function of the reticuloendothelial system in mice, increased the relative weights of the thymus, spleen, and liver, and caused a significant increase in the proportion of helper T cells.	Yonekura et al., 1990; Yamashiki et al., 1992a, 1992b; Kawakita et al., 1990; Matsura et al., 1993; Nagatsu et al., 1989; Sakaguchi et al., 1991; Ito and Shimura, 1985a, 1985b; Tatsuta et al., 1991
	(Table continues)	

TABLE 8.8. *(continued)*		
AGENT	**EFFECT**	**REFERENCE**
Zhu Ling Tang (formula)	Oral and intraperitoneal administration enhanced the function of the reticuloendothelial system in mice, and increased the relative weights of the thymus, spleen, and liver.	Ito and Shimura, 1985a, 1985b
Ziziphus jujuba (da zao)	Contains dammarane-type saponins that are adaptagenic (see *Gynostemma pentaphyllum*).	Shibata, 1985

8.4.2 Melatonin

Melatonin is a hormone produced by the pineal gland. In healthy humans, melatonin is secreted from the pineal gland in a diurnal rhythm, with the highest serum levels occurring during the evening. Melatonin influences a number of biological functions, the most studied of which is its ability to induce sleep. It is becoming increasingly popular as a nontoxic, nonaddictive remedy for jet lag and insomnia. Melatonin is also a potent antioxidant—more potent than glutathione in scavenging the hydroxyl radical and more potent than vitamin E in scavenging the peroxyl radical (reviewed by Reiter et al., 1995; Pieri et al., 1994). Furthermore, it stimulates the main antioxidant enzyme of the brain, glutathione peroxidase (Reiter, 1995). Due to its lipophilic structure, melatonin is readily diffused into all tissues of the body, including intracellular membranes. As such, it protects the DNA against free radical damage (Reiter, 1993).

Recently, investigators have discovered that melatonin inhibits the proliferation of a limited number of cancers in vitro, and a large number of cancers in vivo. One of the mechanisms of in-vitro inhibition appears to be antiestrogenic activity. Melatonin has a direct inhibitory effect on MCF-7 estrogen-responsive human breast cancer cells in vitro (Crespo et al., 1994; Hill et al., 1992; Cos et al., 1994). This effect was reversed by the addition of estradiol, and did not occur in estrogen-unresponsive cell lines. Optimal effects were obtained when melatonin was available on a diurnal cycle. Proliferation was inhibited by 39% at concentrations of 0.3 nM, which is equivalent to the physiologic concentration seen at 2:00 AM in humans (Furuya et al., 1994). Melatonin renders the antiestrogen tamoxifen up to 100 times more effective in inhibiting the proliferation of breast cancer cells in vitro (Wilson et al., 1992). Another study implicated deficient melatonin production in the transformation of endothelial cells in endometrial cancer, due in part, to its antiestrogenic effect (Sandyk et al., 1992). Melatonin also inhibited human M-6 melanoma cells in vitro (Ying et al., 1993). The mechanism by which melatonin affects melanoma cells is uncertain, although it also may be due to an antiestrogen mechanism.

A second mechanism by which melatonin may inhibit cancer is augmentation of the anticancer effects of interleukin-2. In 90 patients with advanced solid neoplasms, the combination of low-dose IL-2 (three million IU) and melatonin (40 mg/day) significantly decreased the proliferation of neoplastic cells as compared to IL-2 alone (Lissoni et al., 1994a). High dose IL-2 is associated with significant adverse effects, and melatonin allows IL-2 to be used at lower, less toxic doses without compromising its immunologic effects. Other clinical studies on melatonin in cancer patients are summarized in Table 8.9.

Melatonin alone has no effect on the number of immune cells and requires the presence of IL-2 to produce an effect. The targets of melatonin activity appear to be helper T lymphocytes and macrophages, both of which are affected by IL-2 (Lissoni et al., 1993c). Melatonin appears to stimulate IL-2-induced T-lymphocyte activity and inhibit IL-2-induced macrophage activity in cancer patients. Inhibition of IL-2-induced macrophage activity may prevent a macrophage-induced inhibition of lymphocytes and NK cells (Lissoni et al., 1991a), such as may occur from a macrophage-induced production of PGE_2.

The relationship between melatonin and IL-2 is complex. Both IL-2 and melatonin levels are commonly abnormal in cancer patients and may affect one another. In seven patients with advanced small cell lung cancer, zero patients had a normal light/dark rhythm of melatonin secretion. However, administering IL-2 produced a normal rhythm in four of the patients.

Possible causes of irregularities in melatonin production include stress (Piccoli et al., 1991), artificial evening light, and extremely low frequency (ELF) electromagnetic fields (Loscher et al., 1994). ELF fields are produced by the 50 to 60 cycle-per-second current used in household electrical equipment. In fact, studies have shown that ELF fields block the ability of melatonin to inhibit the proliferation of breast cancer cells in vitro (Liburdy et al., 1993).

Although it has not been investigated, it may be possible to combine melatonin with *Astragalus membranaceus* or other natural agents that induce IL-2 production to produce clinical benefits. Recall from Table 8.8 that coadministration of *Astragalus membranaceus* allowed the use of lower doses of IL-2.

TABLE 8.9. ANTICANCER EFFECTS OF MELATONIN	
EFFECT	**REFERENCE**
In 14 patients with advanced solid tumors, who received melatonin (40 mg/day orally) in combination with IL-2, partial remission occurred in 3 (21%), and 6 others stabilized.	Lissoni et al., 1994b
In 22 patients with progressing renal cell carcinoma, who received melatonin (10 mg/day orally) in combination with interferon, complete remissions occurred in 3 (14%), partial remissions occurred in 4 (18%) and 9 patients stabilized (41%).	Neri et al., 1994
In 14 patients with metastatic gastric cancer, who received melatonin (50 mg/day orally) in combination with IL-2, complete regression occurred in 1 (7%), partial regression occurred in 2 (14%) and 6 patients (43%) stabilized. Toxicity was low in all cases.	Lissoni et al., 1993a
In 14 patients with hepatocellular carcinoma, who received melatonin (50 mg per orally) in combination with IL-2, complete regression occurred in 1 (7%), partial regression occurred in 4 (25%) and 6 patients (43%) stabilized. Toxicity was low in all cases.	Aldeghi et al., 1994
In 50 patients with brain metastasis due to solid neoplasms, who received either supportive care (steroids and anticonvulsants) or supportive care in combination with melatonin (20 mg/day), the one-year, free-from-brain cancer progression and the one-year survival rate was higher in patients receiving melatonin. In addition, the group that received melatonin experienced reduced side effects from steroid therapy.	Lissoni et al., 1994c
In 63 patients with metastatic non-small cell lung cancer, who received melatonin (10 mg/day orally) or supportive care alone, the patients who received melatonin exhibited increased one-year survival and increased disease stabilization. No toxicity was observed.	Lissoni et al., 1992a
In 20 patients with non-small cell lung cancer, who received melatonin (10 mg/day orally) in combination with IL-2, a partial response occurred in 4 (20%) and 10 patients (50%) stabilized. These results were comparable to those obtained with chemotherapy.	Lissoni et al., 1992b
In 24 patients with a variety of advanced solid tumors, who received melatonin in combination with IL-2, a partial response occurred in three (12%) and 14 patients (59%) stabilized.	Lissoni et al., 1993b
In 40 patients with advanced melanoma who received melatonin, partial responses occurred in 6 patients (15%) and 6 patients (15%) stabilized.	Gonzalez et al., 1991
In 54 patients with mostly lung or colorectal cancer resistant to conventional therapies, who received melatonin (20 mg/day), partial response occurred in 1 (2%), minor response occurred in 2 (4%), and 21 patients (41%) stabilized.	Lissoni et al., 1991b
Note: The dose of IL-2 used in these studies generally was three million IU.	

8.4.3 Thymostimulin

Thymostimulin is a drug derived from calf thymus that contains several thymus peptides. Some carcinomas, such as Kaposi's sarcoma and oat cell carcinoma of the lung, are associated with low levels of plasma T lymphocytes and may respond to treatment with thymus hormones. Trials with isolated thymus hormones have increased the survival of patients with melanoma and small cell lung cancer, and reduced myelosuppression in patients with breast cancer and other cancers (see Table 8.10).

The epithelial cells of the thymus synthesize at least 30 different polypeptides. Numerous immunodeficient diseases are associated with abnormal thymic morphology. In some cases, thymic epithelial cell mass, and hormone production, may be drastically reduced (Linder, 1987). Individual thymus hormones are believed to vary in their effects: some may cause immunostimulation, and some immunosuppression (Oates and Goldstein, 1991).

Other preparations that contain thymus hormones appear to stimulate the immune system. In a series of clinical trials in Poland, over 1,000 patients with immunosuppression related to various diseases were treated with TFX, a semipurified calf thymus extract. In a majority of the patients, long-term treatment with TFX ameliorated signs and symptoms of their disease and normalized disturbed immune parameters (Skotnicki, 1989). In 26 children with acute myeloid leukemia receiving chemotherapy, long-term administration (2 to 3 years) of tactivan, another thymic hormone preparation, reduced concurrent diseases and increased remission periods (Drozdova et al., 1990).

The efficacy of crude thymus extracts, such as those sold as nutritional supplements, is questionable. Von Ardenne (1985) reported that whole thymus extract is nearly as effective as semipure extracts at raising white blood cell counts. However, Giedanowski et al. (1987) reported that, although a crude thymus extract and a

TABLE 8.10. CLINICAL EFFECTS OF THYMOSTIMULIN

EFFECT	REFERENCE
Enhanced NK cell activity ex vivo in peripheral blood of 6 out of 14 patients with bladder cancer.	Molto et al., 1993
Normalized monocyte function ex vivo in peripheral blood obtained from 44 patients with head and neck squamous cell carcinoma.	Tas et al., 1993
Increased lymphocytic response to mitogens in 55% of 29 patients with laryngeal carcinoma treated only with surgery. In the control group, an increase was observed in 30%.	Mantovani et al., 1992
Produced a 50% reduction in leukopenia incidence as compared to controls in a study of 85 breast cancer patients who were also receiving chemotherapy.	Alba et al., 1991
Increased the percentage of disease-free patients as compared to controls in a one-year study of 37 patients with post-surgical malignant melanoma.	Azizi et al., 1984
Reduced myleosuppression, increased complete response rates, and improved survival as compared to controls in a study on 26 patients with small cell lung cancer who were also receiving chemotherapy.	Macchiarini et al., 1989
Reduced infections (37% vs. 77%) and lowered the incidence of myelosuppression as compared to controls in a study of 51 patients with breast cancer who were also receiving chemotherapy.	Iaffaioli et al., 1988
Markedly increased depressed levels of T cells in 16 patients with inoperable squamous cell carcinoma of the head and neck who were also receiving chemotherapy.	Schuff-Werner et al., 1987
Resulted in no difference in mean survival as compared to controls in a study of 22 patients with advanced lung cancer (oat cell excluded) who were also receiving chemotherapy. All 12 patients in the control group died within 12 months. However, two of the 10 patients receiving thymostimulin were alive after 23 and 16 months. In addition, the group receiving thymostimulin suffered from less infections (4 vs. 65) and suffered less bone marrow toxicity from the chemotherapy treatment.	Del Giacco et al., 1984
Resulted in no difference in hematological tolerance to chemotherapy or number and severity of infections in 40 patients with lymphoma or myeloma, as compared to those treated only with chemotherapy.	Canovas et al., 1991

semipure fraction (fraction V) were both able to activate human NK cells in vitro, the crude fraction showed the weakest effect. Fraction V appears to contain the poly-peptides primarily responsible for immune stimulation, and the crude extract contained only 15% of fraction V.

8.4.4 Other Agents that Stimulate the Immune System

Other natural agents that stimulate the immune system include bromelain, certain vitamins and minerals, and glutathione and N-acetyl cysteine (NAC). Bromelain stimulates the production of TNF-alpha in human peripheral blood mononuclear cells cultures. In addition, it may lyse antigen-antibody complexes which can block immune action. These and other activities of bromelain are discussed in more detail in Section 15.3.3. Vitamin D_3 (1,25-dihydroxyvitamin D_3) reduced tumor-induced suppressor T-cell activity in vitro and caused a marked reduction in metastasis in rodents (Rita et al., 1995). The effects of other vitamins and minerals on the immune system and neoplasia are discussed in more detail in Chapter 13.

The amino acid cysteine is a component of the tri-peptide glutathione, which is essential to the liver's detoxification mechanisms. Due to its antioxidant activity, is also involved in a number of immune activities.

Glutathione may be a rate limiting component in IL-2 and LAK immunotherapy. Glutathione-deficient lymphocytes exhibit subnormal activation in response to lectins. Furthermore, exogenous IL-2 cannot restore their activity, although glutathione can (Hamilos et al., 1991). Oral administration of NAC, in conjunction with IL-2 and LAK, reduces the progression of refractory tumors in mice. Complete tumor regression was observed in 11 to 17% (Yim et al., 1994). Glutathione and cysteine are discussed in more detail in Section 12.4.5.

8.5 NATURAL AGENTS THAT SUPPRESS THE IMMUNE SYSTEM

There are a number of mechanisms by which natural agents may suppress the immune system. These include stimulation of glucocorticoid secretion, inhibition of glu-cocorticoid metabolism, inhibition of antibody produc-tion, inhibition of complement action, and inhibition of cytokine production. Studies on the immunosuppressive effects of various natural agents are summarized in Table 8.11. These agents may or may not be appropriate for clinical use, depending on which aspect of the human immune system they inhibit (if any) and the clinical goal. Note that some of these agents, such as *Panax ginseng*, *Codonopsis pilosula*, and the formula *Zhu Ling Tang* are listed in Table 8.8 as stimulating the immune system and

TABLE 8.11. NATURAL AGENTS THAT INHIBIT THE IMMUNE SYSTEM

AGENT	EFFECT	REFERENCE
Aesculus hippocastanum (horse chestnut seeds)	Triterpenoid saponins markedly increased plasma ACTH and corticosterone in animals. The saponins apparently act by stimulating the hypothalamus and/or pituitary, as this action was blocked by removal of the hypothalamus or pretreatment with dexamethasone.	Hiai, 1985
Angelica sinensis (dang gui)	Inhibited antibody formation in animal studies.	Chang and But, 1986:494
Bupleurum falcatum (chai hu)	Contains triterpenoid saponins (see *Aesculus hippocastanum*).	Hiai, 1985
Camellia sinensis (green tea seeds)	Contains triterpenoid saponins (see *Aesculus hippocastanum*).	Hiai, 1985
Codonopsis pilosula (dang shen)	Reduces lymphocyte and total leukocyte populations when administered orally to rabbits.	Chang and But, 1987:975
Cordyceps sinensis (dong chong xia cao)	Inhibited graft rejection of heart allografts in mice. Administration to mice resulted in immunosuppression. In vitro, the herb reduced phagocytic function of peripheral blood leukocytes, spleen lymphocyte response to mitogens, and IL-1 release from macrophages. In vivo, the herb increased survival of mice with skin allografts.	Zhang and Xia, 1990; Zhu and Yu, 1990
Gui Zhi Tang (formula)	Administration to mice resulted in immunosuppression. When added to spleen cell cultures, the formula inhibited production of IL-2.	Lu, 1989
Liquidambar orientalis (styrax, *su he xiang*)	Contains triterpenoid saponins (see *Aesculus hippocastanum*).	Hiai, 1985
Panax ginseng (ren shen)	Total saponins suppressed the delayed hypersensitivity response in mice. Other immune parameters, such as NK cell activity, were not affected. The selective immunosuppression may be related to the steroid-like structure of the saponins. The saponins from ginseng constitute about 2 to 3% of the plant. Some of these saponins are triterpenoid saponins (see *Aesculus hippocastanum*).	Yeung et al., 1982; Hiai, 1985
Perilla frutescens (su zi)	Markedly suppressed IgE production in mice.	Imaoka et al., 1993
Platycodon grandiflorum (jie geng)	Contains triterpenoid saponins (see *Aesculus hippocastanum*).	Hiai, 1985
Polyporus umbellatus (zhu ling)	Eliminated the cytotoxic activity of TNF in mice.	Haranaka et al., 1985a, 1985b
Poria cocos (fu ling)	Eliminated the cytotoxic activity of TNF in mice. Markedly suppressed cytokine production by human peripheral blood mononuclear cells. The herb suppressed production of TNF-alpha, IL-1-beta, IL-6, and GM-CSF.	Haranaka et al., 1985a, 1985b; Tseng and Chang, 1992
Saiboku To (formula)	The formula produced a steroid-sparing effect in asthmatic patients, and inhibited IgE production. IgE inhibition in mice was also reported. The formula suppressed the production of IL-2 in response to antigens in peripheral blood mononuclear cells from patients with bronchial asthma.	Nakajima et al., 1993; Nishiyori et al., 1985; Kabuki et al., 1990
Sophora flavescens (ku shen)	The alkaloid oxymatrine inhibited graft rejection of heart allografts in mice.	Qin et al., 1990
Trichosanthes kirilowii (tian hua fen)	Isolated proteins inhibited the mitogen-induced transformation of mouse spleen lymphocytes.	Yeung et al., 1987
Xiao Chai Hu Tang (formula)	Markedly reduced the cytotoxicity of TNF in mice.	Haranaka et al., 1985a, 1985b
Zhu Ling Tang (formula)	Markedly reduced the cytotoxicity of TNF in mice.	Haranaka et al., 1985a, 1985b

BOX 8.1. CLINICAL EFFECTS OF GLYCYRRHIZA SP.

Glycyrrhizic acid (glycyrrhizin) is a glycosylated saponin that occurs in licorice (*Glycyrrhiza sp., gan cao*) and is thought to be responsible for many of its pharmacologic effects. In the human intestine, bacteria efficiently hydrolyze glycyrrhizic acid to glycyrrhetinic acid, which is the primary active form. Licorice has been shown to exhibit antiulcer, antidiuretic, anti-inflammatory, antitumor, immunosuppressive, antispasmodic, antitussive, hepatoprotective, and antiviral actions (Baker, 1994; reviewed by Chang and But, 1986:304-17; reviewed by Zhang et al., 1990c).

The mechanism by which glycyrrhetinic acid achieves antidiuretic, antitumor, and anti-inflammatory actions appears to be due, in part, to inhibition of cortisol-degrading enzymes (reviewed by Walker and Edwards, 1994; Benediktsson and Edwards, 1994). Glycyrrhetinic acid, and to a lesser extent glycyrrhizic acid, inhibits 11β-hydroxy- steroid dehydrogenase (11β–OHSD), an enzyme present in most human tissues that catalyzes the conversion of cortisol to its inactive metabolites. Inhibition of this enzyme increases serum cortisol concentrations. Excess cortisol produces an anti-inflammatory action, and may inhibit the growth of leukemia and lymphoma cells by affecting glucocorticoid receptors sites on their plasma membranes.

Since both cortisol and the mineralocorticoid aldosterone exhibit similar affinities for mineralocorticoid receptors, a certain level of 11β–OHSD is necessary in mineralocorticoid-sensitive tissues, such as the kidneys, to prevent cortisol from competing effectively with aldosterone for binding sites. When bound to mineralocorticoid sites, cortisone acts as a potent mineralocorticoid and causes hypertension, edema, sodium retention, and other symptoms and signs of mineralocorticoid excess. Licorice is known to produce these effects.

The antiulcer effects of licorice can also be attributed, in part, to inhibition of an enzyme—in this case the enzyme that degrades PGE_2 (reviewed by Baker, 1994). Licorice inhibits the enzyme 15-hydroxyprostaglandin dehydrogenase, which converts PGE_2 to its inactive form. By inhibiting this enzyme, licorice causes a increase in local PGE_2 levels. In the stomach, PGE_2 plays a protective role against ulcer formation by promoting mucus secretion and cell proliferation. (Aspirin and other cyclooxygenase inhibitors can induce ulcers by inhibiting the production of PGE_2 in the stomach.)

In spite of its cortisol-like actions, licorice stimulates NK cell activity, induces interferon production, and inhibits suppressor T-cell activity (reviewed by Suzuki et al., 1992). The effectiveness of some antitumor drugs can be enhanced by administration of agents that inhibit suppressor T cells. Used alone, intraperitoneal administration of glycyrrhizin (20 mg/kg every three days) caused complete remission in 15% of Meth A tumor-bearing mice. Another 45% exhibited delayed tumor growth. At slightly lower dosages (10 mg/kg twice per week), glycyrrhizin significantly increased NK cell activity in tumor-bearing mice, although tumor growth was not affected (Tanaka, 1991).

These studies may be significant in that the dosages used can likely be achieved in humans without adverse effects. Although the antitumor effects of glycyrrhizin were not pronounced in the majority of mice, improved results may be possible by administering the herb daily and in combination with other anticancer therapies.

in Table 8.11 as inhibiting the immune system. This is not necessarily contradictory, since the immune system is complex, and natural agents (which are themselves complex) may affect the immune system in a multitude of ways. Another example of a well-known herb that produces seemingly contradictory effects on the immune system is *Glycyrrhiza sp. (gan cao)*. Glycyrrhiza is discussed in detail in Box 8.1.

8.6 SUMMARY

The human immune system functions along two separate, but interrelated, branches known as humoral immunity and cellular immunity. Cellular immunity includes the actions of T lymphocytes, NK cells, and macrophages, and is the branch most associated with

anticancer activity. The immune system may limit carcinogenesis by destroying newly transformed cells in a process known as immune surveillance, and may also limit the growth of established tumors, depending on their antigenicity and immunogenicity. The majority of human tumors exhibit high antigenicity but low immunogenicity, partly due to their ability to evade detection by producing blocking factors or by other mechanisms. Because of this, the human immune system is generally unable to produce cancer remissions without assistance. Assistance can consist of active or passive immunotherapy. However, even with immunotherapy, remission and cure rates have been rather low. New therapies and combinations of therapies may provide improved results in the future. A large number of natural agents may either stimulate or inhibit various aspects of the immune system, and some agents may be capable of doing both.

9

TREATMENT OF CANCER BY CONVENTIONAL MEDICINE

Surgery, radiotherapy, and cytotoxic chemotherapy are the three primary modalities used in conventional medicine to treat cancer. Surgery has been used as an anticancer treatment throughout this century, and radiotherapy and chemotherapy came into widespread use in the 1960s. This chapter focuses on chemotherapy. Of the three primary anticancer modalities, chemotherapy has the greatest similarity to the use of many natural agents. Because of this, the experience gained with chemotherapy is applicable to future research on natural agents.

9.1 TREATMENT MODALITIES
  9.1.1 Radiotherapy
  9.1.2 Surgery
  9.1.3 Chemotherapy
9.2 SURVIVAL AND MORTALITY
  9.2.1 Mortality Rates
  9.2.2 Relative Survival Rates
9.3 SUMMARY

9.1 TREATMENT MODALITIES

Treatment modalities, in general, can be divided into either local therapies or systemic therapies. Local therapies primarily consist of radiotherapy and surgery, and systemic therapy primarily consists of chemotherapy. Depending upon the type of cancer, tumors that are discovered before metastasis occurs can often be cured with localized treatment. However, early detection is rare for many cancers, and even relatively small tumors may metastasize. Many localized treatments fail because metastasis is undetected. Systemic treatment with chemotherapy is therefore widely used after local treatment, and in this context it is called adjuvant chemotherapy. A brief description of radiotherapy and surgery is provided below, and the remainder of this chapter is devoted to chemotherapy.

9.1.1 Radiotherapy

X rays were first discovered in 1895, and applications in oncology using crude equipment began almost immediately. In the wake of nuclear weapons research in the 1940s, medical radiation technology was rapidly refined, and by the late 1960s, modern radiotherapy was in widespread use.

Radiotherapy uses high-energy x rays, gamma rays, and electrons to damage the DNA of tumor cells. Radiation indirectly causes intercellular water molecules to ionize (split apart), resulting in the formation of free radicals such as superoxide. These radicals damage the DNA within targeted cells and can prevent them from proliferating or cause their death. However, the effects of radiation are not specific to tumor cells and adjacent healthy cells may also be damaged . For this reason, radiation is used primarily to treat localized tumors, rather than tumors that are disseminated. Due to the risk of damage to internal organs, radiotherapy is rarely used to treat tumors located within the abdominal cavity. The effects of administering antioxidants to patients undergoing radiotherapy are discussed in Appendix L.

Radiotherapy is a routine treatment for a number of early stage cancers. (See Box 9.1 for a discussion on staging systems.) These include Hodgkin's disease, neoplasms of the head and neck, brain tumors, lung cancer, esophageal cancer, cancers of the uterus and cervix, and breast cancer. Many of these can be cured with radiotherapy. Radiotherapy is also used as a palliative treatment in other cancers to reduce pain and temporarily inhibit tumor growth.

The direct side effects of radiation are generally limited to the area being treated. These may include lung fibrosis, pneumonitis, neurological abnormalities, dysphagia, colitis, enteritis, malabsorption, diarrhea, hepatitis, and sterility. However, systemic effects, such as fatigue, anorexia, nausea, and vomiting are not uncommon, especially in patients who receive extensive therapy. Secondary effects may follow. For example, gastrointestinal damage may lead to malnutrition and weight loss. Tissues tolerate only a limited amount of radiotherapy, and commonly scar at therapeutic doses. Because of this, treatment of cancers that recur in the same location often is not possible.

One of the long-term side effects of radiotherapy is increased risk of developing a second cancer. Damage to the DNA of healthy cells can greatly increase the probability of neoplastic transformation. Patients who receive radiotherapy may incur a two- to threefold increase in the

---

BOX 9.1. STAGING SYSTEMS

Staging systems are used to describe the extent of progression of a patient's cancer. Several staging systems have been developed, each more or less suitable for a particular type of cancer. The most commonly used staging system is the TNM system, discussed below. Staging systems have been modified over the years as the body of knowledge on cancer has expanded and as international standardization of staging systems has been developed.

The TNM system is anatomically based and derives its name from Tumor-Nodes-Metastasis. The T designation describes the tumor itself (size, location, and potential for invasion). The N designation describes the involvement of regional lymph nodes. The M designation describes the extent of distant metastasis. The TNM system is customized for each type of cancer. For example, in staging stomach cancer, $T_3N_0M_{IHEP}$ describes a cancer in which the primary tumor has penetrated through the stomach lining without invading contiguous structures, no metastasis has spread to regional lymph nodes, and distant metastasis has spread to the liver. Often, TNM stages are condensed into the stages I, II, III, and IV, in order of increasing extent of disease. For example, stage III stomach cancer is less advanced than stage IV stomach cancer.

---

risk of developing secondary cancers. In patients treated intensively with chemotherapy and radiotherapy, the risk of secondary cancers may be as much as 1,000 times greater than normal (reviewed by Calabresi and Schein, 1993:362).

9.1.2 Surgery

Surgery has been used to treat cancer for thousands of years. Today, surgery can often cure localized tumors, depending on the type of cancer. However, many tumors do not lend themselves to surgical cures, either because they are not accessible (such as brain cancers), are not solid tumors that can be removed (such as leukemias), or they are solid tumors that have already metastasized.

Surgery can either be radical, in which a significant amount of surrounding tissue is removed along with the tumor, or conservative, in which only known tumor tissue is removed. In some cases, radical surgery is no more successful than conservative surgery, since a tumor may have metastasized prior to the surgery. This is particularly true for breast cancer, where the trend has been, and continues to be, toward more conservative surgery.

9.1.3 Chemotherapy

Physicians began to use cytotoxic drugs in treating cancer after they observed radiation-like damage in the cells of soldiers exposed to mustard gas. The modern era of chemotherapy began in 1945 when a patient with lymphoma responded to treatment with nitrogen mustard. Many of the chemotherapy agents in common use today were developed in the 1950s and 1960s. Currently, about 35 cytotoxic drugs are licensed for use in North America. As a whole, these agents are cytotoxins that are not specific to cancer cells, but rather target those cells that are rapidly dividing. Recent advances, however, may revolutionize the methods by which cancer is treated. Some of the chemotherapy agents being developed in the 1990s represent a new class of drugs. These agents either specifically target tumor cells or specifically target the newly discovered mechanisms by which tumors grow. Antiangiogenic agents are an example of this new approach. This new generation of anticancer drugs has the potential to act with far greater efficacy and with far fewer side effects. Any number of the natural agents discussed in this book could be among the new agents developed, or could be models on which to develop new agents.

Used alone, chemotherapy provides a cure for a limited number of cancers. Impressive results have been obtained in treating childhood leukemias, however, only about 2% of cancer deaths occur in patients under the age of 30. In adult cancers, chemotherapy has markedly reduced mortality rates for patients with Hodgkin's disease, lymphoma, ovarian cancer, testicular cancer, and a few other, more rare, cancers. As an adjuvant, chemotherapy also provides some clinical benefit in treating breast, colon, and small cell lung cancer. See Table 9.1 for a summary of the responses of various cancers to chemotherapy.

The fact that cytotoxic chemotherapy is not a panacea has great significance for researchers investigating natural agents. In the past, most research on natural anticancer agents in the United States has been devoted to identifying and testing cytotoxic agents. The experience with cytotoxic therapies suggests that research may be more productive if a portion of available resources are directed to the study of natural agents that act by noncytotoxic mechanisms. These mechanisms may include induction of apoptosis or differentiation; inhibition of metastasis, invasion, or angiogenesis; and modulation of the immune system.

CANCER AND NATURAL MEDICINE

TABLE 9.1. THE RESPONSE OF VARIOUS CANCERS TO CHEMOTHERAPY	
ACTIVITY	**CANCER**
Major activity	Acute lymphocytic leukemia, acute myelogenous leukemia, breast*, choriocarcinoma, embryonal rhabdomyosarcoma*, Ewing's sarcoma*, hairy cell leukemia, Hodgkin's disease, small cell lung, Burkitt's lymphoma, diffuse large cell lymphoma, osteogenic sarcoma*, testicular, Wilms' tumor
Moderate activity	Adrenocortical carcinoma, bladder, brain (glioblastoma and medulloblastoma), cervical, chronic lymphocytic leukemia, chronic myelogenous leukemia, endometrial, gastric, head and neck (squamous cell), islet cell carcinoma, Kaposi's sarcoma, mycosis fungoides, myeloma, neuroblastoma, follicular lymphoma
Minor activity	Colorectal, liver, non-small cell lung, melanoma, pancreatic, renal

* Major activity only when combined with surgery, radiotherapy, or both.
Source: Wilson et al., 1991: 1594-97

Mechanism of Action

As mentioned above, cytotoxic agents target those cells that are rapidly dividing.[1] Since cancer cells tend to divide more rapidly than most normal cells, cancer cells are the ones most affected. However, normal cells with a high proliferation rate suffer the same consequences. Rapidly proliferating cells include those from hair follicles, gastrointestinal lining, bone marrow, ovaries, and testicles. This accounts for the common side effects of cytotoxic chemotherapy, such as hair loss, nausea, digestive impairment, immunosuppression, hematological complications, and infertility. Tissues with slower proliferation rates, such as the lung, liver, kidney, endocrine glands, and the lining of the blood vessels, are less susceptible. Tissues with very low proliferation rates, such as the muscles, bones, cartilage, and nerves, are rarely affected.

Cytotoxic drugs interfere with cell mitosis. The mitotic cell cycle can be divided into four phases (see Figure 9.1):

1) A synthesis phase *(S)*, during which DNA, RNA, and proteins are synthesized in preparation for mitosis.
2) A resting or gap phase *(G1)*, during which no mitotic activity occurs.
3) A mitotic phase *(M)*, during which cells divide.
4) A second gap phase *(G2)*.

Cell-cycle-specific agents interrupt the cell cycle during either the synthesis or mitosis phase. Cell-cycle-

nonspecific agents interrupt the cell cycle regardless of which phase the cell is in.

Cells spend most of their lifetime in the two gap phases. Cell-cycle-specific agents are used primarily against rapidly proliferating cancers, such as leukemias, since cells from these cancers enter the *S* or *M* phases more frequently than do cells of slow-growing cancers. Cell-cycle-nonspecific agents are used primarily against slow-growing cancers, such as most solid tumors.

Chemotherapy agents can be divided into the following six categories (see Table 9.2 for indications):

• *Alkylating agents* replace hydrogen atoms in DNA with highly reactive alkyl radicals, causing cross-linking or abnormal pairing of the double strands of

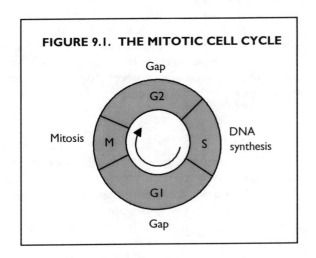

FIGURE 9.1. THE MITOTIC CELL CYCLE

[1] The development of chemotherapy agents that destroy fast-growing cells grew directly out of the use of mouse tumor cell lines in drug-screening assays. Fast-growing mouse tumor lines provide quick turn-around time and minimize animal handling costs. The agents most effective against these cell lines are also most effective against fast-growing human tumors. However, the majority of solid cancers in humans grow relatively slowly, and therefore do not respond well to these agents.

82

DNA molecules. This prevents the tightly bound strands from separating during mitosis. Alkylating agents also react with sulfur, phosphate, and amine groups causing multiple lesions in both dividing and nondividing cells. Therefore, alkylating agents are cell-cycle-nonspecific. Alkylating agents derived from mustard gas were the first cytotoxic anticancer drugs developed.

- *Mitotic inhibitors* interfere with microtubule formation during the *M* phase. Microtubules are elongated tubular structures in the cell that transport substances and help the cell to maintain its structure. Microtubules increase in number during mitosis and assist the duplicate chromosomes in moving to opposite poles of the cell prior to cell division. Mitotic inhibitors include the plant products vincristine and vinblastine (from *Vinca rosea*), and taxanes (from *Taxus brevifolia*). Taxanes inhibit microtubule depolymerization. Agents that inhibit topoisomerase also belong to this category. Topoisomerase I and II

are intracellular enzymes that facilitate the relaxation of supercoiled DNA prior to DNA duplication.

- *Antimetabolites* interfere with various metabolic processes by substituting for other constituents in the formation of cellular compounds and by inhibiting key enzymes. They disrupt nucleic acid synthesis and are specific to the *S* phase.
- *Antibiotics* are drugs isolated from fungal species and are classified solely by their origin. They act by a variety of mechanisms.
- *Hormones* provide a variety of actions. Glucocorticoids suppress lymphocyte proliferation and are used in treating lymphomas and lymphocytic leukemias. Estrogens, androgens, or their inhibitors interfere with hormone receptors on the plasma membrane of tumor cells and are used in treating breast, prostate, and other cancers.
- *Miscellaneous agents* act by a variety of toxic mechanisms other than those specified above.

TABLE 9.2. INDICATIONS FOR COMMON CHEMOTHERAPY DRUGS		
CATEGORY	**AGENT**	**PARTIAL LIST OF INDICATIONS**
DNA alkylating agents: Nitrogen mustards	Cyclophosphamide (Cytoxan)	Lymphomas, Hodgkin's disease, leukemias, breast cancer, ovarian cancer
	Mechlorethamine (Nitrogen mustard; NH_2)	Hodgkin's disease when combined with other agents (MOPP)
	Melphalan (Phenylalanine mustard; L-PAM)	Multiple myeloma, ovarian carcinoma
	Chlorambucil (Leukeran)	Hodgkin's disease when combined with other agents (ChVPP); palliative treatment of leukemias and lymphomas
	Ifosfamide (Ifex)	Testicular cancers
DNA alkylating agents: Nitrosoureas	Carmustine (BCNU)	Palliative treatment of brain tumors, multiple myeloma, Hodgkin's disease, and lymphoma
	Lomustine (CCNU)	Brain tumors, Hodgkin's disease
	Streptozocin (Zanosar)	Endocrine cancers
DNA alkylating agents: Others	Busulfan	Palliative treatment of myelogenous leukemia; included in bone marrow transplant regime
	Thiotepa (Triethylenethiophosphamide; TSPA)	Adenocarcinoma of breast and ovary, superficial bladder cancer
	Cisplatin (CDDP)	Testicular, ovarian, lung, head and neck, and bladder cancers
	Carboplatin	Ovarian cancer and other diseases that respond to platinum
Mitotic inhibitors: Topoisomerase inhibitors	Etoposide	Testicular cancer, lymphomas, lung cancer
	Teniposide	Acute leukemia
Mitotic inhibitors: Microtubule inhibitors *(column continues)*	Vincristine (VCR; LCR)	Acute leukemia, Hodgkin's disease, lymphoma, neuroblastoma, Wilm's tumor
	Vinblastine (VLB)	Lymphomas, testicular carcinoma, Hodgkin's disease, Kaposi's sarcoma, breast cancer
(Table continues)		

	TABLE 9.2. *(continued)*	
CATEGORY	**AGENT**	**INDICATIONS**
Mitotic inhibitors *(continued)*	Taxol	Leukemia; breast, ovarian, and possibly other solid tumors
Antimetabolites	Methotrexate (MTX)	Acute lymphocytic leukemia, choriocarcinoma, breast cancer, lung cancer, lymphomas, bladder cancer
	5-Fluorouracil (5-FU)	Carcinoma of the colon, rectum, breast, stomach, and pancreas
	Cytarabine (Cytosine Arabinoside; ARA-C)	Acute myelogenous leukemia
	Mercaptopurine (6-Mercaptopurine; 6-MP)	Acute myelogenous leukemia
	Thioguanine (6-Thioguanine; TG)	Acute myelogenous leukemia
Antibiotics	Bleomycin Sulfate (BLM)	Squamous cell carcinoma, lymphomas, testicular carcinoma
	Dactinomycin (Actinomycin D; ACT)	Wilm's tumor, choriocarcinoma, testicular carcinoma, Ewing's sarcoma
	Doxorubicin (Adriamycin, ADR)	Acute leukemia, Wilm's tumor, neuroblastoma, sarcomas, breast, ovarian, gastric, thyroid, and bladder carcinoma, lymphomas, bronchogenic carcinoma, Hodgkin's disease
	Mitomycin (Mitomycin-C; MTC)	Adenocarcinoma of pancreas or stomach; colon, lung, and breast cancer
	Fludarabine (Fludara)	B-cell chronic lymphocytic leukemia
Hormones: Estrogens	Diethylstilbestrol diphosphate	Palliative treatment of advanced prostate carcinoma
Hormones: Antiestrogens	Tamoxifen	Estrogen receptor positive breast cancer, uterine cancer
Hormones: Androgens	Testolactone	Breast cancer (inhibits aromatase activity)
Hormones: Antiandrogens	Flutamide	Prostatic cancer
Hormones: Progestins	Megestrol Acetate	Palliative treatment of breast or endometrial cancer
Hormones: Gonadotropin-releasing hormone analogs	Leuprolide	Advanced prostate cancer (LH-RH agonist)
Hormones: Glucocorticoids	Cortisone	Leukemia and lymphoma
Miscellaneous Agents	Mitotane (op'DD)	Adrenocortical carcinoma
	Hydroxyurea	Chronic granulocytic leukemia
	Procarbazine (N-Methylhydrazine; MIH)	Hodgkin's disease, brain tumors

Modified from Olin et al., 1993:2462-2594

Side Effects of Chemotherapy Agents

Cytotoxic chemotherapy agents can cause a host of adverse effects, ranging from short-term, self-limiting adverse reactions to death. Many chemotherapy agents are themselves carcinogenic, or may increase the risk of secondary tumors due to immunosuppression. For example, a 2 to 12% incidence of acute leukemia has been observed 2 to 10 years after treatment of Hodgkin's disease with chemotherapy (reviewed by Calabresi and Schein, 1993:413). A more detailed description of the adverse effects of chemotherapy is provided by Olin et al. (1993:2462-594).

Clinical Use

Cytotoxic chemotherapy drugs are generally more effective if combined with one another. A clinically detectable tumor may contain more than one billion reproducing cells. Such a large and heterogeneous population generates drug resistant variants. Single-agent chemotherapy can result in the survival and subsequent proliferation of resistant populations. Combination chemotherapy lessens the chance that resistant populations will escape destruction. An example of combination chemotherapy is the MOPP regime, used to treat Hodgkin's disease. It consists of the following agents:

- Mechlorethamine: 6 mg/m^2 intravenous, days 1 and 8
- Vincristine: 1.4 mg/m^2 intravenous, days 1 and 8
- Procarbazine: 100 mg/m^2 orally, days 1 through 14
- Prednisone: 40 mg/m^2/day orally, days 1 through 14

The above regime is repeated every 28 days for a minimum of 6 cycles. There are at least 54 other commonly used regimes for various cancers (see Olin et al., 1993:2464).

9.2 SURVIVAL AND MORTALITY

The limits of cytotoxic chemotherapy began to be apparent in the 1980s with the publication of several critical reviews. In 1980, Powles et al. reported that overall survival of patients with breast cancer had not improved in the preceding 10 years and that chemotherapy may even have shortened survival in some patients. In 1985, Cairns stated that "Apart from the success with Hodgkin's disease, childhood leukemia, and a few other cancers, it is not possible to detect any sudden change in death rates for any of the major cancers that could be credited to chemotherapy." Similarly, in 1986, Bailar and Smith from the Harvard School of Public Health and the University of Iowa Medical Center stated, "The main conclusion we draw is that some 35 years of intense effort focused largely on improving treatment must be judged a qualified failure."

Today, the limitations of cytotoxic chemotherapy are not disputed by most oncologists. Based on the knowledge gained over the last four decades, there are cases where chemotherapy is clearly indicated, cases where it is clearly not indicated, and cases where its use is a matter of judgment. Some critics contend that chemotherapy is overprescribed in this latter group of patients (see Braverman, 1991) but, as in other fields, gross errors in judgment are not the norm for good practitioners.

To better understand the successes and failures of chemotherapy, it is useful to review cancer mortality rates and relative survival rates. These are discussed in the following sections.

9.2.1 Mortality Rates

The mortality rate is the ratio between the number of deaths attributed to cancer and the number of deaths due to all other causes. Cancer-related mortality data for the United States has been readily available since 1950 with the advent of national cancer registries. Statistics prior

to about 1955 represent patients who received surgery and possibly radiation therapy, but probably not chemotherapy. Modern radiotherapy and chemotherapy were not applied widely until about 1965 (Calabresi and Schein, 1993:605).

Mortality rates in the chemotherapy era have gone up.[2] Between the years 1950 and 1989, the age- and population-adjusted mortality rate for all races, males and females increased 10%. Overall, the advent of chemotherapy has not greatly affected mortality rates. Figures 9.2 and 9.3 show trends in mortality rates from various cancers from 1930 to 1990 for males and females respectively. However, to more clearly analyze trends in mortality, mortality must be examined in relation to trends in incidence. The incidence rate for most cancers has increased during the last 40 years. Changes in incidence rates for various cancers between the years 1950 and 1989 are shown in Figure 9.4. An analysis of mortality and incidence trends for selected cancers is provided below:

Melanoma. As can be seen from Figure 9.4, the incidence of melanoma in the white population increased 321% since 1950—more than that for any other cancer. The causes of the drastic increase in melanoma are not well understood, although increased exposure to the sun and artificial tanning devices may play a role. Depletion of the earth's ozone layer may have an impact on future incidence rates, but as yet, research has not correlated depletion of the polar ozone layer with an increase in ultraviolet radiation in the U.S., and therefore, the past rise in melanoma has not been attributed to damage to the ozone layer. In the white population, mortality from melanoma has increased 152% since 1950. The difference between the high increase in incidence and the relatively lower increase in mortality is due primarily to increased early detection. This contributes to a greater percentage of cures (small localized tumors can be successfully cured with surgery).

Lung cancer. Lung cancer has the second highest increase in incidence (263%), which is primarily due to delayed results of past increases in the number of people smoking cigarettes, particularly women. Mortality in white males and females has kept pace by increasing 245%.[3] These comparable increases reflect the inability of current therapies to cure lung cancer. The 44% increase in all-cancer incidence and the 10% increase in all-cancer mortality since 1950 can be attributed, in large part, to tremendous increases in lung cancer incidence. Although the incidence for melanoma has grown faster than that of lung cancer, the prevalence of lung cancer is much greater.

---

[2] The source mortality and survival data for Section 9.2 is the National Cancer Institute (Miller et al., 1992) unless stated otherwise.

[3] Mortality rates for males began to decrease slightly starting around 1990.

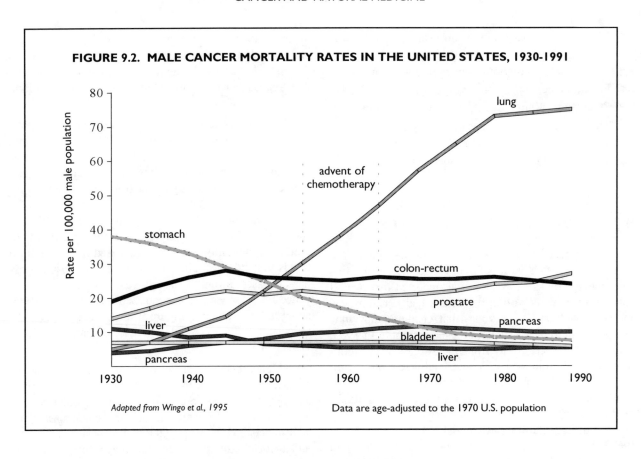

FIGURE 9.2. MALE CANCER MORTALITY RATES IN THE UNITED STATES, 1930-1991

Adapted from Wingo et al., 1995

Data are age-adjusted to the 1970 U.S. population

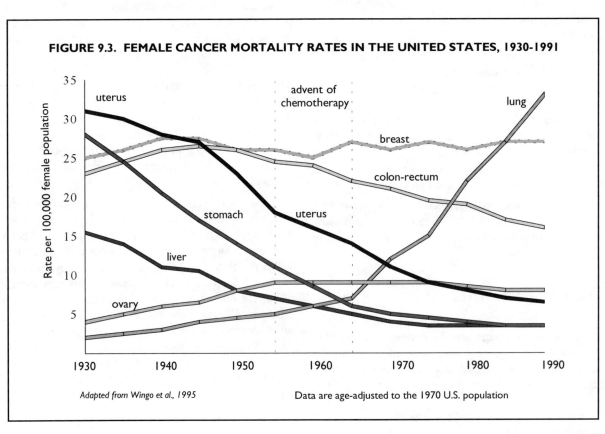

FIGURE 9.3. FEMALE CANCER MORTALITY RATES IN THE UNITED STATES, 1930-1991

Adapted from Wingo et al., 1995

Data are age-adjusted to the 1970 U.S. population

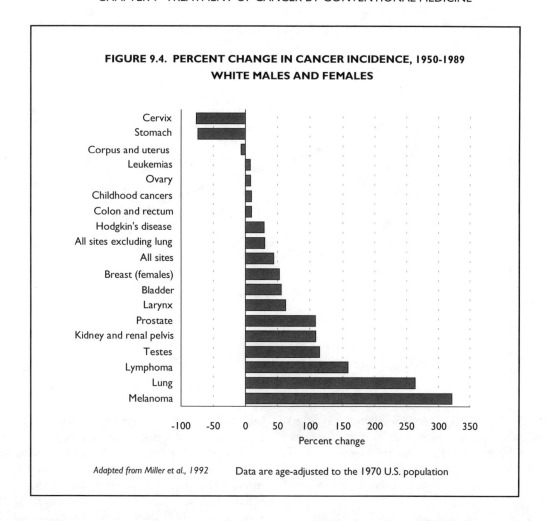

**FIGURE 9.4. PERCENT CHANGE IN CANCER INCIDENCE, 1950-1989
WHITE MALES AND FEMALES**

Percent change

Adapted from Miller et al., 1992   Data are age-adjusted to the 1970 U.S. population

Stomach cancer. Since 1950, the incidence of stomach cancer has decreased by 73% in the white population. The reasons for this decline are uncertain, but increased access to refrigeration, decreased use of salt, and the addition of vitamin C to nitrite-containing products are all suspected. Mortality rates have kept pace, declining by 76%.

Cervical cancer. The incidence of cervical cancer has declined 76% since 1950 in the white population, primarily due to improved standards of living and a high rate of hysterectomies. Although incidence rates are going down, early detection has improved due to the use of PAP smears. Mortality from cervical cancer has declined by 74%, mostly as a result of successful local treatment of preneoplastic lesions, early detection of neoplastic lesions, and decreasing incidence.

Colorectal cancer. The incidence of colorectal cancer has increased 10% since 1950 in the white population, and mortality has decreased by 25%. The difference between these rates may be due to better diagnostic procedures and improvements in surgical treatment. Further decreases in mortality are expected following widespread application of effective adjuvant chemotherapy.

Prostate cancer: The incidence of prostate cancer has increased 108% in the white population since 1950, in part, due to improved diagnostic techniques. Mortality rates have increased approximately 23% (Wingo et al., 1995). The difference between the two rates is due to greater surgical and radiological cure rates with early diagnosis.

9.2.2 Relative Survival Rates

Bailar and Smith (1986) argue that age-adjusted mortality rates are the single best indicator of success of treatment. Other measures—in particular, relative survival rates—are more problematic. Survival rate, often reported as the five-year relative survival rate, is the ratio between the observed survival of the cancer patients and the expected survival of the general population measured after five years. As such, it is always higher than the observed survival rate.

Figure 9.5 shows the difference between observed and relative survival rates based on data for female colon cancer patients in Norway in the 1950s and 1960s, prior to the advent of chemotherapy (Cairns, 1985). The data

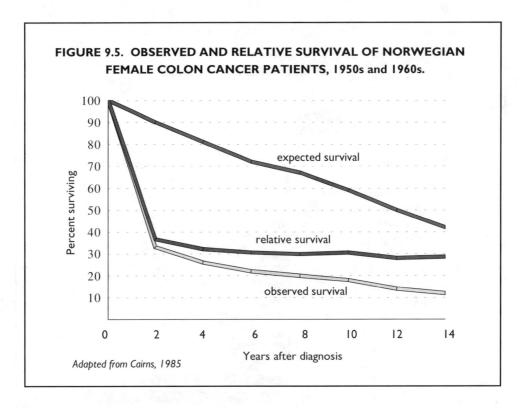

FIGURE 9.5. OBSERVED AND RELATIVE SURVIVAL OF NORWEGIAN FEMALE COLON CANCER PATIENTS, 1950s and 1960s.

expected survival

relative survival

observed survival

Percent surviving

Years after diagnosis

Adapted from Cairns, 1985

indicate that almost 70% of the female colon cancer patients died within 2 years. However, the data also shows that the remaining 30% died at approximately the same rate as the general population. That is, having cancer did not limit the life span of a significant minority of patients.

A plot of the relative survival rate that parallels the horizontal axis signifies that the mortality rate is the same as that for the general population. Not all cancers show this pattern of leveling (see Appendix H).

Prostate cancer provides a good example of the complications involved in interpreting relative survival rates. In the United States, 25% of all males over the age of 70 who have died from other causes can be shown on autopsy to have small cancers of the prostate. However, fewer than 10% of these would have grown to a size that produces symptoms. With improved diagnostic techniques and screening programs, the number of new prostate cancers discovered has increased, but these new cases include many that would never have actually produced symptoms or fatality. Accordingly, five-year survival rates for prostate cancer have increased from 43% to 77% between 1950 and 1985.

Early detection increases survival rates for any cancer. For example, breast cancer mortality rates in the white population have not changed appreciably since 1950 (they have increased 5%). Incidence rates have risen 52% and five-year survival rates have increased about 20% (from 60% to 79%). The rise in five-year survival rates is due primarily to improvements in screening programs, which increases the chances for early diagnosis and cure, and to a lesser extent, improvements in chemotherapy. If a cancer is detected an average of six months earlier than in the past, more women will live through the first five years because they started with smaller tumors. In addition to increasing relative survival rates, early diagnosis also increases incidence rates. Early detection of breast cancer results in an additional population of women with small lesions, who are, therefore, identified as having cancer.

With these issues in mind, Figure 9.6 illustrates the changes in relative five-year survival rates between 1950 and 1988. As shown, five-year survival rates increased for all cancers during this period. The maximum increase was 60% (from 19% to 79%) for bladder cancer, and the minimum increase was 4% (from 12% to 16%) for stomach cancer. The increase in survival for bladder cancer is due primarily to improved detection and improved surgical techniques. Transurethral resection and fulguration of the bladder (TURB) can produce relative five-year survival rates as high as 77% for stage I disease, the stage during which many bladder cancers are detected.

Appendix C provides additional data on current incidence rates, mortality rates, five-year relative survival rates, and median age at diagnosis and death for a variety of cancers.

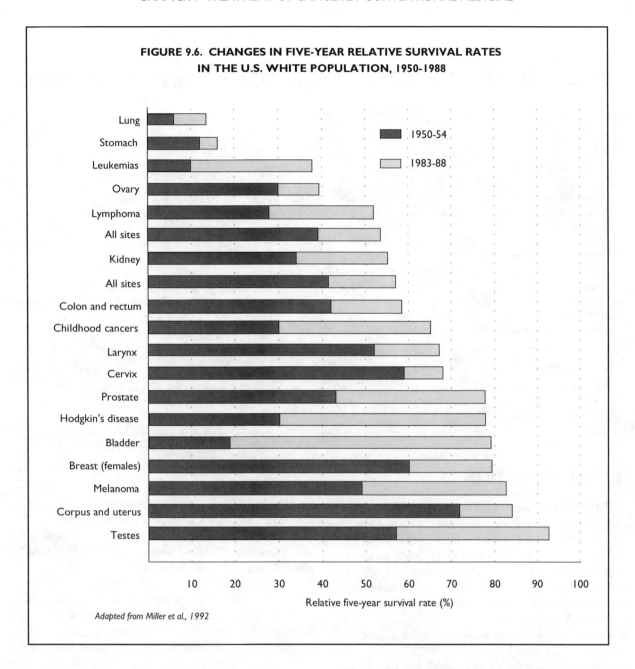

FIGURE 9.6. CHANGES IN FIVE-YEAR RELATIVE SURVIVAL RATES IN THE U.S. WHITE POPULATION, 1950-1988

Adapted from Miller et al., 1992

9.3 SUMMARY

The three primary therapies used to treat cancer are surgery, radiotherapy, and chemotherapy. Of these, chemotherapy is most similar to the use of many natural agents. Although cytotoxic chemotherapy is able to produce cures or increase survival in a number of childhood cancers and in some adult cancers, it is not highly effective in a majority of common adult cancers.

The experience gained with cytotoxic chemotherapy is valuable for investigators of natural agents. The limited, although important, success of cytotoxic chemotherapy suggests that research on natural agents may be most fruitful if it is divided between the search for new cytotoxic agents (especially tumor-specific cytotoxic agents) and the search for agents that act through noncytotoxic mechanisms.

10
THE THEORY OF TRADITIONAL CHINESE MEDICINE

Many of the natural agents discussed in this book are Chinese herbs, and this chapter is intended to aid the reader in understanding their traditional use. Chinese medicine views disease from a fundamentally different vantage point than that of conventional medicine. This view does not contradict conventional medical theory, but rather complements it in the same way that a northern view of a building complements a southern view. One of the strengths of Chinese medical theory is that it affords insight into the relationships between disparate signs and symptoms. It provides unifying theories with which to view the body, the emotions, and the spirit as a whole.

10.1 INTRODUCTION

The roots of Chinese medicine reach back more than 2,500 years to shamanistic healers of the early Zhou Dynasty (1100 to 403 B.C.). In the later Zhou Dynasty (403 to 221 B.C.), the ideas of Taoism and Confucianism developed, along with the concepts of *yin-yang* duality and the Five Phases.[1] All of these have a great impact on the current practice of Chinese medicine. The first major materia medica, the *Shen Nong Ben Cao Jing (Divine Husbandman's Classic of the Materia Medica)* was written in the latter Han Dynasty (25 to 220 A.D.). The foundations of modern Chinese medicine theory were firmly established by the seventh century A.D., with the compilation of the cornerstone work, *Huang Ti Nei Ching (Yellow Emperor's Classic On Internal Medicine)*, by Yang Shang-Shan and other unknown authors from the second century B.C. to the seventh century A.D.

Since its conception, Chinese medicine has evolved dynamically as new techniques, theories, and medicinal substances have been incorporated and inferior ones have been eliminated. Evolution continues to this day with the current emphasis in China on integrating conventional and Chinese medicine. Nevertheless, throughout the last 1,400 years the basic core of Chinese medicine has remained surprisingly stable.

The term Traditional Chinese Medicine (TCM) actually refers to a rather recent evolutionary stage. The Communist Chinese government made a decision in the 1940s to promote China's native medicine rather than replace it entirely with Western conventional medicine. Before this time, the knowledge to practice Chinese medicine passed from generation to generation informally by family lineage, rather than through formal instruction at universities. Each lineage stressed different aspects, causing differences to exist between lineages. In the 1940s committees appointed by the Communist government conducted a survey of the entire tradition, deleted what they believed was superfluous, and standardized the rest. The term Traditional Chinese Medicine refers to this reorganized system. Although some elements were lost during the reorganization, overall it has fostered a consistency in practice and teaching that has allowed TCM to flourish internationally.

TCM was introduced to the United States in 1971 when *New York Times* correspondent James Reston was successfully treated for postsurgical pain after having his appendix removed while on assignment in China. Since that time, TCM has grown rapidly in the United States.

---

[1] This period is called the Warring States due to the bitter and widespread warfare between feudal lords that preceded the unification of China in the Qin Dynasty (221 to 206 B.C.).

Currently there are over 25 colleges of Oriental medicine that are accredited or soon to be accredited by the National Accreditation Commission for Schools and Colleges of Acupuncture and Oriental Medicine (NAC-SCAOM). Seventeen of these offer masters degrees. Doctorate programs are expected to begin by 1996. Approximately 30 states now license practitioners of acupuncture and oriental medicine. The majority of these states require that applicants successfully complete the acupuncture competency exam administered by the National Commission for the Certification of Acupuncturists (NCCA) or an equivalent exam. The NCCA has also recently developed a national competency exam covering the practice of herbal medicine.

Traditional Chinese Medicine includes the modalities of acupuncture, herbal medicine, moxibustion (heat therapy), *tui na* (massage), *qi gong* (exercises for internal energy), diet therapy, and meditation. In addition to TCM, other traditions exist within acupuncture and Oriental medicine. For example, the Japanese have developed their own system, and specific schools of thought within China have developed their own systems. This chapter addresses Chinese medicine within the framework of TCM.

The theory of Traditional Chinese Medicine differs significantly from that of conventional medicine. Conventional medicine tends to emphasize the biochemical and cellular aspects of pathology, whereas TCM emphasizes the macroscopic relationships present between different bodily systems. TCM views the body, mind, and spirit as interconnected. Any change in one part of the organism necessarily affects the whole.

10.2 ELEMENTS OF TRADITIONAL CHINESE MEDICINE

To understand Traditional Chinese Medicine, it is first necessary to understand some of the basic terms and concepts it uses. Major terms and concepts include the *eight principles, qi, blood, phlegm, toxins,* the *twelve channels,* and the *twelve organs.*[2] Each of these are defined in the following sections.[3]

10.2.1 The *Eight Principles*

The *eight principles* provide a structure by which to group related symptoms and are the foundation for diagnosis of symptom patterns in TCM. The *eight principles* are:

- *Internal* or *external*
- *Vacuous* or *replete*
- *Yin* or *yang*
- *Hot* or *cold*

A symptom pattern is classified as *internal* if the *organs* are affected, and *external* if the superficial layers of the body (such as the muscles) are affected. A pattern is classified as *replete* if it is due to a problem of local or systemic excess (such as the excess heat of a high fever), or *vacuous* if it is due to a problem of local or systemic deficiency (such as deficient *blood,* which can manifest as anemia). The remaining four principles are discussed below.

Yin and Yang

The concepts of *yin* and *yang* have played a fundamental role in Chinese philosophy since at least 700 B.C. and form a theoretical cornerstone of TCM. *Yin* and *yang* can be thought of as a set of qualities that exist in opposition to, yet in support of, one another. *Yin* qualities can be conceived of as cooling, moistening, nutritive, and quiet. *Yang* qualities, on the other hand, can be conceived of as warming, drying, energetic, and active. They are opposites of each other, yet they complement and balance each other. Indeed, they cannot exist without one another. To enjoy good health, *yin* and *yang* must be in dynamic balance. For example, rest must follow activity, and coolness holds back heat. *Yin* and *yang* are always in motion. They support each other and transform into each other.

In relationship to disease, there are four imbalances of *yin* and *yang.* These imbalances can cause a disease, or alternately, the imbalances can result from disease. The imbalances are *vacuity* of *yin* or *yang,* and *repletion* of *yin* or *yang.* These four imbalances are illustrated in Figure 10.1.

Chinese medicine generally views the balance between *yin* and *yang* as it occurs within the *organs.* Therefore, one can speak of the *lung yin vacuity* or *liver yang repletion. Yin* and *yang* will be discussed again under the topic of internal *organs* below.

Hot and Cold

Hot and *cold* refer to temperature abnormalities associated with a symptom pattern. Signs of *cold* in the body can include fixed pain, numbness, stiffness, sluggishness, chill, lack of thirst, a pale or purple tongue body, a white tongue coat, and a slow pulse. *Cold*

---

[2] TCM gives specialized meaning to some common conventional terms. To distinguish between the common usage and the TCM usage, all references to the specialized TCM terms are italicized. Terms in Pinyin are also italicized.

[3] The sources for the information in this chapter are Maciocia (1989) and Zmiewski and Feit (1989) unless stated otherwise.

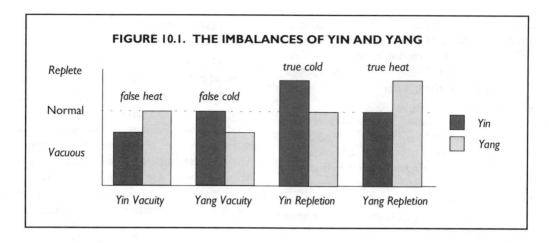

FIGURE 10.1. THE IMBALANCES OF YIN AND YANG

symptoms can occur in the patterns of either *yin reple-tion* or *yang vacuity*. In the former, there is an excess of cooling energies, and the *cold* is called *true cold* (see Figure 10.1). In the later, there is a lack of warming energies, and the *cold* is called *false cold*. Patterns of *true cold* and *false cold* are similar in that they may have many of the same symptoms (chill, slow pulse, and so on), but differ in that they also exhibit symptoms that are specific to *yin repletion* and *yang vacuity* respectively. For example, in addition to general *cold* symptoms, a patient with *yin repletion* will exhibit symptoms of *repletion*, such as a strong pulse and acute onset of symptoms. In contrast, a patient with *yang vacuity* will exhibit general symptoms of *cold*, and also symptoms of *vacuity*, such as a weak pulse and slow onset of symptoms.

Signs of *heat* in the body can include bleeding disorders (hot blood becomes "reckless" and spills out of the vessels), fever, thirst, infection, redness, a red tongue body, a yellow tongue coat, and a fast pulse. *Heat* is associated with the patterns of *yang repletion* and *yin vacuity*. In *yang repletion* there is an excess of *heat*, and it is called *true heat*. In *yin vacuity* there is an deficiency of cooling energies and the *heat* is called *false heat*. *False heat* is like the heat that forms when a tea kettle is left on the stove until all the water (the *yin* fluid) boils out. Once the water evaporates, the pot gets extremely hot, even though the heat of the burner has not increased. The *false heat* of *yin vacuity* tends to manifest most during the *yin* hours (the evening and nighttime). Table 10.1 provides a list of symptoms that distinguish *true cold* from *false cold*, and *true heat* from *false heat*.

10.2.2 *Qi*

Energy, or vital force, is called *qi* (pronounced "chee") in TCM. Energy and matter are viewed as a continuum, rather than as opposites; as energy condenses it becomes matter. There are at least 15 different types of *qi* that are important in Chinese medicine. These include

the *qi* of each *organ (zangfu zhi qi)*, the *qi* that circulates in the *twelve channels (jingluo qi)*, the *qi* of food and air *(gu qi* and *da qi)*, and the defensive *qi (zheng qi)* that protects the body from pathologic or *evil qi (xie qi)*. *Zheng qi* is similar in some respects to the immune system.

Because the nature of energy is motion, healthy *qi* is never stagnant. This point is very important, for the stagnation of *qi* is one of the primary causes of disease. Among other things, *stagnant qi* causes pain. An axiom in TCM equates stagnation with pain. In other words, the cause of pain is stagnation.

There are three sources of *qi* in the body. They are the *qi* passed on to us from our parents that is stored in the *kidneys*, called *prenatal qi (yuan qi)*; the *qi* we obtain from the air we breathe; and the *qi* we obtain from the food we eat. Although the latter two can be replenished through proper living habits, the *yuan qi* cannot be replenished.

Yuan qi is closely related to congenital essence, called *jing*. *Jing* can be thought of as the potential energies obtained through inheritance, and *yuan qi* can be thought of as actualized *jing*. Our parents provide us with a limited supply of *jing*, and once it is used up our life is over. *Jing* can be likened to a car battery. It provides the spark to start the engine, but is exhausted quickly if the engine runs on it. If we do not obtain adequate *qi* from air and food, or we burn energy faster than we replenish it, we will begin to draw more *qi* from our *jing* stores. To conserve the loss of *jing*, one must maintain healthy eating and breathing habits, obtain adequate rest, and not waste *qi* on unproductive thoughts, actions, or emotions. The aging process is closely related to the slow loss of *jing*.

Qi has many functions in the body. General functions and examples of each are listed below:

- *Qi* transforms. For example, *stomach qi* transforms food into nutrients (see Box 10.1).

BOX 10.1. DIGESTION AND *SPLEEN AND STOMACH QI*

In TCM, the treatment of chronic disease may include measures to assure proper digestion. Without proper digestion, the body will not be able to produce enough *qi* from the food to overcome the disease.

Digestion is often compared to the process of cooking soup. Foods are "cooked" in the stomach until they break down, after which the energies of the food are fully available to the body. Patients are often cautioned not to eat icy or cold foods, since cold foods cause the temperature of the "soup" to drop and the

body must work extra hard to raise it back up. For the same reason, patients are often cautioned not to eat too many raw foods, as raw foods require excessive amounts of "cooking" before they can be assimilated.

The primary *organs* of digestion are the *stomach* (which "rots" the food) and the *spleen* (which "transforms" the food). Disorders of these *organs* may result in symptoms such as abdominal distention, abdominal pain, loose stools, diarrhea, constipation, belching, gas, and sinus and lung congestion.

TABLE 10.1. GENERAL SIGNS OF *YIN* AND *YANG* IMBALANCES			
COLD SYMPTOMS ***YIN REPLETION* OR *YANG VACUITY***		**HEAT SYMPTOMS** ***YIN VACUITY* OR *YANG REPLETION***	
YIN REPLETION *(TRUE COLD)*	*YANG VACUITY* *(FALSE COLD)*	*YANG REPLETION* *(TRUE HEAT)*	*YIN VACUITY* *(FALSE HEAT)*
chill	chill	high fever	low-grade fever, especially in the afternoon
strong and slow pulse	weak and slow pulse	strong and fast pulse	weak and fast pulse
lack of thirst	lack of thirst	high thirst	high thirst
pain worse with pressure	pain better with pressure	pain worse with pressure	pain better with pressure
acute disease	chronic disease	acute disease	chronic disease
metabolism unchanged	slow metabolism	metabolism unchanged	fast metabolism
no fatigue	fatigue	excess energy	restlessness
loose stools	loose stools	constipation	dry stools
pale tongue body	pale tongue body	crimson tongue body	red tongue body
expression unchanged	inexpressive	angry	irritable
speech unchanged	slow speech	manic	fast speech
clear and abundant urination	clear and abundant urination	scanty urination	scanty urination
no sweating	daytime sweating	continuous sweating	nighttime sweating
poor local circulation	poor systemic circulation	excessive circulation	normal or excessive circulation

- *Qi* transports. For example, *lung qi* transports fluids to the skin.
- *Qi* holds. For example, *bladder qi* holds in urine.
- *Qi* raises. For example, *spleen qi* prevents prolapse by holding the *organs* in their proper upright positions.
- *Qi* protects. For example, *zheng qi* protects against invasion of external pathogenic factors.

The functions of *qi* are similar to the functions of *yang*. The primary distinction between *qi* and *yang* is that *yang* has the additional function of warming the body. Two primary pathological patterns of *qi* are recognized. These are *qi vacuity* and *qi stagnation*. Symptoms of *qi vacuity* are similar to those of *yang vacuity*

(low energy, weak pulse, and so on), except that the patient does not exhibit *cold* symptoms. Symptoms of *qi stagnation* may include distended pain, purplish tongue body, poor circulation, and suppressed emotions.

10.2.3 *Blood*

Blood in TCM is similar to, but not the same as, blood in conventional medicine. TCM considers *blood* to be a denser form of *qi*. The close relationship between *blood* and *qi* is signified by the axiom "*blood* is the mother of *qi,* and *qi* is the commander of *blood*." If the *blood* becomes *vacuous,* the *qi* will lose its strength. Similarly, if the *qi* stagnates for too long, the *blood* will

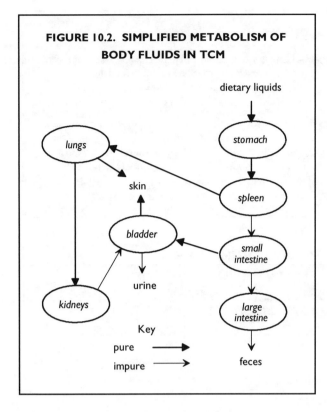

FIGURE 10.2. SIMPLIFIED METABOLISM OF BODY FLUIDS IN TCM

dietary liquids

lungs

skin

stomach

spleen

bladder

small intestine

urine

kidneys

large intestine

Key

pure ⟶

impure ⟶

feces

10.2.4 *Phlegm*

Phlegm is a type of *body fluid*. *Body fluids* include all watery substances in the body other than *blood*. *Fluids* are categorized as either *liquids* or *humors*. *Liquids* are thin and mobile, such as sweat and urine. *Humors* are thick and less mobile and include cerebrospinal fluid and the fluids that lubricate joints. The four disorders of *fluids* are:

- *Damage to liquid.* This includes minor *fluid depletion*, such as that caused by heavy sweating.
- *Humor desertion.* This is a more serious form of *fluid depletion*, which may result after a prolonged *heat* illness, such as some infectious diseases.
- *Water swelling.* This includes most types of edema.
- *Phlegm.* *Phlegm* involves excessive production or buildup of either *liquids* or *humors*. *Phlegm* can be either *substantial*, which means its has form, or *nonsubstantial*, which means it does not have form. Sputum is an example of *substantial phlegm*, whereas lymph node swelling can be an example of *nonsubstantial phlegm*. When *nonsubstantial phlegm* settles in the *channels*, it can cause numbness (such as in stroke patients). If it settles in the joints it can cause pain and deformity (such as in arthritis). The main cause of *phlegm* is *spleen vacuity*, as discussed below.

Body fluids originate from the food we eat and the liquids we drink. After fluids are absorbed in the *stomach*, they move to the *spleen*, which transforms the liquids into "pure" and "impure" fractions (see Figure 10.2). The pure fraction moves upward to the lungs, and from there is dispersed to the skin, the *kidneys*, and other areas of the body. The impure fraction is sent to the *small intestine*, which also separates the pure from the impure. This time, the pure is sent to the *bladder*, and the impure is sent to the *large intestine*. In the *bladder*, the fluids are separated yet again with the pure moving upward to form sweat, and the impure moving downward as urine. The energy of the *spleen* provides the primary force behind the transformation of fluids, and disorders of the *spleen* often result in fluid disorders.

Symptoms of *phlegm* include a sticky tongue coat, lung and sinus congestion, lipomas, fibroids, edema, numbness of the limbs, and swelling of the lymph nodes and thyroid.

10.2.5 *Toxins*

The word *toxin (du)* has a variety of meanings in Traditional Chinese Medicine, including poison, venom, fevers, and other symptoms associated with infectious disease. With respect to cancer, its most important meaning is that of purulent tissue decay. This is referred

also stagnate. Since *qi* is more refined than *blood*, a disease often affects the *qi* first. The affected *qi*, in turn harms the *blood*.

As each *organ* has its own *qi*, certain *organs*, such as the *heart* and *liver*, are said to have their own *blood*. Three *organs* are in close relationship with the *blood*. *Blood* is "governed" by the *heart*, "managed" by the *spleen*, and "stored" by the *liver*. The *liver* also functions to maintain a smooth and even flow of *blood* (and *qi*). Because of the effect the *liver* has on *blood*, disorders of the *liver* are responsible for a wide range of menstrual problems.

The sources of *blood* are the same as the sources of *qi*. They are *jing*, air, and food. The functions of *blood* are similar to the functions of *yin*. *Blood* nourishes the *qi*, and keeps body tissues moist.

Three pathological conditions of *blood* are recognized. These are *blood vacuity*, *blood stagnation*, and *blood heat*. *Blood vacuity* is somewhat similar to anemia. Its symptoms may include dry skin, weakness, dizziness, and a pale face and tongue. *Blood stagnation* symptoms may include boring pain, clotted menstrual blood, and a purplish tongue. Because *blood* is denser than *qi*, *blood stagnation* is considered a more serious condition then *qi stagnation*. *Blood heat* symptoms may include hemorrhage, skin rashes, fever and other *heat* signs, and excessive menstrual bleeding.

TABLE 10.2. THE SIX *YIN ORGANS* AND THEIR FUNCTIONS							
YIN ORGAN	ASSOCIATED *YANG ORGAN*	EFFECT ON *QI*	EFFECT ON *BLOOD*	EFFECT ON *BODY FLUIDS*	EFFECT ON FOOD	ASSOCIATED EMOTION (in pathology)	OTHER EFFECTS
Lungs	*large intestine*	"governs" the *qi*	aids the heart	moves *fluids*	—	sadness and worry	—
Spleen	*stomach*	—	holds *blood* in the vessels	transforms *fluids*	controls digestion	compulsive thought	"houses" thought
Heart	*small intestine*	—	"governs" the *blood*	—	—	excess joy	"houses" the mind
Kidneys	*bladder*	stores the *prenatal jing*	—	"governs" water	—	fear	produces bone marrow and fills the brain; houses will power
Liver	*gall bladder*	ensures the smooth flow of *qi* and *blood*	stores the *blood*	—	—	anger	—

to as *hot toxins (re du)* or *fire toxins (huo du)* and is a by-product of excess *heat* and *damp*. This type of *toxin* includes infections such as mastitis, lung abscesses, appendicitis, and infected cancerous lesions. It also includes dysentery and certain viral infections, such as mumps. Fetid discharges of blood, pus, or tissue are general signs of *fire toxins.*

10.2.6 The *Twelve Channels*

In order to bring energy and nourishment to all tissues, *qi* and *blood* are constantly moving. Whereas *blood* travels through the blood vessels, *qi* is said to travel through the *channels.* The *channels* can be thought of as a fixed network of invisible energy pathways that cover the body from head to toe. There are twelve primary *channels,* and each one is connected internally with one of the twelve primary *organs.* Superficially, portions of the *channels* transverse the body just below the skin.

Diseases that occur in the *channels* are called external, or superficial, diseases. For example, the pain of physical trauma or arthritis may be due to a blockage of *qi* in the *channels.* Since each *channel* connects internally with an *organ,* diseases that occur in the *organs* (internal diseases) may also reflect superficially as symptoms in the *channels.* A classic example is the arm pain associated with myocardial infarction, which radiates down the arm along the *heart channel.* The *heart channel* originates in the chest, runs down the medial aspect of the arm, and ends in the little finger.

Acupuncture is the insertion of fine needles into specific points on the *channels* to affect the flow of *qi.*

Because each *channel* connects to an *organ,* acupuncture can also affect the flow of *qi* in the *organs.* *Channels* can be likened to a system of waterways, reservoirs, and gates used for irrigation. In this analogy, acupuncture acts on the gates (the acupuncture points) to equalize the water levels by altering the inward or outward flow.

10.2.7 The *Twelve Organs*

There are twelve primary internal *organs* in TCM. These are the *lungs, large intestine, spleen, stomach, heart, small intestine, kidneys, bladder, pericardium, triple burner, liver,* and *gall bladder.* Six of these are considered *yang* (or hollow) *organs,* and six are considered *yin* (or solid) *organs.* Five *yin organs* are of primary importance in TCM disease theory, and only these *organs* will be discussed in detail in this book. These *organs* are the *lungs, spleen, heart, kidneys,* and *liver.* Table 10.2 lists their functions.

The way TCM views *organs* is significantly different from the way conventional medicine views organs. TCM generally ascribes a much larger energetic and physiologic function to each organ. There are two reasons for this:

- TCM may group a number of physiologic systems under one organ name. For example, the *spleen* of TCM probably also includes the pancreas of conventional medicine. This may explain the *spleen's* central effect on digestion, since the pancreas produces digestive enzymes. As a second example, the *kidneys* of TCM probably include the sex glands, which explains the *kidneys'* role in metabolism and sexual function.

• *Organs* are viewed from an energetic standpoint, and both mental faculties and emotions are associated with individual *organs*. This is particularly true for the *yin organs*. Examples of this are the *heart*, which "houses" the mind, and the *spleen*, which controls concentration. The heart is also associated with joy, and the spleen is also associated with the ability to concentrate. *Organ* diseases can be caused from excessive or inappropriate emotions, and conversely, emotional excesses can also be caused by *organ* diseases. Emotion-*organ* associations are very important clinically, as disturbances of the emotions are considered to be one of the primary causes of disease. The five primary *yin organs* are discussed below.

The *Lungs*

The *lungs* aid the *heart* in circulating the *blood*. The *lungs* also "govern" the *qi*. They extract the *qi* of the air, and mix it with the *qi* of the food that the *spleen* sends up to the *lungs*. The *lungs* then spread the enriched *qi* to the entire body. They also disperse fluids to the skin, *kidneys*, and other areas of the body. Each *yin organ* is given the title of a ruling official to signify its most important role. Because of the *lungs'* vital work in circulating *qi* and *blood*, the *lungs* are likened to a "minister who issues policies." Breathing exercises are sometimes prescribed in TCM to stimulate the *lungs*. The emotions associated with the *lungs* are grief, sadness, and worry. Excesses of these emotions can stagnate the *qi* of the *lungs*.

The *Spleen*

The *spleen* performs a variety of functions. The *spleen* is compared to a "granary official" because of its influence on digestion—it transforms food into *qi*. In this way the *spleen* nourishes the body and gives muscles their strength. The *spleen* also transforms dietary liquids into *body fluids*. The *spleen qi* holds the *blood* in the blood vessels. If *spleen qi* is weak, epistaxis, menorrhagia, or other forms of bleeding may occur. The *spleen* is the *organ* associated with the ability to concentrate. If *spleen qi* is disturbed, a person may experience compulsive thought or an inability to concentrate.

The *Heart*

The *heart* is considered the "ruler" of all the internal *organs*. The *heart* pumps the *blood* through the vessels so that all tissues can be nourished. The *heart* is the residence of the mind and provides the capacity to feel joy. In this way the *heart* affects mental and emotional activity, consciousness, memory, and sleep. Disturbances of the heart can manifest as circulatory problems, agitation, insomnia, restlessness, or anxiety.

The *Kidneys*

The *kidneys* are considered the "root of life." By storing the *jing* passed on to us from our parents, the *kidneys* provide the energetic base for the body. As *jing* is consumed during the aging process, we lose our vitality and warmth. The *kidneys* also have a variety of other functions and attributes. They control the excretion of water, they "rule" the lower back, and they create the bone marrow and the gray matter of the brain (called the *sea of marrow*). The *kidneys* are said to *root*, or draw down, the breath. Therefore, a *vacuity* of *kidney qi* can result in asthma and shortness of breath. The emotion associated with the *kidneys* is fear, and the *kidneys* "house" or contain the will. In this regard, a disturbance of the *kidneys* can cause panic attacks, phobias, and lack of will power.

The *Liver*

The *liver* maintains the smooth flow and proper direction of *qi* as it moves through the *channels*. For this reason it is compared to an "army general from whom strategy is derived." Since *qi* is the "commander" of *blood*, a smooth flow of *qi* assures a smooth flow of *blood*. The *liver* stores the *blood* and the *liver* meridian passes through the genital area. For these reasons, disorders of the *liver* are at the root of many gynecological problems.

Anger and frustration, the emotions associated with the *liver*, easily stagnate or disturb the flow of *qi*. They affect the *liver* whether or not they are expressed outwardly. Because the lives of so many Americans are stressful, *liver qi stagnation* is a common symptom pattern in this country.

10.3 DIAGNOSIS IN TRADITIONAL CHINESE MEDICINE

10.3.1 Methods of Diagnosis

The techniques of diagnosis in TCM were already ancient by the time conventional medicine developed its laboratory diagnostic equipment. In the integrated practice of TCM, as currently practiced in China, diagnosis is based on both laboratory data and, more traditionally, the *four methods* of examination as listed below:

• *Looking*. Looking includes observation of the facial color, vitality, demeanor, health of the hair, color of the nails, firmness of the flesh, and other physical parameters. Looking also includes observations of the tongue, such as the color and shape of the tongue body and the color and texture of the tongue coating.

- *Hearing (and smelling).* Hearing includes listening to the sound of the voice, the rhythm of breathing, and the characteristics of any cough.
- *Asking.* Asking involves questions regarding bowel function, menstruation, chills, fever, sweating, health of the skin, taste, appetite, diet, digestion, urination, sleep, hearing, thirst, emotional health, pain, and primary complaints.
- *Feeling.* Feeling includes palpation of the radial pulse and palpation of tender areas of the body.

Using the *four methods,* the practitioner makes both subtle and gross observations. For example, on a gross level, the practitioner palpates the pulse to determine its rate and strength. On a more subtle level, palpating the pulse can determine a host of other qualities. TCM recognizes at least 28 different types of pulses. Pulses may be fast, slow, superficial, deep, empty, full, slippery, choppy, tight, long, short, thin, hollow, wiry, knotted, hesitant, or one of twelve other types. Pulse diagnosis is an art that takes many years of experience for a practitioner to master.

10.3.2 Symptom Patterns

TCM does not base treatment solely on a diagnosis from conventional medicine. Rather, TCM also bases treatment on the chief complaint and the discrimination of symptom patterns.[4] This is called *bian zheng lun zhi* in Chinese. Symptom patterns are derived from the entire constellation of pathological symptoms that a given imbalance may exhibit.[5] Disease patterns incorporate the relationship between pathological states of different *organs* and systems. In this way, TCM diagnoses and treats the whole person.

TCM symptom patterns can, at times, take into account a more encompassing view of a patient's symptoms than does the disease names of conventional medicine. For example, in conventional medicine, the disease of primary hypertension is associated almost singularly with the sign of elevated blood pressure. In contrast, TCM recognizes at least eight disease patterns associated with primary hypertension (Huang BS, 1993:148). Taking one of these as an example, the pattern *flaring-up of liver fire* may be associated with the symptoms of irritability, anger, tinnitus, deafness, temporal headache, red face,

red eyes, bitter taste in the mouth, dizziness, thirst, constipation with dry stools, epistaxis, red tongue with a yellow coat, and a rapid pulse.

As illustrated in the previous example, numerous patterns can be associated with one disease name of conventional medicine. The opposite is also true; numerous diseases may be associated with one TCM pattern. For example, the disease of primary dysmenorrhea is associated with at least five different symptom patterns in TCM, one of which is called *qi and blood vacuity.* This particular pattern can also be associated with the diseases of rheumatic heart disease, pancreatitis, iron deficiency anemia, chronic leukemia, and others (Huang BS, 1993:136-164).

The arrangement of symptoms into recognized symptom patterns does not manifest haphazardly. The arrangement can be explained by TCM's theories of pathophysiology. These theories describe the relationships between pathological symptoms and the physiologic functions of the involved *organs* or bodily substances. In fact, patterns are named for the affected *organ* or substance. As an example, Table 10.3 relates the symptoms of the pattern *liver qi stagnation* to the specific liver functions that produce them.

10.4 CAUSES OF DISEASE

In TCM, diseases arise from one or more of three types of causes: *internal, external,* and *other* causes. Each of these are discussed separately below.

10.4.1 *Internal* Causes of Disease

The *internal* cause of disease is emotional upset. The seven emotions that are subject to upset are anger, joy, worry, pensiveness, sadness, fear, and shock. Any emotional imbalance affects the movement of *qi.* However, the excessive and long-standing imbalances manifest most clearly in disease patterns. Emotional factors are not to be taken lightly, as they are one of the most frequent causes of disease.

Excesses of the seven emotions affect the *qi* in the following ways:

- Excess anger affects the *liver* and makes the *qi* rise upward
- Excess joy (excessive excitement) affects the *heart* and slows the *qi* down

---

[4] In TCM, the chief complaint is considered the diagnosis. For example, a diagnosis might be headache or dysmenorrhea. The symptom pattern describes the environment in which the chief complaint occurs. In the integrated practice of TCM and conventional medicine as practiced currently in China, treatment is based on both conventional disease names and symptom patterns.

[5] Over 340 common disease patterns have been identified (Huang BS, 1993).

TABLE 10.3. SYMPTOMS OF LIVER *QI* STAGNATION AND RELATED *LIVER* FUNCTIONS

SYMPTOMS OF *LIVER QI STAGNATION*	RELATED *LIVER* FUNCTIONS
Depression or moodiness, feeling "wound-up," anger	The *liver* is responsible for the smooth flow of *qi*. Because emotions are a form of *qi*, the *liver* is also responsible for the smooth flow of emotions. Tension or moodiness result when the *qi* (and emotional energy) is constrained or moves erratically. Depression may result when the *qi* stagnation reduces the amount of *qi* available for circulation, thereby creating a relative *qi vacuity*. Stagnant *liver qi* can heat up, much like water overheats in a pressure cooker. If enough pressure develops, the *qi* can release suddenly and express itself as an explosion of anger (the emotion associated with the *liver* is anger).
Pain or distention in the flank, chest, or just below the ribcage; premenstrual breast distention	The *liver channel* criss-crosses the flank and chest. *Stagnation of liver qi* causes distention and pain along its *channel*.
Frequent sighing	Since the *lungs* are the primary force behind moving the *qi*, sighing is a natural way to release some of the stagnant *qi* of the *liver*.
Nausea, vomiting, poor appetite, belching, or diarrhea	In Five Phases theory, the *liver* (a *wood element*), is said to "control" the *stomach* and *spleen* (the *earth elements*). When the *liver qi* is stagnant, the *liver* has a tendency to "overcontrol" or "invade" the *stomach*. This can cause a host of digestive disturbances. See Maciocia (1989:15-34) for further discussion on the Five Phases.
Irregular or painful menstrual periods	The *liver* "stores" the *blood* prior to menstruation and releases the *blood* during menstruation. Because the flow of *qi* is stagnant, the flow of *blood* out of the *liver* is not smooth. Pain is caused by *stagnant qi and blood*.
Cold hands and feet	*Qi* is the "commander" of *blood*. If the *qi* does not move freely neither does the *blood*. This results in lack of circulation to the extremities.

Note: *Liver qi stagnation* can be divided into the patterns of *liver qi stagnation*, in which physical symptoms predominate, and *liver qi depression*, in which emotional symptoms predominate.

- Excess worry affects the *spleen* and *lungs* and stagnates the *qi*
- Excess pensiveness affects the *spleen* and stagnates the *qi*
- Excess sadness affects the *lungs* and weakens the *qi*
- Excess fear affects the *kidneys* and descends the *qi*
- Excess shock affects the *kidneys* and *heart* and scatters the *qi*

Emotional imbalances cause aberrations in the movement of *qi*, which in turn, leads to a variety of physical symptoms. For example, excessive upward movement of *qi* can result in vomiting or headaches. Excessive downward movement of *qi* can result in diarrhea or incontinence. Excessive scattering of *qi* can result in weakness and palpitations. Excessive stagnation of *qi* can result in pain. In the case of *stagnant liver qi*, the pressure of *stagnant qi* can build to the point of an *qi* explosion. This may occur when someone holds anger and frustration inside rather than expressing or resolving it. If the anger is intense, and the person holds it inside for too long, he or she can reach a point where the *qi* can no longer be contained and it explodes upward in a red-faced rage, a migraine headache, or some other symptom of *heat* and *repletion*.

Emotion-based *qi* diseases cannot be prevented simply by expressing emotions freely, although in some cases, this may be a necessary step. The most profound preventive medicine is self-cultivation through meditation, whereby a sense of peace and ease is developed. To the degree that we have inner peace, the comings and goings of the world do not upset us and our capacity to be engaged in the world increases. In TCM and in many Eastern spiritual cultures, various meditation techniques are used to calm the mind to accomplish this goal. In China, some hospitals use meditation techniques to treat patients with cardiovascular disease and other diseases.

10.4.2 *External* Causes of Disease

External causes of disease are TCM's six climatic factors: *wind, cold, dampness, summer heat, dryness,* and *fire*. These may affect a patient either singularly or in combination. Under normal circumstances, exposure to these climatic influences do not result in pathology. However, if the exposure is excessive, the climatic factor is particularly strong, or the patient is weak, a disease pattern can develop. In addition to causing disease, climatic factors characterize the patterns of disease that arise from exposure. For example, exposure to wind and cold weather can manifest as a *wind cold* pattern, with symptoms similar to that of the common cold. Climatic factors may also develop into patterns other than their namesake. For example, a *wind cold* pattern, left untreated, may evolve into a *wind heat* pattern, with flu-like symptoms. In the former, chills may prevail, and in the later, fever may prevail.

The six climatic factors produce symptoms that are symbolically akin to themselves:

- *Wind* symptoms act like the wind. They arise suddenly, move freely around the body, vibrate, and change rapidly. The wind is said to act as a carrier, for bringing *heat, cold, and dampness* into the body (hence *wind cold, wind heat,* and *wind damp* disease patterns). *Wind* symptoms include tremors, convulsions, stiffness, paralysis, and itching.
- *Cold* symptoms act like cold. They are slow, cold, and cause contractions and pain. *Cold* symptoms include a slow pulse, chills, pain, and muscle contractions.
- *Heat* symptoms act like heat. They are red, hot, dry, and overactive. *Heat* symptoms include fever, skin rashes, fast pulse, red face, delirium, and irritability.
- *Damp* symptoms act like dampness. They are wet, heavy, slow, and often recalcitrant. *Damp* symptoms include turbid and sticky discharges, lethargy, and edema.
- *Dry* symptoms act like dryness. They are dry and brittle. *Dry* symptoms include constipation, dry mucus membranes, and dry skin.
- *Fire* symptoms act like fire. They are very hot, intense, and dry. *Fire* symptoms include high fever, acute infection, and any intense *heat* sign.
- *Summer heat* symptoms are like the heat of midsummer. *Summer heat* symptoms include heat exhaustion and digestive upset related to heat exhaustion.

10.4.3 *Other* Causes Of Disease

The third type of causative factor of disease is called *other, neither internal nor external* causes. These include genetic weakness (a weak constitution), overexertion, excessive sexual activity (which depletes the *jing*), poor diet, trauma, parasites, poisons, and the improper treatment of a condition.

10.5 SYMPTOM PATTERNS AND CANCER

10.5.1 Symptom Patterns Associated with Cancer

According to TCM, cancer can develop from any of the three primary causes of disease. These primary causes produce a variety of symptom patterns. Cancer patients commonly exhibit one or more of four broad categories of patterns: *phlegm, toxins, qi* and *blood vacuity,* and *qi* and *blood stagnation.* In essence, these four categories include most of the commonly diagnosed patterns found in the general population. In other words, cancer may be associated with most TCM symptom patterns. Some of the more commonly observed patterns are listed in Table 10.4. A patient need not present with every symptom listed to be diagnosed with a given pattern and patients may be diagnosed with more than one pattern.

To some degree, the association between symptom patterns and cancer may be causative. For example, *stagnant qi* often leads to *stagnant blood.* The initiation or progression of cancer due to *stagnant qi* and *stagnant blood* could be facilitated, in part, by impairment of local blood and lymph circulation, causing an imbalance of nutrients, antioxidants, hormones, eicosanoids, and/or growth factors. Likewise, *qi* and *blood vacuity* could facilitate carcinogenesis, in part, by deficiencies of immune factors, antioxidants, and nutrients.

TABLE 10.4. PATTERNS ASSOCIATED WITH CANCER IN GENERAL	
PATTERN	**SYMPTOMS**
Yin vacuity (general symptoms)	○ *False heat* symptoms, which may be worse in the afternoon or evening, include thirst, rapid pulse, facial flush, warm palms, warm feet, warm chest, scanty-dark urine, lack of tongue coat, irritability, and night sweats ○ Emaciation ○ *Dryness* symptoms such as dry mouth, dry stools, and dry skin
— *Stomach yin vacuity*	○ General *yin vacuity* symptoms, plus lack of appetite, stomach pain, and feeling of fullness after eating
(Table continues)	

PATTERN	SYMPTOMS
— *Liver yin vacuity*	○ General *yin vacuity* symptoms, plus dry eyes, dream-disturbed sleep, insomnia, scanty menstruation, numbness in the extremities, and sallow complexion
— *Kidney yin vacuity*	○ General *yin vacuity* symptoms, plus vertigo, dizziness, tinnitus, deafness, poor memory, low back pain, nocturnal emissions, and pain in the bones (especially the knees)
— *Lung yin vacuity*	○ General *yin vacuity* symptoms, plus unproductive cough, dry sticky sputum, and blood-tinged sputum
Yang vacuity (general symptoms)	○ *Cold* symptoms, including cold limbs, aversion to cold, body aches, body stiffness, lack of thirst, bright-white complexion, white tongue coat, slow pulse, and a pale, swollen, and moist tongue body ○ Low energy ○ Loose stools
— *Kidney yang vacuity*	○ General *yang vacuity* symptoms, plus sore lower back, edema, weak knees, impotence, premature ejaculation, and clear urination
— *Spleen yang vacuity*	○ General *yang vacuity* symptoms, plus lack of appetite, abdominal distention after eating, and weakness in the extremities
— *Stomach yang vacuity*	○ General *yang vacuity* symptoms, plus discomfort in the stomach that is improved after eating warm foods, lack of appetite, and desire for warm foods and liquids
Liver yang repletion	○ Anger or irritability, dizziness, tinnitus, deafness, insomnia, dream-disturbed sleep, scanty menstruation, numbness in the extremities, sallow complexion, dry eyes, red tongue body, and also headache on the temples, eyes, or sides of the head
Upward rising heat	○ *Upward rising heat* is usually due to the *heat* of *liver yang repletion, stomach heat,* or any type of *yin vacuity.* The symptoms are *heat* in the upper portion of the body, such as a red face or neck, headache, red tongue body, dry throat, and thirst.
Stomach fire	○ Burning sensation and pain in the stomach, thirst for cold liquids, strong hunger, bleeding gums, sour regurgitation, constipation, nausea, bad breath, rapid pulse, red tongue body, and a thick, yellow and dry tongue coat. If *phlegm* is involved, there may be less thirst, fullness in the stomach, mucus in the stools, and mental derangement.
Qi vacuity (general symptoms)	○ Weak voice, spontaneous sweating, lack of appetite, loose stools, fatigue, shortness of breath, facial pallor, and a pale tongue
— *Lung qi vacuity*	○ General *qi vacuity* symptoms, plus cough, and a tendency to catch colds frequently
— *Kidney qi vacuity*	○ General *qi vacuity* symptoms, plus soreness of the lower back, clear and frequent urination, dribbling after urination, incontinence, night time urination, nocturnal emissions not associated with dreams, premature ejaculation, spermatorrhea, chronic vaginal discharge, asthma, and cold limbs.
— *Heart qi vacuity*	○ General *qi vacuity* symptoms, plus palpitations
— *Spleen qi vacuity*	○ General *qi vacuity* symptoms, plus abdominal distention after eating and weak extremities
Qi stagnation (general symptoms)	○ Feeling of distention, distended pain, abdominal masses, mental depression, irritability, mood swings, and sighing
— *Liver qi stagnation*	○ General *qi stagnation* symptoms, plus hiccup, irregular periods, painful periods, premenstrual tension, and premenstrual breast distention; if *liver Qi invades the stomach,* then also nausea, vomiting, lack of appetite, sour regurgitation, diarrhea, and abdominal distention
— *Blood vacuity*	○ Sallow or pale complexion, poor memory, numbness in the extremities, blurred vision, insomnia, scanty menstrual periods, depression, dry skin, itchy skin, dry hair, and a pale tongue
— *Blood stagnation*	○ Purple lips and tongue, sharp, boring, or stabbing pain, fixed masses, clotted menstrual blood, dark colored menstrual blood, and purple nails

TABLE 10.4. (continued)

(Table continues)

TABLE 10.4. *(continued)*

PATTERN	SYMPTOMS
Blood heat	○ Feelings of heat, red eruptions on the skin, dry mouth, red tongue, and rapid pulse. Also excessive menstrual bleeding, epistaxis, bleeding gums, or other forms of bleeding.
Phlegm accumulation (general symptoms)	○ Sticky and greasy tongue coating, sputum, lumps under the skin, masses, numbness in the extremities, mental disease, gall stones or kidney stones, and arthritic bone deformities
— Phlegm accumulation in the lungs	○ General *phlegm accumulation* symptoms, plus cough, chest congestion, and sinus congestion
Damp heat (general symptoms)	○ Infection, yellow discharge, fever, thirst without desire to drink, feeling of heaviness in the body, scanty urine, fast pulse, red tongue with a yellow and moist coat
— Lung damp heat	○ General *damp heat* symptoms, plus cough, yellow sputum, shortness of breath, asthma, and stuffy chest
— Large intestine damp heat	○ General *damp heat* symptoms, plus abdominal pain, diarrhea, burning in the anus, and mucus and blood in the stool
— Liver damp heat	○ General *damp heat* symptoms, plus fullness and pain in the chest and abdomen, jaundice, bitter taste in the mouth, nausea, vomiting, loss of appetite, distention of the abdomen, vaginal discharge, and pain and swelling in the scrotum
Toxins (general symptoms)	○ Green discharge from lesions, tissue decay, stench of tissue or discharge, fever, and fast pulse
— Toxins in the large intestine	○ General *toxin* symptoms plus symptoms of *large intestine damp heat*

10.5.2 Symptom Patterns Associated with Specific Cancers

Groups of symptom patterns may be associated with specific cancers. For example, *phlegm stagnation, kidney qi vacuity, kidney yin vacuity,* and *kidney yang vacuity* may all be associated with brain cancer. Patterns reported to be associated with other cancers are provided in Table 10.5. The strengths of these associations are uncertain, as the original epidemiologic studies could not be located.

According to TCM, it is important to address these symptom patterns in cancer patients. The presenting pattern may have played an etiological role in the develop-

ment of the cancer, and/or may be facilitating the growth of the cancer. However, both of these relationships are unverified. At the very least, the presenting pattern may cause the patient distress, which consumes the patient's strength.

In addition to their use in devising appropriate treatment plans, symptom patterns may also be relevant as indicators of survival. For example, in a study of 254 patients with cervical cancer treated with radiotherapy and followed for over three years, those diagnosed as having *qi stagnation* exhibited a significantly reduced survival rate as compared to those diagnosed as having *liver and kidney yin vacuity* (Yu et al., 1991a).

TABLE 10.5. SYMPTOM PATTERNS ASSOCIATED WITH SELECTED CANCERS

CANCER	PATTERNS	CANCER	PATTERNS
Esophageal	*phlegm-qi blocking the throat*	Stomach	*liver qi stagnation invading the stomach*
	injury to the stomach and spleen		*stomach yang vacuity*
	qi and blood stagnation		*phlegm stagnation and food retention*
	phlegm accumulation		*blood stagnation due to qi stagnation*
(column continues)	*toxins*	(column continues)	*stomach yin vacuity due to stomach fire*
(Table continues)			

TABLE 10.5. (continued)			
CANCER	**PATTERNS**	**CANCER**	**PATTERNS**
Esophageal (continued)	yin vacuity	Stomach (continued)	qi and blood vacuity
	qi and blood vacuity	Liver	liver qi stagnation causing blood stagnation
Colorectal	damp heat in the large intestine		damp heat and toxins
	toxins		liver and kidney yin vacuity
	spleen and kidney yang vacuity		liver yang repletion
	liver and kidney yin vacuity	Nasopharyngeal	upward rising heat
	qi and blood vacuity		yin vacuity
Lung	lung yin vacuity and phlegm accumulation		toxins
	lung and kidney qi vacuity		lung and stomach damp heat
	toxins	Breast	liver qi stagnation
	blood stagnation due to qi stagnation		phlegm accumulation
	qi and blood vacuity		blood stagnation and toxins
	lung qi and yin vacuity		qi and blood vacuity
	lung and kidney yin vacuity		spleen qi vacuity and phlegm accumulation
	phlegm damp in the lung	Lymphoma	liver qi stagnation
Cervical	toxins		phlegm accumulation
	liver and kidney yin vacuity		toxins
	liver qi stagnation		yin vacuity
	heart and spleen qi vacuity	Chronic leukemia	blood stagnation
Acute leukemia	blood stagnation causing heat		qi and blood vacuity
	qi and yin vacuity		blood heat
Brain	phlegm accumulation		toxins
	kidney qi vacuity		stomach and spleen qi vacuity
	kidney yin vacuity		spleen and heart qi vacuity

Sources: Huang BS, 1993:147-164; Zhang, 1989:45-89; Zhang E, 1990:402-408

10.6 CLINICAL USE OF CHINESE HERBS

In TCM, herbs are rarely prescribed individually, and the patterns described in Table 10.5 are treated, instead, with herbal formulas.[6] Formulas typically contain from 4 to 12 herbs and are can be taken in a variety of ways, including decoctions, pills, powders, and lozenges.

Approximately 400 historic formulas are in common use today, 20% of which originated from the text *Shan Han Za Bing Lun (Discussion of Cold-induced Disorders and Miscellaneous Diseases)* written in the third century A.D. Contemporary formulas have also been devised, many of which are based on pharmacological studies. Whether historic or contemporary, formulas are commonly altered to suit the needs of each individual patient.

---

[6] The TCM materia medica contains a wide range of natural substances, including plants (roots, stems, bark, branches, leaves, and fruits), minerals, sea products (fish bones and shells), fungus and mushrooms, insects, and mammal products (bones, hair, horns, etc.). Plant products are, by far, the most common substances used. For convenience, this book considers all of these products as herbal agents. Currently, over 5,500 substances are listed in comprehensive materia medicas (such as the *Encyclopedia of Traditional Chinese Medicinal Substances* written by the Jiansu College of New Medicine in 1977). However, only about 500 of these are in common use.

TABLE 10.6. CATEGORIES AND ACTIONS OF CHINESE HERBS	
CATEGORY	**ACTION**
Herbs that *resolve the exterior*	These herbs treat superficial conditions, such as the common cold or flu, often by making the patient sweat. This category is further divided into *cooling herbs that resolve the exterior* (which are used in *heat* patterns), and *warming herbs that resolve the exterior* (which are used in *cold* patterns).
Herbs that *clear heat*	These herbs reduce *true heat*, and *false heat*. They treat fevers, infections, the heat of *yin vacuity*, and other *heat* conditions. Many of these herbs have antibacterial or antiviral activity. Some have cytotoxic and antitumor activity and have been used traditionally as anticancer agents. Herbs that *clear heat* can be divided into herbs that *quell fire*, which treat extreme *true heat*, herbs that *cool blood*, which treat *heat in the blood*, herbs that *clear damp heat*, which treat mixtures of *heat and dampness* (such as that found in bacterial infections), and herbs that *clear heat toxins*, which treat *toxin* patterns (including viral infections). Traditional anticancer agents commonly come from this last category.
Herbs that *drain precipitation*	These herbs induce bowel movements. They treat constipation and some forms of *heat*.
Herbs that *percolate damp*	These herbs are used to remove excess *dampness* from the body. Many of these herbs have diuretic actions. They treat edema and other forms of *dampness*.
Herbs that *dispel wind dampness*	These herbs treat arthritic-like conditions. Many have anti-inflammatory actions.
Herbs that *transform phlegm and stop coughing*	These herbs *clear phlegm* from the lungs and other areas. Many of these herbs have antitussive actions.
Aromatic herbs that *transform dampness*	These are aromatic herbs that treat *dampness*. They can also treat digestive disturbances due to *dampness*. Many of these herbs are rich in volatile oils.
Herbs that *relieve food accumulation*	These herbs improve digestion. Many contain digestive enzymes such as amylase.
Herbs that *rectify the qi*	These herbs treat *qi stagnation*, and also correct the flow of *qi* if it is flowing the wrong direction (such as the upward rising *qi* associated with hiccups). These herbs tend to be rich in volatile oils.
Herbs that *regulate the blood*	These herbs treat *blood stagnation*. Many of these herbs have anticoagulant actions. A subset of this category treats bleeding problems.
Herbs that *warm the interior and expel cold*	These herbs *warm* a patient who is suffering from a *cold* pattern.
Herbs that *supplement*	These herbs strengthen the *yin, yang, qi, or blood*. Many have a beneficial effect on the immune and hematologic systems and have been used to treat the side effects of chemotherapy and radiation therapy.
Herbs that *astringe*	These herbs stop excessive sweating or diarrhea. Many are rich in tannins.
Herbs that *quiet the spirit*	These herbs calm nervousness and anxiety and treat insomnia. Many have sedative or tranquilizing actions.
Aromatic herbs that *open the portals*	These herbs revive a patient from delirium. Some have an action similar to smelling salts.
Herbs that *extinguish wind and stop tremors*	These herbs treat *wind* conditions, such as epilepsy. Many of these herbs have antihypertensive or antispasmodic actions.
Herbs that *expel parasites*	These herbs rid the body of parasites.
Herbs for topical application	These herbs tend to be poisonous and treat a wide range of skin infections and other skin diseases. Some of these herbs are used in cancer treatment.

In general, formulas are designed to antagonize the symptom pattern. Patterns that involve *heat* are treated with *cooling* herbs, patterns that involve *dampness* are treated with *drying* herbs, and so on. There are 18 functional herb categories, as listed in Table 10.6. Although any given herb may have several functions applicable to several categories, each is categorized according to its primary function. For example, the functions attributed to the herb *Panax ginseng (ren shen)* are to *supplement the qi, generate fluids and stop thirst,* and *quiet the spirit.* However, ginseng is normally categorized according to its primary function, *supplement the qi.*

The roles of individual herbs in a formula are described by analogy to positions within a royal court. One or two are considered the "ruler" or "chief" herbs. These are chosen to have the greatest effect on the symptom pattern or complaint. Other herbs may be "deputies," which assist the chief herbs; "assistants," which help the chief or deputy herbs or treat less important aspects of the pattern; and "envoys," which guide the effects of the formula to a specific region in the body or harmonize the actions of the other herbs. Licorice *(Glycyrrhiza sp., gan cao)* is one of the most commonly used envoy herbs.

For further information regarding the use of herbal formulas, the reader is referred to Bensky and Barolet (1990) and Huang and Wang (1993). For information regarding formulas intended specifically for cancer patients, the reader is referred to Pan (1992) and Kun (1985).

Traditional herbal treatment of cancer relies heavily on herbs from two categories of action: herbs that *supplement,* and herbs that *clear heat.* Their function, in Chinese, is *fu zheng qu xie,* which literally means to "support the correct and eliminate the pathogen." This strategy attempts to strengthen the patient (and his or her immune system) while concurrently attacking the cancer with herbs that *clear heat.* Herbs that "reduce accumulations" are also used. Herbs that reduce accumulations include some herbs from the categories *regulate the blood, transform phlegm,* and *rectify the qi.* These herbs are used to "soften the accumulation of hard masses" *(ruan jian san jie),* which may be accumulations of *blood, phlegm,* or *qi.*

10.7 SUMMARY

The foundation for diagnosis in Traditional Chinese Medicine is the *eight principles.* These are *yin* and *yang, hot* and *cold, replete* and *vacuous,* and *internal* and *external.* The *eight principles,* along with the concepts of *qi, blood, phlegm, toxins,* and the *twelve channels* and *twelve organs* constitute the core of TCM theory. In TCM, diseases are viewed in terms of symptom patterns, which relate a constellation of symptoms with the terms and concepts of TCM theory. A select number of symptom patterns may be common in patients with cancer. Patients may benefit from the use of herbal formulas designed to treat these patterns.

11
ANTITUMOR AND ANTICANCER EFFECTS OF BOTANICAL AGENTS

In the last four decades, antitumor activity has been verified in thousands of plants. However, only one botanical compound, taxol, has received marketing approval by the U.S. Food and Drug Administration. This chapter discusses the research conducted on plants in the search for anticancer compounds, and explains why so few botanical compounds have been developed into useful drugs. It also discusses results of Chinese clinical trials using crude herbal extracts.

11.1 INVESTIGATIONS OF PLANT EXTRACTS AT THE NATIONAL CANCER INSTITUTE

11.1.1 Plant Screening Program

An intensive program to screen plant extracts and other natural materials for anticancer activity began in 1955 with funding from the United States National Cancer Institute (NCI) through the Cancer Chemotherapy National Service Center (CCNSC). The original mission of the CCNSC was to develop new agents acquired from outside sources, but by 1956 the CCNSC was procuring and screening their own samples. Even so, they investigated relatively few plant samples up through 1960. Prior to this time their primary focus was on investigating fermentation products. In 1960, CCNSC entered into an agreement with the U.S. Department of Agriculture Medicinal Plant Resources Laboratory (MPRL), in which the MPRL would collect plants for screening.[1] MPRL has since collected plants from over 60 countries. Since its inception, the CCNSC has screened over 114,000 plant samples representing 4,000 species (Suffness and Pezzuto, 1991; Lien and Li, 1985:2). This

represents 2% of the world's approximately 250,000 plant species. Although the NCI screening program is the largest of its type in the world, it is by no means the only screening program. Nonaffiliated research centers and research centers sponsored by other governments are also actively searching for botanical anticancer agents.

One of the first decisions that had to be made in NCI's plant collection program was the method for selecting which plants to test. After considering methods based on the use of plants in folklore and traditional medical systems, and methods based on botanical relationships, NCI decided to select plants on a basis of diversity. That is, plants were selected to be representative of existing biodiversity. There were a variety of considerations in making this choice (reviewed by Suffness and Douros, 1979). For example, Hartwell (1970, 1971a, 1971b) identified over 3,000 species of plants used in traditional medicines to treat cancer. Although selection based on traditional medicine may have provided a high ratio of active plants to inactive plants, there were also perceived disadvantages. These included issues of secrecy within primitive cultures, difficulty obtaining an accurate botanical identification based upon folklore, and the possibility of missing plants that are active, but not

---

[1] The MPRL was called the New Crops Research Branch prior to 1972. The office was headed by Dr. Robert Perdue and Dr. James Duke for many years.

used in traditional medicines. In addition, most plants used in traditional medicines were used against skin cancers, since skin cancer is one of the few cancers that is easily diagnosed. Internal cancers can be very difficult to diagnose, even with the aid of modern technology. Therefore, there are fewer reports of effective agents against these cancers in traditional medicines. Lastly, many of the plants used to treat skin cancer were applied superficially and are too toxic to be used internally.

The difficulty of successfully conducting a search for anticancer agents within the world's flora is monumental. Listed below are issues that NCI faced:

- *Cancer is not a single disease.* There are more than 100, and possibly as many as 300, distinct types of cancer, and each type behaves quite differently (Suffness and Pezzuto, 1991). An ideal screen therefore would include multiple human cancers. However, this would be expensive and time-consuming, and for many years was technologically unfeasible.

- *Cancer cells resemble normal cells in many important respects.* It has been very difficult to identify properties unique to cancer cells that can be exploited as treatment targets. For this reason, the most common target has simply been cells that proliferate rapidly.[2] However, this has resulted in a lack of agents active against the most common human tumors, which are relatively slow-growing. It has also resulted in agents that are toxic to the gastrointestinal lining, bone marrow, and other normal cells that proliferate rapidly. Only recently have researchers identified some of the more subtle differences between cancer cells and normal cells.

- *When active agents are identified, the mechanism by which they work may remain unknown.* This limits the ability to identify new agents that act by similar mechanisms. Furthermore, many agents appear to work by multiple mechanisms, which further complicates the development of rational screening procedures.

- *Individual cancers are not comprised of homogenous cells.* Mutant lines allow resistant subpopulations to survive treatment and continue their growth. This phenomenon can quickly render active anticancer agents useless, and also makes it difficult to breed appropriate experimental cell lines for testing purposes. For example, the classic P388 and L1210 leukemia cell lines have been grown for 30 to 40 years and have lost much of their heterogenicity. They are less able to mimic human cancers and may now be of minimal value in discovering new agents

active against human cancers (Suffness and Pezzuto, 1991).

- *The majority of human cancers grow very slowly.* For example, the lag time between starting to smoke tobacco and a diagnosis of lung cancer may be 20 to 30 years. It would be very expensive and time-consuming to use these types of experimental tumors.

- *Many animal assays are very expensive and require special facilities.* In some cases, this has resulted in the use of less expensive in-vitro prescreens, followed by in-vivo testing of effective agents. However, the in-vitro prescreen is not effective at identifying agents that act by mechanisms other than cytotoxicity, such as stimulation of immune function.

- *Plants may contain very small amounts of an active constituent, and large amounts of the plant material may be required for advanced testing.* For example, to meet the needs of clinical trials, 31,000 pounds of *Maytenus buchananii* were purchased in Kenya in 1976. This allowed the purification of 15 grams of maytansine, which was enough for several thousand patients (Suffness and Douros, 1979). Procurement of adequate samples can be difficult and expensive if the plant is rare.

- *A large amount of existing data are now obsolete.* When the screening program began, investigators had no way of knowing what types of compounds they were looking for, what extraction procedures would yield the active compounds, and what assays would point out the active compounds. Through the years, as information became available, the extraction and assay systems were modified. As of 1979, the data for as much as one-third of the total extracts screened were considered incomplete and in need of recollection (Suffness and Douros, 1979).

Taken together, these difficulties suggest that no single screening procedure is optimal. In the end, NCI designed a program that was a compromise between the various extremes. Because of this, the NCI data, although useful, is probably incomplete. As will be discussed shortly, in almost 40 years of research, the NCI program has discovered less than a half-dozen agents that demonstrate acceptable clinical efficacy, and only one of these has received marketing approval by the Food and Drug Administration. However, this does not necessarily mean that other botanical agents may not be of some use.

To illustrate the changes in screening protocols over time, the evolution of the extraction procedures and assay methods is discussed in the following two sections.

---

[2] To some degree, this target evolved due to the use of fast-growing mouse tumors in the screening program. Fast-growing tumors were selected for study because they provided rapid assay results and minimized animal holding costs.

TABLE 11.1 STEPS IN THE DEVELOPMENT OF BOTANICAL ANTITUMOR AGENTS AT NCI

MAJOR STEPS	SUBSTEPS
Preparation	Plant collection and extraction
Prescreen	In-vitro and/or in-vivo assays against one or two cell lines
Screen	In-vivo assays against multiple cell lines
Monitor	Fractionation studies to isolate and characterize active compounds
Secondary testing (also called detailed evaluation)	In-vivo testing of active compounds against multiple cell lines; large-scale production; pharmacokinetic and toxicology studies
Clinical trials	○ Phase I: Toxicology studies ○ Phase II: Limited trials to evaluate activity against specific cancers ○ Phase III: Larger trials against a greater variety of cancers to compare the activity of the new agent with standard therapy. Agents are chosen for phase III studies if they show activity in phase II trials.

11.1.2 Extraction Methods

The ability to successfully isolate a botanical compound from its parent material is largely dependent on the type of solvent used in the extraction procedure. Ideally a number of different extracts, each obtained with a different solvent, would be tested for each plant. However, the expense of this approach is prohibitive. The first method NCI used involved a two-fraction extraction, one obtained with water and one obtained with 95% ethanol. The water-soluble fraction resulted in a moderate percentage of active confirmations in the in-vivo sarcoma 180, adenocarcinoma 755, and Walker 256 carcinoma models, which were the primary prescreens in use at the time.[3] However, NCI eventually learned that these cell lines were, for some reason, overly sensitive to tannins and that some active agents were identified as such only due to their tannin content.[4] Tannins, which are common constituents in plants, are soluble in water but do not possess the type of activity that NCI was looking for. For this reason, the sarcoma 180 and adenocarcinoma 755 lines were discontinued as prescreens in 1962, the extraction method was modified in 1964, and the Walker 256 line was discontinued as a prescreen in 1969.

The next extraction method used a solvent comprised of 50% water and 50% ethanol to produce a single fraction. The reasoning behind this choice of solvent was that highly polar solvents (such as pure water) might yield too many compounds that lack biologic activity due to their lipophobic nature. Conversely, highly nonpolar solvents (such as hexane or petroleum ether) might yield too many compounds that lack biologic activity due to their hydrophobic nature. The water-ethanol solvent was of intermediate polarity and was thought to be a good compromise. However, this method resulted in a very low percentage (0.8%) of active confirmations in the

P388 leukemia line (which replaced the Walker 256 line). Therefore, the NCI changed this method in 1974 to a two-fraction procedure as follows:

1) The plant material was extracted with petroleum ether to remove highly lipophilic compounds, and this extract was discarded.

2) The redried plant material was extracted with ethanol, after which, a portion of the ethanol extract was dried to obtain Fraction A.

3) The remaining portion of the ethanol extract was partitioned between water and chloroform. The water-soluble portion was discarded (to remove highly hydrophilic compounds), and the chloroform-soluble portion was dried to obtain Fraction B. Chloroform is a solvent of intermediate polarity.

Although this system improved performance, it did not yield a number of compounds, such as polysaccharides, that later became of interest. Polysaccharides are water-soluble compounds, and as such were discarded (see step 3 above). For similar reasons, this method would not yield taxol, a polar compound with anticancer activity. Because of these problems, the extraction system has since been further refined.

11.1.3 Assay Methods

Before proceeding with a discussion of assays, it is first necessary to clarify the meaning of some terms that investigators in the NCI program use. *Cytotoxic* refers to agents that are toxic to cells in vitro. *Antitumor* refers to agents that inhibit tumor growth in animals. *Anticancer* refers to agents that inhibit tumor growth in humans. Cytotoxic agents can be further divided into those that are cytostatic (those that stop cell growth) and those that are cytocidal (those that kill cells). According to the NCI

---

[3] Walker 256 is a rat tumor. Most of the other animal lines mentioned in this chapter are mouse tumors.

[4] The sarcoma 180 and adenocarcinoma 755 lines were also overly sensitive to phytosterols.

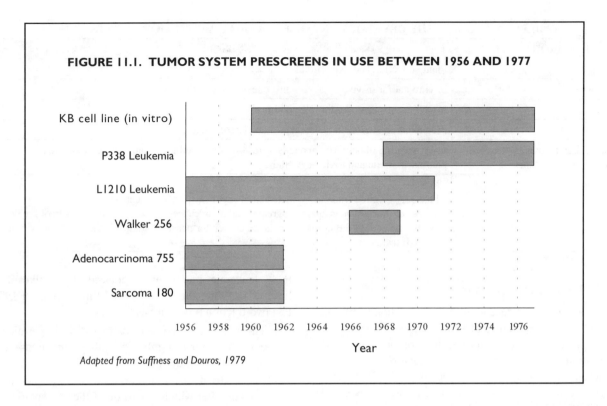

FIGURE 11.1. TUMOR SYSTEM PRESCREENS IN USE BETWEEN 1956 AND 1977

Adapted from Suffness and Douros, 1979

data, many plant extracts possess cytotoxic activities. Of these, a small number possess antitumor activities, and of these, a very few possess anticancer activities.

To accommodate this ever-narrowing selection process, NCI used a screening procedure as outlined in Table 11.1 (for various reasons, some compounds may have followed a slightly different screening procedure). Simple in-vitro or in-vivo prescreens were used to identify extracts with potential activity. Active extracts were further screened against multiple cell lines in vivo. Extracts that were successful in this screen advanced to the monitoring stage, where they were fractionated to obtain the pure, active compounds. The pure compounds were tested further using in-vivo assays. Successful compounds advanced to secondary testing to determine whether they were suitable for clinical trials. Clinical trials are the final step in the screening process.

As mentioned above, the tumor systems used in the prescreens have changed over time. In addition to discontinuing the sarcoma 180, adenocarcinoma 755, and Walker 256 carcinoma lines for their sensitivity to tannins, NCI discontinued the L1210 leukemia prescreen in 1971, because it identified too few active substances. Changes to the prescreen lines prior to 1977 are shown in Figure 11.1. From 1977 to 1986, the prescreen remained the P338 leukemia and KB cell line (in vitro).

It is important to recognize the weaknesses of these lines. The international literature contains many references to botanical agents that are active in one or more of the discontinued prescreens, and caution must be used in interpreting their activities.

Starting in 1977, NCI began to incorporate human tumor cell lines into its in-vivo screening program. Although in-vitro human cell lines had been available for some time, in-vivo lines were not available due to lack of a suitable host animal. NCI overcame this problem in 1968 with the discovery of genetically athymic mice (also called nude mice because they lack fur). Since these mice lack a thymus gland, they are immunodeficient and cannot readily reject a transplant of foreign tissue, such as a human tumor xenograft (Vlietinck and Dommisse, 1985; Crommelin and Midha, 1992).[5] Between 1980 and 1986 the NCI protocol employed a variety of human cancer xenografts, but still relied on a mouse tumor model as a prescreen. Since agents that were not effective in the prescreen did not receive further testing, the screening protocol continued to emphasize the discovery of agents that were active against fast-growing cancers. Table 11.2 provides a list of the tumor lines used by NCI prior to 1986.

The method used to select the dose, route of administration, and administration schedule for in-vivo testing has also changed over time. The purpose of the in-vivo prescreen is to determine, in general terms, whether or not any activity is present. If activity is found, then dosage parameters in future studies can be adjusted to optimize the antitumor effect. The NCI protocol for many years was to administer large doses (100, 200, and 400

---

[5] A xenograft is an interspecies tissue transplant.

TABLE 11.2. PRE-1986 NCI CELL LINES			
NCI CELL LINE CODE	**DESCRIPTION**	**NCI CELL LINE CODE**	**DESCRIPTION**
B1	B16 melanoma	M5	M-5076 ovarian carcinoma
CA	Adenocarcinoma 755	NH	Novikoff hepatoma
CD	CD8F1 mammary tumor	P-4	P-1534 leukemia
C6	Colon 26	PA	P-338 Adriamycin resistant
C8	Colon 38	PV	P-338 vincristine resistant
CY	Colon 36	P6	P-338 L-alanosine resistant
CZ	Colon 51	PS	P-388 lymphocytic leukemia
DL	Dunning leukemia	SA	Sarcoma 180 (S-180)
EA	Ehrlich ascites	WA	Walker carcinosarcoma 256
EM	Ependymoblastoma	CX-1	Human colon cancer
KB (in vitro)	Carcinoma of nasopharynx	CX-5	Human colon cancer
LE	L-1210 lymphoid leukemia	LX-1	Human lung cancer
LL	Lewis lung carcinoma	MX-1	Human mammary tumor

Note: Cell lines are used in vivo unless specified.
Adapted from: Lien and Li, 1985:2; Suffness et al., 1989; Crommelin and Midha, 1992

mg/kg) on a daily schedule for either 5 or 9 days. Both the agent and tumor implant (generally P388 leukemia cells) were administered by intraperitoneal (i.p.) injection, with treatment starting one day after tumor cell implant (Suffness, 1995, personal communication).[6] The reasoning behind this protocol was to provide the agent with every possible chance of success—the protocol uses a highly sensitive tumor line, employs high doses and relatively frequent administration of the test agent, and places both test agent and cell implant into the same compartment. If test agents do not show activity under these conditions, it is assumed that they will not have activity under more rigorous conditions. Drawbacks of this approach include the need for high quantities of test agents, and the fact that placing both test agent and implant into the same compartment bypasses physiological barriers—such as absorption, distribution, and excretion—that would otherwise be encountered.

The criteria used to judge the effectiveness of an extract are assay-specific. Examples of criteria for selected assays are shown in Table 11.3. As can be seen, active extracts produced either a tumor inhibition of approximately 60% or an increase in survival of 120 to 140%. The P338 prescreen used a low criteria (120% survival) to help assure that all active extracts would pass into the full screen. In-vivo assays using mouse tumors are generally evaluated after 20 to 60 days, and assays involving human xenografts are generally evaluated after 11 to 15 days (Suffness et al., 1989).

The assay system changed dramatically in 1986, when NCI began to use a "disease-oriented" screen. This system differs from older ones in two major respects. First, it is based on human tumors rather than animal tumors. And second, it uses a large number of human tumors, which are divided into panels of organ specific cancers. The disease-oriented system is designed to identify those agents that have specific action on a particular type of cancer. For example, the lung cancer panel contains multiple types of human lung cancer and is designed to identify agents that are effective specifically on one or more of these types. The prescreens used in this system are panels of human tumor cells in vitro. Since this system relies on initial in-vitro screens it identifies only those anticancer agents that act by cytotoxic mechanisms. In this system, anticancer agents that act by non-cytotoxic mechanisms are inactive. Some of the cell lines used in the disease-oriented screens are listed in Table 11.4.

Dosages for in-vivo testing are determined through the use of range-finding studies in healthy mice, which identify the maximum safe dosage. The agent is then tested in mice bearing human tumor xenografts that are known to be sensitive to the agent in vitro. Administration is usually intermittent, but may be modified according to the chemical nature of the test agent. For example, agents with short half-lives may be administered more frequently.

---

[6] Matthew Suffness, Ph.D. is the Program Director of the Natural Products Grants, Grants and Contracts Operations Branch in the Division of Cancer Treatment at NCI.

TABLE 11.3. CRITERIA USED TO EVALUATE SELECTED ASSAYS		
TUMOR	**PARAMETER ***	**CRITERIA ***
Adenocarcinoma 755 (CA)	Tumor inhibition	T/C $\leq$ 42%
B16 melanosarcoma (B1)	Survival	T/C $\geq$ 125%
CD8F1 mammary tumor (CD)	Tumor inhibition	T/C $\leq$ 20%
Colon 38 (C8)	Tumor inhibition	T/C $\leq$ 42%
Human colon cancer xenograft (CX-1)	Tumor inhibition	T/C $\leq$ 20 or 42%
Human lung cancer xenograft (LX-1)	Tumor inhibition	T/C $\leq$ 20 or 42%
Human mammary tumor xenograft (MX-1)	Tumor inhibition	T/C $\leq$ 20 or 42%
KB cell line (in vitro)	Growth inhibition	ED_{50} at <20 µg/ml for crude extracts; <4 µg/ml for pure substances
L1210 leukemia (LE)	Survival	T/C $\geq$ 125%
Lewis lung carcinoma (LL)	Survival	T/C $\geq$ 140%
P338 leukemia (PS)	Survival	T/C $\geq$ 120%
Sarcoma 180 (SA)	Tumor inhibition	T/C $\leq$ 42%
Walker 256 carcinosarcoma (WA)	Tumor inhibition	T/C $\leq$ 42%

* Tumor inhibition is measured as the median tumor weight change between test and control animals.
** T/C is the ratio of the results of test animals to the results of control animals.
Adapted from: Suffness and Douros, 1979; Suffness et al., 1989; Douros and Suffness, 1981

In recent years, a wide assortment of in-vitro and in-vivo assays have been developed in addition to those mentioned previously. They are not used within the NCI screening program as a matter of course, but are widely used by NCI or at-large investigators to study specific activities of an agent. These can be divided into cellular-based assays, which measure the overall effect on the cell, and mechanism-based assays, which measure only certain aspects of cell life. Examples of cellular-based assays include measurement of an agent's cytotoxic effect against isolated stem cells, and measurement of an agent's cytotoxic effect under both aerobic and hypoxic conditions. Examples of mechanism-based assays include measurement of angiogenesis inhibition and measurement of invasion inhibition.

11.1.4 Results of the NCI Screening Program

Less than 0.004% of the plant materials tested in the NCI screening program contained compounds that demonstrated clinical efficacy as anticancer agents. Of the approximate 114,000 plant extracts studied, 11,000 exhibited antitumor activity in the P338 prescreen. Of these, approximately 500 exhibited antitumor activity in panel testing, and of these, only about 26 proceeded to

TABLE 11.4. CELL LINES USED IN THE DISEASE ORIENTED SCREEN	
DESCRIPTION	**NCI CELL LINE CODE**
Human lung cancer	NCI-H23, NCI-H226, NCI-H322M, NCI-H522, A549/ATCC, EKVX, HOP-18, HOP-62, HOP-92, LXFL-529, DMS-114, DMS-273
Human renal cancer	UO-31, SN12C, A498, CAKI-1, RXF-393, RXF-631, ACHN, 786-0, TK-10
Human colon cancer	HT29, HCC-2998, HCT-116, SW-620, COLO-205, DLD-1, HCT-15, KM12, KM20L2
Human melanoma	LOX IMVI, MALME-3M, SK-MEL-2, SK-MEL-5, SK-MEL-28, M-19-MEL, UACC-62, UACC-257, M14
Human CNS cancer	SNB-19, SNB-75, SNB-78, U251, SF-268, SF-295, SF-539, XF-498
Human ovarian cancer	OVCAR-3, OVCAR-4, OVCAR-5, OVCAR-8, IGR-OV-1, SK-OV-3
Human leukemia	CCRF-CEM, K-562, MOLT-4, HL-60, RPMI-8226, SR

Adapted from: Crommelin and Midha, 1992

TABLE 11.5. COMPOUNDS SELECTED FOR ADVANCED DEVELOPMENT FROM WITHIN THE NCI SCREENING PROGRAM

COMPOUND	CHEMICAL FAMILY	PLANT SOURCE
4-beta-hydroxy-withanolide E	triterpene	*Withania sp.*
Acronycine	alkaloid	*Acronychia baueri*
Aphidicolin glycinate	diterpene	*Cephalosporium aphidicola*
Aristolochic acid	alcohol	*Aristolochia sp.**
Baccharin, Isobaccharin	trichothecane	*Baccharis megapotamica*
Bruceantin	diterpene	*Brucea sp.**
Camptothecin, 10-hydrocamptothecine	alkaloid	*Camptotheca acuminata**
Ellipticine	alkaloid	*Ochrosia moorei*
Eriofertopin	sesquiterpene lactone	*Eriophyllum confertiflorum*
Fagaronine	alkaloid	*Fagara macrophylla*
Harringtonine, Homoharringtonine	alkaloid	*Cephalotaxus harringtonia*
Indicine N-Oxide	pyrrolizidine alkaloid	*Heliotropium indicum**
Lapachol	quinone	*Tabebuia sp.*
Maytansine	ansa macrolide	*Maytenus ovatus*
Nitidine	alkaloid	*Zanthoxylum nitidum**
Pancratistatin	alkaloid	*Pancratium littorale*
Phyllanthoside	sesquiterpene	*Phyllanthus brasiliensis*
Podophyllotoxin derivatives	lignan	*Podophyllum sp.**
Psorospermin	xanthone	*Psorospermum febrifugum*
Taxol	taxane type diterpene	*Taxus brevifolia*
Tripdiolide	diterpene triepoxide	*Tripterygium wilfordii*
Tylocrebrine	alkaloid	*Ficus sp.**

* Used in Chinese herbal medicine.
Sources: Suffness, 1994, personal communication; Suffness and Pezzuto, 1991; Crommelin and Midha, 1992; Suffness et al., 1989; Vlietinck and Dommisse, 1985; Lien and Li, 1985; Hsu et al., 1986; Hsu et al., 1985; Hsu et al., 1982

secondary testing. Isolated compounds that proceeded to advanced development (secondary testing or clinical trials) are listed Table 11.5. Of these, four progressed to clinical trials and demonstrated efficacy. These compounds are taxol, homoharringtonine, camptothecin, and ellipticine (Suffness and Pezzuto, 1991; Suffness, 1994, personal communication). Of these, only taxol has received marketing approval by the U.S. Food and Drug Administration, although camptothecin and its derivatives are probably not far behind.

Not all plant-derived anticancer agents were discovered in the NCI screening program. The anticancer properties of vinblastine and vincristine (derived from *Catharanthus roseus,* or Madagascar periwinkle) were discovered by accident when researchers were testing this plant for antidiabetic activity. The test animals became susceptible to bacterial infections due to a lowered leukocyte count, which led to its testing as an antileukemic

agent. Other active botanical agents that were not products of the NCI screening program include etoposide and teniposide (from *Podophyllum peltatum*). Active agents obtained from microorganisms include doxorubicin (Adriamycin), actinomycin D, and mitomycin C, all produced by *Streptomyces* species; and bleomycin, derived from a fungal culture.

11.2 ANTITUMOR COMPOUNDS SELECTED FOR ADVANCED DEVELOPMENT IN CHINA

Antitumor compounds isolated from plants (or insects) that have proceeded to advanced development as anticancer agents in China are listed in Table 11.6. Other compounds that have demonstrated antitumor activity in vivo, but have not proceeded to advanced

TABLE 11.6. COMPOUNDS TESTED IN CHINESE CLINICAL TRIALS OR SELECTED FOR FURTHER DEVELOPMENT IN CHINA

COMPOUND	CHEMICAL FAMILY	PLANT SOURCE
Camptothecin, 10-hydroxycamptothecin	alkaloid	*Camptotheca acuminata (xi shu)*
Cantharidin	not specified	*Mylabris phalerata (ban mao)* (insect)
Harringtonine, Homoharringtonine	alkaloid	*Cephalotaxus harringtonia*
Indirubin	alkaloid	*Isatis tinctoria (da qing ye* or *qing dai)*
Monocrotaline	alkaloid	*Crotalaria sessiliflora (ye bai he)*
Oridonin	diterpene	*Isodon sp.*
Ponicidin	diterpene	*Isodon sp.*
Vinblastine, vincristine, vindesine	alkaloid	*Catharanthus roseus (chang chun hua)*

Sources: Lien and Li, 1985; Hsu et al., 1986; Hsu et al., 1985; Hsu et al., 1982

development are listed in Appendix F. A number of these compounds may not be desirable candidates for anticancer agents because they are either overly toxic to normal cells or cause excessive immunosuppression. Other compounds have not been studied in sufficient depth to comment on their utility. Therefore, the majority of these compounds will not be discussed further. However, there are a few compounds listed in Table 11.6 and Appendix F that do hold some clinical promise, or are otherwise worthy of further discussion. These include indirubin, rhein, emodin, psoralen, matrine, and oxymatrine. These compounds are discussed in more detail below.

11.3 ANTITUMOR COMPOUNDS OF INTEREST

A number of antitumor compounds isolated from natural agents either do not cause excessive adverse side effects, or are otherwise worthy of discussion. Some of these are listed in Table 11.7. Other antitumor compounds that are dietary components, such as quercetin, genistein, green tea polyphenols, and eicosapentaenoic acid (EPA), will be discussed in the following chapters.

Much of the data discussed in this section was obtained from animal models. Before continuing, it may be useful to review the methods by which animal data are extrapolated to human use.

11.3.1 Extrapolation of Animal Data

Extrapolation of data between species is difficult to perform with accuracy. A number of methods have been used, but the two most common are to base extrapolation on surface area or on metabolic weight. Small animal species often require higher doses of an agent per unit body weight than humans, and simple body weight extrapolation (such as mg/kg per day) can overestimate the equivalent human dose.

Extrapolation based on surface area requires an estimate of the surface area for the human and animal in

TABLE 11.7. ANTITUMOR COMPOUNDS OF INTEREST

COMPOUND	SOURCE
Berberine	*Coptis chinensis (huang lian)*, *Hydrastis canadensis* (goldenseal) and *Berberis aquifolium* (Oregon grape).
Indirubin	*Isatis tinctoria (da qing ye* or *qing dai)*
Limonene and perillyl alcohol	*Citrus reticulata* (orange oil)
Matrine and oxymatrine	*Sophora flavescens (ku shen)*, *S. subprostrata (shan dou gen)*
Psoralen	*Psoralea corylifolia (bu gu zhi)*, *Glehnia littoralis (sha shen)*, *Angelica pubescens (du huo)*, *A. dahurica (bai zhi)*, *Ledebouriella seseloides (fang feng)*, and *Ficus carica* (fig)
Rhein and emodin	*Rheum palmatum* and other *Rheum sp. (da huang)*; *Cassia tora* and *C. obtusifolia (jue ming zi)*, *C. angustifolia* and *C. acutifolia (fan xie ye*, senna); *Polygonum multiflorum (he shou wu)*, and *P. cuspidatum (hu chang)*; *Rumex crispus (yellow dock)*; *Rhamnus purshiana* (cascara sagrada) and *R. frangula* (alder buckthorn)

TABLE 11.8. EFFECTS OF BERBERINE IN VITRO

CELL LINE	EFFECT	REFERENCE
Human U-251 MG, SF-210, SF-188, U-87 MG, U-373 MG, SF-126 brain	Average of 91% cell kill at 150 µg/ml (446 µM)	Zhang RX, 1990
Human HepG2 hepatoma	Marked growth inhibition starting at 10 µg/ml (30 µM)	Chi et al., 1994
Human Hela	50% cytotoxicity at 3.5 µg/ml (10.4 µM)	Hladon et al., 1978
Ehrlich and NK/Ly lymphoma	50% growth inhibition at 50 µg/ml (148 µM)	Shvarev and Tsetlin, 1972

question. For adult humans and animals, this can be accomplished using the formula:

$$\text{Surface area (m}^2) = \frac{(K \cdot BW^{0.66})}{100}$$

K is a species-specific factor and BW is the body weight in kilograms. The value of K is approximately 9 for mice and rats, and 10.6 for a 70-kilogram (154 pound) human (reviewed by Amdur et al., 1991:991-2). The ratio of the human-to-animal surface area is then used to calculate the appropriate human dose. For example, the surface area ratio between a 70-kilogram human and a 20-gram mouse is 1.8/0.0068, or 260. If the dose of an agent for a 20-gram mouse is 0.025 grams, then the equivalent human dose is approximately 0.025 x 260, or 6.5 grams.

Extrapolation based on metabolic mass uses the ratio of body weights raised to an exponential factor, K:

$$\left(\frac{BW_{human}}{BW_{animal}}\right)^K$$

The value K ranges from 0.08 to 1.31, depending on the drug effect being measured (reviewed by Hayes, 1984:717). For extrapolating data for noncarcinogenic agents, a value of K between 0.74 and 0.76 may be appropriate in a variety of situations (Van Miert, 1989, Watanabe et al., 1992).[7] Using the data from the surface area example, and a K of 0.75, the ratio of the body weight of human to mouse is $(70/0.02)^{0.75}$ or 450. Therefore, the estimated equivalent dose for humans is 450 x 0.025, or 11 grams.

As is apparent from the above examples, different extrapolation techniques do not always produce identical results. These techniques provide only a rough estimate of the equivalent human dose. Only human clinical trials can determine an actual, effective dose.

11.3.2 Berberine

Plants containing berberine have been used for centuries to treat infections, and recent research has verified that berberine is cytotoxic to a variety of pathogenic bacteria (reviewed by Chang and But, 1987:1029-40). Berberine also produces an antitumor effect, although the mechanism by which it acts has not been fully determined. Berberine inhibits oxygen uptake by neoplastic cells in vitro (reviewed by Zhang RX, 1990) and induces differentiation in human teratocarcinoma cells in vitro (Chang et al., 1990). Although berberine was more potent than vitamin A in inducing differentiation, a relatively high concentration of berberine was required (100 µg/ml, or 297 µM), which was approximately 20% of the toxic concentration. Achieving this concentration in humans without adverse effects may be difficult. Studies reporting a cytotoxic effect for berberine in vitro are summarized in Table 11.8.

A limited number of in-vivo studies have also been conducted. Intraperitoneal administration of 10 mg/kg berberine to rats bearing 9L brain tumors resulted in an 81% cell kill as demonstrated on autopsy (Zhang RX, 1990).[8] The berberine was administered in a single dose and animals were sacrificed 24 hours after treatment. In contrast Bodor and Brewster (1983) reported that berberine did not penetrate the blood-brain barrier when injected intravenously into rats as determined on autopsy. In their experiments, intraperitoneal administration of 10 mg/kg berberine three times per day increased the life span of rats bearing P338 lymphocytic leukemia by 12%, but did not prolong their life span when the P338 cells were implanted intracerebrally. At 2.5 to 7.5 mg/kg per day, intraperitoneal administration of berberine did not inhibit Ehrlich ascites tumor growth in mice (Shvarev and Tsetlin, 1972).

It is possible that the antitumor effects of berberine are related, in part, to its effects on the immune system. At 0.15 µg/ml (0.45 µM) berberine markedly activated macrophages against EL4 leukemic cells in vitro (Kumazawa et al., 1984).

From the above data, it does not appear that berberine, on its own, will produce significant anticancer effects. However, it may be useful when used in combination with other agents that reinforce its effects. For

---

[7] A value of 0.67 roughly corresponds to extrapolations based on surface area.

[8] This dose is approximately one-half the toxic dose. The LD_{50} of berberine in rats and mice is 205 mg/kg and 24.3 mg/kg intraperitoneal respectively (Chang and But, 1987:1034).

example, DMSO and vitamin A may reinforce its effect on differentiation. However, this approach has not yet been studied clinically.

11.3.3 Indirubin

Indirubin is a compound found in *Isatis tinctoria* (*qing dai* or *da qing ye*). Its effects were first reported in 1978, when Chinese investigators observed that indirubin was the active agent in *Dang Gui Lu Hui* pills, which had previously been reported to be effective against chronic myelocytic leukemia (CML) in humans. It is not yet known how indirubin may exert its antileukemic effect. It inhibits DNA synthesis in neoplastic cells, and its actions appear to be specific to immature leukemic cells in the bone marrow. Indirubin may increase the membrane fluidity of leukocytes (Gan et al., 1987), secondary to altering their surface charge (Wang et al., 1984b).

Indirubin has been shown to inhibit DNA synthesis in a variety of cell lines, including human chronic and acute granulocytic leukemic cells, Walker 256 cells, ascitic hepatic carcinoma, and Ehrlich ascites carcinoma cells (reviewed by Chang and But, 1987:695). A derivative of indirubin, meisoindigo (methylisoindigo), exhibited greater activity in rodent models than did indirubin itself, primarily because the rodents absorbed meisoindigo better (Ji et al., 1991).

Some investigators think the antileukemic effects of indirubin are due, in part, to stimulation of the immune system. Administration of indirubin to patients with CML normalized cellular and humoral immune parameters, possibly in response to a normalization of cAMP levels (Chang and But, 1987:695).

Indirubin has been tested clinically in China. In a study of 314 patients with chronic myelocytic leukemia treated with synthetic indirubin (150 to 200 mg orally), the partial remission rate was 33%, and the complete remission rate was 26%.[9] Optimal effect was seen after approximately 72 days of treatment. Although the complete remission rate is higher in those patients treated with conventional drug therapy (Myleran), indirubin has the advantage of lower toxicity and mild side effects. Unlike Myleran, indirubin does not suppress bone marrow function (Ma and Yao, 1983; Chang, 1985).

Indirubin exhibits a low water solubility and is poorly absorbed. Not surprisingly, most of its side effects are due to irritation of the gastrointestinal lining. These side effects include mild abdominal pain, diarrhea, nausea, vomiting, and blood in the stool. Severe gastrointestinal reactions have occurred in 5 to 7% of treated patients, thrombocytopenia occurred in 20%, and mild marrow suppression occurred in 5% (Ma and Yao, 1983). Three cases of reversible pulmonary arterial hypertension and cardiac insufficiency were reported in patients on long-term indirubin therapy (Jiang et al., 1986). Indirubin may be as toxic as hydroxyurea, which is commonly used in the United States to maintain CML patients.

11.3.4 Limonene and Perillyl Alcohol

Limonene

The anticarcinogenic and antitumor effects of limonene and other monoterpenes have been studied for the last 10 years at the University of Wisconsin by Michael Gould, Ph.D. Limonene, which comprises up to 96% of orange oil, has been shown to inhibit stomach, lung, skin, and liver cancers in rodent models.[10] None of the evidence suggests that the effects of limonene are specific to certain tumor lines and, therefore, a wide variety of cancers may respond to limonene treatment. Oral administration of limonene (10% of diet) for three weeks caused reversible regression of tumors in 89% of rats with chemically-induced mammary tumors. This effect was observed in rats with both small and advanced tumors, and the majority of tumor regressions were complete. Regression was maintained as long as limonene administration was continued. Little or no toxicity was observed (Haag et al., 1992).[11]

At lower doses (less than 1% of diet), limonene inhibits rat mammary carcinogenesis induced by a variety of carcinogens. Limonene's anticarcinogenic effects are probably due to its ability to stimulate hepatic drug metabolism, thereby effectively detoxifying carcinogens. Terpenes induce a wider spectrum of detoxification enzymes than does the classic enzyme inducer, phenobarbital (Gould, 1993).[12]

---

[9] The standard definition of a complete response is the disappearance of all disease for a period greater than 30 days. A partial response is a 50% reduction in all measurable disease, sustained for greater than 30 days, as determined by the sum of products of the perpendicular diameters of all lesions. Special criteria are made for leukemias. It is not always clear in the Chinese studies if this criteria is being used.

[10] Midseason sweet orange oil may contain 80 to 96% limonene, with the remainder being other terpenes. However, analysis of some commercial orange oil revealed a zero limonene content (Gould, 1994, personal communication).

[11] Although limonene causes kidney damage in male rats, this effect is specific to rats and is not relevant to humans (Flamm and Lehman-McKeeman, 1991).

[12] This suggests that low doses of limonene could be used to stimulate detoxification pathways in appropriate patients.

At larger doses, the antitumor activity of limonene is probably due to its ability to inhibit the synthesis of isoprenylated proteins, such as members of the p21 *ras* family. This prevents them from assuming their correct location and function. It also inhibits the synthesis of coenzyme Q (ubiquinone), which contains a condensation of a long isoprene chain. Limonene may also induce the secretion of transforming growth factor-β (Gould, 1993; Jirtle et al., 1993), an effect quercetin and a variety of other ligands also induce (discussed in Section 14.4.4)

Limonene is currently undergoing phase I (toxicity) trials in pancreatic and colorectal cancer patients in London (McNamee, 1993). In a phase I trial, the dosage is generally increased, in stepwise fashion, from 1/10th the maximally tolerated dose to the point that toxic effects are observed or a desired dosage is achieved. As of December, 1994, the current dose administered in this trial is 8 grams/m^2 per day (roughly 14 grams/day for 70-kilogram human). The dose necessary to induce tumor regression in humans is expected to be roughly 90 to 100 grams/day for a 70-kilogram human, based on extrapolation from rodent studies. According to Dr. Gould, this large dosage may cause local irritation of the stomach tissues (1994, personal communication). Limonene can also be expected to reduce cholesterol biosynthesis (Elegbede, 1985).

Perillyl Alcohol

Due to the high dosages of limonene required for tumor regression, Dr. Gould and colleagues have been investigating related monoterpenes and have discovered that perillyl alcohol, a naturally occurring analog of limonene is 5 to 10 times more potent than limonene itself (Haag and Gould, 1994). Perillyl alcohol (at 2.0 to 2.5% of diet) induced regression of 81% of small mammary tumors and 75% of advanced, chemically-induced mammary tumors in rats. The majority of these regressions were complete, and secondary tumors were also prevented. No toxic effects were observed at a 2.0% diet. A 2.5% diet resulted in weight loss in rats, which may have been due to food aversion. A 3.0% diet resulted in several deaths. A minimum of 1.0% was required to produce a significant number of complete tumor regressions (regression rate 55%). A 1.0% perillyl alcohol diet in rats corresponds to a dose of approximately 10 grams/day in a 70-kilogram human. Dr. Gould hopes to receive an investigational new drug (IND) permit and be administering perillyl alcohol to patients in 1995 (Gould, 1994, personal communication).

Both limonene and perillyl alcohol are rapidly metabolized to terpene derivatives. Within one hour of administration of limonene to rats, more than 80% is metabolized to limonene derivatives, the most common of which is perillic acid and dihydroperillic acid (Crowell et al., 1992). Complete metabolism occurs within 24 hours. Perillyl alcohol produces the same metabolites in a shorter amount of time. No perillyl alcohol was detected in the plasma of rats within 15 minutes of administration, although perillic and dihydroperillic acids were detectable in the serum after 24 hours (Haag and Gould, 1994). These metabolites may, in fact, account for the antitumor effects of both limonene and perillyl alcohol.

Perillyl alcohol produces local irritation of the gastric mucosa, and sufficiently large doses produces reversible renal damage. It is not known if, or when, tumor resistance to limonene or perillyl alcohol will develop during long-term administration.

Other monoterpenes may be even more potent than perillyl alcohol. Preliminary studies on the monoterpene geranoil suggest that it may be effective at 1/6th the concentration of perillyl alcohol (Anderson et al., 1993). Toxicity data on geranoil is not yet available.

11.3.5 Matrine and Oxymatrine

Matrine and oxymatrine are alkaloids found in *Sophora subprostrata (shan dou gen)* and *Sophora flavescens (ku shen)*. These alkaloids show cytotoxic activity in vitro and antitumor activity in vivo. The antitumor effects of *S. subprostrata* and its alkaloids are summarized in Table 11.9. Crude extracts of *S. subprostrata* also possess antiarrhythmic, antibacterial, antiasthmatic, antileukopenic, and antiulcer activities in vivo (reviewed by Chang and But, 1986:108-16). For example, 25 patients with radiotherapy-induced leukopenia were treated with 200 to 400 mg of an extract that contained primarily oxymatrine. The blood counts of 84% of the patients improved. In 30 patients with radiotherapy-induced leukopenia, 93% improved. In 20 patients with chemotherapy-induced leukopenia, 65% improved (reviewed by Chang and But, 1986:108-16).

Oxymatrine was shown to be 7.8 times stronger than mitomycin C against sarcoma 180 (Kojima et al., 1970). Mice treated with matrine and oxymatrine gained weight during treatment, suggesting that the treatment was not toxic. In contrast, mice treated with mitomycin C lost weight. The effects of oxymatrine were not dose-dependent, as maximal effects were sometimes seen at less than maximal dosages. Crude extracts of a variety of *Sophora sp.* have been shown to be moderately effective against sarcoma 180, lymphoid leukemia 1210, and melanoma at 250 to 400 mg/kg intraperitoneal (reviewed by Kojima et al., 1970).

Although a number of clinical trials of *Sophora subprostrata* or its alkaloids have been conducted in China,

TEST ANIMAL	CANCER	DOSE	EFFECT	REFERENCE
	TABLE 11.9. ANTITUMOR EFFECTS OF *SOPHORA SUBPROSTRATA* AND ITS ALKALOIDS			
Mice	U14 cervical carcinoma	60 g/kg of the aqueous extract	Marked inhibition	Reviewed by Chang and But, 1986:108-16
	Sarcoma 180		25% inhibition	
	Ascitic type lymphosarcoma L1		No effect	
Rats	Ascitic Jitian sarcoma	500 mg/kg i.p. of aqueous extract of the herb powder	Complete remission > 60%	
	Solid ascitic carcinoma of the liver		Complete remission > 60%	
Mice	Ehrlich ascites carcinoma	2.5 mg/kg matrine	effective	
	Sarcoma 180		effective	
Mice	Ehrlich ascites	0.5 mg i.p. of matrine daily	40% survival rate (0% in controls)	Kojima et al., 1970
Mice		0.5 mg i.p. of oxymatrine daily	0% survival	
Mice	Sarcoma 180 (Bulgaria strain)	0.25 mg i.p. of oxymatrine daily	Reduction in tumor size by 58%	
	Sarcoma 180 (Hokken strain)	0.5 mg i.p. of oxymatrine daily	Reduction in tumor size by 9 to 20%	
		0.25 mg i.p. of matrine daily	Reduction in tumor size by 54%	

results have not clearly demonstrated a positive effect (reviewed by Chang and But, 1986:112).

11.3.6 Psoralen

Psoralen and related compounds (psoralens) are furocoumarins originally derived from *Psoralea sp.* (including *Psoralea corylifolia, bu gu zi*) that have been used in dermatology since the 1950s to treat psoriasis and other skin disorders.[13] Psoralens are used in conjunction with ultraviolet-A light (long-wave ultraviolet, 320 to 400 nm) to potentiate their effect. The combined treatment is referred to as PUVA therapy. Since PUVA therapy may be carcinogenic, it is usually reserved for moderate to severe forms of psoriasis (Stolk and Siddiqui, 1988). Because of its effects on cell proliferation, PUVA therapy is also used to treat mycosis fungoides, a type of cutaneous T-cell lymphoma.

Purified psoralen may be more appropriate than crude psoralea extract as an anticancer agent. The discussion of psoralens is included here since a number of furocoumarin-containing herbs have been investigated for their anticancer effects, and the reader may desire a review of psoralen studies.

PUVA therapy causes an exaggerated sunburn reaction and inhibits cell proliferation. In the presence of ultraviolet radiation, the psoralen molecule converts to an electronically excited state that is capable of binding directly to cellular proteins (including DNA), and is also capable of generating superoxide anions. Both of these events may be involved in PUVA-induced cytotoxicity.

PUVA therapy inhibits the growth of a variety of tumor cells in vitro. Photoactivated psoralens, at concentrations of 20 µg/ml (107 µM), inhibited K562, human HL-60 and human Raji leukemic cell lines in vitro by 86%, 35%, and 35% respectively (Lu et al., 1993). Psoralen or UV-A light alone did not inhibit growth of sarcoma 180 cells, but photoactivated psoralen in biologically attainable concentrations (0.01 to 50 µM) inhibited the cells by 50% (Yurkow and Laskin, 1991).

In addition to its antiproliferative effects, photoactivated psoralens also produce immunosuppression. Administration of high doses of photoactivated psoralens to mice inhibited delayed-type hypersensitivity (DTH) skin reactions to sheep red blood cells (Potapenko et al., 1994). Human psoriasis patients also exhibit reduced DTH reactions after PUVA treatment (Grekin and Epstein, 1981).

Although pharmacokinetic data are not available on psoralen itself, the naturally occurring psoralen derivative 8-methoxypsoralen (8-MOP) has been used clinically and studied extensively. The standard oral dose is 0.5 to

---

[13] Psoriasis is a chronic inflammatory condition marked by uncontrolled epidermal cell growth and rapid cell death, which leads to the formation of thick scales or plaques of epidermal tissue.

0.6 mg/kg per day.[14] Peak serum levels normally occur within one to four hours of administration, and commonly reach a concentration of 200 µg/l (1.1 µM), which is less than that required for cytotoxic effects. The half-life is about one hour. In treating psoriasis, UV-A treatment is given to skin tolerance two hours after psoralen administration. The treatment is repeated two to four times per week. Side effects may include nausea and patchy skin pigmentation (Stolk and Siddiqui, 1988).

Some studies suggest that nonphotoactivated psoralens may also produce a cytotoxic effect. Nonactivated psoralen, at a concentration of 8.6 µg/ml (46 µM), inhibited human salivary mucoepidermoid carcinoma (MEC-1) cells by 50% (Wu et al., 1992).[15] Nonactivated psoralen has also demonstrated in-vivo activity. In nude mice inoculated with MEC-1 cells, an intraperitoneal dose of 3.3 mg/kg once per day reduced tumor weights by 79% (Wu et al., 1992). Treated mice exhibited a 5% weight loss as compared to tumor-bearing controls, suggesting mild systemic toxic effects.

11.3.7 Rhein and Emodin

Rhein

Rhein is an anthraquinone found in a number of common purgative herbs (see Table 11.7) and is responsible, in large part, for their effects. Rhein-induced purgative effects occur through two distinct mechanisms: 1) an increase in intestinal fluid transport, and 2) an increase in intestinal motility. These effects are probably due to stimulation of PGE_2 synthesis and alteration of calcium transport in colon cells (Yamauchi et al., 1993; Geboes et al., 1993). In addition to laxative actions, rhein also has antibacterial, antitumor, and anti-inflammatory properties (reviewed by Anton and Haag-Berrurier, 1980; reviewed by Freidmann, 1980).

Cytotoxic and Antitumor Activities

Rhein inhibits protein synthesis in neoplastic cells by decreasing the rates of cellular respiration and glycolysis. A variety of neoplastic lines are susceptible to rhein concentrations of approximately 65 µM, including Ehrlich ascites, sarcoma 180, Yoshida ascites, and AS-30D hepatoma (Castiglione et al., 1990). The decrease in glycolysis may be due to a decrease in glucose uptake by neoplastic cells, which is caused by alterations in the functional properties of the plasma membrane (Castiglione, et al., 1993). Rhein induces a marked increase in plasma membrane rigidity, possibly due to increased lipid peroxidation (Iosi et al., 1993). The fluidity of the plasma membrane plays a role in regulating glucose uptake and many other cellular activities. Rhein, at 100 µM, maximally reduced aerobic lactate production in Ehrlich ascites cells in vitro. Under anaerobic conditions, such as found in many solid tumors, maximal reduction occurred at 220 µM (Floridi et al., 1990a).

Rhein may be most effective when exposure is prolonged. Human A431 epithelial cells are reversibly inhibited at 50 µM when exposed for 8 hours, and irreversibly inhibited after 12 hours (Iosi et al., 1993). Exposure for 24 hours at 53 µM, and 48 hours at 18 µM both produced a 50% cell kill in human glioma cells. Exposure for 4 hours produced little cytotoxicity (Floridi et al., 1990b). Similarly, rhein produced a 50% cell kill of human glioma cells at a concentration of 20 µM after 12 hours (Delpino et al., 1992). Prior to 20 hours, the effect of exposure time on cell kill is exponentially related to rhein concentration. After about 20 hours, the relationship is linear.

Rhein has also shown an antitumor effect in vivo. Intraperitoneal administration of 40 mg/kg per day for seven days increased the survival time of P388 leukemia-bearing mice by 61% (Lu and Chen, 1989). Administration of 5 mg/kg inhibited melanoma in mice by 76% (reviewed by Chang and But, 1986:77). According to NCI data generated in 1959 and 1960, rhein is inactive in the intraperitoneal CA755, L1210, and sarcoma 180 models (Suffness, 1995, personal communication). As was mentioned previously, negative NCI data do not necessarily prove that an agent is devoid of antitumor activity. Rhein may turn out to be a case in point. Contemporary investigators are actively pursuing further studies.

Pharmacology

Although plants that contain rhein have been used for millennia to treat constipation, the biochemistry and action of rhein and related anthranoid compounds is complex and not yet fully elucidated. Rhein is found in plant materials in a variety of forms, including rhein anthrone, rhein anthraquinone, rhein dianthrones (two rhein molecules bound together, called sennosides and sennidins), and rhein anthraquinone glucosides (rhein anthraquinone bound to a sugar molecule). It appears that the primary form responsible for the purgative action of rhubarb and senna is rhein anthrone. The sennosides are not absorbed in the intestinal tract, and therefore enter the large intestine after oral administration (see Figure 11.2). In the large intestine, bacteria quickly degrade them to form sennidins, which further degrade to form rhein anthrone and rhein anthraquinone.

---

[14] In contrast, Wu et al. (1992) report that a standard dose of psoralen is 5.5 mg/kg per day.

[15] MEC-1 cells exhibit some biological characteristics of squamous cell carcinoma.

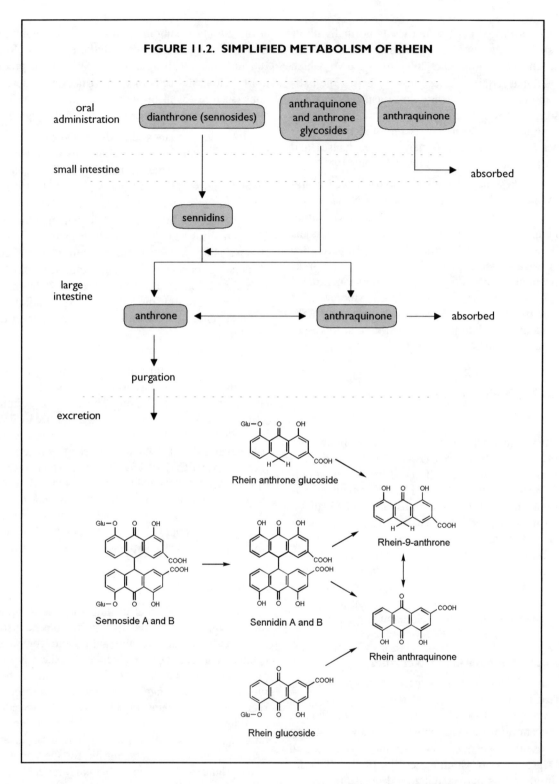

FIGURE 11.2. SIMPLIFIED METABOLISM OF RHEIN

Bacteria reduce rhein anthraquinone to form rhein anthrone. Similar to sennosides, rhein glycosides are poorly absorbed and are also degraded by bacteria to form rhein anthrone and rhein anthraquinone (reviewed by Lemli and Lemmens, 1980; reviewed by De Witte, 1993).

A significant portion of the rhein anthraquinone present in the original plant material or formed by bacterial action is absorbed through the gastrointestinal lining and enters the blood. In tests using radiolabeled ^{14}C-rhein anthraquinone, 50 to 60% of the orally administered anthraquinone is absorbed in rats (Lang, 1988).[16] Other

---

[16] Note that the intestines of small mammals tend to absorb a greater variety of compounds than do the intestines of humans.

CELL LINE	PERCENT INHIBITION	EMODIN CONCENTRATION	REFERENCE
Transformed human bronchial epithelial cells *	50%	4.2 µg/ml (15 µM)	Chan et al., 1993
	90%	100 µg/ml (370 µM)	
Normal human bronchial epithelial cells *	minimal		
Human promyelocytic leukemia HL-60	50%	5 µg/ml (19 µM)	Yeh, 1988
Human lung A-549	50%	10 µg/ml (37 µM)	Chen et al., 1991
Mouse mammary carcinoma FM3A	varied	1 to 10 µg/ml (3.7 to 37 µM)	Morita et al., 1988
Ehrlich ascites	50%	20 µg/ml (74 µM)	Chen et al., 1980

TABLE 11.10. INHIBITION OF TUMOR LINES IN VITRO BY EMODIN

* Assays comparing cytotoxicity in transformed cells versus nontransformed cells of the same line are primarily used to determine if the cytotoxic activity of an agent is specific to neoplastic cells.

investigators have reported slightly lower values. After intracaecal administration of radiolabeled rhein anthraquinone to rats, ^{14}C recovery in the urine was only 37% (De Witte and Lemli, 1988a, 1988b).

In contrast to rhein anthraquinone, rhein anthrone is poorly absorbed. After administration of rhein anthrone, ^{14}C recoveries in the urine and feces were 2.8 % and 95% respectively (De Witte and Lemli, 1988a, 1988b).[17] Rhein anthrone, and to a lesser extent rhein anthraquinone, accumulate in rat kidney tissues.

Rhein anthrone also produces a greater purgative action than the anthraquinone. The effective oral dose of rhein anthraquinone in mice is 97.5 mg/kg, whereas the effective dose of the sennosides (which form the anthrone and anthraquinone) is 13.3 to 16.1 mg/kg (Natori et al., 1981:424).

From the above discussions, it can be seen that the optimum form of rhein for the treatment of cancer is rhein anthraquinone. The anthraquinone is readily absorbed and causes the least purgative effect. To some degree, simply boiling the crude drug will favor its formation. For example, it is well known that rhubarb *(Rheum palmatum, da huang)* loses much of its purgative effect by boiling. Boiling the ground herb for 1.5 hours reduces the purgative effect by 50% (Natori et al., 1981:422). Rhubarb contains a number of natural acids, and boiling the herb appears to facilitate hydrolysis of the dianthrones. This allows the small intestine to absorb the released anthraquinones, thereby reducing the purgative effect in the large intestine. In addition, rhein anthrone is quite unstable. In the presence of oxygen, such as found in boiling water, rhein anthrone is readily converted to its anthraquinone form. It is interesting to note that in Chinese medicine, rhubarb is traditionally treated with vinegar to increase its ability to treat *blood stagnation.* One explanation of this may be that the acids in vinegar promote hydrolysis of the dianthrones and, therefore, reduce the purgative effects. This would allow the herb to be used at higher doses for its other effects.

Emodin

Like rhein, emodin is an anthraquinone found in a number of purgative herbs. It too exhibits numerous biologic activities. Studies indicate that emodin has vasorelaxive, immunosuppressive, immunostimulant, antibacterial, antitumor, anti-inflammatory, antiulcer, and hypolipidemic properties (Huang et al., 1991, 1992a; Goel et al., 1991; reviewed by Anton and Haag-Berrurier, 1980; reviewed by Freidmann, 1980). Herbs that contain emodin have been used in various aspects of cancer treatment in China. For example, in one study, 67 patients with leukopenia who received radiotherapy also received crude extracts of *Polygonum cuspidatum (hu chang)* or its anthraquinones. Both significantly increased leukocyte counts, often by more than 1,000/mm^3 (reviewed by Chang and But, 1987:783).

Cytotoxic and Antitumor Activities

Emodin is mildly cytotoxic to a number of human and animal cancer cell lines in vitro. Proliferation is inhibited by 50% at concentrations ranging from 4 to 20 µg/ml (15 to 74 µM), as shown in Table 11.10. The cytotoxic activity of emodin may be specific to neoplastic

[17] The ^{14}C recovered in these studies was not necessarily associated with rhein anthraquinone or anthrone. In previous studies reviewed by De Witte and Lemli, as much as 20 to 57% of administered rhein was not recovered as rhein. Much of this loss was likely due to the formation of unknown rhein metabolites.

cells, as cultures of normal human bronchial epithelial cells were minimally affected even at high concentrations.

Emodin has also shown an antitumor effect in a small number of animal studies. Emodin, at 40 mg/kg per day intraperitoneal, increased the survival time of P388-bearing mice by 47% (Lu and Chen, 1989). Administration of 5 mg/kg inhibited melanoma in mice by 73% and administration of 75 mg/kg intraperitoneal inhibited mammary cancer in mice by 45% (reviewed by Chang and But, 1986:77). According to NCI data, emodin shows weak activity in the intraperitoneal P388 system, but is not active in the B16, CA755, L1210 or sarcoma 180 systems.[18] Therefore, although emodin would be officially classified as an active agent by NCI, few investigators consider it to be a realistic candidate for further development (personal communication, Suffness, 1995). However, like rhein, the study of emodin is continuing.

Pharmacology

Emodin possesses a similar absorption rate to rhein anthraquinone. Like rhein, emodin is retained in kidney tissue. It is also retained in adipose tissue (Bachmann and Schlatter, 1981). Emodin is a much less active purgative agent than rhein. The effective oral dose of emodin in mice is greater than 500 mg/kg, more than 5 times that of rhein (Natori et al., 1981:424).

11.4 CHINESE HERBS THAT EXHIBIT ANTITUMOR ACTIVITY

Crude extracts of a large number of Chinese herbs have been shown to exhibit antitumor activity. Studies on these agents are summarized in Table 11.11.[19] Studies on the in-vitro effects of these agents are not discussed further, since in-vitro cytotoxic activity is by no means rare and does not necessarily imply that the agent possesses suitable in-vivo activity.

Many of the agents listed in Table 11.11 may produce their antitumor effects by stimulating the immune system. Herbs that contain high molecular weight polysaccharides are examples. The applicability of these studies to human tumors is dependent on a number of factors, one of which is the tumor model used to obtain the data. Four types of tumor models, and their applicability to human anticancer immunity, are listed below (Tannock and Hill, 1992:243):

- Long-established transplantable tumor lines, such as many of those listed in Table 11.2, may be valid for studying transplantation immunity in humans, but probably are not valid for studying anticancer immunity. This is because the genetic makeup of either the tumor line or the "syngeneic" animal strain that hosts the tumor line may drift over time.[20] If such a "nonself" tumor is transplanted into an animal, the animal will readily reject the transplant due to its major histocompatibility complex products rather than due to recognition of tumor-specific antigens. Tumors in human cancer patients are truly syngeneic and this model is not applicable. For similar reasons, models using allogeneic tumor transplants are also not applicable.

- Animal tumors induced by viruses are strongly immunogenic and the immune response is virus-specific. These models may be applicable to human tumors if both are caused by the same virus. However, few human tumors are virally-induced.

- Animal tumors induced by high levels of carcinogens are usually strongly immunogenic and tumors induced with low levels of carcinogens are usually less immunogenic. Since many human tumors are thought to be caused by chronic exposure to low levels of carcinogens, and are weakly immunogenic, animal models that use low levels of carcinogens are most applicable to humans.

- Spontaneous animal tumors are usually weakly immunogenic or nonimmunogenic. The applicability of this model to humans varies depending on the cause and nature of the transformation (such as unrecognized chemicals or viruses).

Because of the differences in immunogenicity between experimental animal tumors and human tumors, immunostimulants that produce antitumor effects in animals may not necessarily produce the same effects in humans.

For descriptions of tumor lines mentioned below, see Table 11.2.

---

[18] In the P388 system, the T/C was 127 to 154% at doses of 20 to 100 mg/kg.

[19] Appendix G lists additional herbs with reported antitumor effects. This data was obtained from summaries of other works.

[20] Syngeneic tumors are grown and transplanted in the same animal strain, and allogeneic tumors are grown in one strain and transplanted into another. Syngeneic tumors express the same major histocompatibility complex products as the animal host.

TABLE 11.11. ANTITUMOR EFFECTS OF SOME CHINESE HERBS		
HERB	**EFFECT**	**REFERENCE**
Acanthopanax sp. (*wu jia pi, ci wu jia*)	Administration of *A. giraldii* polysaccharides to SA-bearing mice inhibited tumor growth by up to 67% and prolonged the survival by up to 71%. Up to 33% of the mice obtained complete remission. The extract also enhanced the phagocytosis and chemiluminescence of mouse macrophages in vitro. Although *A. giraldii* is not commonly used in Chinese medicine, similar results were obtained with *A. senticosus* and *A. obovatus*.	Wang et al., 1992a; Xie, 1989; Shen et al., 1991; Wang et al., 1993a; Williams, 1993
Actinidia chinensis (teng li)	Intraperitoneal administration of a polysaccharide extract to tumor-bearing mice inhibited the growth of EA and hepatoma A (ascites form) by 89%, and hepatoma S (solid form) by 49% as compared to controls. The compound prolonged the life of EA- or PA-bearing mice. In addition, the extract enhanced the antitumor effect of 5-fluorouracil.	Lin, 1988
Agrimonia pilosa (*xian he cao*)	Intraperitoneal administration of the methanol extract prolonged the survival of SA, Meth-A fibrosarcoma, and MM-2 mammary carcinoma-bearing mice. The extract also elevated peripheral leukocyte counts.	Koshiura et al., 1985
Aloe vera	Polysaccharide fractions (acemannan) increased antibody-dependent cellular cytotoxicity (ADCC) and stimulated the proliferation of thymic cells. Acemannan also increased the survival of sarcoma-bearing mice. The tumors in acemannan-treated animals exhibited vascular congestion, edema, leukocyte infiltration, central necrosis with hemorrhage, and peripheral fibrinolysis. The authors report that these effects may be due to stimulation of the production of IL-1 and TNF by macrophages. Intraperitoneal or intralesional administration of acemannan to 43 dogs and cats with spontaneous tumors resulted in histopathologic evidence of immunologic attack as demonstrated by marked necrosis or lymphoid infiltration in 60% of the animals. Twelve animals (30%) showed obvious clinical improvement. These included five of seven cases of fibrosarcoma. *Aloe vera* gel also inhibits metastasis in numerous animal models.	Peng et al., 1991; Harris et al., 1991; Gribel and Pashinskii, 1986; Ralamboranto et al., 1982
Aloe vahombe	Administration of a polysaccharide fraction decreased the growth rate of fibrosarcoma and melanoma tumors in mice. The compound also protected mice against bacterial, parasitic, and fungal infections.	Ralamboranto et al., 1982
Angelica sinensis, A. acutiloba (dang gui)	Administration of a polysaccharide fraction increased the life span of SA-bearing mice by up to 180%, increased the life span of IMC-bearing mice by up to 274%, increased the life span of Meth-A fibrosarcoma-bearing mice by up to 170%, and increased the life span of solid MM-46-bearing mice by up to 99%. Crude extracts inhibited transplanted EA tumors in mice and increased the cytotoxic activity of TNF.	Yamada et al., 1990; Haranaka et al., 1985a, 1985b
Arctium lappa (burdock root)	Various fractions that are not water-soluble inhibited EA and Yoshima sarcoma in mice by as much as 61%.	Dombradi and Foldeak, 1966
Artemisia capillaris (*yin chen hao*)	Aqueous extracts inhibited Meth-A tumors in mice. *A. capillaris* acted through direct cytotoxic action with no associated immunosuppression.	Mori et al., 1989
Astragalus membranaceus (*huang qi*)	Fractions improved the function of T lymphocytes obtained from 13 cancer patients by 260%, as compared to untreated cells, and by 160% as compared to cells from normal healthy donors. T-cell function was measured by observing the degree of in-vitro reaction to foreign cells.	Chu et al., 1988a, 1989
Astragalus membranaceus (*huang qi*) and *Ligustrum lucidum* (*nu zhen zi*)	Ex-vivo, extracts reversed macrophage suppression caused by renal cell carcinoma in mice. Intraperitoneal administration of the extract inhibited renal cell tumor growth in mice, reaching a 100% cure rate in mice with small tumor loads.	Rittenhouse et al., 1991, Lau et al., 1992
(Table continues)		

TABLE 11.11. *(continued)*		
HERB	**EFFECT**	**REFERENCE**
Atractylodes macrocephala (bai zhu)	The volatile oil inhibited EA and SA, although results were conflicting.	Reviewed by Chang and But, 1986:376
Bu Zhong Yi Qi Tang (formula)	Intraperitoneal administration suppressed the growth of EA carcinoma in mice.	Ito and Shimura, 1985a, 1985b
Bupleurum chinense (chai hu)	Crude extracts inhibited EA tumors in mice and increased the cytotoxic activity of TNF.	Haranaka et al., 1985a, 1985b
Cinnamomum cassia (rou gui)	Crude extracts inhibited EA tumors in mice and increased the cytotoxic activity of TNF.	Haranaka et al., 1985a, 1985b
Cordyceps sinensis (dong chong xia cao)	Oral administration of the crude extract reduced tumor size and increased survival times of mice implanted with EL-4 lymphoma cells. In untreated mice, peritoneal macrophage activity decreased markedly within a few days of injection of the lymphoma cells, which lasted until death. In treated mice, macrophage activity increased to levels approximately four times greater than controls. In other experiments, macrophage activity in mice was restored to normal levels after being suppressed by cyclophosphamide treatment. The ethanol extract reduced the growth of B1 melanoma cells implanted in mouse lungs. The hot-water extract prolonged survival of mice with EA carcinoma by 316%, and mice with Meth-A fibrosarcoma by 312%, as compared to controls. No cytotoxic effects were observed in vivo, suggesting that the response was due to immune modulation. The antitumor effect of the extract decreased significantly when the mice were pretreated with radiotherapy.	Yamaguchi et al., 1990; Xu et al., 1992; Yoshida et al., 1989
Crocus sativa (saffron)	Oral administration of the crude extract increased the life span of EAC, SA, and Dalton's lymphoma ascites (DLA)-bearing mice by 183 to 212%. In vitro, the extract was cytotoxic to P38B, SA, EA and DLA cells. The mechanism of action was inhibition of DNA synthesis. Toxicity studies indicated that hematological and biochemical parameters of the treated mice were normal. Human tumor cells were more sensitive to treatment than healthy cells. Liposome encapsulation enhanced the antitumor activity against SA and EA carcinoma in mice. *C. sativa* exhibited antioxidant activity as demonstrated by increased intracellular reduced glutathione levels in treated SA cells in vitro.	Nair et al., 1991, 1992; Abdullaev and Frenkel, 1992
Curcuma aromatica (yu jin or *e zhu)*	The volatile oil of *C. aromatica* exhibited marked antitumor activity against mouse EA carcinoma and rat ascitic reticulum cell sarcoma. Antitumor activity was also observed against SA in mice and Yoshida sarcoma in rats. During treatment, 13% of the tumor-bearing animals experienced diarrhea or weight loss, which suggests that there may be some toxicity to the host. Extracts of *Curcuma sp.* inhibited Dalton's lymphoma cells in vitro and in vivo. The active component was found to be curcumin. Ethanol extracts of *Curcuma longa (yu jin)* provided symptomatic relief in humans with external cancerous lesions.	Shi, 1981; Kuttan et al., 1985, 1987
Ganoderma lucidum (ling zhi)	High molecular weight polysaccharide compounds obtained from water extracts markedly inhibited SA in mice. Injection of the aqueous extract into LL-bearing mice increased life spans up to 195%. This effect was observed when the extract was administered alone or in conjunction with chemotherapy drugs. The extract was nontoxic to cell cultures, and the antitumor action was believed to occur through T-cell activation.	Maruyama et al., 1989; Furusawa et al., 1992
(Table continues)		

HERB	EFFECT	REFERENCE
Liu Wei Di Huang Tang (formula)	Administration of the formula to SA-bearing mice, in conjunction with the chemotherapy agents Adriamycin, cyclophosphamide, cisplatin, vincristine, and 5-fluorouracil, resulted in increased survival rates, leukocyte counts, platelet counts, NK cell activity, and increased T- and B-lymphocyte transformation rates, as compared to controls receiving only the chemotherapy agents. The formula decreased the incidence of stomach and lung cancers in chemically treated mice, and enhanced macrophage activity and prolonged the life span of U14-bearing mice.	Xu, 1992; Jiang et al., 1984
Panax ginseng (ginseng, *ren shen*)	In SA-bearing mice, administration of the immunostimulant saponins for 8 days reduced tumor weights by as much as 75%, although inhibition decreased when tumor loads were large. Oral administration of the 70% methanol extract inhibited the growth of solid ascites hepatoma AH-130 in rats, inhibited metastasis to the lung, and decreased the elevated platelet and fibrinogen levels induced by the tumor cells. In combination with mitomycin, the extract produced a greater antitumor effect than mitomycin alone. The extract promoted the uptake of mitomycin into the tumor cells in vitro and enhanced the cytotoxicity of mitomycin. Administration of the crude extract to rats with chemically-induced hepatocellular cancer significantly inhibited tumor growth and prolonged survival times.	Hau and You, 1990; Yang and Yu, 1988; Kubo et al., 1992; Li and Wu, 1991
Pseudostellaria heterophylla (tai zi shen)	Fractions of the herb stimulated mouse spleen cell growth in vitro, stimulated the release of TNF in mice, and inhibited EA carcinoma tumor cells in vivo, but not in vitro. These results suggest that the antitumor effect is due to stimulation of the immune system, rather than due to cytotoxic mechanisms.	Wong et al., 1992
Ren Shen Tang (formula)	Intraperitoneal administration suppressed the growth of EA carcinoma in mice. The formula derives its name from, and contains, *Panax ginseng (ren shen)*.	Ito and Shimura, 1985a, 1985b
Rubia cordifolia (qian cao gen)	An isolated peptide inhibited tumor growth in vivo in several experimental tumor systems. The compound produced a 100% cure rate (8/8) in C8-bearing mice compared with a cure rate of 1/8 with mitomycin.	Hamanaka et al., 1987
Schisandra chinensis (wu wei zi)	Administration of the isolated compound schizophyllan to rats with chemically induced bladder cancer decreased weight loss in the body and thymus, increased survival time, and postponed malignant changes in the bladder tissue.	Horii et al., 1991
Scutellaria baicalensis (huang qin)	Crude extracts inhibited cyclophosphamide- and 5-fluorouracil-induced myelotoxicity and decreased tumor growth in tumor-bearing mice and rats. An extract of the herb produced a normalizing effect on platelet-mediated hemostasis in rats with Pliss' lymphosarcoma. Disorders of platelet-mediated hemostasis (either lowered or increased aggregation activity) were associated with tumor advancement and metastatic activity. The extract produced a normalizing effect on hemostasis whatever the pattern of alteration. The authors believe that this activity may be responsible for the drug's metastasis-inhibiting effects.	Razina et al., 1987, 1989
Shi Quan Da Bu Tang (formula)	This formula consists primarily of herbs that *supplement qi* and *blood*. As such, it may stimulate immune function and hematopoiesis. The formula inhibited EA tumors in mice. It inhibited tumor growth and increased the survival rate of mice with chemically-induced bladder tumors treated with the chemotherapy agent cisplatin. *(column continues)*	Haranaka et al., 1985a, 1985b; Ebisuno et al., 1989; Yamada, 1989; Aburada et al., 1983; Ito and Shimura, 1985a, 1985b

(Table continues)

	TABLE 11.11. *(continued)*	
HERB	**EFFECT**	**REFERENCE**
Shi Quan Da Bu Tang (formula)	*(continued)* The formula also protected mice against renal and hepatic toxicity and bone marrow suppression caused by cisplatin. The formula increased the survival of PA-bearing mice treated with mitomycin, as compared to those treated only with mitomycin. The formula decreased the leukopenia, thrombocytopenia, and weight loss associated with mitomycin treatment. The formula prolonged the survival of PS-bearing mice treated with mitomycin. In tumor-free mice, the formula reduced the leukopenia and loss of body weight caused by mitomycin treatment, and delayed death due to a lethal dose of mitomycin. Intraperitoneal administration suppressed the growth of EA carcinoma in mice. Oral administration prolonged the survival of the mice.	See previous page
Solanum indicum (huang shui qie)	Purified extracts exhibited cytotoxic actions in seven cell lines in vitro and inhibited C6 glioma in vivo.	Chiang et al., 1991
Viscum album (sang ji sheng)	Anticancer therapy with viscum extracts has been conducted in Europe for over 60 years with thousands of patients. More than 40 clinical trials have been conducted and most of these have shown a positive effect. However, the studies were, in general, poorly designed and the efficacy of viscum has remained uncertain. Studies on the standardized extract suggest that it produces marked anti-inflammatory and immune-stimulating effects. Macrophages obtained from treated mice inhibited tumor cells in vitro. Injection of the macrophages lengthened the survival of tumor-bearing mice.	Bocci, 1993; Bruseth and Enge, 1993; Kuttan, 1993
Xiao Chai Hu Tang (formula)	Intraperitoneal administration suppressed the growth of EA carcinoma in mice. Oral administration prolonged the survival of the mice. The formula inhibited the growth of LL cells implanted in the footpads of mice. Administration of the formula to tumor-bearing mice treated with 5-fluorouracil increased their life span by 56%, as compared to controls receiving only 5-fluorouracil. Administration of the formula to mice with chemically-induced colon cancer prevented body weight loss and reduced the number of carcinomas by 29%, as compared to controls. Body weight loss was 0.05% in the mice receiving the formula, as compared to 15.9% for controls.	Ito and Shimura, 1985a, 1985b, 1986; Ohta et al., 1983; Sakamoto et al., 1993
Yi Kang Ling (formula)	The formula inhibited the growth of tumors, and potentiated the antitumor effects of cyclophosphamide and mitomycin in SA- and EA-bearing mice. The formula also prevented weight loss, increased thymus weight, and enhanced peritoneal macrophage phagocytosis. Toxicological experiments indicated that the formula was free from serious side effects.	Zhang and Qi, 1992
Zhu Ling Tang (formula)	Intraperitoneal administration suppressed the growth of EA carcinoma tumors in mice. Oral administration prolonged the survival of the mice. The formula derives its name from the fungus *Polyporus umbellatus* (zhu ling).	Ito and Shimura, 1985a, 1985b

11.5 CHINESE HERBS THAT EXHIBIT ANTICANCER ACTIVITY

This section discusses human clinical trials using Chinese herbs as anticancer agents. Trials were conducted in China (unless stated otherwise). Unfortunately, the majority of the clinical studies conducted in China suffered design problems. Many did not use double-blind methods, and the formula being tested was often varied to meet the needs of the individual patient.

In some cases, results were compared against historic controls rather than a randomized control group. If controls were provided, they were often not clearly chosen to match the extent of disease, performance status of the patient, or the type of conventional treatment given. In many cases, the information published on the study agent, study protocol, or study results was inadequate to allow sufficient review. Therefore, most of these studies are impossible to interpret and the validity of their results is questionable. Studies with particularly gross inadequacies are omitted from the discussion below.

Most of the formulas and single herbs discussed below contain, or are, herbs that *supplement the qi.* Among other actions, these can be expected to have a beneficial effect on the immune system. Herbs that *clear heat, regulate the blood,* and *supplement the blood, yin, and yang* are represented with a lesser frequency.

11.5.1 Colon Cancer

In a study of 176 patients with cancer of the digestive tract, who were undergoing chemotherapy, one group received injections of *Astragalus membranaceus (huang qi)* and *Panax ginseng (ren shen)* extracts. The injections inhibited a reduction in leukocyte count and macrophage activity produced by the chemotherapy, and increased the patients' body weight, as compared to patients in the control group (Li NQ, 1992).

11.5.2 Esophageal and Nasopharyngeal Cancer

In a study of 272 patients with nasopharyngeal cancer, half of the patients were treated with radiation therapy, and half were treated with radiation combined with the formula *Yi Qi Yang Yin Tang.* The five-year relapse rate was more than 3 times lower for those patients who received the combined therapy (12% vs. 38%). Three- and five-year survival rates also significantly improved in the group that received the combined treatment (87% vs. 66% at 3 years, and 67% vs. 48% at 5 years) (Li et al., 1992a). The formula contains herbs that *supplement the qi and yin,* and herbs that *clear heat toxins.*

In a study on 197 patients with stage III and IV nasopharyngeal cancer, approximately half received radiotherapy in combination with Formula #1 and half received radiotherapy alone. After 1 year, survival was 91% in the group receiving the combined treatment and 80% in the group receiving only radiotherapy. After 3 years the survival rates were 67% and 33% respectively. After 5 years the survival rates were 52% and 24% (Li PP, 1992; Sun, 1988). Although Formula #1 contains the *qi* supplement *Astragalus membranaceus (huang qi),* most of the other herbs in the formula are herbs that *reduce blood stagnation.*

In a study on 69 patients with esophageal cancer, who received the formulas *Mieai* powder and *Mieai* decoction, 9 survived over 3 years, and 3 of these did not relapse within 7 to 13 years. The overall three-year observed survival rate was 13% (Zhang, 1986). These formulas contain herbs that reduce *qi* and *blood stagnation,* and herbs that *clear heat toxins.*

For rough (and not statistically valid) comparison, the relative three-year survival rate for esophageal cancer in the U.S. is approximately 14%. Relative survival rates are, by definition, equal to or greater than the observed rates, and therefore, the relative survival rate in the above Chinese study would be somewhat greater than 13%. It is difficult to say how much greater the relative rate might be.

In a study on 150 patients with nasopharyngeal cancer treated with the formula *Fu Zheng Sheng Jin* decoction, in combination with radiotherapy and other supportive measures (symptomatic herb treatment, vitamins, etc.), the 5-year observed survival rate was 58%, and the 10-year observed survival rate was 31%. For rough (and not statistically valid) comparison, 5- and 10-year relative survival rates in the U.S. for cancers of the oral cavity and pharynx are 51% and 40%. The formula contains herbs that *supplement the yin,* herbs that *clear heat toxins,* and herbs that *supplement the qi.*

11.5.3 Leukemia

Li XM (1989) has reviewed a number of studies on acute leukemia. In a study of 32 patients treated with an alcohol extract of the skin of *Bufo bufo gargarizans (chan su),* the partial remission rate was 50% and the complete remission rate was 25%. The longest remission period was 71 months. The protocol was 15 to 30 milliliters of the extract 3 times per day until improvement, then 15 days of treatment and 15 days of rest. In a study of six patients treated with realgar (arsenic sulfide, *xiong huang*) and processed *Isatis tinctoria* (indigo, *qing dai*) complete remissions occurred in three patients, and two of these patients lived over four years. The protocol used was 8 to 18 grams 3 times per day in liquid when acute, and 2 to 6 grams twice per day for maintenance.

Prior to the 1930s, arsenic (as potassium arsenite) was widely used in the West for controlling blood counts in patients with chronic myeloid leukemia (CML) (Treleaven et al., 1993; Chang, 1985). The most common form was in Fowers solution. In portions of India, where chemotherapy drugs are scarce, traditional (Ayurvedic) arsenic-containing drugs are still used with success for this purpose. According to Treleaven et al., the effect is similar to hydroxyurea or busulfan. Some patients taking these agents show signs of chronic arsenic poisoning.

Arsenic sulfide (as in realgar) is less toxic than potassium arsenite. In four of seven cases of CML, realgar (at 9 to 18 grams/day) induced complete remissions. No obvious neurotoxicity, hepatotoxicity, or renal toxicity occurred. Although realgar contains arsenic sulfide, no detrimental effects on hemopoiesis were seen in mice injected with dosages corresponding to 35 times the human dose for 35 days.

In a study on 58 patients with CML, 28 patients were treated with Myleran and 30 were treated by alternating Myleran with the formula CML pills. The mean survival time for those treated with Myleran and herbs was 61 months, while the survival time for those treated only with Myleran was 40 months. Results from outside China indicate Myleran commonly produces mean survival rates of 37 to 43 months. The active ingredients in the CML pill appears to be indirubin, derived from processed *Isatis tinctoria* (indigo, *qing dai*), and arsenic sulfide, from realgar. However, some patients who were not responsive to indigo or realgar singularly or in combination were responsive to the CML pill (Zhang et al., 1985a, 1985b; Chang, 1985). CML pills also contain other herbs to *clear heat toxins* and *reduce blood stagnation.*

In a study of 17 patients with CML treated with indigo, the mean survival time was 47 months (Ma and Yao, 1983). In a study of 22 patients treated with indigo (6 to 12 grams per day orally), 36% achieved complete or partial remission (Chang, 1985). When indigo was used in combination with realgar (9:1 by weight), complete remission rates were as high as 72%.

In a study of 58 patients with CML, 30 received alternating administration of *Manli* Pill and busulfan, and 28 controls received busulfan alone. In the treatment group, mean survival was 61 months. In the control group, mean survival was 40 months. The average time to onset of acute blastic transformation was also greater in the treatment group (53 vs. 34 months) (Zhang et al., 1985a, 1985b). *Manli* pills primarily contain herbs that *clear heat toxins.*

11.5.4 Liver Cancer

In a study on 124 medium-stage liver cancer patients treated with radiotherapy in combination with the herbal formula *Si Jun Zi Tang*, the five-year observed survival rate was 43% (Zhang, 1988). For purposes of rough (and not statistically valid) comparison, the five-year relative survival rate for liver cancer patients in the United States is approximately 6% (Miller et al., 1992:I25-6). The formula is comprised of *qi supplement* herbs such as *Panax ginseng (ren shen).*

11.5.5 Lung Cancer

In a study on 62 lung cancer patients, the two-year survival rate was 21% for those patients receiving radiation therapy in combination with irisqunone (isolated

from *Iris pallasii*), and 14% for those treated with radiation only.[21] There was a 37% complete response rate in the group receiving the combined therapy, and a 13% complete response rate in the group receiving only radiation. In addition to increased survival rates, the authors also report that irisqunone decreased the side effects of radiation, protected the bone marrow, and enhanced the patient's immune function, thereby improving the patient's quality of life (Sun, 1988).

In a study of 81 patients with small cell lung cancer receiving either chemotherapy or radiotherapy, half the patients were randomly assigned to receive either a formula that *supplements the kidney yin (Liu Wei Di Huang Tang)* or a formula that *supplements the kidney yang (Jin Gui Shen Qi).* The overall response rate (complete response plus partial response) was 91.5% for the group that received the combined treatment, and 46.9% for control group. The median survival was 16 months for the group that received the combined treatment, and 10 months for the control group. Four patients in the group that received the combined treatment, and one in the control group, lived for more than seven years. Hematologic toxicity was observed more frequently in the control group (Liu and Ang, 1990).

In a study of 40 patients with terminal primary bronchogenic carcinoma, administration of the formula *Fei Liu Ping* resulted in mean survival of 7.5 months as compared to 6 months in control patients treated with cytotoxic chemotherapy. Body weight, immunologic indices, gastrointestinal reactions, and toxicity reactions were more normal in the group treated with the formula (Cheng et al., 1991). The formula is comprised of herbs that *supplement the qi* (such as *Astragalus membranaceus, huang qi)*, and herbs that *clear heat toxins.*

11.5.6 Lymphoma

In a study of 47 patients with lymphoma, 31 were treated with *Salvia miltiorrhiza (dan shen)* in conjunction with the COP chemotherapy protocol (Zhang YW et al., 1989). The control group consisted of 16 patients treated only with COP protocol. In the treatment group, 9 patients experienced complete remission and 22 experienced partial remission (total remission rate 100%). In the control group, 2 patients experienced complete remission and 10 experienced partial remission (total remission rate 75%). The authors conclude that salvia works synergistically with the COP protocol. *Salvia miltiorrhiza* is an herb that *regulates the blood.*

---

[21] Although irisqunone is not a crude extract, it is discussed here as a matter of convenience.

TABLE 11.12 OBSERVED SURVIVAL RATES FOR PATIENTS WITH STOMACH CANCER TREATED WITH *LI WEI HUA JIE TANG*			
PATIENT CLASS	THREE-YEAR SURVIVAL RATE (%)	FIVE-YEAR SURVIVAL RATE (%)	10-YEAR SURVIVAL RATE (%)
Radical operation (N=76)	61	47 *	18
Palliative operation (N=177)	44	23	5

* The observed five-year survival rate for patients with radical operations treated with conventional therapy in China is reported to be 11 to 22%.

11.5.7 Stomach Cancer

In one study, 158 patients with late-stage, postoperative stomach cancer received both chemotherapy and Formula #2. Some patients took the formula for more than four years. The observed five-year survival rate was 30%, with 7 patients living longer than 11 years. The 10-year survival rate was 12%. Immunological studies of the survivors revealed an enhancement of both humoral and cellular immunity, including an increase in NK cell function (Wang et al., 1988; Wang, 1990). The formula contains primarily herbs that *supplement the qi* and herbs that *clear heat toxins.*

Some of the better-designed Chinese studies were conducted on the formula *Pishen Fang* (also known as *Jian Pi Yi Shen*). In a study of 81 patients with stage III stomach cancer who received chemotherapy, those who also received the formula *Pishen Fang* experienced increased five-year observed survival, as compared to controls (20% vs. 46%). Digestive and hematopoietic functions also improved (Pan, 1992:34). The formula contains herbs that *supplement the qi* and *yang.*

The effects of the formula *Pishen Fang* were investigated in 669 patients that were receiving chemotherapy for late stage stomach cancer. Of these, 365 had radical surgical operations. The patients were randomly divided into the treatment group (414 patients), which received the formula, and the controls (255 patients). Improvements in body weight and appetite, and reductions in nausea and vomiting, were observed in the group that received the formula. The leukocyte count fell below 4,000/mm^3 in 7% of the treatment group and in 33% of the controls. Macrophage activity increased 21% in the treatment group over that of controls. Five-year observed survival among 303 stage III and 63 stage IV patients who received follow-up were 53% and 10% respectively. After 10 years, 47% of the stage III patients were still alive (Yu et al., 1993).

One study on postoperative stomach cancer followed 216 patients at stage III, and 110 patients at stage IV who received chemotherapy treatment. Approximately half also received the formula *Pishen Fang*. In the control group, 75% were able to finish the complete course of chemotherapy, as compared to 95% in the treatment group. In addition, more patients in the treatment group gained weight (23% vs. 8%), fewer lost weight (6% vs. 14%), fewer lost their appetites (10% vs. 32%), and fewer suffered from vomiting (4% vs. 12%) (Zhang, 1992, Ning et al., 1988).

In a study of 81 stage III and IV stomach cancer patients treated with chemotherapy, approximately 75% also received the formula *Shen Xue Tang*. After six weeks of treatment, 0% of the patients who received the formula suffered from diarrhea, as compared to 33% in the control group. Nineteen percent suffered from vomiting as compared to 33% of the controls; and 14% suffered a loss of appetite as compared with 22% of controls (Rao, 1987). The formula contains herbs that *supplement the qi, yin, blood,* and *yang.*

In a study on 67 patients with stomach cancer, who received the formulas *Mieai* powder and *Mieai* decoction, 4 did not relapse within 7 to 13 years, and 12 survived over 3 years. The overall three-year observed survival rate was therefore 24% (Zhang, 1986). These formulas contain herbs that *reduce qi and blood stagnation* and *clear heat toxins.*

In a study of 320 patients with stomach cancer treated with both conventional medicine and the formula *Li Wei Hua Jie Tang*, the observed survival rates were as shown in Table 11.12 (Pan et al., 1986). The formula is composed primarily of herbs that *supplement the qi.*

Thirty-nine patients with postsurgical gastrointestinal cancer, who received the formula *Shi Quan Da Bu Tang*, experienced a marked elevation of NK cell activity measured at three and six months after treatment, as compared to pretreatment levels. A concomitant drop in serum cholesterol was also observed (Okamoto et al., 1989). The formula is composed primarily of herbs that *supplement the qi* and *blood.*

11.5.8 Other Studies

A study on 62 patients undergoing chemotherapy for various cancers investigated the effects of the formula *Ye Qi Sheng Xue Tang* on the patient's leukocyte counts. Each patient received two daily doses of the formula.

During the 6-week trial, the patients who received the formula before breakfast and lunch experienced a less drastic decrease in leukocyte counts than the patients who received the formula before lunch and supper (11% vs. 26%). The incidence of leukopenia was also less frequent in the group that received the formula before breakfast and lunch (13% vs. 48%). The authors suggest the difference in response between the two groups is due to the natural circadian rhythm of DNA synthesis in bone marrow. DNA synthesis is at a maximum in the morning, and it appears that agents that stimulate the bone marrow may be more effective if administered early in the day (Li and Yu, 1993). NK cell activity is also highest in the morning or early afternoon (Whiteside and Herberman, 1989). The formula primarily contains herbs that *supplement the qi and blood*.

In a study of 242 patients with a variety of cancers and *spleen qi vacuity*, treatment with the formula *Shen Xue Tang* significantly improved a number of immune indices. Macrophage activity improved 16%, helper T-lymphocyte populations increased 50%, and NK cell function increased 81% (Rao et al., 1991). The formula contains herbs that *supplement the qi, yin, blood, and yang*.

In a study of 40 patients with various types of cancers and depressed immune systems, administration of the herbs *Gynostemma pentaphyllum (jiao gu lan)* and *Astragalus membranaceus (huang qi)* increased lymphocyte transformation rates by 46% and 26% respectively as compared to pretreatment levels (Hou et al., 1991).

11.6 SUMMARY

This chapter has reviewed studies related to the antitumor and anticancer effects of botanical agents. For the past 40 years the National Cancer Institute has been screening plant extracts in search of anticancer compounds. The complexity of this task required that compromises be made in screening methodology. The program thus far has introduced of one drug, taxol, into the market. However, since the screening program in many ways was not comprehensive, other botanical agents may also be useful in treating cancer. Crude extracts and isolated compounds from a number of plants may deserve further study.

Clinical trials have been conducted in China with some crude extracts. Unfortunately, the trials have generally not been well-designed, and the accuracy of the results is questionable. The formulas used in these studies often contained herbs that *supplement the qi and yang*, herbs that *clear heat*, and herbs that *regulate the blood*.

12

DIETARY MACRONUTRIENTS AND THEIR EFFECTS ON CANCER

Dietary factors may play a significant role in both preventing and promoting carcinogenesis and the progression of neoplasia. For the purposes of this book, dietary components are divided into three categories: macronutrients, such as fat, fiber, amino acids, and sugar; micronutrients, such as vitamins and minerals; and non-nutrient factors, such as flavonoids and isoflavones. Macronutrients are discussed in this chapter, and micronutrients and non-nutrient factors are discussed in the following two chapters.

12.1 TYPES OF DIETARY FAT

12.2 MECHANISMS BY WHICH DIETARY FATS
MAY PROMOTE CANCER
12.2.1 Increased Bioavailability of Sex Hormones
12.2.2 Decreased Immune Response
12.2.3 Increased Production of PGE$_2$
12.2.4 Enhanced Membrane Fluidity

12.2.5 Increased Production of Free Radicals
12.2.6 Reviews of Animal Studies

12.3 MECHANISMS BY WHICH DIETARY FATS
MAY INHIBIT CANCER
12.3.1 Increased Membrane Fluidity
12.3.2 Increased Free Radical Damage
12.3.3 Increased PGE$_3$ Production
12.3.4 Reduced Platelet Aggregation
12.3.5 Decreased Production of Angiogenic
Factors
12.3.6 Decreased Cachexia
12.3.7 Other Fatty Acids

12.4 MACRONUTRIENTS OTHER THAN FATS
12.4.1 Total Calories
12.4.2 Sugar
12.4.3 Fiber
12.4.4 Vegetarian Foods
12.4.5 Amino Acids

12.5 SUMMARY

12.1 TYPES OF DIETARY FAT

The average American consumes approximately 38% of dietary calories as fat, a 25% increase since 1910 (reviewed by Linder, 1991:51). Increased intake of fat has been associated with increased incidence of breast, prostate, and other cancers. In response to these and other concerns, the United States National Research Council has recommended that fat consumption be reduced to no more than 30% of calories.

There are three forms of fat in the diet: glycerides (principally triglyceride), phospholipids, and sterols (principally cholesterol). Triglycerides account for approximately 96% of all dietary fats, and are the form in which the body stores fat for fuel. The remaining 4% are phospholipids, from the cell membranes of plants and animals, and cholesterol, from animal sources.

The fatty acid moieties of glycerides are categorized as being either essential fatty acids (EFAs) or nonessential fatty acids. EFAs cannot be synthesized in the human body and must be obtained through the diet. Humans require EFAs for the proper development and function of numerous tissues, including the brain, retina, and sperm. In addition, EFAs are required for prostaglandin synthesis.

EFAs are characterized by an unsaturated bond within the last 7 carbons of the methyl end of the fatty acid chain (the "omega" end). There are two groups of EFAs that are of primary interest here: omega-3 fatty acids, which have their first unsaturated bond between carbons three and four from the omega end, and omega-6 fatty acids, which have their first unsaturated bond between the sixth and seventh carbons.

Adults require a minimum of 2% of calories as omega-6 EFAs, and the optimum amount may be 12 to 14% (reviewed by Linder, 1991:56). Higher levels of omega-3 fatty acids may be needed. Some investigators suggest that the ratio of omega-3 to omega-6 fatty acids should be as high as 10 to 4 and that lower ratios may lead to an omega-3 depletion in vital organs. A high ratio may be difficult to achieve without supplementing the diet with fish, fish oil, or flaxseed oil, all of which are high in omega-3 fatty acids (see Table 12.1). Most vegetable oils are poor sources of omega-3 fatty acids, but are good sources of linoleic acid (an omega-6 fatty acid).

Linoleic acid and linolenic acid (an omega-3 fatty acid) are two common polyunsaturated EFAs. Polyunsaturated fatty acids (PUFAs) are fatty acids with more than one unsaturated double bond. Linoleic acid and linolenic acid are metabolized in unrelated pathways through the actions of the elongase and desaturase

TABLE 12.1. PERCENT FATTY ACID CONTENT OF VARIOUS FATS AND OILS						
OIL	**SATURATED**	**OMEGA-9 MONOUNSATURATED**	**OMEGA-6 POLYUNSATURATED**		**OMEGA-3 POLYUNSATURATED**	
		Oleic (18:1)*	Linoleic (18:2)	Arachidonic (20:4)**	Linolenic (18:3)	EPA and DHA (20:5 and 22:6)
Safflower oil	9	11	74	—	0.5	—
Corn oil	13	31	39	—	1	—
Peanut oil	19	55	26	2.2	1	—
Flaxseed oil	13	17	13	—	55	—
Salmon oil	26	—	1	—	1	13
Cod liver oil	19	23	2	0.7	1	24
Soybean oil	15	22	53	—	8	—
English walnut oil	11	—	55	—	11	—
Human milk fat	50	—	7	0.2	0.7	1
Lard (pork)	36	46	9	—	0.5	—
Chicken fat	33	47	22	—	1.5	—
Coconut oil	88	7	1	—	—	—
Olive oil	14	72	8	—	1	—
Butter	62	25	2	—	1	—
Wheat germ oil	>16	27	42	—	—	1
Sesame seed oil	>12	40	42	—	0.4	—
Sunflower seed oil	10	22	55	—	0.5	—
Canola (rapeseed) oil	>6	24	15	—	5.2	7.4
Shark oil	>38	16	0.3	5	—	20

 * This code represents the number of carbon atoms in the fatty acid chain and the number of unsaturated double bonds it contains. For example, 18:1 represents 18 carbon atoms and one unsaturated double bond.
** The primary source of arachidonic acid is animal products.
Adapted from: Linder, 1991:74; and Murray and Pizzorno, 1991:163

enzymes (see Figure 12.1). Linoleic acid is metabolized to PGE_1, PGE_2 and, to a lesser degree, arachidonic acid (an omega-6 fatty acid). Linolenic acid is metabolized to eicosapentaenoic acid (EPA), docosahexaenoic acid (DHA) and PGE_3. Both EPA and DHA are omega-3 fatty acids.

PUFAs affect the metabolism of one another. For example, the following observations have been made in studies on mouse fibrosarcoma cells and in other experimental systems (Rubin and Laposata, 1992; reviewed by August, 1995):

- Omega-6 fatty acids enhance the transformation of EPA to DHA, thereby reducing the substrate material for PGE_3 production.
- Omega-6 fatty acids redistributed cellular EPA from the phospholipid layer into storage as triglycerol. This reduces the bioavailability of EPA as a substrate for PGE_3 production.

- Omega-3 fatty acids inhibit delta 6 desaturase, and the production of both PGE_1 and PGE_2 by linoleic acid. (Delta 6 desaturase is also decreased by dietary carbohydrates and is increased by protein.)
- Omega-3 fatty acids inhibit delta 5 desaturase and the conversion of DGLA to arachidonic acid, which may result in a reduction of PGE_2 production. (Delta 5 desaturase is also stimulated by carbohydrates via insulin-mediated effects).
- Omega-3 fatty acids reduce kinin-induced PGE_1 and PGE_2 release.

In summary, omega-3 fatty acids, such as EPA, inhibit PGE_1 and PGE_2 production; and omega-6 fatty acids, such as most vegetable oils, inhibit PGE_3 production and EPA bioavailability.

These observations may have important clinical implications. As will be discussed shortly, EPA may possess some anticancer activity. However, it has proven difficult to increase cellular levels of EPA to the degree

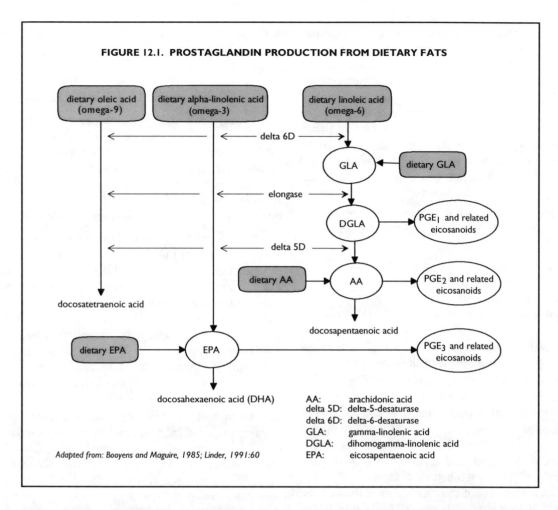

FIGURE 12.1. PROSTAGLANDIN PRODUCTION FROM DIETARY FATS

Adapted from: Booyens and Maguire, 1985; Linder, 1991:60

required to exert a physiologic effect. This difficulty may be due, in part, to the inhibition of EPA (and PGE$_3$) by omega-6 fatty acids. Therefore, to achieve sufficient EPA concentrations, it may be necessary to severely restrict the intake of omega-6 fatty acids.

12.2 MECHANISMS BY WHICH DIETARY FATS MAY PROMOTE CANCER

In 1982 the National Research Council identified fats as the single dietary component most strongly related to carcinogenesis. There is a strong correlation between fat consumption and incidence of gastrointestinal, prostate, and breast cancers. A correlation also exists with cancers of the testis, ovary, uterus (Creasey, 1985:86-102). In a study of 905 cases of colorectal cancer in North America and in China, saturated fat intakes above 10 grams/day, particularly in physically inactive people, may have accounted for 40 to 60% of colorectal cancer incidence (Whittemore et al., 1990). The average American consumes approximately 65 grams/day of saturated fat (Linder, 1991:52). In rodent studies, a low-fat

diet reduced the growth of established human prostate tumors. The lower the fat content, the greater the growth reduction (Wang et al., 1995).

A number of mechanisms exist by which some dietary fats may promote the development and growth of cancer. These include increased bioavailability of sex hormones, decreased immune response, increased production of PGE$_2$, increased membrane fluidity, and increased production of free radicals (Broitman and Cannizzo, 1992). Each of these mechanisms are discussed below. Not all types of fat appear to promote cancer however, and the beneficial effects of omega-3 fatty acids will be discussed later in this chapter.

12.2.1 Increased Bioavailability Of Sex Hormones

Dietary fat may promote carcinogenesis by increasing the bioavailability of sex hormones (reviewed by Dwyer, 1992; Fernandes and Venkatraman, 1992). This may account for the association between high fat intake and high incidence of estrogen-responsive cancers such as breast and endometrial cancers, and androgen-responsive cancers such as prostate cancer. For example, excessive exposure to estrogen can produce endometrial cancer in laboratory animals. Low fat (10%), high fiber diets reduce circulating estrogen levels in premenopausal women (Bagga et al., 1995). Fat tissue is a major source of estrogen production in postmenopausal women, and high intake of dietary fat can lead to increased fat tissue. Increased estrogen production by fat tissue may partially account for the association between high body weight and decreased survival in breast cancer patients (Albanes, 1990).

In addition to increasing estrogen production by fat tissue, dietary fat may increase sex hormone bioavailability by the following mechanisms:

- *By decreasing the levels of sex hormone binding globulin (SHBG).* SHBG is a serum protein that binds (and reduces the bioavailability of) estrogen. Its levels are inversely correlated with body weight.
- *By decreasing estrogen metabolism in the liver.* Obesity increases the bioavailability of estrogen by altering estrogen metabolism in favor of removal of metabolites with low estrogenic effects (Rose, 1993).
- *By increasing enterohepatic circulation of estrogen.* Estrogen is metabolized in the liver and secreted in conjugated form into the small intestine through the bile. Under the action of intestinal bacteria, estrogen can be deconjugated and recirculated back into the liver through the enterohepatic circulation. This decreases the amount of estrogen excreted through the feces and increases the overall estrogen load in the body. Dietary fats increase the ability of intestinal bacteria to deconjugate estrogen.

As mentioned above, one patient group that may benefit from a reduction in dietary fat is women with breast cancer. Seventy percent of women with breast cancer have estrogen-responsive tumors at diagnosis, and of these, one-third to one-half appear to respond to anti-estrogen drugs such as tamoxifen (Dwyer, 1992). To this end, the Women's Health Trial Vanguard Group has studied 303 women at increased risk for breast cancer to determine the feasibility of reducing dietary fat to 20% of calories. Results indicate that cholesterol and serum estradiol levels can be decreased, and that patients will comply successfully with dietary fat restrictions (Dwyer, 1992; Boyar et al., 1988). Other large clinical studies are underway. Smaller studies have reported similar results. For example, studies show that eating a 10% fat diet can reduce plasma estradiol levels in postmenopausal women by 50% (Heber et al., 1991). Diets that contain less than 20% of calories in fat can reduce the incidence of mammary cancer in animal models (Cohen et al., 1986a, 1986b). In light of these results, Wynder et al. (1992) proposed a diet with 15% of calories from fat as an adjuvant therapy for postmenopausal breast cancer patients,

and a diet of 20 to 25% of calories from fat for the population at large.

12.2.2 Decreased Immune Response

High fat diets may decrease immune function. In a study of 17 men who reduced their fat intake to less than 30% of calories, NK cell activity markedly increased as compared to baseline levels. An inverse linear relationship was observed between dietary fat and NK cell activity—NK cell activity increased 0.53% for every 1% reduction in calories as fat (Barone et al., 1989).

However, the effect of omega-3 fatty acids on the immune system is still uncertain. Some investigators have reported that omega-3 fatty acids inhibit certain aspects. For example, EPA reduces the production of interleukin-1 and tumor necrosis factor (TNF) by immune cells (reviewed by Linder, 1991:77). EPA also suppresses NK cell activity in vitro (Barone and Hebert, 1988). Recall that NK cells are a primary source of TNF. DHA inhibits macrophage tumoricidal activity in vitro (Lu et al., 1992). Omega-3 fatty acids may also reduce free radical production by macrophages (Dyerberg, 1991). In contrast, other investigators report that EPA augments free radical production by macrophages and increases the respiratory burst of neutrophils (Das, 1990). Furthermore, fish oil (18 grams/day) has been shown to decrease the number of suppressor-T cells in patients with solid tumors (Gogos et al., 1995). In spite of any suppressive effect on the immune system, omega-3 fatty acids appear to have an overall inhibitory effect on cancer, as will be discussed shortly.

12.2.3 Increased Production Of PGE$_2$

As discussed at the beginning of this chapter, the type of fat consumed may affect the preferential production of prostaglandins. Excessive consumption of omega-6 vegetable oils and animal fats increase the arachidonic acid content in the cell membranes of normal and neoplastic cells (Karmali et al., 1984). In turn, this increases the capacity of malignant cells to synthesize PGE$_2$, a prostaglandin produced in excessive quantities by many types of tumors. Mammary and lung cancer cells also have an increased percentage of arachidonic acid compared to normal cells. In human non-small cell lung cancer cells, up to 40% of the fatty acid composition of the membrane has been reported to be arachidonic acid (Bockman et al., 1987). This is a much larger percentage of arachidonic acid than found in normal cells, such as the normal erythrocytes shown in Table 12.3. Table 12.3 also shows that some neoplastic cells, such as HL-60 cells, do not exhibit increased levels of arachidonic acid.

TABLE 12.3. PERCENT OF FATTY ACIDS IN PLASMA MEMBRANES OF NORMAL ERYTHROCYTES AND HUMAN LEUKEMIC HL-60 CELLS

FATTY ACID *	UNMODIFIED HL-60 CELLS **	HL-60 CELLS SUPPLEMENTED WITH 22:6 (DHA) **	NORMAL ERYTHROCYTES ***
18:1 (includes oleic acid)	38.62	22.00	13
18:2 (includes linoleic acid)	1.15	2.00	9
20:4 (includes arachidonic acid)	4.79	3.49	13
22:6 (includes DHA)	2.37	9.91	4
Mean number of unsaturated double bonds	1.00	1.22	—

   * The number of different membrane phospholipids present may exceed 100.
  ** *Source: Burns et al., 1989*
*** *Source: Cullis and Hope, 1991*

12.2.4 Enhanced Membrane Fluidity

One method by which PUFAs may promote cancer is by enhancing the fluidity of the plasma membrane surrounding tumor cells. Incorporation of unsaturated fatty acids into the plasma membrane promotes greater freedom of molecular motion and reduces membrane order. The order parameter S is a measure of membrane fluidity. A low value of S reflects greater fluidity. Increased membrane fluidity is associated with increased metabolism and a greater capacity for division, characteristics present in neoplastic cells. Excessive increases in fluidity, however, can cause cell death.

Membrane fluidity is controlled by numerous factors, including the saturation index (SI), which is the ratio of saturated to unsaturated fatty acids in the membrane (Aclimandos et al., 1992). The saturation index is commonly reduced in neoplastic cells, and also may be reduced in the membranes of red blood cells and platelets of patients with a variety of cancers (Copland et al., 1992; Kelly et al., 1990; Persad et al., 1990).[1] PUFAs, in sufficient amounts, may further lower the saturation index, increase membrane fluidity, and stimulate tumor cell proliferation.

12.2.5 Increased Production of Free Radicals

Polyunsaturated fatty acids are readily oxidized. There are at least two ways in which lipid oxidation, or peroxidation, can promote cancer.[2] First, the body uses antioxidants to counteract the oxidation process. Depletion of body stores of antioxidants increases the possibility of carcinogenesis. Second, free radicals, which play a role in oxidation, can stimulate cellular proliferation. An example of this is the stimulation of immune cell proliferation after a phagocyte-induced discharge of hydrogen peroxide.

12.2.6 Reviews of Animal Studies

Numerous animal studies indicate that omega-6 fatty acids (most vegetable oils) promote tumor development, and saturated and omega-3 fatty acids inhibit tumor development. In a review of numerous animal studies, Welsch (1992) reported the following:

- The amount of dietary fat has a profound effect on the development of mammary tumors. A threshold level may exist above which tumor development is no longer linearly related to fat intake and begins to increase exponentially. This threshold may be as low as 10% total calories of fat, including no more than 4.4% linoleic acid.
- Diets high in linoleic acid promote tumor development.
- It is not clear if the type of fat ingested affects the initiation stage of carcinogenesis, but it is clear that the type of fat affects the promotional stage.
- High levels of saturated fats, compared to unsaturated fats, can inhibit tumor development. However, this effect can be reversed by modest intake of linoleic acid.
- Oleic acid, such as found in olive oil, has not been reported to inhibit or promote tumor growth. The same is true for whole olive oil (Lasekan et al., 1990).
- The few studies conducted on linolenic acid (e.g., evening primrose oil) indicate that it may inhibit

---

[1] A reduced saturation index of red blood cells has been proposed as a marker of malignancy. However, it is not consistently seen in patients with cancer (Zaridze et al., 1990) and can also be present in patients with diseases other than cancer.

[2] Lipid peroxidation is free radical-induced damage of lipid membranes.

tumor development, although not in a dose-dependent fashion.

- Marine oils (omega-3) consistently inhibit tumor development in animals. However, this inhibition can be blocked by administering modest amounts of linoleic acids (e.g., 75% fish oil, 25% corn oil).
- A definitive effect of dietary fats on metastasis has not been established.

12.3 MECHANISMS BY WHICH DIETARY FATS MAY INHIBIT CANCER

Studies on allograft or chemically-induced tumors in mice have reported that omega-3 marine lipids, such as EPA:

- inhibit the development of colon and pancreatic cancers (Carrol, 1991; Butrum and Messina, 1991)
- inhibit the growth and metastasis of mammary tumors (Karmali, 1985; Istfan et al., 1992; Butrum and Messina, 1991)
- inhibit the growth of colon tumors (Broitman and Cannizzo, 1992)
- inhibit the growth of prostatic and pancreatic tumors (Butrum and Messina, 1991)
- inhibit the growth of human breast cancer xenografts (Pritchard et al., 1989)

In addition to their effects on cancer, omega-3 fatty acids may protect against cardiovascular disease by inhibiting platelet aggregation and altering cholesterol levels. They may also lessen the severity of autoimmune diseases by suppressing the immune system and by inhibiting eicosanoid-induced inflammation (Fernandes and Venkatraman, 1992). Three grams daily each of EPA and DHA increased the proportion of omega-3 fatty acids and decreased the proportion of arachidonic acid in platelets from healthy subjects (Sanders and Roshanai, 1983). The oils also prolonged bleeding time, lowered plasma triglycerides, slightly lowered plasma cholesterol, and slightly raised plasma HDL cholesterol. Administration of nine grams daily of linolenic acid from flaxseed oil, another omega-3 fatty acid, produced minimal effects on these parameters. Administration of two to six grams of EPA daily reduced serum triglycerides, reduced total cholesterol, and increased HDL cholesterol in humans (Saynor, 1984; Sanders and Roshanai, 1983; Simons et al., 1985). Although effective dosages of EPA/DHA are still uncertain, 2 to 4 grams/day may be adequate to inhibit platelet aggregation, 4 grams/day may be adequate to suppress inflammation, and 4 to 24 grams/day may be adequate to lower plasma lipids (reviewed by Linder,

1991:78). The various effects become apparent within four weeks of administration.

There are a number of mechanisms by which omega-3 fatty acids may inhibit cancer initiation and progression. These mechanisms include increased membrane fluidity, increased free radical damage, increased PGE_3 production, reduced platelet aggregation, decreased production of angiogenic factors, and decreased cachexia. Each of these mechanisms is discussed separately below.

12.3.1 Increased Membrane Fluidity

It was mentioned in Section 12.2.4 that PUFAs increase membrane fluidity of tumor cells and stimulate proliferation. However, under certain conditions, increased membrane fluidity can also inhibit tumor cell proliferation:

- Increased fluidity increases the capacity for drug transport across the membrane. In-vitro studies confirm that the incorporation of PUFAs into the plasma membrane of mouse leukemia cells increases the uptake of a variety of cytotoxic drugs (Burns and Spector, 1990). PUFAs can also modify intracellular membranes, such as nuclear membranes and mitochondria.
- Excessive fluidity destabilizes the membrane, and interferes with essential cellular processes. This leads to a cytotoxic effect. Linoleic acid is cytotoxic to Ehrlich ascites cells in vitro (Norman et al., 1988), and omega-3 and omega-6 fatty acids are cytotoxic to human breast, lung, and prostate cancer cells in vitro, but not to normal cells (Begin et al., 1986). In-vitro tests have demonstrated that PUFAs are cytotoxic to at least 16 different human cell lines derived from 11 different organs, but are not cytotoxic to normal cells (reviewed by Begin et al., 1986). The selective inhibition of neoplastic cells by PUFAs may account for the low incidence of cancers originating in the small intestine (Norman et al., 1988).

This selectivity may be explained by the fact that plasma membranes of tumor cells tend to be inherently unstable (Booyens, 1985), possibly due to their increased arachidonic acid content, as was discussed previously. Further increases in the PUFA content may destabilize membranes to the point where cell function is no longer supported. Since normal cells do not contain excessive PUFA levels initially, they are not as susceptible to PUFA treatment.

12.3.2 Increased Free Radical Damage

The cytotoxic effects of PUFAs discussed above may also be due to an increase in the susceptibility of cancer cell membranes to free radical damage (Das, 1990). For example, P815 cells obtained from tumor-bearing mice were more susceptible to hydrogen peroxide than were normal cells (Nathan and Chon, 1981). Similarly, a variety of human tumor cells lines were more susceptible to ozone-induced oxidative damage in vitro than were normal cells (Sweet et al., 1980). PUFAs contain multiple unsaturated double bonds, and each double bond is a target for free radical damage.[3] Saturated and monounsaturated fatty acids account for approximately 62% of the phospholipid content of normal (erythrocyte) cell membranes (Cullis and Hope, 1991). However, as mentioned above, cancer cells have an increased content of arachidonic acid (four double bonds), which makes them more susceptible than normal cells to lipid peroxide damage. Incorporation of EPA, which has five double bonds, and DHA, which has six double bonds, into the membrane further increases the susceptibility to lipid peroxide damage.[4] As shown in Table 12.3, the introduction of DHA into a culture of leukemia cells increases the number of unsaturated double bonds in the plasma membrane by 31%.

Agents that augment free radical damage, such as iron and copper salts, increase the cytotoxic effects of EPA and gamma linolenic acid (GLA). In contrast, free radical scavengers, such as vitamin E, uric acid, glutathione peroxidase, quercetin, and SOD, decrease cytotoxicity (Das, 1991, 1987; Begin et al., 1989, 1986; Ramanathan et al., 1994a; Cantrill et al., 1993). GLA and EPA inhibited the proliferation of three human colon cancer cell lines in vitro. The addition of vitamin E at 10 μM decreased the cytostatic effect and reversed the PUFA-induced increase in membrane fluidity (Mengeaud et al., 1992). This concentration of vitamin E is present in normal serum, which suggests that radical-induced cytotoxicity may be difficult to achieve in vivo.

12.3.3 Increased PGE$_3$ Production

As was illustrated in Figure 12.1, omega-3 fatty acids provide a source for the production of PGE$_3$. At the same time, omega-3 fatty acids inhibit the production of PGE$_2$ by successfully competing with arachidonic acid as a substrate for cyclooxygenase, the enzyme that synthesizes prostaglandins from fatty acids. Omega-3 fatty acids also displace arachidonic acid in the cell membrane, thereby decreasing the amount of arachidonic acid available for PGE$_2$ production; and inhibit the desaturase enzymes that allow PGE$_2$ production from linoleic acid.

Tumor cells produce excessive quantities of PGE$_2$. High PGE$_2$ levels increase inflammation, and have been linked with tumor metastasis to bone and poor survival in breast cancer patients (Karmali, 1985). PGE$_2$ also inhibits NK cell activity, presumably, in part, by elevating intracellular cAMP (Barone and Hebert, 1988).

A number of investigators have reported that omega-3 supplementation decreases PGE$_2$ production by tumor cells and inhibits their growth. An EPA and DHA mixture inhibited the growth of human lung tumors in mice by 45%. The mixture reduced the content of arachidonic acid in the tumor cells by 50%, and increased the content of omega-3 fatty acids three- to five-fold. PGE$_2$ levels in the tumor were reduced over seven-fold (De Bravo et al., 1991). EPA/DHA mixtures also decreased the production of PGE$_2$ and decreased the growth of human prostate cancer xenografts in mice (Karmali et al., 1987). PGE$_2$ is required for the invasive and metastatic activity of certain tumors, and the addition of EPA to mouse melanoma and human fibrosarcoma cell cultures inhibited invasiveness and inhibited collagenase production. EPA also reduced the ability of mouse melanoma cells to metastasize to the lung after intravenous injection to mice (Reich et al., 1989).

12.3.4 Reduced Platelet Aggregation

As discussed in Chapter 5, platelet aggregation facilitates the process of metastasis. Omega-3 fatty acids may inhibit metastasis by inhibiting platelet aggregation. EPA inhibits platelet aggregation both in vitro and in vivo (Sanders and Roshanai, 1983), which may account for the low incidence of ischemic heart disease in populations that consume diets rich in cold-water fish (reviewed by Karmali et al., 1984).

12.3.5 Decreased Production of Angiogenic Factors

Solid tumors must induce angiogenesis to create an adequate blood supply to survive. One factor that stimulates angiogenesis is platelet activating factor (PAF). The production of PAF appears to depend on the cyclooxygenase products of arachidonic acid (PGE$_2$ etc.). DHA competes for cell uptake with arachidonic acid and decreases PAF production in vitro (Shikano et al., 1993). PGE$_1$ and PGE$_2$ both stimulate angiogenesis (Folkman and Klagsburn, 1987), and EPA and DHA may inhibit angiogenesis by favoring the production of PGE$_3$.

---

[3] Saturated fats have no double bonds present, and monounsaturated fats have one double bond. The lack of double bonds in saturated fats (such as animal fats) allows them to withstand high cooking temperatures and long storage without degrading.

[4] The uptake of EPA in tumor cells is about half the uptake of EPA in normal cells (Begin et al., 1986).

12.3.6 Decreased Cachexia

Causes Of Cachexia

Cachexia is a complex metabolic syndrome characterized by malnutrition and tissue wasting that causes greater than 10 to 15% weight loss. It is responsible for 4 to 23% of all cancer-related deaths (reviewed by Calabresi and Schein, 1993:1149). Patients with tumors of the digestive tract are particularly vulnerable to cachexia, where tumor-induced physical interference of gastrointestinal function is common. However, systemic mechanisms of cachexia also exist, as evidenced by the relatively high rates of cachexia in patients with lung cancer. However it is induced, cachexia is associated with poor clinical outcome—patients without weight loss tend to survive substantially longer. Not all cancers are associated with cachexia. For example, cachexia is relatively rare in patients with breast cancer and sarcoma.

Systemic causes of cachexia are related to dysfunctions in the metabolism of carbohydrates, proteins and fats. As such, the cachectic patient may not be able to gain weight, even with adequate nutrition. Changes in glucose metabolism are often central to cachexia. Tumors can produce factors that decrease the sensitivity of normal cells to insulin, resulting in hyperglycemia and the production of more insulin. Recall from Chapter 7 that insulin stimulates cell proliferation. Increased cell proliferation leads to an increased demand for glucose, which is aggravated by the fact that cancer cells metabolize glucose in an inherently inefficient anaerobic process. The high glucose demand is met, in part, by the conversion of fat and muscle into glucose. It is also met by gluconeogenesis, a process by which the byproduct of anaerobic metabolism, lactic acid, circulates back to the liver and is metabolized into glucose. Gluconeogenesis itself is an energy-intensive process that further depletes energy stores and causes additional tissue wasting.

A second metabolic change that leads to tissue wasting is altered lipid metabolism caused by production of tumor necrosis factor (TNF). Due to its affect on cachexia, tumor necrosis factor was originally termed cachectin. Macrophages secrete TNF in an attempt to destroy cancer cells or other foreign cells. At the same time, TNF has a secondary effect of mobilizing fat and protein energy stores, possibly for use as an energy source for immune cells. In short-term diseases such as infection, TNF-induced lipid catabolism does not lead to a critical loss in tissue mass. However, in chronic diseases such as cancer, ongoing catabolism eventually depletes fat and muscle stores and leads to cachexia. To counteract excessive wasting, a negative-feedback loop appears to exist in which the hyperlipidemia caused by excessive mobilization of fat stores inhibits macrophage activity and TNF secretion (recall that PUFAs inhibit macrophage activity). However, in cancer-induced cachexia, this feedback loop is inadequate to stop tissue wasting, possibly because the growing tumor mass and its metastatic cells continually stimulate macrophages.

In the absence of frank cachexia, malnutrition is also common in the cancer patient. Malnutrition may result from physical obstruction of the gastrointestinal tract, chemotherapy-induced gastrointestinal disturbance, mental-emotional depression, changes in the central nervous system, or changes in taste. In general, nutritional support for the malnourished patient does not appear to stimulate tumor growth or increase the rate of metastatic spread (Istfan et al., 1992). However, certain nutrients, such as the amino acids tyrosine and phenylalanine, may stimulate the growth of some tumors. These amino acids are discussed in more detail later in this chapter.

Inhibition of Cachexia by EPA

EPA effectively reverses cachexia induced by MAC16 colon adenocarcinoma in mice (Tisdale, 1993). Other omega-3 or omega-6 fatty acids were not effective. Cachexia appeared to be blocked at the level of the adipocyte and was associated with reductions in cAMP production. The anticachexic effect was observed at doses of 1.2 to 5.0 grams/kg (Beck et al., 1991; Tisdale and Beck, 1991). When extrapolated on a surface area basis to humans, this corresponds to a dose of approximately 6.4 to 25.6 grams of pure EPA per day. Muscle protein degradation in cachexia is associated with a rise in PGE_2 content, and EPA inhibited both of these in healthy mice injected with serum from cachectic mice (Smith and Tisdale, 1993).

In addition to inhibiting cachexia, EPA inhibits tumor growth in a dose-dependent manner. In mice treated with EPA, survival was approximately double that of controls and no cachexia was apparent (Tisdale and Beck, 1991; Beck et al., 1991). The anticachexic effects appeared to be due to inhibition of tumor lipolytic activity, and the study suggested a correlation may exist between inhibition of cachexia and inhibition of tumor growth. The effects of GLA were considerably less and may have been due to production of PGE_1. Administration of DHA resulted in increased weight loss and a slight stimulation of tumor proliferation. For this reason, the authors suggest that pure EPA should be used in future studies (fish oil products contain a mixture of EPA and DHA). EPA at 2.0 grams/kg prevented weight loss and delayed tumor growth in MAC16-bearing mice (Hudson et al., 1993). Oral administration of pure linoleic acid reversed the antiproliferative effect, but not the anticachexic effect. EPA alone or in combination with linoleic acid did not increase incorporation of EPA into tumor cell lipids. The authors suggest that the antiproliferative effects of EPA may be due to the blocking of adipose catabolism that normally supplies the fatty acids essential for tumor growth.

Tumor characteristics may determine the success of EPA treatment. For example, mice bearing the poorly differentiated fast-growing rat ascites hepatoma AH-130, which also induces cachexia, did not respond to EPA treatment (Costelli et al., 1995). The authors suggest that EPA may be most effective in well-differentiated, slower-growing tumors, such as the MAC16.

It appears that a number of mechanisms may be involved in EPA-induced inhibition of cachexia and tumor growth. These may include a reduction in tumor necrosis factor production secondary to immune inhibition, direct blocking effects on fat cells, reduction in PGE_2 production, and increased membrane fluidity.

Other Agents that May Treat Cachexia

Certain agents may protect the gastrointestinal lining from physical trauma induced by chemotherapy and, thereby, prevent cachexia. For example, plantain has shown significant promise as an antiulcer agent. It increases the thickness of the gastric mucosa (Best et al., 1984; Goel et al., 1986). A preparation of plantain sap inhibited the acute toxic effects of 5-fluorouracil on the gut mucosa in tumor-bearing mice. In addition to reducing gastrointestinal toxicity, the combined treatment produced a greater reduction in tumor cell viability than did treatment of 5-fluorouracil alone (Borovskaia et al., 1987). A second natural agent that may protect the gastrointestinal lining is N-acetyl glucosamine (NAG), or its alternative, glucosamine sulfate. Glucosamine is a component of connective tissue and mucus secretions.

In 1968, Dr. Joseph Gold proposed the use of hydrazine sulfate for treating cachexia. In theory, hydrazine sulfate inhibits cachexia by inhibiting gluconeogenesis, thus eliminating an energy-intensive biochemical reaction and depriving the cancer of glucose. Although once on the American Cancer Society's "Unproven Methods" list, it was taken off in 1979, due to promising results in preliminary studies. However, recent clinical trials indicate that the compound has no effect on cachexia and may even lower the quality of life (Kosty et al., 1994; Loprinzi et al., 1994a, 1994b).

Although the efficacy of hydrazine sulfate is questionable, the mechanism behind its use remains of interest. Studies have shown that a small number of natural agents inhibit gluconeogenesis and lower blood sugar in animal models. These include two Indian plants in the Cucurbitaceae family, *Coccinia indica* and *Momordica*

charantia (Shibib et al., 1993; Hossain et al., 1992), and a formula that contains *Nigella satvia, Boswellia carterii (ru xiang), Commiphora myrrha (mo yao), Ferula assafoetida, and Aloe vera* (Al-Awadi et al., 1991).

12.3.7 Other Fatty Acids

Other lipid substances, such as glycerol-derived ether lipids, have been tested for their antitumor effects. One natural source of these is Greenland shark liver oil. An increased regression of tumor growth was reported in patients with cervical cancer who received extracts of Greenland shark liver oil prior to radiotherapy (Brohult et al., 1986). The active constituents in the oil are thought to be alkoxyglycerols, which are natural components of human bone marrow and mother's milk.

12.4 MACRONUTRIENTS OTHER THAN FATS

12.4.1 Total Calories

High calorie intake has been associated with increased cancer risk, independent of high fat content. In a review of data from 100 animal experiments, Freedman et al. (1990) reported that both high calorie and high fat diets independently increase spontaneous mammary tumor incidence. The effect of a high fat diet was two-thirds the magnitude of the high calorie effect. Other investigators have reported that small reductions in calorie consumption (e.g., 12%) substantially reduce mammary tumor development in animals, whereas large reductions of fat are required to reach the same effect. In addition, caloric restriction, even in animals fed a high fat diet, significantly suppressed mammary tumor development (Welsch, 1992; Weindruch, 1992). Diets high in fat or calories have been associated with five of the six most common cancers: breast, colorectal, pancreatic, prostatic, and uterine (Schapira, 1992; Albanes, 1990).

One mechanism by which high calorie diets may increase cancer incidence is by increasing metabolism, and therefore increasing free radical generation. Long-term calorie restriction is associated with an inhibition in lipid peroxidation in animals (Koizumi, 1991).

12.4.2 Sugar

Sucrose intake has been associated with increased risk of colon cancer in humans and animals (Bostick et al., 1994; La Vecchia et al., 1993; Stamp et al., 1993). Apparently, sucrose directly affects colon cell proliferation. Sucrose may also increase liver tumor development in mice, independently of caloric contribution (Rogers et al., 1987), and promote chemically-induced liver cancer in rats (Hei and Sudilovsky, 1985). In a two-year study, mice fed diets containing either 30% fat or moderate amounts of sucrose exhibited a higher incidence of spontaneous mammary tumors than mice fed other experimental diets (Gridley et al., 1983). Dietary sugar may also reduce the survival of tumor-bearing mice. For example, administration of glucose to EA-bearing mice increased tumor growth and lowered survival (Demetrakopulos and Brennan, 1982).

Two possible mechanisms by which sugar may increase tumor cell proliferation are by increasing blood glucose levels, and by increasing insulin secretion. As discussed in Chapter 7, tumor cells exhibit a three- to fivefold increase in glucose uptake compared to normal cells. Glucose is the preferred source of energy for tumor cells, since they do not metabolize fat as easily (Rossi-Fanelli et al., 1991). One mechanism by which tumors may ensure a source of glucose is by secreting factors that prevent glucose uptake by normal cells, thus leading to cachexia and hyperglycemia. Hyperglycemia appears to be common in cancer patients, with incidence reported as high as 60% (Rossi-Fanelli et al., 1991). Dietary sugar intake may further increase hyperglycemia and may stimulate tumor proliferation by providing additional glucose.

A hyperglycemic state causes secretion of additional insulin. Recall from Chapter 7 that insulin stimulates cell proliferation. Insulin is involved in a variety of other biochemical processes, including glucose uptake; metabolism of carbohydrates, amino acids, and lipids; and amino acid transport. Insulin also activates phospholipase A_2, the enzyme that frees arachidonic acid from cell membranes for PGE_2 synthesis. Yam (1992) reported that cancer-promoting effects of insulin have been observed in animal cell lines and in human breast cancer cells. He suggests that elevated insulin may activate dormant cancer cells, initiate the development of preneoplastic lesions, or stimulate the growth of existing tumors. He further reported that sucrose, glucose, fructose, and omega-3 and omega-6 fatty acids all increase insulin secretion (fats are high in calories). In addition, omega-6 fatty acids and saturated fatty acids lead to insulin resistance of normal cells and hypoglycemia, an effect omega-3 fatty acids prevent.

In addition to the above mentioned effects, sugar may have other general negative effects. Ingestion of moderate levels of sucrose or glucose have been shown to inhibit neutrophil and lymphocyte activity, possibly by competing with vitamin C for insulin-dependent membrane transport (reviewed by Murray and Pizzorno, 1991:63). For example, the uptake of ascorbic acid by neutrophils is inhibited by moderate glucose levels (Henson et al., 1991). Inhibition of lymphocyte activity may

play a role in sucrose-induced tumor growth in animal models.

12.4.3 Fiber

Fiber-rich diets have been reported to reduce the risk of colorectal cancer (reviewed by Clifford and Kramer, 1993). Fiber may reduce the risk of colorectal cancer by decreasing the length of time the stool remains in the bowels; by decreasing the concentration of carcinogens in the stool; and by increasing intestinal bacterial populations that may destroy carcinogenic metabolites (Doll and Peto, 1981). Fiber also increases the excretion of fiber-bound steroids such as cholesterol, and allows for the production of butyric acid, which may induce differentiation and apoptosis.

Fiber-rich diets may reduce the incidence of breast cancer by reducing estrogen levels (Clifford and Kramer, 1993). As stated previously, estrogen is conjugated in the liver and secreted via the bile into the small intestine. High-fiber, low-fat diets suppress the ability of fecal bacteria to deconjugate estrogen and thereby increase estrogen loss through fecal excretion. This may account for the observation that vegetarian women tend to have fewer estrogen-induced menstrual irregularities than nonvegetarians (Rose, 1993). A number of studies have shown that within a two- to three-month period, a high-fiber, low-fat diet may significantly reduce blood estrogen levels (reviewed by Rose, 1993). In a Canadian cohort study of 56,837 women, 519 eventually developed breast cancer. Those who consumed high amounts of fiber exhibited a 30% reduction in risk of breast cancer compared to those who consumed low amounts of fiber (Rohan et al., 1993). Dietary fiber may affect other sex hormone-dependent cancers in a similar manner.

12.4.4 Vegetarian Foods

A number of studies have shown that cancer risk is lower and immune competence is higher in individuals who consume a vegetarian diet. Epidemiological studies almost unanimously report a strong correlation between a diet high in fruits and vegetables and low cancer risk. In a study on 22 German vegetarians, NK cell activity was 4 times higher than omnivorous controls. However, lifestyle habits other than vegetarianism may have affected the results (Malter et al., 1989).

Vegetarian diets may inhibit neoplastic cells by altering the fatty acid content of their cell membranes (Siguel, 1983). In humans, arachidonic acid is produced only to a limited extent from linoleic acid, and therefore the production of PGE_2 (from arachidonic acid) is limited by vegetarian diets.[5] Ingestion of animal products provides a source of arachidonic acid independent of linoleic acid, and therefore may allow increased PGE_2 production. In a study of 25 subjects, a vegetarian diet resulted in a marked increase in platelet linoleic acid concentration and a decrease in arachidonic acid concentration (Fischer et al., 1986). In addition to limiting PGE_2 production, an increased ratio of linoleic-to-arachidonic acid may alter membrane fluidity by depriving cell membranes of higher carbon fatty acids (Siguel, 1983).

Vegetarian diets may also inhibit the growth of some tumors by reducing prolactin levels. Blood levels of prolactin appear to be lower in vegetarians (reviewed by Linder, 1991:488), and increased prolactin levels are associated with enhanced breast tumor growth in postmenopausal women (Ingram et al., 1992). Dietary fat promotes prolactin secretion, and low prolactin levels in vegetarians may be due to a low fat diet. Prolactin levels are higher in nonvegetarian men, which may explain, in part, the connection between high fat intake and prostate cancer (reviewed by Linder, 1991:488).

12.4.5 Amino Acids

Amino acids are the building blocks of protein in the body. A number of amino acids are particularly relevant to the treatment of cancer. These include phenylalanine, tyrosine, cysteine, glutathione, methionine, arginine, glutamine, and tryptophan. Each of these are discussed separately below.

Phenylalanine

The essential amino acid phenylalanine is the direct precursor of tyrosine (which is necessary for the synthesis of thyroid hormones) and of dopamine, epinephrine, and other adrenal catecholamines. Dietary restriction of phenylalanine may inhibit the growth of some cancers. Melanomas and certain adenocarcinomas appear to require excessive amounts of phenylalanine (Lawson et al., 1985). In contrast, oral administration of phenylalanine has been reported to inhibit the development of gastric cancers in mice (Iishi et al., 1990).

Tyrosine

Similar to phenylalanine, dietary restriction of tyrosine may inhibit the growth of some cancers. Cultured melanoma and glioblastoma multiforme cells require high amounts of tyrosine, and withholding tyrosine can inhibit the growth of these tumors (reviewed by Braverman and Pfeiffer, 1987:55). Since the synthesis of melanin requires tyrosine, tyrosine starvation theoretically may be useful in treating melanomas, although this has not been well investigated.

Cysteine

Cysteine is thiol-containing amino acid. Cysteine molecules bond to one another to form cystine, a protein that acts as a glue to hold insulin and many other proteins together. In the liver, cystine (in the form of the tripeptide glutathione) facilitates drug metabolism by forming conjugates with lipophilic substances to render them water-soluble. On its own, and incorporated into glutathione, cysteine is a free radical scavenger.

Cysteine (or its derivative N-acetyl cysteine (NAC)) may protect humans from the toxic side effects of a variety of chemotherapy agents, including doxorubicin and cyclophosphamide (Yarbro et al., 1983). Presumably this is due to its free radical scavenging effects. NAC also protects dogs from doxorubicin-induced heart damage (Unverfeth et al., 1983). It is currently being studied in European clinical trials as a chemopreventive agent in curatively treated patients with oral, laryngeal, and lung cancer (De Vries and De Flora, 1993). The major clinical use of NAC is to facilitate drug metabolism in the treatment of acetaminophen overdose. It is also use as a mucolytic agent in the treatment of chromic bronchitis.

Glutathione

Glutathione is an amino acid that contains cysteine, glycine, and glutamic acid. Because of cysteine, it contains a thiol group that provides antioxidant activity. Glutathione is a component of glutathione peroxidase, an enzyme that converts hydrogen peroxide to water. It is also a component of glutathione-S-transferase, an enzyme that assists drug metabolism in the liver. Glutathione is also essential in several immune-related processes and protects the integrity of red blood cells. Glutathione is present in all cells of the body. Levels decrease with age, and the aging process itself may be due to low levels of glutathione (Ames et al., 1993; Richie et al., 1994; Fletcher and Fletcher, 1994; Stio et al., 1994). Serum levels of selenium and glutathione peroxidase tend to decrease after the sixth decade of life in healthy adults, and tend to be lower in patients with malignant cancers (Kuroda et al., 1988).

---

[5] The production of PGE_2 from dietary linoleic acid may be greater in rodents than in humans. This may explain why PUFAs have been more clearly linked to cancer progression in rodents than in humans. This may also explain in part why meat has been more clearly linked to human cancer than PUFAs.

Glutathione may inhibit carcinogenesis and/or cancer progression by a number of mechanisms:

- As an antioxidant, glutathione may reduce free radical damage to DNA and prevent depletion of other antioxidants.
- Glutathione is required for the metabolism of some carcinogenic substances.
- Glutathione is involved in the synthesis and repair of DNA.
- Glutathione is required for optimal activation of T lymphocytes.
- Thiol-containing substances may inhibit angiogenesis (discussed in Section 3.4).

Other investigators have reported additional benefits. Glutathione may prevent radiation-induced damage, presumably due to its antioxidant functions (Kuna et al., 1978). It may also partially protect patients from the adverse effects of treatment with fluorouracil and cisplatin (Cascinu and Catalano, 1995; Gebbia et al., 1992). In vitro, tumor cells that are glutathione-depleted are excessively susceptible to fluorouracil cytotoxicity, presumably because their detoxification capabilities are restricted (Chen et al., 1995; Bravard et al., 1994). In vivo, glutathione administration does not appear to limit the effectiveness of fluorouracil.

Few studies have investigated the potential antitumor/anticancer activity of glutathione in animals or humans. In one study on rats, administration of glutathione caused partial or complete regression in 81% of established aflatoxin B1-induced liver tumors (Novi, 1981).

Methionine

Some cancers appear to require methionine for growth, and dietary restriction may inhibit their proliferation (reviewed by Braverman and Pfeiffer, 1987:149). For other cancers, the opposite may be true. Dietary supplementation of the lipotropic factors methionine and choline increased survival in mice with aflatoxin B1-induced hepatocarcinomas (Newberne et al., 1990).[6]

Arginine

Numerous investigators have reported that arginine inhibits the growth of a variety of experimental animal tumors (Weisburger et al., 1969; Takeda, 1975; Milner and Stepanovich, 1979; Barbul et al., 1977; reviewed by Braverman and Pfeiffer, 1987:174-6). In contrast, other investigators have reported that arginine stimulates tumor growth. Arginine increased metastasis of mouse colon tumors to the liver by 55% as compared to controls,

and an arginine-deficient diet inhibited tumor growth by 78% (Yeatman et al., 1991). Arginine supplementation stimulated the growth of breast cancer tumors in humans (Park et al., 1992).

The reason for these contradictory results may be that arginine stimulates T-lymphocyte production and action, presumably through its effects on the thymus gland. Therefore, an inhibition of immunogenic tumors, such as many experimental animal tumors, could be expected. Similarly, an inhibition of human tumors, which are generally weakly immunogenic, would not be expected (or they may even be stimulated). In support of this, administration of arginine to mice on low protein diets inhibited the growth of an immunogenic neuroblastoma, but stimulated growth of a weakly immunogenetic neuroblastoma (Bourut et al., 1988). Arginine also stimulates the release of insulin and in this way may stimulate tumor growth.

Glutamine

One of the dose-limiting adverse side effects of cytotoxic chemotherapy and abdominal radiotherapy is small bowel injury. Therapy-induced enteritis affects a significant number of cancer patients and in some cases may require surgical intervention and/or total parenteral nutrition. Glutamine is a principal fuel used by intestinal mucosal cells, and supplementation with glutamine may inhibit intestinal injury caused by a variety of noxious agents. In studies on rats treated with abdominal radiation, methotrexate, and fluorouracil, oral glutamine supplementation reduced bowel perforation, bloody diarrhea, and endotoxemia, and increased survival (Klimberg et al., 1990; Fox et al., 1987, 1988; O'Dwyer et al., 1987; Jacobs et al., 1987).

However, glutamine supplementation may also be detrimental to the cancer patient. Glutamine acts as a prominent fuel for lymphocytic and other tumor cells. In fact, an enzyme that degrades glutamine has been tested as an anticancer drug against childhood leukemia (Holcenberg and Kien, 1985). Further research is needed to determine the end effect of administering glutamine to cancer patients.

Tryptophan

Tryptophan supplementation may stimulate the growth of some tumors. Tryptophan depletion has been shown to inhibit leukemia cells in vitro, and chemotherapy agents that deplete tryptophan stores have been investigated in humans (Covington et al., 1990; Wallerstein et al., 1990). Nicotinamide (niacinamide), a form

---

[6] Lipotropic factors are compounds that promote the transportation and utilization of fats, and help prevent the accumulation of fat in the liver. They include methionine, choline, folic acid, and vitamin B12.

of vitamin B_3, is synthesized in the body from the amino acid tryptophan. As discussed in Chapter 3, nicotinamide may stimulate angiogenesis.

12.5 SUMMARY

The amount and type of dietary fat consumed may affect cancer growth through numerous mechanisms. High-fat diets, in particular those rich in omega-6 fatty acids, may promote cancer growth. Mechanisms include increasing sex hormone bioavailability, decreasing the immune response, increasing production of PGE_2, increasing membrane fluidity, and increasing the production of free radicals. On the other hand, diets rich in omega-3 fatty acids, in particular EPA, may inhibit cancer growth. This may occur by markedly increasing membrane fluidity, markedly increasing free radical damage, increasing PGE_3 production, decreasing PGE_2 production, reducing platelet aggregation, decreasing the production of angiogenic factors, and decreasing cachexia.

Modification of other macronutrients may inhibit the growth of some cancers. These include reducing total calorie intake, reducing sugar intake, increasing fiber intake, and reducing the intake of animal products. Certain amino acids may either stimulate or inhibit the growth of some cancers.

13
DIETARY MICRONUTRIENTS AND THEIR EFFECTS ON CANCER

Dietary micronutrients, such as vitamins and metals, appear to play a significant role in preventing the development of various cancers. The study of the effects of micronutrients on cancer is hampered by the variability of micronutrients in foods, the variability of human diets, the difficulty in long-term dietary recall, and the modest effect that these micronutrients generally produce. Even more controversial is how useful micronutrients may be in treating established cancers.

13.1 VITAMINS

Fourteen vitamins are known to be essential to human health and must be obtained through the diet. Although specific roles of some of these vitamins have been identified, many of their functions are still poorly understood. The majority of epidemiological studies on vitamins and cancer have been conducted through investigations of dietary habits rather than through investigations of vitamin supplementation. Therefore, with respect to vitamin supplementation, the conclusions of the majority of these studies are only presumptive. Even with respect to dietary habits, the results of these studies are open to criticism, since eating habits are complex and variable, and foods contain multiple micronutrients (Creasey, 1985:110). The vitamins A, C, E, B6, and folic acid are especially pertinent to a discussion of cancer. Studies on these vitamins are discussed separately below.

13.1.1 Vitamin A and Beta-Carotene

Data from animal and in-vitro experiments almost uniformly support the role of vitamin A in preventing cancer (reviewed by Creasey, 1985:116). The preventive role is probably due to the vitamin's ability to support normal differentiataion of epithelial cells (Van Poppel, 1993). Vitamin A also probably plays a part in regulating apoptosis. Its main functions are in supporting vision, differentiation of epithelial cells, growth (especially in bones), and reproduction (reviewed by Linder, 1991:153-6). High doses of vitamin A, such as those theoretically necessary to cause differentiation of cancer cells, are toxic to the liver, and therefore the role of

vitamin A in cancer treatment is limited to modest supplementation. Clinical studies on the effects of vitamin A and beta-carotene (provitamin A) on cancer are summarized in Table 13.1.

13.1.2 Vitamin C (Ascorbic Acid)

A number of studies suggest that an inverse association exists between vitamin C intake and cancer incidence. For example, low intake of vitamin C has been linked to increased incidence of stomach and esophageal cancers (Kolonel et al., 1981; Mettlin et al., 1981), and colorectal cancer (Ferraroni et al., 1994) Theoretically, vitamin C may inhibit carcinogenesis or tumor growth through at least four mechanisms:

1) Vitamin C is necessary for maintenance of the extracellular matrix, and therefore may inhibit tumor invasion. Low levels of vitamin C produce scurvy, a disease characterized by destruction of the matrix, vascular disorganization, and undifferentiated cellular proliferation.

2) Vitamin C intake can stimulate the immune system by increasing natural killer cell activity and the proliferation of lymphocytes in response to mitogens. Leukocytes contain a relatively high percentage of vitamin C, possibly to protect them from auto-oxidation during activation. The ability of neutrophils to kill bacteria is reduced when vitamin C is deficient (Henson et al., 1991).

3) Vitamin C is a potent antioxidant, and therefore may inhibit carcinogenesis.

4) Vitamin C has an antihistamine effect, which may be due to an inhibition of lipoxygenase activity and

TABLE 13.1. SUMMARY OF SELECTED CLINICAL STUDIES ON THE EFFECTS OF VITAMIN A AND BETA-CAROTENE ON CANCER

EFFECT	REFERENCE
Based on data obtained from 25,000 volunteers, high serum beta-carotene levels were associated with decreased risk of lung cancer.	Comstock et al., 1991
In a review of prediagnostic serum levels of beta-carotene, selenium, vitamin A, and vitamin E from 10 study populations for 10 cancer sites, serum levels were slightly lower for all four micronutrients among those who were diagnosed with cancer in comparison to those who were not. The strongest association was between low levels of beta-carotene and the subsequent development of lung cancer. Results indicate that it is unlikely that any one of these micronutrients is associated with protection against all cancer types. Other epidemiological studies of the cancer preventive effects of antioxidants have been inconclusive, partially because the beneficial effects have been small and thus may be due to other confounding factors	Comstock et al., 1992; Hennekens et al., 1994
In a study of 29,133 Finnish male smokers 50 to 69 years of age, administration of beta-carotene (20 mg/day) for 5 to 8 years increased the rate of lung cancer by 18%. Vitamin E at 50 mg/day had no effect on incidence of lung cancer. However, fewer cases of prostate cancer were diagnosed in the group receiving vitamin E. Since no other studies have reported a harmful effect of beta-carotene, but instead have reported beneficial effects, the authors state that "In light of all the data available, an adverse effect of beta-carotene seems unlikely... therefore, this finding may well be due to chance."	Alpha-tocopherol, beta carotene cancer prevention study group, 1994
Administration of vitamin A (350,000 to 500,000 IU) significantly increased response rates, duration of response, and projected survival in postmenopausal patients with metastatic breast cancer who were treated by chemotherapy.	Israel et al., 1985
In a crossover study on 18 patients with mucosal dysplasia of the head and neck region (a recognized premalignant lesion), supplementation with beta-carotene and cis-retinoic acid resulted in improvement in 61% of the subjects, and a complete response in 33%.	Malaker et al., 1991
A review of epidemiologic studies consistently associated beta-carotene with a reduced risk for a number of human cancers, especially epithelial cancers (such as lung cancer).	Mayne et al., 1991
In a review of data for 439 patients with oral and pharyngeal cancers and 2106 hospital controls, low beta-carotene intake accounted for 24% of the cancers in males and females. (Smoking and alcohol accounted up to 87% and 60%, respectively, of the oral cancers in males.)	Negri et al., 1993
In a 14-month trial of vitamin A in 181 patients with postsurgical non-small cell lung cancer, relapses were lower in the group receiving vitamin A (300,000 IU daily) as compared to controls (18% vs. 28%). Mild signs of toxicity were seen in some patients. After 46 months, the rates for tumor recurrence or the development of new primary tumors were 37% in the treated group and 48% in the controls. Daily administration of 300,000 IU of retinol palmitate (in aqueous emulsion) is reasonably safe for a period up to 2 years. Increases in serum triglycerides and gama-glutamyltransferase were observed in some treated patients.	Pastorino et al., 1988, 1993; Infante, 1991
Administration of retinol palmitate was effective as a salvage therapy in three of four patients undergoing chemotherapy for acute nonlymphocytic leukemia. Retinol palmitate may act by inducing differentiation and slowing the proliferation of leukemic cells after conventional chemotherapy.	Tsutani, 1991
In a study of 532 men with oral leukoplakia and/or chronic esophagitis (risk factors for cancers of the mouth and esophagus), administration of retinol, beta-carotene, and vitamin E reduced the prevalence of leukoplakia after 6 months, and reduced the risk of progression of chronic esophagitis after 20 months.	Zaridze et al., 1993
Blood samples were stored for 25,802 adults in Maryland, 28 of whom later developed oral or pharyngeal cancer. Analysis of blood samples revealed that high levels of beta carotene and vitamin E (alpha-tocopherol) were associated with decreased cancer risk. Persons with the highest tier of total carotenoids exhibited approximately a 66% reduction in risk compared to the lowest tier.	Zheng et al., 1993

an associated decline in leukotriene B_4 production (reviewed by Linder, 1991:149). In animal studies, histamine release and inflammation are associated with tumor promotion.

Animal studies support a protective role for vitamin C. For example, in studies on several tumor lines in mice, a combination of vitamins C and B12 inhibited tumor growth in up to 50% of the treated animals. The effects may be due to release of the cobalt nucleus in the presence of B12, and its attachment to ascorbic acid. This treatment did not inhibit normal cells. Vitamin C also reduced the toxicity and increased the effectiveness of a variety of chemotherapy and radiotherapy regimes in animals (Henson et al., 1991).

Linus Pauling and colleague Ewan Cameron have been long-time proponents of the use of vitamin C in treating cancer patients. In a study on 100 terminal cancer patients, Cameron and Pauling (1976) reported that administration of approximately 10 grams of vitamin C daily resulted in a 4-fold increase in survival (210 vs. 50 days) as compared to 1,000 patients treated without vitamin C. However, this study has been criticized for lack of randomization, lack of placebo controls, and other design flaws (Comroe, 1978). Other investigators have reported positive effects. In a trial of 99 cancer patients in Japan, the average time of survival after a terminal diagnosis was 43 days for 44 patients given low levels of ascorbic acid, and 246 days for 55 patients given high levels of ascorbic acid (Murata et al., 1982). In a second trial by these authors, 19 control patients with a terminal diagnosis survived for 48 days, and 6 patients administered high levels of ascorbic acid survived for 215 days.

In two studies sponsored by the United States government, the life span of patients treated with high doses of vitamin C did not increase (Creagan et al., 1979; Moertel et al., 1985). Pauling objected that these clinical trials were flawed (Pauling and Moertel, 1986). Cameron (1991) claimed that the patients in the first study had already been treated unsuccessfully with chemotherapy or radiation therapy, and such immune compromised patients would be the least likely to obtain any benefit from vitamin C. In the second study, Cameron contends that patients did not receive vitamin C therapy for a sufficient period of time. The patients received vitamin C only until tumor progression was detected, a median period of 10 weeks. In addition, he contends that the few controls used in the study were self-medicating with vitamin C.

Cameron (1991) suggests that in vitamin C therapy, vitamin C should be administered intravenously for the first 10 days, and orally afterwards. The desired plasma level of vitamin C is 3 mg/dl, which can be achieved on a oral dose of 10 to 30 grams daily. Other researchers have suggested a possible ceiling to vitamin C absorption of about 3 grams daily. It may be difficult to obtain higher

serum levels by increasing the dose above this level (reviewed by Linden, 1991:147-9). Vitamin C is rapidly excreted in the urine, and administration must be continuous or at frequent intervals (every six hours when taken orally). High doses of vitamin C (even 1 gram/day) induce increased levels of vitamin C-degrading hepatic enzymes, which persist for some time after discontinuation of treatment. For this reason, abrupt cessation of treatment can deplete serum vitamin C to levels well below nonsupplemented values. This rebound effect can reportedly produce a sharp decline in immunocompetence and may explain the decline in survival after patients were removed from vitamin C treatment in Moertel's 1985 study.

According to Cameron, side effects of intravenous administration of sodium ascorbate (the form of vitamin C used intravenously) commonly include transient fluid retention due to sodium overload, which may be dangerous in patients with cardiac impairment. Side effects may rarely include life-threatening septicemic shock caused by sudden necrosis of the tumor load. This may require the patient's transfer to an intensive care unit. The danger of kidney damage due to oxalate stone formation is not well-founded and has not been observed in over 1,000 cancer patients using this high dosage regime (Cameron, 1991). Dosages near or above 10 grams/day can cause diarrhea.

Cameron states that the common response to vitamin C treatment is either retardation or stasis of tumor growth, but not cure (Cameron, 1991). Oral administration is continued indefinitely and, Cameron states that patients commonly enter an extended period of many months or even years of comparative well-being. Patients may then enter an abrupt downhill phase with explosive metastasis. Intravenous "booster" treatment is used at this time.

In a study of 1,826 terminal cancer patients in Scotland, 294 patients who had received supplemental doses of vitamin C (10 grams/day) exhibited a median survival almost double that of controls (343 days vs. 180 days) (Cameron and Campbell, 1991). Cytotoxic chemotherapy treatment is used sparingly in the treatment of adult cancers in Scotland. Due to its effects on the immune system and the likely interference with response to vitamin C, the authors chose to exclude from the study any patients receiving cytotoxic chemotherapy. Plasma vitamin C levels associated with optimum survival were greater than 3 mg/dl.

13.1.3 Vitamin E

A primary function of vitamin E is to prevent the oxidation of fatty acids in cell membranes. For this reason, the most obvious sign of vitamin E deficiency in humans is red blood cell fragility. Vitamin E may also inhibit thromboxane A_2 and increase PGI_2 formation in platelets (thereby reducing platelet aggregation). And it may inhibit lipoxygenase activity (thereby reducing leukotriene production and associated inflammation) (reviewed by Linder, 1991:167-76). Vitamin E may possess anticarcinogenic activities through its ability to scavenge free radicals. The average American may be deficient in vitamin E, probably due to low dietary intake, high intake of polyunsaturated fatty acids (which undergo free radical damage and deplete antioxidant reserves), and low intake of selenium. Selenium has a vitamin E-sparing effect through selenium-dependent production of the antioxidant glutathione peroxidase.

13.1.4 B6 (Pyridoxine)

Vitamin B6 is a cofactor in more than 100 enzyme reactions, the majority of which are concerned with amino acid metabolism. For this reason, B6 deficiency has been implicated in "Chinese restaurant syndrome," in which monosodium glutamate (a form of the amino acid glutamine) is ingested in quantity and must be metabolized. Since the American diet contains many refined foods that lack B6, the average American may suffer from a marginal B6 deficiency (reviewed by Linder, 1991:127-37).

Vitamin B6 deficiency may be involved in carcinogenesis, since vitamin B6 is required for DNA repair. In established cancers, however, B6 supplementation may be detrimental. A number of animal and in-vitro studies have indicated that B6 may increase the proliferation of various cancer cell lines. Conversely, B6 deficiency inhibits proliferation (Demetrakopoulos and Brennan, 1982). Several human tumors xenografts in mice exhibit increased growth with B6 administration, and reduced growth with B6 deficiency (Fortmeyer et al., 1988; Stone, 1989). In a study of 248 patients with ovarian epithelial cancer, administration of B6 significantly reduced the neurotoxicity of cisplatin and hexamethylmelamine, presumably by facilitating the repair of drug-induced DNA lesions. However, it adversely affected the survival of these patients (Wiernik et al., 1992).

In contrast to other tumor lines, B6 may inhibit cell proliferation of human melanoma cells in vitro (Shultz et al., 1988) and B16 melanoma in mice (Di Sorbo et al., 1985). In part, the inhibitory effects of B6 on melanoma may be due to the strong immunogenicity of melanoma cells. Administration of B6 to nude mice bearing human melanoma xenografts did not inhibit tumor growth, but did increase immune functioning as evidenced by increased oxygen radical production by splenic phagocytic cells, and increased mitogen-induced cell proliferation of spleen cells (Gebhard et al., 1990). The authors speculate that the tumor-inhibiting effects of B6 supplementation in mouse melanoma reported elsewhere may be mediated by T-lymphocyte-dependent mechanisms that are genetically lacking in the nude mice. Similarly, Hofsli and Waage (1992) reported that B6 administration enhanced tumor necrosis factor-induced cytotoxicity in mouse fibrosarcoma cells in vitro.

13.1.5 Folic Acid

Folic acid is a cofactor in numerous biochemical processes in the body, and shares many of the same functions of vitamin B12. One of these functions is protein synthesis. In particular, folic acid (folate) is required in the formation of thymidylate, which is the rate-limiting step in DNA synthesis. Therefore, deficiency of folate inhibits DNA synthesis. The chemotherapy drugs methotrexate and aminopterin are synthetic analogs of folate that inhibit tumor cell growth by interfering with DNA synthesis. These drugs are most effective against fast-growing tumors, since cells of these tumors are sites of rapid DNA synthesis.

Although folate inhibitors are used to treat cancer, adequate folic acid is necessary to prevent some cancers. Low folic acid intake, or low erythrocyte levels, are associated with increased risk of developing colorectal and cervical cancers (Bernardi and Pace, 1994; Liu et al., 1993b; Lashner, 1993). Folic acid may reduce the risk of cervical cancer by inhibiting the incorporation of human papilloma virus genes into fragile chromosomal sites in affected cells (Butterworth, 1992). Low erythrocyte levels are a risk factor for abnormal cytologic smears in both benign atypia and more advanced lesions (Harper et al., 1994). The mechanism by which folate reduces the risk of colorectal cancer is not well understood.

13.1.6 Coenzyme Q-10

Coenzyme Q10 (ubiquinone) is a vitamin-like substance that plays an essential role in mitochondrial energy production. It is also a potent antioxidant, and declining tissue concentrations may play a role in the aging process. Among other uses, coenzyme Q10 (CoQ10) has been studied as an adjunct therapy in individuals with heart disease. Due to its high metabolic activity, the heart may require large amounts of CoQ10. Similarly, CoQ10 has been administered to cancer patients to successfully reduce chemotherapy-induced heart toxicity (Okuma et al., 1984, Takimoto et al., 1982).

More recently, CoQ10 has been studied as an anticancer agent. In a study on 32 node-positive breast cancer patients treated with conventional therapy and with 90 mg/day of CoQ10 and other nutritional supplements,

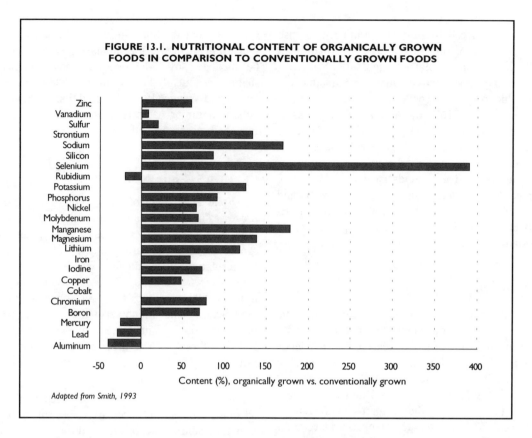

FIGURE 13.1. NUTRITIONAL CONTENT OF ORGANICALLY GROWN FOODS IN COMPARISON TO CONVENTIONALLY GROWN FOODS

Content (%), organically grown vs. conventionally grown

Adapted from Smith, 1993

all survived at least 24 months. During this period about six deaths would have been expected. A partial response was observed in six patients. Two of these were later given high doses (300 to 400 mg/day) and experienced complete remissions (Lockwood et al., 1994a, 1994b; Folkers et al., 1993). Three new positive high-dose case studies have been published (Lockwood et al., 1995).

13.2 METALS

Metals are important in a wide variety of biological processes in humans, including bone formation, nervous system function, antioxidant synthesis, hormone action, and blood clotting. The metals selenium, zinc, and calcium are particularly important with respect to cancer and are discussed separately below.

13.2.1 Selenium

Numerous studies suggest that an inverse association exists between selenium levels and cancer incidence (Hocman, 1988; Willett and Stampfer, 1986; Milner, 1985). Associations appear to be particularly strong with cancers that are also associated with high-fat, low-fiber diets (i.e., breast, colon, prostrate, etc.). The mechanism for selenium's reported protective effects is likely due to its function in antioxidant synthesis. Glutathione

peroxidase, the primary enzyme that converts hydrogen peroxide to water (and thus prevents lipid peroxidation) is selenium-dependent. Inhibition of lipid or bile acid oxidation may account for its protective role (reviewed by Linder 1991:496-7). Selenium may also act as an immune stimulant. Selenium deficiency inhibits macrophage-mediated tumor destruction, and inhibits tumor necrosis factor-alpha production in animals (Kiremidjian-Schumacher et al., 1992). Dietary supplementation with selenium produced the opposite effects.

In a study on 111 subjects who later developed cancer, those with the lowest selenium levels were twice as likely to develop cancer as those with the highest levels. The association was strongest for cancers of the gastrointestinal tract and prostate (Willett et al., 1983). Serum selenium levels were lower in patients with malignant oral cavity lesions as compared to healthy controls, and as compared to patients with premalignant lesions. Twenty-two patients with premalignant lesions were treated with selenium supplements and, after 12 weeks, 39% of the subjects improved (Toma et al., 1991). In a five-year study conducted in Qidong county, China, an area with a high incidence of primary liver cancer, selenium supplementation significantly reduced the incidence of liver cancer (Yu et al., 1991b). In a study on women over 50 years old, serum selenium in the range of 1.00 to 1.2 μmol/L provided a significant preventive effect against breast cancer (Hardell et al., 1993).

In contrast to these studies, other investigators have reported no association or a positive association between selenium deficiency and cancer, and the anticarcinogenic activity of selenium is still a matter of debate (Neve, 1985; Yan et al., 1991).

The intake of selenium and other nutrients from plant foods may be influenced by the type of farming practices used. In a preliminary investigation, organically grown foods were, in some cases, nutritionally superior to conventionally grown foods (Smith, 1993). This comparison was conducted on foods purchased in the Chicago area, and the results are illustrated in Figure 13.1. Other preliminary studies have reported similar results. Sharon Hornick, a soil scientist with the U.S. Department of Agriculture has reported that the vitamin C content in crops decreases as available nitrogen fertilizer increases. In kale, vitamin C was reduced by as much as 50% by high-nitrogen fertilizers (Hornick, 1992). In a German study, organically grown spinach, cabbage, and lettuce contained 59 to 91% more vitamin C (Hildenbrand, 1989). These studies are not adequate to prove that organically grown foods contain higher nutrition, but they do suggest that additional research in this area is warranted.

In addition to the potential for providing superior nutrition, organically grown foods also reduce the risk of pesticide exposure. Low-level exposure to certain pesticides, such as DDT, has been associated with high rates of breast cancer (Lewis, 1994; Key and Reeves, 1994; Westin, 1993), although other studies question the association (Taubes, 1994). Pesticides such as DDT and hexachlorobenzene accumulate in fat tissues, and possibly endocrine tissues, of humans and animals (Foster et al., 1993).[1] Chlorinated organics and triazine herbicides appear to act as xenoestrogens, affecting estrogen production and metabolism in humans, and inducing mammary cancer in mice. These, and similar environmental contaminants may be responsible for the feminization of reptiles and fish seen in Florida and the Great Lakes region (Ginsburg, 1994). Epidemiologic studies indicate that the breast fat and serum lipids of women with breast cancer contain significantly elevated levels of some chlorinated organics, as compared to noncancer controls (Davis et al., 1993). Xenoestrogens may also be associated with increased risk of endometriosis, testicular cancer, and lowered sperm quality (Ginsburg, 1994). Two possible sources of xenoestrogen exposure are ingestion of plant foods treated with pesticides and herbicides, and ingestion of the fat (butter, meat, etc.) of animals that consume plants treated with pesticides and herbicides. Further investigation is needed to determine the level of risk that pesticide- and herbicide-treated foods may pose.

13.2.2 Zinc

Zinc is required by more than 100 enzymes such as those involved with the metabolism, function, and maintenance of the skin, pancreas, and male reproductive organs. Along with copper, zinc is necessary for the synthesis of superoxide dismutase (SOD), an ubiquitous enzyme that degrades superoxide to form hydrogen peroxide. Zinc is also required for proper function of T lymphocytes. Zinc deficiency can lead to atrophy of the thymus gland, depression of NK cell and lymphocyte activity, and other immunodeficiencies. The average American may be deficient in zinc, as intake is about 10 mg/day and the Recommended Daily Allowance is 15 mg/day. Symptoms of severe zinc deficiency include growth retardation, anorexia, skin lesions, hair loss, diarrhea, loss of taste, loss of smell, and, since zinc is a cofactor for collagenase, impaired wound healing (Linder, 1991:226-31). Severe zinc deficiency is uncommon in the United States.

The effects of zinc on the initiation and progression of cancer are not well established, although the negative effects of zinc deficiency on the immune system are clear (Linder, 1991:499, 512). In an evaluation of 261 patients with breast cancer and 261 controls, the cancer patients had significantly higher mean zinc blood levels. The higher levels were thought to be due to a release of tissue zinc stores (Cavallo et al., 1991). The effect of this release on cancer growth is uncertain.

13.2.3 Calcium

Numerous animal studies indicate that calcium may inhibit colon cancer, and human studies indicate that calcium may reversibly inhibit hyperproliferation of colon cells (Arlow, 1989; Wargovich, 1988; Buset et al., 1986; Lipkin and Newmark, 1985). Calcium is likely to reduce colon cancer risk by complexing fat in the stool, thereby reducing lipid damage (Wargovich et al., 1991).

13.3 SUMMARY

Although certain vitamins and minerals may be important in preventing the development of some cancers, the efficacy of using these micronutrient factors to treat cancer is uncertain. In many cases a reasonable theoretical framework suggests that some micronutrients may be useful, but further clinical investigation is necessary before definitive statements can be made.

---

[1] Although DDT has been banned in the United States since 1972, U.S. manufacturers continue to produce and export the product. It can return to the U.S. as residue on imported foods.

14

DIETARY NON-NUTRIENT FACTORS AND THEIR EFFECTS ON CANCER

Evidence is accumulating that non-nutrient dietary factors—factors other than macro-nutrients and micronutrients—may play a significant role in preventing cancer. Non-nutrient compounds include phytoestrogens, saponins, flavonoids, protease inhibitors, isoflavones, and lignans. In-vitro and in-vivo studies suggest that some of these compounds also may be useful in treating established cancers.

14.1 NON-NUTRIENT ANTICARCINOGENS

Epidemiological studies from around the world have consistently reported that a high intake of fruits and vegetables is associated with a low incidence of most types of cancer (Weisburger, 1991). Although the content of vitamins, minerals, and other micronutrients in these foods is likely a factor, recent evidence suggests that there are a host of non-nutritive constituents in foods that also may play a significant anticarcinogenic role.

Wattenberg (1992) identified two basic mechanisms by which non-nutritive dietary constituents may inhibit carcinogenesis: by blocking the action of carcinogens and/or tumor promoters, and by suppressing the evolution of initiated cells. A partial list of non-nutrient factors that act by these mechanisms are listed in Table 14.1. Blocking agents act by at least four methods:

- Inhibiting the metabolism of noncarcinogenic compounds into carcinogenic compounds.
- Inducing enzyme systems that detoxify carcinogens (such as glutathione S-transferase and the P_{450} enzyme system).[1]
- Scavenging free radicals.
- Preventing tumor promoters from reaching or reacting with their cellular targets.

It is apparent from Table 14.1 that certain plants, such as those of the *Brassica* and *Allium sp.*, contain a variety of anticarcinogens. Regular consumption of cruciferous vegetables (cabbage, broccoli, etc.) is associated with reduced rates of colon, lung, and other cancers in humans. In addition, they may have a role in cancer treatment. Orally administered indoles from cruciferous vegetables prevent the development of multidrug resistance in chemotherapy-treated mice (Christensen and Le-Blanc, 1996).

Some non-nutrient factors may inhibit both carcinogenesis and the growth of established tumors. For example, ingestion of cabbage and collards decreased lung metastasis in animals injected intravenously with mammary tumor cells (Scholar et al., 1989). Limonene is another example of a non-nutrient compound that inhibits both carcinogenesis and tumor growth.

Non-nutritive food constituents apparently have been protecting humans from cancer since the beginning of history. Steinmetz and Potter (1991) hypothesized that in light of the many non-nutrient food components that prevent cancer, cancer may be a disease of maladaption to diets lacking a rich variety of these compounds. They state, "It appears extremely unlikely that any one substance is responsible for all the associations seen. ... Cancer may be the result of reducing the intake of foods that are metabolically necessary."

---

[1] The P_{450} enzyme system oxidizes lipophilic drugs and other compounds to a more polar form, which increases their water solubility and excretion through the urine. The major site of P_{450} and glutathione S-transferase activity is in the liver.

TABLE 14.1. NON-NUTRIENT DIETARY CONSTITUENTS THAT INHIBIT CARCINOGENESIS

COMPOUND	SOURCE
Agents that Block Carcinogen Activation	
Aromatic isothiocyanates (benzyl isothiocyanate, phenethyl isothiocyanate)	cruciferous vegetables
Glucosinolates (glucobrassin, glucotropaeolin)	cruciferous vegetables
Monoterpenes (d-limonene, d-carvone)	citrus fruit oils, caraway seed oil
Organosulfur compounds (diallyl sulfide, diallyl disulfide, allyl mercaptan, allyl methyl disulfide)	*Allium sp.*
Blocking Agents that Increase Carcinogen Detoxification	
Aromatic isothiocyanates	cruciferous vegetables
Organosulfur compounds	*Allium sp.*
Agents that Block the Action of Tumor Promoters	
Aromatic isothiocyanates	cruciferous vegetables
Beta-carotene	numerous plants
Conjugated dienoic linoleic acids	numerous plants
Coumarins	numerous plants
Curcumin	*Curcuma sp.*
Dithiolethiones	cruciferous vegetables
Ellagic acid	numerous plants
Flavones	numerous plants
18-beta-Glycyrrhetinic acid	*Glycyrrhiza sp.*
Indoles	cruciferous vegetables
Nucleophiles	numerous plants
Organosulfur compounds	*Allium sp.*
Phenols	cruciferous vegetables
Tannins	numerous plants
Terpenes	numerous plants
Glucarates	numerous plants
Suppressing Agents	
Aromatic isothiocyanates	cruciferous vegetables
Inhibitors of the arachidonic acid cascade	numerous plants
Inositol hexaphosphate	numerous plants
Protease inhibitors	soy and other legumes
Terpenes	numerous plants
Source: Wattenburg, 1992	

14.2 PHYTOESTROGENS

Phytoestrogens are estrogen-like compounds produced in human intestines by bacterial action on precursors present in a variety of seeds and vegetables. One phytoestrogen, equol, has a low affinity for estrogen receptors, but is produced in high quantity from diets rich in soy foods (Setchell et al., 1984). Equol has a biologic estrogen activity approximately 0.2% that of estradiol. However, by sheer numbers, equol may compete with estrogen receptors, and thus lower the bioavailability of circulating estrogen. Soy products appear to have an estrogenic effect on postmenopausal women, and an antiestrogenic effect on premenopausal women who have relatively high estrogen levels (Messina and Barnes, 1991).

Due to their antiestrogenic effect, phytoestrogens derived from soy may protect against breast cancer (Rose, 1993). In fact, tamoxifen, which has shown some effectiveness in treating breast cancer, is structurally related to some phytoestrogens (Messina and Barnes, 1991). Vegetarian and Japanese diets contain approximately 4.5 times the phytoestrogens of the average American diet (Messina and Barnes, 1991), which may account, in part, for the relatively low level of breast cancer in the Japanese population. In rodent studies, consumption of soy inhibited the growth of chemically-induced mammary cancer. These effects were associated with a decrease in available tumor estrogen receptors (Barnes et al., 1990).

14.3 PHYTOSTEROLS AND SAPONINS

Phytosterols and saponins are common constituents of legumes and other plants. Plant sterols, such as beta-sitosterol, reduce tumor yields when given orally to tumor-bearing animals (Nair et al., 1984). Beta-sitosterol inhibited neoplastic transformation in chemically induced colon cancer in mice (Deschner, 1982).[2] Plant sterols are structurally similar to cholesterol, and oral administration of phytosterols have been shown to bind cholesterol and reduce its absorption in humans.

Saponins are plant compounds that have surfactant properties and, like phytoestrogens, bind to cholesterol and bile acids. Research suggests that various saponins stimulate the immune system, inhibit sarcoma 37 cells in vitro, decrease the growth of human epidermoid and cervical cancer cells in vitro, inhibit Epstein-Barr virus expression, and, like phytoestrogens, reduce abnormal colonic cell proliferation induced by carcinogens (reviewed by Messina and Barnes, 1991).[3] Because of their surfactant properties, herbs that contain saponins may help to increase the absorption of plant constituents that are not water-soluble.

---

[2] A wide variety of Chinese herbs contain beta-sitosterol. These include *Magnolia liliflora (xin yi), Cassia tora (jue ming zi), Rehmannia glutinosa (shu di huang), and Isatis indigotica (da qing ye)* (Hsu et al., 1985; Bensky and Gamble, 1993).

[3] Chinese herbs that contain saponins include *Glycyrrhiza uralensis (gan cao), Dioscorea opposita (shan yao), Pseudostellaria heterophylla (tai zi shen), Codonopsis pilosula (dang shen), Bupleurum chinense (chai hu)* and many others (Bensky and Gamble, 1993).

14.4 FLAVONOIDS

Flavonoids (or bioflavonoids) are a group of over 4,000 naturally occurring phenolic compounds (polyphenols) sharing a similar chemical structure.[4] They are found in a wide variety of plants, including most common fruits and vegetables. In citrus fruit, they may represent up to 1% of fresh material. Beverages such as beer, wine, tea, and coffee also contain considerable amounts of flavonoids. The average daily dietary consumption of flavonoids may be as high as one gram (Kuhnau, 1976). Flavonoids appear to be the active constituents in numerous medicinal plants, and plants that contain flavonoids are widely used in herbal medicine traditions around the world.

Flavonoids can be divided into five categories (Harborne and Baxter, 1991:324):

1) *Anthocyanins, anthochlors, and aurones.* Anthocyanins are red-blue pigments in plants (such as found in red to blue fruits). Anthochlors and aruones are yellow pigments found in flowers.

2) *Minor flavonoids.* Minor flavonoids include flavanones, flavan-3-ols, dihydroflavones, and dihydrochalcones. These are categorized as minor flavonoids due to their limited natural distribution. Two flavan-3-ols that will be discussed below include (+)-catechin and epigallocatechin 3-gallate (EGCG). Some authors have argued that, due to their unique properties, flavan-3-ol (flavanol) compounds should be considered as an independent class rather than a subcategory of flavonoids (Schwitters and Masquelier, 1993:13-5). Certain flavanols are sometimes referred to by the trademark term pycnogenols, coined by the French researcher Professor Jack Masquelier. The term pycnogenol means "that which creates condensation," and refers to the tendency of flavanols to create dimers (two identical compounds joined together), oligomers (a few joined together), and polymers (many joined together). One group of flavanol dimers and oligomers are termed proanthocyanidins, and are discussed below in item 5.

3) *Flavones and Flavonols.* Flavones and flavonols are the most widely occurring flavonoids. Although several hundred flavonol aglycones are known, only quercetin, kaempferol, and myricetin are widely distributed.[5] The other known flavonols are structural variants on these three and occur in limited distribution. More than 135 different glycosides of quercetin have been isolated, the most common of which is rutin, a flavonol that has been used to treat capillary fragility. Flavones also occur as glycosides, but in a more limited fashion than flavonols. Baicalin, such as found in *Scutellaria baicalensis (huang qin),* is a common flavone *O*-glycoside used in Chinese medicine.

4) *Isoflavonoids.* Isoflavonoids are found mostly in the Leguminosae family (legumes), and can be divided into isoflavones, isoflavanones, pterocarpans, isoflavans, and rotenoids. Common isoflavonoids include genistein, daidzein, and biochanin A.

5) *Tannins.* Tannins include proanthocyanidins and gallic acid phenolics (the gallo- and ellagi-tannins). They are characterized by their ability to bind with proteins. Proanthocyanidins are dimers of flavanols. In France, where much of the basic research on flavanols has taken place, they are termed "procyanidols" or in French "oligomeres procyanidoliques", or OPC. The abbreviation OPC is now used in many countries to refer to proanthocyanidins.

The distribution of these compounds vary between plant species. For example, citrus fruits contain high levels of flavones and flavanones; green tea contains high levels of catechins (17 to 30% of dry weight) and gallic acid phenolics; red, blue, and purple fruits such as berries, grapes, and pomegranates contain high levels of anthocyanins; and pine bark and grape seeds contain high levels of OPC. Small molecular weight flavonoids are responsible for the tartness and bitterness of many fruits, whereas large molecular weight flavonoids (tannins), are responsible for their astringency.

Some researchers question the bioavailability of flavonoids. Approximately half of the ingested flavonoids are absorbed into the bloodstream through the gastrointestinal tract lining, and half are metabolized to other compounds by gastrointestinal microflora (reviewed by Leibovitz, 1994). However, this varies, depending on the flavonoid. For example, flavonoids found in citrus fruits are poorly metabolized by the microflora (reviewed by Leibovitz, 1994), rutin is poorly absorbed in mice (Schwitters and Masquelier, 1993:26), and quercetin is not absorbed in humans (Gugler et al., 1975).[6] In

---

[4] The phenolic structure is an aromatic ring bearing one or more hydroxyl groups. The majority of polyphenol compounds are water-soluble and occur combined with sugar in their glycoside form. A smaller number of polyphenols are lipid-soluble, occurring with the phenolic group masked by *O*-methylation. There are approximately 8,000 plant polyphenols, approximately half of which are flavonoids. Other nonflavonoid polyphenols include phenolic acids, lignins, melanins, coumarins, chromones, benzofurans, xanthones, and quinones (Harborne and Baxter, 1991:324).

[5] Quercetin is found in *Crataegus cuneata (shan zha), Pueraria thunbergiana (ge gen), Glycyrrhiza glabra (gan cao), Morus alba (sang ye),* and many other herbs and fruits (Hsu et al., 1982:454).

[6] A water-soluble quercetin product may soon be available in nonprescription form. This form should be more easily absorbed.

contrast, OPCs are readily absorbed by mice (Schwitters and Masquelier, 1993:24-58).[7]

Research on flavonoids began in 1936 when Szent-Gyorgi and colleagues discovered that crude extracts of vitamin C from lemon juice were more effective than pure vitamin C in treating guinea pigs with experimentally-induced scurvy. Since that time, researchers have identified a number of biochemical actions of flavonoids and polyphenols, including the following:

• Antiallergy actions
• Immunomodulating actions
• Inhibition of platelet aggregation
• Antitumor actions

The first three of these are discussed briefly below, followed by a more detailed discussion of antitumor actions.

14.4.1 Antiallergy Actions

Flavonoids can inhibit allergic reactions by inhibiting the production of histamine, the primary agent responsible for allergic reactions (Berg and Daniel, 1988).[8] This is accomplished in part by the inhibition of two enzymes that increase histamine release from mast cells and basophils: cyclic AMP phosphodiesterase and calcium-dependent ATPase. Cyclic AMP phosphodiesterase is an enzyme that degrades cAMP (see Box 6.1). High cAMP levels block the release of histamine from cellular storage granules. Calcium-dependent ATPase is an enzyme that degrades ATP to obtain energy to pump calcium into the cell. High intracellular calcium levels cause the release of histamine from intracellular storage granules.

A standard pharmaceutical drug used to treat asthma and allergies is disodium cromoglycate, a synthetic flavonoid based upon khellin, a flavonoid found in *Amni visnaga*. Its mechanism of action appears to be identical to those described above. Some flavonoids may be more potent than disodium cromoglycate in inhibiting histamine release. Phenolic glycosides from *Acanthopanax sp. (ci wu jia, wu jia pi)* were 6,800 times stronger than disodium cromoglycate in inhibiting histamine release from rat mast cells in vitro (Umeyama et al., 1992), and quercetin was 5 to 10 times stronger (Amellal et al., 1985).

14.4.2 Immunomodulating Actions

Flavonoids may affect immune function by inhibiting eicosanoid-mediated inflammation (Welton et al., 1988), by inhibiting histamine-induced inflammation (as described above), and by conserving vitamin C and other antioxidants. The effects of flavonoids on the immune system are complex and poorly understood. In high concentrations, some flavonoids inhibit lymphocyte proliferation and function (possibly by scavenging phagocyte-induced free radicals). In lower concentrations, they may act as immunostimulants, especially in immunodeficient individuals (Berg and Daniel, 1988). Immunostimulation has also been reported in vitro. For example, (+)-catechin stimulates interleukin-1 production and lymphocyte proliferation and function in vitro at concentrations less than 64 µg/ml, but inhibits them at higher concentrations (Daniel et al., 1988). Similar results were shown with epigallocatechin 3-gallate (EGCG) (Sakagami et al., 1992).

Flavonoids such as quercetin and those found in *Ginkgo biloba* extract (GBE) are free radical scavengers that decrease the proliferation of rat lymphocytes in vitro in a dose-dependent manner (Pignol et al., 1988). These two actions may be related. Stimulated neutrophils and macrophages produce a marked and transient increase in oxygen consumption, called a respiratory burst (or chemiluminescent burst). This burst involves the production of superoxide ($O_2\cdot$). The superoxide radical, along with hydrogen peroxide and hydroxyl radicals (OH $\cdot$) are highly toxic and are responsible for the bactericidal action of these cells. Hydrogen peroxide also accumulates intracellularly and ultimately may be responsible for inducing cell division. In this way, increased immune cell activity may induce increased immune cell proliferation. Hydroxyl radical scavengers, such as urea, can inhibit lymphocyte proliferation in response to mitogens. Some flavonoids produce a similar effect.

In addition to inhibiting cell proliferation, free radical scavengers can directly inhibit phagocyte activity by scavenging radicals produced during the respiratory burst. For example, GBE decreases the respiratory burst in human neutrophils in a dose-dependent manner ex vivo. Quercetin and kaempferol decrease the cytotoxicity of natural killer cells in vitro, presumably through a similar free radical scavenging effect (Pignol et al., 1988).

The flavonoid-induced immune suppression demonstrated in-vitro may not occur in vivo, at least at some

---

[7] OPC has shown efficacy in clinical studies for improving capillary fragility. In radiolabeled studies in mice, OPC demonstrated a marked affinity for vascular tissue (Schwitters and Masquelier, 1993:24-58).

[8] Leukotriene production from arachidonic acid plays a secondary role in facilitating allergic reactions. In the case of asthma, leukotriene production plays a primary role (by causing bronchoconstriction and inflammation), and histamine plays a secondary role.

doses. Neutrophil chemiluminescence was markedly increased in human subjects who received GBE (360 mg orally) (Pignol et al., 1988). Green tea extract (GTE), which contains EGCG, stimulated the proliferation of T lymphocytes and increased NK cell activity in SA-bearing mice (Yan, 1992). Intraperitoneal administration of GTE (80 mg/kg) stimulated the proliferation of T lymphocytes in SA-bearing mice by roughly 300%, and increased NK cell activity by 30% as compared to controls.

14.4.3 Inhibition of Platelet Aggregation

Flavonoids appear to influence a number of steps in both coagulation and fibrinolysis. Many flavonoids inhibit platelet adhesion and aggregation, most likely through inhibition of cAMP phosphodiesterase. Inhibition of cyclooxygenase activity (and associated inhibition of thromboxane synthesis) may also be involved. Green tea polyphenols inhibit thromboxane formation and inhibit platelet aggregation (Ali et al., 1990; Sagesaka-Mitane et al., 1990). Other flavonoids, such as those in apple cider, have been shown to inhibit fibrinolysis and may enhance thrombosis formation (Anderson et al., 1983).

14.4.4 Antitumor Actions

Various flavonoids inhibit carcinogenesis and/or tumor growth. Mechanisms by which this may occur include the following:

1) inhibition of mitosis
2) blocking or competing for receptor sites
3) stabilizing collagen
4) binding with laminin
5) inducing the production of transforming growth factor-β_1
6) altering gene expression
7) inhibiting tumor blood supply
8) reducing free radical damage and inflammation

Each of these mechanisms is discussed below. In many studies, the actual mechanism inhibiting tumor growth is not clear, since one or more of the above mechanisms may occur in unison and their effects may be interrelated.

Inhibiting Mitosis

A number of investigators have reported that flavonoids inhibit tumor growth by inhibiting some phase of the cell cycle. Green tea extract and quercetin have been the most extensively studied agents.

Selected in-vitro studies are summarized in Table 14.2. As can be seen, cell lines vary widely as to their sensitivity to flavonoid treatment.

Blocking or Competing for Receptor Sites

Green tea extract produced a 50% growth inhibition of PC-9 and PC-14 lung cancer cell lines at up to 36 μg/ml (67 μM as EGCG), and MCF-7 and BT-20 mammary cancer lines at up to 420 μg/ml (780 μM as EGCG). The authors suggest that growth-inhibiting actions of GTE may be due to a blocking effect, either on growth factor and hormone receptor sites or on the action of tumor promoters. This "sealing" effect would account for the reversible growth inhibition observed. GTE and EGCG inhibited the growth of lung and mammary tumor cell lines with similar potencies (Komori et al., 1993). Similarly, EGCG and GTE inhibited the growth of estrogen-dependent mammary cancer (MCF-7) cells and other mammary and lung cancer cell lines in vitro (Suganuma et al., 1993). The authors suggest that these effects are due in part to the "sealing" effect.

Numerous investigators have reported that 10 μM quercetin concentrations reversibly inhibit a number of human tumors cell lines in vitro by competing for type II estrogen binding sites (type II EBS).[9] These data are summarized in Table 14.3. Inhibition was dose-dependent and occurred within hours or days. Type II EBS were identified on all of the tumors listed in Table 14.3. Rutin, a flavonoid that does not bind to type II EBS did not inhibit the growth of these tumors.

Stabilizing Collagen

The basement membrane surrounding capillaries presents a major obstacle to tumor invasion and metastasis. It is composed primarily of collagen, fibronectin, and laminin. Agents that inhibit collagen breakdown may inhibit invasion and metastasis. The flavonoid (+)-catechin stimulates collagen synthesis and changes its functional properties by making it less susceptible to the action of collagenase (Beretz and Cazenave, 1988).[10] In

---

[9] Type II estrogen binding sites differ from "true" estrogen binding sites by their higher concentration and lower affinity for estrogen. Type II estrogen binding sites are present in a wide range of human tumors. Their actual purpose may be to bind an endogenous flavonoid-like ligand that has growth-inhibitory activity rather than to bind estrogen (Piantelli et al., 1993).

[10] Chinese herbs that contain (+)-catechin include *Cinnamomum cassia (rou gui), Polygonum multiflorum (he shou wu), Areca catechu (da fu pi), Sargentodoxa cuneata (hong teng), Rheum palmatum (da huang)*, and *Crataegus oxyacantha (shan zha)* (Scutt et al., 1987; Hsu et al., 1985:351-2; Hsu et al., 1982:566-7; Ficarra et al., 1990; Rucker et al., 1991).

TABLE 14.2. IN-VITRO CYTOTOXIC EFFECTS OF FLAVONOIDS			
FLAVONOID	**CELL LINE**	**EFFECT**	**REFERENCE**
Quercetin	Mouse L929	61% growth inhibition at 250 µM, significant inhibition as low as 50 µM.	Ramanathan et al., 1994b
	Chago lung cancer, S102 hepatoma, SW620 colon cancer, and BT474 human lung cancer	50% inhibition between 2.2 and 18.3 µM.	Moongkarndi et al., 1991
	Human gastric cancer	Reversible G1 (gap) phase arrest—50% inhibition at 32 to 55 µM. DNA synthesis was suppressed by 86% at concentrations of 70 µM for two days.	Matsukawa, 1990; Yoshida et al., 1990
	HTB-43 and 0023 (human squamous cell carcinoma ex vivo)	Dose-dependent inhibition; complete growth inhibition of both lines at 110 µM; inhibition of normal lung cells at 200 µM.	Castillo et al., 1989
	Human squamous cell carcinoma HTB-43	45% growth inhibition at 4.4 µM in the presence of 2 µg/ml ascorbic acid. Ascorbic acid potentiated the cytostatic effects of quercetin.	Kandaswami et al., 1993
	Human Raji lymphoma and Hela carcinoma	46% and 77% inhibition at 100 µM respectively.	Ramanathan et al., 1994a
Baicalein from *Scutellaria baicalensis*, quercetin, and EGCG	Human CEM leukemia, Daudi lymphoma, and HeLa cervical carcinoma	Induced substantial (10 to 50%) enzymic DNA damage (topoisomerase II-dependent cleavage) at concentrations of 17 to 175 µM. Baicalein and quercetin produced a 50% growth inhibition at 13 to 25 µM. EGCG slightly stimulated growth.	Austin et al., 1992
EGCG	Mouse lung carcinoma	Inhibited cell survival by 36% at 1,000 µM.	Isemura et al., 1993
	DS19 mouse erythroleukemia and HTC rat hepatoma	Nearly complete growth inhibition at 218 µM and 436 µM respectively.	Lea et al., 1993a, 1993b
	MT-4	50% inhibition at 10 µM.	Nakane and Ono, 1990
GTE	HTC rat hepatoma and DS19 mouse erythroleukemia	Inhibited DNA synthesis at concentrations of 100 to 200 µg/ml.	Lea et al., 1993a, 1993b

one study catechin compounds from green tea strongly inhibited the collagenolytic effects of *Porphyromonas gingivalis,* the bacteria associated with periodontal disease (Osawa et al., 1991). Purified tannins or (+)-catechin from *Areca catechu (da fu pi)* increased collagen resistance to both human and bacterial collagenases (Scutt et al., 1987). (+)-Catechin promoted the cross-linking of collagen in the connective tissue of arthritic animals (Rao et al., 1983). Of the green tea catechins, EGCG and (-)-epicatechin gallate may be the most potent inhibitors of collagenase derived from mammalian cells. Optimal concentrations are approximately 218 µM (Makimura et al., 1993). OPC also inhibits collagenase activity against vascular collagen (reviewed by Schwitters and Masquelier, 1993:43).

Other flavonoids, in particular anthocyanins and proanthocyanidins, also promote collagen synthesis and stability. Anthocyanins from *Vaccinium myrtillus* (bilberry) protect cartilage (a collagen-rich substance) by stimulating collagen cross-linking, inhibiting free radical

damage and inflammation, inhibiting enzymatic degradation, and stimulating collagen synthesis (reviewed by Murray, 1992:224-5; Monboisse et al., 1983).

Binding with Laminin

Laminin is a glycoprotein in the extracellular matrix that may regulate invasion. Laminin accumulates at the front of invading cells and accumulates between invading cells and host tissue (reviewed by Bracke et al., 1988a, 1988b). It promotes adhesion of a number of tumor cell types to collagen via specific laminin receptors on the cell's membranes.

(+)-Catechin inhibits the invasion of a variety of tumor cells in vitro at concentrations of 0.5 µM. The anti-invasive activity of (+)-catechin may be related to its ability to bind tissue-type plasminogen activator (t-PA) to laminin, leading to partial inactivation of tPA (Bracke et al., 1991, 1988a, 1988b, 1986, 1985, 1984; Mareel and

TABLE 14.3. EFFECT OF QUERCETIN ON CELL LINES EXHIBITING TYPE II ESTROGEN BINDING SITES

CELL LINE	EFFECT *	REFERENCE
Human transitional cell bladder carcinoma tumor ex vivo	67% growth inhibition	Larocca et al., 1994
Multidrug-resistant MCF-7 human breast cancer	50% growth inhibition	Scambia et al., 1994b
Estrogen receptor positive and ER-negative human breast cancer cells	65% growth inhibition	Scambia et al., 1993
MCF-7-ADRr multidrug-resistant, ER-negative human breast cancer cells	53% growth inhibition**	Scambia et al., 1991
Human ovarian cancer cells OVCA 433	Synergistically increased the cytotoxicity of cisplatin	Scambia et al., 1990a, 1990b
Human meningioma cells ex vivo	80% growth inhibition	Piantelli et al., 1993
HT-29, WiDr, COLO 210, and LS-174T human colon cancer cells	50% growth inhibition at 0.06 to 3.1 μM	Ranelletti et al., 1992
Human acute myeloid leukemia (AML) and acute lymphoid leukemia (ALL) ex vivo	Greater than 50% inhibition at 2 μM in 12 of 14 AML, and 4 of 4 ALL ex vivo ***	Larocca et al., 1991
HL-60 human acute leukemia	Acted synergistically with the chemotherapy agent Ara-C	Teofili et al., 1992

* The concentration of quercetin was 10 μM unless stated.

** The antiestrogen tamoxifen also competed for type II estrogen binding sites, but was not as effective as quercetin in securing binding sites or in producing tumor inhibition.

*** Normal bone marrow cells were less sensitive to quercetin (less than 50% inhibition at concentrations higher than 20 μM.

De Mets, 1989). Recall from Chapter 4 that tPA is an enzyme that facilitates invasion.

Citrus flavonoids also exhibit anti-invasive activity in vitro. Tangeretin has been shown to inhibit both invasion and proliferation of malignant tumor cells, but appears to act by a different mechanism. Tangeretin shows poor affinity to the extracellular matrix and does not bind enzymes to laminin (Bracke et al., 1991).

Inducing the Production of Transforming Growth Factor-β_1

Transforming growth factor-beta (TGF-β_1) is present in a variety of normal and neoplastic cells and is involved in regulating normal growth and differentiation. It also has been found to inhibit the growth of several human cancer cell lines. The production of TGF-β_1 is stimulated by a number of antitumor agents such as retinoids, vitamin D, antiestrogens (including tamoxifen), and interferons, and may account, in part, for their antitumor effects (reviewed by Scambia et al., 1994a). Quercetin produced dose-dependent growth inhibition in human ovarian cancer cells (OVCA 433) in vitro, apparently by stimulating the cells to produce TGF-β_1. Quercetin concentrations of 10 μM inhibited growth by 32% as compared to controls (Scambia et al., 1994a).

Altering Gene Expression

Quercetin (at 100 μM) inhibited the expression of the multidrug resistance gene MDR1 in human hepatocarcinoma cells (HepG2) in response to the toxic compound arsenite (Kioka et al., 1992). MDR1 is expressed in HepG2 and other neoplastic cells in response to stress and conveys resistance to the cells against a variety of chemotherapy drugs. Multidrug resistance is associated with overexpression of a membrane protein called P-glycoprotein.

Quercetin may inhibit P-glycoprotein overexpression (and multidrug resistance) through inhibiting activation of heat shock factor (HSF). HSF is activated in cells in response to heat and other stressors (such as chemotherapy), and quercetin inhibits the activation of HSF in a variety of neoplastic cell lines (see Section 7.3.1).

Quercetin concentrations of 1 to 10 μM potentiated the cytotoxicity of Adriamycin against Adriamycin-resistant human breast cancer cells (MCF-7). Adriamycin resistance is associated with the expression of high levels of P-glycoprotein, and quercetin (at 10 μM) inhibited this expression. These cells contain type II EBS and the effects of quercetin on P-glycoprotein expression may be related to its ability to bind to these sites. Quercetin did not potentiate Adriamycin cytotoxicity against nonresistant MCF-7 cells (Scambia et al., 1994b).

Quercetin may also induce apoptosis by altering gene expression. Quercetin inhibited human breast cancer cells (MDA-MB468) in vitro by strongly and specifically inhibiting the expression of the mutated p53 plasma membrane protein (50% inhibition at 16 µM). The normal p53 protein is a tumor suppressor protein that has been identified as a key regulator of apoptosis in normal and malignant hematopoietic cells. Recall from Chapter 2 that DMSO induces apoptosis in human leukemic cells by the same process. P-glycoprotein expression was not altered by the quercetin treatment (Avila et al., 1994).

Quercetin also induced apoptosis in heat-stressed human leukemia and Burkitt's lymphoma cells by inhibiting the activation of HSF (and the resulting synthesis of heat shock protein-70). The concentration for inducing maximal apoptosis was 200 µM. Apoptosis was also observed in heat-stressed gastric, colon, and lung carcinoma cells (Wei et al., 1994).

Inhibiting Tumor Blood Supply

Flavone acetic acid (FAA) is a synthetic flavonoid that has been heavily studied as an antitumor agent. It appears to stimulate an immune response, the debris of which clogs the capillaries within established tumors, thereby causing hypoxic necrosis. Quercetin also induced a blockage of tumor blood flow in mice (Teicher et al., 1991). In animal studies, FAA has been highly effective in treating chemotherapy-resistant animal tumors, and shows greater activity against advanced solid tumors than against either leukemias or small tumors. Necrosis occurs within as little as four hours of administration (Zwi et al., 1989; Armand et al., 1988). Unfortunately, FAA is not effective against human tumors, presumably due to differences in tumor immunogenicity.

Reducing Free Radical Damage and Inflammation

Inflammation is intimately involved with carcinogenesis. Flavonoids inhibit inflammation by a number of mechanisms, as discussed previously. One of these mechanisms is free radical scavenging. In-vitro testing demonstrates that many flavonoids are potent free radical scavengers. For example, condensed tannins from *Rheum palmatum (da huang)*, *Camellia sinensis* (green tea leaves), and persimmon have a free radical scavenging ability markedly greater than vitamin E (Uchida et al., 1988). OPCs have been shown to have an antioxidant potency up to 18 times greater than that of vitamin C, and 50 times greater than that of vitamin E. Flananol dimers were more potent than monomers or flavonoids

(Schwitters and Masquelier, 1993:28-35). Quercetin and catechins possess marked antioxidant activity, as exhibited by their ability to inhibit hydrogen peroxide-induced lipid peroxidation in red blood cells (Affany et al., 1987).

Numerous investigators have reported that oral or intravenous administration of green tea extract inhibits the development of animal neoplasms in a variety of tissues (tongue, lung, stomach, skin, etc.) by a variety of chemical inducers (PAH, N-nitrosamines, aflatoxin, aromatic amines, etc.) and promoters (TPA, etc.) (Katiyar et al., 1992, 1993a, 1993b, 1993c, 1994; Komori et al., 1993; Tanaka et al., 1993; Luo and Li, 1992; Heur et al., 1992; Agarwal et al., 1992; Fujita et al., 1989). These effects presumably are due to inhibition of free radical damage and inflammation. Established tumors may also be affected. Oral doses of GTE (500mg/kg) inhibited the proliferation of EA carcinoma by 32% in vivo. Intravenous administration inhibited EA carcinoma and HAC, and prolonged the survival of SA-bearing mice by 128% (Yan, 1992).

Similarly, topical application of quercetin and other flavonoids inhibits the development of chemically-induced skin cancer in mice (Cassady, 1990). Topical application of the flavonoids kaempferol, quercetin, and rutin to mice with DMBA-induced and TPA-promoted skin cancers significantly reduced the number of tumors per mouse and the number of mice with tumors (Yasukawa et al., 1988). Tannic acid, derived from a number of plants, also inhibited TPA-promoted skin cancers in mice. Tannic acids from sumac leaf were the most potent (Gali et al., 1993). Oral administration of quercetin (5 mg/kg) reduced tumor yields by 50% in mice with chemically-promoted tumors (Wattenberg and Leong, 1970).[11]

In addition to inhibiting carcinogenesis, free radical scavenging effects may also account for the reported ability of flavonoids to inhibit invasion. Superoxide radicals have been reported to potentiate the invasive capacity of rat ascites hepatoma cells in vitro (Shinkai et al., 1986). Oral administration of EGCG, a potent superoxide scavenger, inhibited invasion in vitro and metastasis in vivo (Taniguchi et al., 1992). In Taniguchi's study, EGCG was administered in drinking water (approximately 160 mg/kg per day) to mice injected with B16 melanoma and Lewis lung carcinoma cells. The number of lung tumors in each group decreased by 50% and 29% as compared to controls. Tumor volume also decreased. The authors suggest that the inhibition of invasion and metastasis may be due to a free radical scavenging effect.

---

[11] Although humans do not absorb orally administered quercetin (Gugler et al., 1975), rats absorb approximately 20% of the dose (Ueno et al., 1983). Quite likely, quercetin is also absorbed, to some extent, by mice.

14.4.5 Adverse Effects of Flavonoids

A number of flavonoids, such as quercetin, kaempferol, and galangin have shown some genotoxicity in Salmonella assays (MacGregor, 1988) and hamster cells (Hirono et al., 1981) in vitro. However, due to the artificial nature of these tests, many antioxidants, including vitamin C, have produced genotoxic effects under these conditions (reviewed by Leibovitz, 1994).

In-vivo testing generally has not confirmed a carcinogenic effect, but has instead indicated a possible anticarcinogenic effect (Fujiki et al., 1986). Numerous in-vivo studies have been conducted on the carcinogenicity of quercetin, and results suggest that the compound is not carcinogenic. In rats fed diets containing up to 5% quercetin for two years, no effects on survival were observed, although benign tumors of the kidneys did appear in some male rats (Dunnick and Hailey, 1992; Ito et al., 1989). Similar effects were seen in hamsters and rats on a 10% quercetin diet for up to two years (Morino et al., 1982; Hirono et al., 1981). However, quercetin enhanced the carcinogenic activity of 3-methylcholanthrene in mice (Ishikawa et al., 1985). In a review of a Japanese National Toxicology Program report concerning the long-term carcinogenic effect of quercetin in rats, Ito (1992) states "Therefore, although the data of [the program] do indicate possible carcinogenic activity, its risk potential for man on the basis of our present knowledge must be considered to be negligible." In fact, some studies have demonstrated an anticarcinogenic effect for quercetin. Oral administration of quercetin (2 to 5% of diet) inhibited the incidence and the number of palpable mammary cancers in rats injected with N-nitrosomethylurea (Verma et al., 1988).

Severe side effects have been associated with (+)-catechin (also known as cianidanol). These include acute intravascular hemolysis, acute renal failure, and thrombocytopenia (Beretz and Cazenave, 1988; Jaeger et al., 1988).

14.5 PROTEASE INHIBITORS

A number of natural protease inhibitors, such as those found in soy and other seeds, have been reported to prevent cancer. Seeds may contain protease inhibitors as a survival mechanism, since protease inhibitors prevent the seeds from being destroyed by proteolytic enzymes in the digestive tract of animals who consume them.

The Bowman-Birk protease inhibitor (BBI) derived from soybeans has been shown to inhibit or prevent experimentally induced cancers of the colon, oral cavity, lung, liver, and esophagus in animals. However, the ability of BBI to irreversibly suppress carcinogenesis may, in part, be due to unidentified factors that are not protease inhibitors (Messina and Barnes, 1991). BBI is nontoxic and does not appear to compromise cellular immune functions (Maki and Kennedy, 1992).

A concentrate of the Bowman-Birk inhibitor (BBIC) inhibits malignant transformation, probably through an inhibition of chymotrypsin activity (Kennedy et al., 1993). Trypsin inhibition may also be involved. The authors propose that this concentrate may be useful as an agent to prevent human cancer in several different organs. The dosage suggested would provide a level of protease inhibitors equivalent to that found in the high soybean diets of the Japanese. Although protease inhibitors may prevent conversion of malignant cells even in late stages in carcinogenesis, they have no effect on established neoplastic cells (Messina and Barnes, 1991). However, soybeans contain an agent other than BBI that is capable of inhibiting later stages of cancer. An autoclave-resistant factor in soy reduced the metastasis of lymphosarcoma in mice and prevented weight loss (Evans et al., 1992).

Soybeans may contain a number of anticarcinogenic or antitumor agents in addition to protease inhibitors. Some of these are discussed in the following sections. Epidemiological studies indicate that soybean consumption may be responsible for the decreased incidence of a number of cancers seen in Chinese and Japanese populations. For example, Japanese who consume miso soup daily have significantly reduced risk of cancers of all types, compared with those who consume miso less often.[12] Asian women who consume soy products regularly have lower rates of breast cancer than American women who do not consume soy (Messina and Barnes, 1991). Colon cancer incidence is reduced by 50% in those subjects who consume miso soup frequently (Billings et al., 1990). Animal studies also support an anticarcinogenic activity. A diet supplemented with miso reduced the incidence and delayed the appearance of DMBA-induced mammary adenocarcinomas in rats. However, miso supplementation did not result in a decreased growth rate of the cancers (Baggott et al., 1990).

14.6 ISOFLAVONES

Isoflavones are flavonoid compounds found in a variety of legumes, such as soy, and other plant sources. The volume of isoflavone research has exploded in the last four years, especially with respect to the isoflavone genistein.

[12] Miso is a paste made from fermented soybeans.

Genistein has several characteristics that make it very promising as an anticancer agent. For example, genistein:

- inhibits platelet aggregation
- induces apoptosis
- inhibits DNA topoisomerase II
- inhibits leukotriene production
- inhibits angiogenesis
- reduces the bioavailability of sex hormones
- induces differentiation in cancer cells

Many of these characteristics may be related to genistein's ability to inhibit protein tyrosine kinase (see Section 6.3).

In addition to the above, genistein is a natural component of the diet and is relatively nontoxic.[13] Genistein is found in soy, *Cytisus* and *Genista sp.* (broom), *Stellaria sp.* (chickweed), *Trifolium sp.* (clover), *Pueraria lobata* and *P. thunbergiana (ge gen), Sophora japonica (huai hua mi),* and *Sophora subprostrata (shan dou gen)* (Duke, 1994; Hsu et al., 1982:508).

Studies regarding the effects of isoflavones on tyrosine kinase inhibition and other anticancer mechanisms are discussed below. It should be noted that all of these studies have been conducted in vitro. The results of in-vivo studies are expected soon.

14.6.1 Inhibition of Platelet Aggregation

As discussed in Chapter 5, platelet aggregation may facilitate the process of metastasis. Tyrosine kinases are important signaling enzymes in inducing platelets to aggregate in response to soluble factors produced at sites of blood vessel injury. As an inhibitor of tyrosine kinase, genistein inhibits platelet aggregation. For example, genistein inhibited the aggregation of rabbit platelets stimulated by vasopressin (Akiba et al., 1993). The action was thought to be due to tyrosine kinase inhibition of vasopressin-induced phospholipase A_2 activity on the platelet cell membranes. Genistein completely blocked aggregation of human platelets stimulated by thrombin (Asahi et al., 1992; Furman et al., 1994).

Other mechanisms besides inhibition of tyrosine kinases may be involved in inhibiting platelet aggregation. Genistein inhibited the aggregation of human platelets in response to thromboxane analogs by antagonizing the thromboxane receptor rather than by inhibition of tyrosine kinases (McNicol, 1993; Nakashima et al., 1991).

14.6.2 Induction of Apoptosis and Inhibition of Mitosis

Numerous investigators have reported that genistein induces cell death, either through apoptosis or by inhibiting mitosis. Some investigators have reported that genistein inhibits mitosis by inhibiting topoisomerase II (see Section 9.1.3). Table 14.4 summarizes these studies. The study by Hirano and colleagues listed in Table 14.4 is remarkable due to the very low concentration of genistein (10 ng/ml) that was effective against human leukemia cells. This was similar to the IC50 (the dose that inhibits growth by 50%) for a variety of conventional cytotoxic drugs, such as methotrexate and vincristine (2 to 15 ng/ml). In this study 100% cell death occurred at approximately 10 µg/ml.

14.6.3 Inhibition of Leukotriene Production

Leukotriene production (and inflammation) are associated with the stimulation of tumor growth by tumor promoting agents. Inhibitors of leukotriene production may suppress the action of tumor promoting agents.

Genistein inhibited leukotriene production by leukemia and mastocytoma cells stimulated by growth factors in vitro. The inhibition appeared to be due to tyrosine kinase inhibition by genistein (Hagmann, 1994).

14.6.4 Inhibition of Angiogenesis

Isoflavones may inhibit angiogenesis. In one study, fractions of the urine of healthy subjects who consume a plant-based diet inhibited the proliferation of vascular endothelial cells and inhibited angiogenesis in vitro. The most potent fractions contained isoflavones, of which the most potent isoflavone was genistein. Endothelial cell proliferation in culture was inhibited by 50% at a concentration of 5 µM, and completely inhibited at 50 µM. Angiogenesis was inhibited by 50% at 150 µM. Genistein also inhibited the production of plasminogen activator and plasminogen activator inhibitor-1 in response to stimulation by basic fibroblast growth factor. The urine of subjects eating a western-type diet contained over 30 times less genistein (Fotsis et al., 1993).

---

[13] Dietary soy isoflavones are 85% degraded in the intestines. However, sufficient isoflavones may enter the plasma to exert some health effects. The isoflavone daidzein was more bioavailable than genistein (Xu et al., 1994).

TABLE 14.4. INDUCTION OF APOPTOSIS AND INHIBITION OF MITOSIS BY GENISTEIN IN VITRO

CELL LINE	EFFECT	REFERENCE
T-lymphocyte leukemia (Jurkat)	Induced apoptosis at 18 to 110 μM; inhibited tyrosine kinase activity at 111 μM.	Spinozzi et al., 1994
Rat lymphoma (Nb2)	Inhibited growth by 50% at 15 to 25 μM.	Buckley et al., 1993
Human gastric carcinoma (AGS)	Inhibited growth by 50% at 10 to 23 μM.	Piontek et al., 1993
Human gastric carcinoma	Dose-dependent inhibition of growth (28 to 89%) between 10 and 60 μM; 50% inhibition at 20 μM (after 4 days).	Matsukawa et al., 1993
Human myelogenous leukemia (HL-60)	At 110 μM induced apoptosis in cells stimulated with growth factors (IL-3 and GM-CSF). The action was primarily due to inhibition of tyrosine kinase activity, but genistein may also act as an inhibitor of topoisomerase II.	Bergamaschi et al., 1993
Rat ovarian granulosa	Completely blocked the ability of epidermal growth factor, transforming growth factor-alpha, and basic fibroblast growth factor to suppress apoptosis in cells.	Tilly et al., 1992
Ten human gastrointestinal cell lines	Genistein and the isoflavone biochanin A strongly inhibited some cell lines and moderately inhibited others. The compounds were cytostatic at low concentrations (approximately <37 and <74 μM respectively), and induced apoptosis at high concentrations (>74 and >150 μM respectively).	Yanagihara et al., 1993
Human myelogenous leukemia (HL-60) and human lymphocytic leukemia (MOLT-4)	Induced apoptosis in 50% of cells at 31 to 48 μM. Genistein did not induce apoptosis in normal human lymphocytes.	Traganos et al., 1992
Human prostate cancer (LNCaP and DU-145)	Inhibited growth by 50% at 16 to 100 μM.	Peterson and Barnes, 1993
Human neuroblastoma cells	50% growth inhibition at 5 to 10 μM.	Schweigerer et al., 1992
ER-positive and ER-negative human breast cancer cell lines	50% inhibition at 24 to 44 μM. The effects were not reduced by overexpression of the multidrug-resistance gene.	Peterson and Barnes, 1991
Human myelogenous leukemia (HL-60), human T lymphocytic leukemia (MOLT-4)	50% growth inhibition of HL-60 at 0.04 μM; 100% cell death at 37 μM; 50% growth inhibition of MOLT-4 at 11 μM; nontoxic to normal lymphocytes.	Hirano et al., 1994

14.6.5 Reduction of Sex Hormone Bioavailability

High levels of urinary lignans and isoflavones, particularly genistein, are associated with a low incidence of breast and prostate cancers—two cancers that can be responsive to sex hormones. In vitro, genistein increased the production of sex hormone-binding globulin (SHBG) by human hepatocarcinoma cells, and also suppressed the proliferation of these cells (Mousavi et al., 1993). Sex hormones are tightly bound by SHBG and are rendered unavailable to stimulate the growth of hormone responsive cancers.

In a study on 30 postmenopausal women, higher levels of plasma SHBG were found in women with high urinary excretion of estrogen, lignans, and isoflavones. The authors suggest that lignans and isoflavones may inhibit tumor growth by increasing SHBG and by competing with estradiol for estrogen binding sites (isoflavones exhibit weak estrogenic activity) (Adlercreutz et al., 1992).

Japanese men consuming high quantities of soy products exhibit a low mortality rate from prostatic cancer. Total isoflavone content in the plasma in 14 Japanese men were 7 to 110 times higher than in Finnish men who consumed a low-soy diet. Genistein was the most prominent isoflavone (Adlercreutz et al., 1993).

TABLE 14.5 EFFECTS OF ISOFLAVONES ON DIFFERENTIATION

ISOFLAVONE	EFFECT	REFERENCE
Genistein	Induced differentiation in five human melanoma cell lines.	Kiguchi et al., 1990
	Inhibited the growth of mouse leukemia cells, in part, by inducing cell differentiation.	Kanatani et al., 1993
	Induced differentiation in HL-60 and human erythroid K-562 clones. DNA damage was an early event, occurring after 1 hour of treatment with 110 to 740 μM.	Constantinou et al., 1990
	Kinase inhibitors suppressed the inhibition of differentiation in mouse neuron cells caused by the protease thrombin. (Thrombin is an inhibitor of neuron differentiation.)	Jalink and Moolenaar, 1992
	Induced differentiation in a human medulloblastoma and neuroblastoma cell lines, probably through inhibition of tyrosine kinases.	Matsumoto, 1991
	Induced differentiation in mouse embryonal carcinoma cells, probably by inhibiting topoisomerases.	Kondo et al., 1991
Daidzein	In a study of more than 1,000 synthetic and natural compounds thought to induce differentiation, the isoflavone daidzein was highly potent in inducing differentiation in human leukemia HL-60 cells. Differentiation was induced at approximately 40 μM.	Jing et al., 1993
	Induced differentiation in HL-60 cells.	Han, 1994
	Induced differentiation in B16 melanoma cells at a concentration of approximately 40 to 150 μM.	Jing and Han, 1992

14.6.6 Induction of Differentiation

Studies of the effects of the isoflavones genistein and daidzein on differentiation are summarized in Table 14.5.

14.7 LIGNANS

Lignans are alcohols that derive from the same biosynthetic pathway as lignins and, indeed, may be intermediates in the biosynthesis of lignins. Lignins are a group of polysaccharides that combine with cellulose to form the cell walls of plants. A number of lignans exhibit cytotoxic or antiviral activity. For example, podophyllotoxin is a cytotoxic lignan occurring in the *Podophyllum* species. Lignans are primarily found in the woody tissues of plants.

The two major mammalian lignans, enterodiol and enterolactone, are produced by the actions of colonic bacteria on plant lignan and other dietary precursors. These mammalian lignans are structurally similar to estrogens, and produce weak estrogenic and antiestrogenic activities. Their production in the gut may serve to protect against breast cancer in humans, presumably by competing with estrogen for estrogen binding sites (Serraino and Thompson, 1992). Due to their limited estrogenic activity, those lignans that do successfully bind produce a lower estrogenic response than would estrogen.

Flax seed *(Linum usitatissimum)* is an abundant source of dietary plant lignans, 100 to 800 times greater than 67 other common plant foods. Flax seed has demonstrated anticarcinogenic effects in animal studies. In one study, mice bearing DMBA-induced mammary tumors were fed a high-fat diet (including 20% corn oil). The addition of flax seed (5% of diet) during the 21-week promotional stage reduced tumor sizes by 67% (Serraino and Thompson, 1992). However, the antitumor mechanisms involved may be complex, since the number of tumors per mouse was greater in the group fed a high-fat, high-flax diet as compared to mice fed a high-fat diet. The lowest number of tumors per animal were observed in mice fed a normal-fat, high-flax diet. Flax seed contains omega-3 fatty acids, which may also inhibit cancer growth and metastasis.

The seed of *Arctium lappa (niu bang zi)* contains a number of lignans, including arctigenin. Methanol extracts of the seed induced differentiation of mouse myeloid leukemia (M1) cells (Umehara et al., 1993). Arctigenin has also demonstrated potent cytotoxic effects against HL-60 human lymphocytic leukemia. The IC50 was 0.067 μg/ml, a concentration nearly as low as the IC50 values of a variety of conventional cytotoxic drugs such as methotrexate and vincristine. In addition, arctigenin was found to be nontoxic to normal lymphocytes. Arctigenin was relatively less potent at inhibiting the growth of MOLT-4 human T lymphocytic leukemia cells, and exhibited an IC50 of 0.53 μg/ml (Hirano et al.,

BOX 14.1. ESSIAC AND HOXSEY FORMULAS

Two herbal mixtures reported in the lay press to possess anticancer properties are the Hoxsey and Essiac formulas. The Hoxsey formula was promoted by Harry Hoxsey (1901-1974), and the Essiac formula was promoted by Rene Caisse (1888-1978), a Canadian nurse (reviewed by Walters, 1993:95-119). Both formulas continue to be prescribed to this day by certain practitioners of complementary medicine. The formulas are also commonly self-prescribed by cancer patients.

The Hoxsey formula was developed by Harry Hoxsey's great grandfather when he observed a cancer-bearing horse apparently cure itself by feeding on certain plants. By 1950, Harry Hoxsey had established one of the world's largest private cancer clinics (in Dallas, Texas), where he used the formula extensively. Although a number of physicians testified in various courts on behalf of Hoxsey, the FDA labeled the treatment as ineffective and, under pressure, Hoxsey closed his Dallas clinic in 1960.

The Hoxsey formula may contain *Trifolium pratense* (red clover), *Arctium lappa* (burdock root), *Glycyrrhiza glabra* (licorice), *Mahonia repens* (Oregon grape root), *Rhamnus purshiana* (cascara sagrada), *Rhamnus frangula* (buckthorn), *Phytolacca decandra* (poke root), *Xanthoxylum americanum* (prickly ash), *Baptisia tinctoria* (wild indigo), and potassium iodide. These herbs contain the potentially active compounds genistein, berberine, emodin, and possibly arctigenin (it is not clear if arctigenin occurs in burdock root).

The Essiac formula was based upon a formula passed down to Rene Caisse by a woman who had supposedly used it to cure herself of breast cancer. The woman had learned of the formula from an Ontario Indian healer. Caisse refined the original formula and developed oral and injectable components. Caisse treated thousands of patients, some of whom reported cures or remissions. The former physician to President John F. Kennedy, Dr. Charles Brusch, testified that he had cured himself of colon cancer using only the Essiac formula. In 1939, the Ontario parliament came within three votes of legalizing the formula for use by doctors. Over 55,000 people signed a petition supporting the bill. Despite her popularity, Caisse practiced under constant harassment by the Canadian authorities. In part, this was due to her unwillingness to divulge the ingredients of the formula.

Although the exact composition of the formula was only known by Caisse, the principle herbs are believed to be *Arctium lappa* (burdock root), *Rheum sp.* (Indian rhubarb), *Rumex acetosella* (sheep's sorrel), and *Ulmus fulva* (slippery elm bark). These herbs contain the potentially active compounds rhein, emodin, high molecular weight polysaccharides, and possibly arctigenin.

As discussed in Chapter 17 and Appendix K, it may be possible to optimize the dose of the active ingredients to improve efficacy over that of the original formulas. Further study with more concentrated and well-defined extracts is warranted.

1994). Further information regarding the historic use of *Arctium sp.* in treating cancer is provided in Box 14.1.

bioavailability, inhibiting mitosis, inhibiting invasion, inhibiting angiogenesis, and inducing differentiation.

14.8 SUMMARY

Numerous non-nutrient dietary factors, such as those from the *Allium sp.* and cruciferous vegetables, may play key roles in preventing cancer. Since anticancer compounds may be widely distributed, it may be prudent for humans to maintain a diverse diet.

A number of non-nutrient dietary factors may also be useful in treating cancer. These include certain phytoestrogens, phytosterols, saponins, flavonoids, protease inhibitors, isoflavones, and lignans. Some of the more promising compounds include the phytoestrogen equol; the flavonoids quercetin, (+)-catechin, and epigallocatechin 3-gallate (EGCG); the isoflavone genistein; and lignans obtained from flax seed and *Arctium lappa*. These compounds may act by a variety of mechanisms to inhibit cancer growth, such as by reducing estrogen

15

OTHER NATURAL AGENTS

15.1 DMSO

Dimethyl sulfoxide (DMSO) was initially discovered by the Russian scientist Dr. Alexander Saytzeff in 1866 in a byproduct from the wood processing industry. Since the 1950s, DMSO has been used widely in the United States as an industrial solvent. It was not until the early 1960s that it began to be used medically. Although its major clinical use is in treating inflammation, DMSO has a number of other biologic activities (reviewed by De la Torre, 1983; reviewed by Walker, 1993):

- DMSO is a potent solvent that carries molecules of low molecular weight through intact membranes (including the blood-brain barrier).
- It stimulates various aspects of the immune system and increases interferon production.
- It is a potent scavenger of hydroxyl radicals.
- It is bacteriostatic and virostatic.
- It reduces the incidence of thrombus formation.
- It has a tranquilizing effect.
- It softens collagen due to its cross-linking effect and may be useful in treating scar tissue.
- It is a potent diuretic when given intravenously.
- It causes differentiation in a number of human cancer cell lines in vitro.

In spite of its many biological effects and its low toxicity, the use of DMSO is approved for only one medical condition by the U.S. FDA.[1] This condition is interstitial cystitis, a relatively rare type of bladder disease. However, it is used with some frequency for a variety of other health problems, both by prescription and by patient self-medication.

Although DMSO may affect the initiation and development of cancer in a variety of ways, only two are discussed here: its solvent activity and its ability to scavenge hydroxyl radicals. The effect of DMSO on differentiation was discussed in Chapter 2.

15.1.1 Solvent Activities

Effects on Membrane Permeability

A number of investigators have suggested that DMSO may carry chemotherapy drugs through cell membranes and, therefore, allow chemotherapy drugs to be used at lower, less toxic doses. Oral administration of a DMSO-cyclophosphamide mixture has been shown to double cyclophosphamide concentrations in the plasma, brain, and liver tissue in rats, and increase the drug's therapeutic action. However, a therapeutic effect was not seen in patients with brain tumors (Thuning et al., 1983). Intraperitoneal administration of a DMSO-mitoxantrone mixture to P388 leukemia-bearing mice increased survival by 46 to 61% compared to mice receiving only mitoxantrone (Pommier et al., 1992). Intravesical administration of a DMSO-doxorubicin mixture to rats bearing bladder tumors dramatically increased the concentration of doxorubicin in bladder and lymph tissues and reduced tumor weights as compared with controls receiving only doxorubicin (See and Xia, 1992).

Effects on Drug Solubility

DMSO can dissolve a number of compounds that are not soluble in water or in other common solvents and laboratories regularly use it for this purpose. The ability of DMSO to dissolve hematoxylin, a common biological

---

[1] One reason approval has not been granted for additional medical uses is that the unique smell of DMSO presents an obstacle to designing placebo-controlled studies. Without placebo-controlled studies, the FDA is reluctant to approve any drug for market.

dye, serendipitously led to the discovery of the reported anticancer effects of a DMSO-hematoxylin mixture.

Dr. Eli Jordan Tucker, a orthopedic surgeon from Texas, has used DMSO in combination with hematoxylin to treat patients with a variety of cancers (Tucker and Carrizo, 1968). Hematoxylin is a biological dye obtained from *Haematoxylon campechianum* that has been used for over a hundred years to stain animal cells. It has also been used in humans as an astringent for diarrhea.[2] It readily oxidizes to a red substance called hematein and appears to have an affinity for neoplastic tissue. Presumably, hematoxylin damages tumor cells by generating free radicals during its oxidation. However, it stands to reason that the radical scavenging effect of DMSO may attenuate this effect.

The DMSO-hematoxylin solution used by Dr. Tucker was prepared by mixing 25 grams of hematoxylin in 75 cc of DMSO. The dosage used was 1 cc of the hematoxylin solution given intravenously for each 75 pounds of body weight (or approximately 0.7 grams hematoxylin per person) (Tucker and Carrizo, 1968). The treatment was repeated approximately every 48 hours. Some patients also received the mixture topically. Febrile reactions were common during early treatment. The authors suggest that this may have been due to dissolution of the tumor mass. Alternatively, cytokine production or toxic reactions could have been involved. Of 37 preterminal patients who received the hematoxylin solution in combination with conventional treatment (i.e., surgery, radiation, 5-fluorouracil, etc.), 71% improved (the criteria used for judging improvement was not specified). In contrast, only 5% improved when conventional agents were used alone. Of those patients treated only with the hematoxylin solution, 38% improved—mostly on a symptomatic level.

Controlled studies are needed to better determine the effects of the DMSO-hematoxylin solution. Unfortunately, no studies have been published on the subject since Dr. Tucker's original work. In an unpublished study, Stanley Jacob, M.D. was not able to reproduce Dr. Tuckers work (Jacob, 1995, personal communication).[3] Some alternative cancer clinics continue to use the DMSO-hematoxylin solution (Walker, 1993; Sessions and Walker, 1985), although no studies on the results have been published.

15.1.2 Hydroxyl Scavenger Action

DMSO is a potent scavenger of the hydroxyl radical (OH·) and as such may improve the survival of cancer patients. In a five-year double-blind study, 228 patients with postsurgical gastric cancer received a 10% DMSO-water solution (500 mg orally, 4 times per day) (Salim, 1992b). In the group treated with DMSO, five-year patient survival was 33%, whereas survival was 11% in the control group. In addition, DMSO may have reduced cancer recurrence. Death due to recurrence was 67% in the group treated with DMSO and 89% in the control group. Since similar results were observed in a group of patients taking allopurinol, which is also a free radical scavenger, the authors suggest that free radicals mediate the aggressiveness of gastric cancer and that DMSO may increase survival by inhibiting free radical damage. A similar increase in survival was reported in a study of 198 patients with postsurgical colon cancer taking the same dose of DMSO (Salim, 1992a). Recall from Chapter 14 that EGCG (from green tea) also inhibited invasion, presumably due to free radical scavenging effects.

15.2 CARTILAGE

Cartilage is naturally resistant to both angiogenesis and cancer invasion. Human cartilage contains a number of collagenase inhibitors, such as tissue inhibitors of metalloproteinases (in particular TIMP-2).[4] TIMP-2 is currently in preclinical evaluation at the National Cancer Institute as a possible chemotherapeutic agent. Human TIMP compounds appear to prevent the invasion of cancer cells (Banda et al., 1992) and inhibit angiogenesis (Stetler-Stevenson, 1992). Cartilage obtained from numerous species may contain TIMP-like compounds and may exhibit anticancer activity. For example, angiogenesis is markedly inhibited in vitro by agents present in the cartilage of chicks (Pepper et al., 1991).

Cartilage products have a long history of use in China. Shark cartilage, in the form of shark fin soup, has long been considered a food delicacy. A number of materials that contain collagen, gelatin, or keratin are used in Chinese herbal medicine.[5] As a group, these materials exhibit anti-inflammatory, hemostatic, immunostimulating, and analgesic properties. Some may also possess anticancer properties and have been used in TCM to treat cancer patients. Examples include the scales of

---

[2] The dose used to treat diarrhea is approximately 0.6 to 2.0 grams.

[3] Dr. Jacob is Gerlinger professor of Surgery at Oregon Health Sciences University and one of the original medical investigators of DMSO.

[4] Human cartilage is composed of types II, IX, and X collagen (45 to 75%), hyaluronate (0.5 to 2%), proteoglycans such as chondroitin-4-sulfate, chondroitin-6-sulfate, and keratin sulfate (15 to 50%), and other minor constituents (Wilson et al., 1991:1861).

[5] Gelatin is a protein derived from collagen.

Manis pentadactyla (anteater, *chuan shan jia*), and the shell of *Chinemys reevesii* (turtle, *gui ban*).

Two types of cartilage products investigated as anticancer agents in the United States are bovine cartilage and shark cartilage. Each is discussed separately below.

15.2.1 Bovine Cartilage

Dr. John Prudden initiated cartilage research in the United States in 1958 when he began studying bovine cartilage to accelerate postsurgical wound healing (Prudden and Allen, 1965; Allen and Prudden, 1966; Alexander and Prudden, 1966; Wolarsky et al., 1966; Prudden and Wolarsky, 1967; Prudden and Wolarsky, 1969; Prudden et al., 1970). The product Prudden and colleagues investigated was bovine tracheal cartilage (BTC or Catrix), a nontoxic prescription drug.[6] The principal wound-healing constituent of BTC was reported to be N-acetyl glucosamine (Prudden, 1985). During his investigations, Dr. Prudden also reported positive results using BTC to treat acne, arthritis, ulcerative colitis, dermatitis, psoriasis, and other inflammatory diseases (Prudden and Balassa, 1974).

The use of BTC on human cancer patients began in 1972, after BTC was administered to a woman to treat ulcerative skin lesions secondary to breast cancer. The product not only healed her lesions but also appeared to inhibit her cancer. Treatment of other cancer patients followed. Prudden (1985) reported that 31 patients with various cancers received BTC (approximately 9 grams/day orally) over a several year period. Thirty-five percent of the patients showed disappearance of all clinical evidence of active tumors. An additional 26% exhibited tumor remission with a subsequent relapse, and an additional 20% exhibited a reduction in tumor size of 50% or more.

Since 1972, Dr. Prudden has used BTC to treat approximately 110 patients with advanced cancer. He has been treating some of these patients for up to 15 years. Dr. Prudden reports an overall partial and complete response rate of approximately 30% within a 7-month treatment period (Prudden, 1994, personal communication).

In addition to inhibiting tumor growth, stimulating wound healing, and inhibiting inflammation, BTC also stimulates the immune system. Prudden (1985) reported that administration of BTC to cancer patients resulted in enhanced lymphocyte proliferation ex vivo in response to mitogens. Similar immunostimulant effects were observed in mice (Rosen et al., 1988).

In support of Prudden's results, local administration of a calf cartilage extract prevented the growth of tumor-induced blood vessels in rabbit corneas. The extract also strongly inhibited protease activity, which is responsible for tumor invasion (Langer et al., 1976). Regional perfusion of calf cartilage extract inhibited the growth of both mouse melanoma and V2 carcinoma transplants in mice and rabbits (Langer et al., 1980). No toxic effects were observed. At concentrations achievable in vivo, BTC inhibited breast ovarian, pancreatic, colon, and testicular cancer, and sarcoma biopsy specimens ex vivo (Durie et al., 1985; Sadove and Keuttner, 1977). In human studies, nine patients with progressive, advanced malignancy were given BTC injections. One patient with metastatic renal cell carcinoma to the lungs showed a complete response. The disease progressed in the remaining eight patients. No toxicity was reported (Romano et al., 1985). Although this study reported a low response rate, the BTC dosages used were significantly lower than those recommended by Dr. Prudden.

A single macromolecule has been identified in bovine cartilage (cartilage-derived inhibitor or CDI) which inhibits angiogenesis in vivo as measured in the chick chorioallantoic assay (Moses et al., 1990). In-vitro studies by the same authors revealed that CDI inhibited proliferation and migration of capillary endothelial cells. CDI was also shown to be a collagenase inhibitor.

15.2.2 Shark Cartilage

Following an early suggestion by Dr. Prudden, shark cartilage has also been investigated as an anticancer drug. Due to their larger size, higher cartilage content, and higher grade cartilage, on a per animal basis, sharks may contain 1,000 times more antiangiogenesis factor than do calves (Lee and Langer, 1983).[7]

Researchers at MIT have reported that an extract of shark cartilage significantly inhibits blood vessel growth at ocular tumor sites in rabbit models. At the end of a 20-day experiment, the average maximum blood vessel length at the tumor site was 75% shorter in treated animals as compared to controls (Lee and Langer, 1983). In a similar study, researchers in Japan have reported that an extract of shark cartilage significantly inhibited blood vessel growth at tumor sites in rabbit models, and inhibited the growth of new blood vessels in chicken eggs (Oikawa et al., 1990a).

Shark cartilage has been tested for TIMP-2 activity at the National Cancer Institute. Although preliminary experiments suggest that there are TIMP-like inhibitors

---

[6] Bovine cartilage is now available in nonprescription form.

[7] This does not infer that, per gram, processed shark cartilage is more potent then processed calf cartilage. However, it does imply that sharks may offer a rich supply of antiangiogenesis factor.

in shark cartilage, TIMP-2 itself was not found. This result was as expected, since the bioassay used in the study is specific for detecting human TIMP-2 (Stetler-Stevenson, 1994, personal communication).[8]

Charles Simone, M.D., an oncologist, author, and past investigator at the National Cancer Institute, has treated approximately 100 cancer patients with shark cartilage since spring of 1993 (Simone, 1994, personal communication, Mathews, 1993). All of these patients had advanced (stage IV) cancers and were not receiving chemotherapy or radiotherapy. Dr. Simone reported that, on the average, 20 to 25% of these patients have exhibited a partial response. Commonly, an anti-inflammatory response is observed within 2 to 4 weeks, and the maximum response is observed within 16 weeks. Some tumors, such as prostate, breast, primary brain, and ovarian cancers, appear to have higher response rates. Dr. Simone reports an 80 to 90% response rate in 20 patients treated for prostate cancer. As with BTC, shark cartilage appears to be completely nontoxic.

Dr. Simone's patients ingest approximately 90 to 110 grams/day of cartilage (based on a 70-kilogram adult). Dosages below 90 grams/day may be less effective or ineffective. It should be noted that this is a very large dose of cartilage, much greater than the recommended dose printed on many cartilage products. Dr. Simone estimates that 10,000 to 15,000 people are purchasing shark cartilage in health food stores in the United States, and that 80% of these patients may be ingesting a dose inadequate to affect tumor growth. In addition, he reports that up to 80% of the cartilage on the market has been adulterated and may be ineffective. The carbohydrate content of whole, dry shark cartilage is about 6 to 8% and higher levels may represent the addition of sugar or other products.

Many investigators have questioned whether the large peptides contained in cartilage can pass through the stomach and small intestine without digestion, then further pass through the intestinal lining to enter the circulation. Gardner (1988, 1984) reviewed evidence that demonstrates large polypeptides do pass through the stomach and intestines undigested and that the terminal stages of protein digestion occur intracellularly in the mucosal absorptive cells of the intestinal lining. In addition, small amounts of intact proteins and peptides do enter the circulation under normal conditions. Peptide transport systems, as distinct from free amino acid transport, have been identified in the intestinal brush-border membranes.[9] However, the degree to which peptides are able to enter the circulation is thought to be limited.

Digestion of cartilage compounds may not destroy the active proteins. Stetler-Stevenson (1993, personal communication) reported that digestion of cartilage materials may alter, but not completely inhibit, TIMP activity, if present.

The recommended dosage for shark cartilage is considerably higher than that for BTC. Since cows are biologically more similar to humans than sharks, it is possible, and likely, that protease inhibitors in calf cartilage may have additional domains that facilitate binding to human metalloproteinases (Stetler-Stevenson, 1994, personal communication). This may explain why lower doses of BTC appear to be as effective as higher doses of shark cartilage. However, all of the human data is speculative at this point and must be confirmed.

15.3 DIGESTIVE ENZYMES

A number of investigators have suggested that digestive enzymes may be useful in treating cancer patients. Discussed below are the work or Dr. Nicholas Gonzalez, the multienzyme product Wobe-Mugos, and the single enzyme bromelain.

15.3.1 The Gonzalez Program

Based on early work by Beard (1911), Kelley (1972), and his protégé, Dr. Nicholas Gonzalez (Gonzalez, 1993, taped lecture), have suggested that digestive enzymes may be used as anticancer agents. The heart of the Gonzalez program consists of high doses of multiple proteolytic enzymes, although the program also includes patient-specific dietary modifications and vitamin and mineral supplementation. Gonzales has recently presented a series of case studies to the National Cancer Institute, who has encouraged him to pursue further study. With supervision from NCI, Gonzalez is currently conducting a clinical trial in New York on patients with pancreatic cancer.

In Kelley's program, patients receive a protease/amylase mixture orally, in incremental doses, until a noticeable effect is seen (Richards, 1988). Often this effect is severe, and can include flu-like symptoms, fever, perspiration, shivering, headache, and nausea. Inflammation commonly appears at known tumor sites and other locations. At this point treatment is suspended until the patient's condition stabilizes, and then treatment is resumed. Coffee enemas are advised to relieve severe reactions. Coffee enemas are reported to stimulate the

---

[8] William Stetler-Stevenson, M.D., Ph.D. is Chief of the Extracellular Matrix Pathology Section at NCI's Laboratory of Pathology.

[9] Intestinal permeability to macromolecules may be increase in a variety of diseases and by chemotherapy. Tests are now available by which gut permeability can be measured by quantifying the amount of a specific, orally-ingested macromolecule that has passed through the intestinal lining and entered the urine.

release of bile from the liver, thereby facilitating the transport of waste metabolites into the intestines for excretion (Gonzalez, 1993, taped lecture).[10]

Other doctors have used multienzyme formulas to treat cancer patients. For example, in the 1960s Frank Shively, M.D. treated more than 96 advanced or far advanced patients using a combination of chymotrypsin, trypsin, amylase, pepsinogen, and desoxyribonuclease. The enzymes were administered intravenously. More than 3,000 infusions were given to these patients. Case studies of some of these patients, and information on cautions and contraindications of the treatment, are available (Shively, 1969). According to Dr. Shively, many of these patients responded favorably to the enzyme treatment. In many cases, the tumors apparently became necrotic, detached from their surrounding tissue, and were easily removed by surgery. The most commonly treated tumors were carcinomas of the breast, gastrointestinal tract, and genitals.

15.3.2 Wobe-Mugos

Max Wolf, M.D. has treated over 1,000 cancer patients in Germany using a multiple-enzyme product named Wobe-Mugos or similar single or multienzyme products (Wolf and Ransberger, 1972:184-204). Wobe-Mugos contains approximately 40 mg chymotrypsin (40,000 USP), 40 mg trypsin (6,000 USP), 100 mg papainases (6X), and calf thymus extract.[11] Dr. Wolf began treating patients in about 1949 with a variety of enzyme formulations and Wobe-Mugos was used exclusively after 1959. Early treatment protocols used oral doses of 200 mg/day. This was increased over the years to 2 to 4 grams/day. Enzyme treatments were often combined with surgery, vitamins, heparin, or other agents. Where possible, treatment included intratumor injection or topical application of the enzymes. With colon cancer, retention enemas were employed. Although it is difficult to evaluate the success of this therapy based on the data provided (Wolf and Ransberger, 1972:184-204), the following conclusions are suggested:

1) Enzyme therapy was generally not curative, but appeared to inhibit metastasis and moderately prolong survival. For example, breast cancer was the most common cancer treated. Of 107 postmastectomy patients, the five-year observed survival rate was 84%. The authors report that observed survival rates for conventional therapy at the time

were 43 to 48%. The benefits gained with other types of cancers were less clear, although the authors assert that patients generally benefited to some degree.

2) Systemic treatment was less successful than localized treatment. Intratumor injections, topical salves, bladder infusions, or other localized treatments were employed.

3) Therapy must be continued long-term (or indefinitely) for best results in inhibiting metastasis.

Two points were made by the authors. First, higher doses provided better results; and second, mixed plant and animal enzymes provided better results than single enzymes.

The dose recommended by the manufacturer is 12 to 20 tablets/day. Although each capsule contains the same amount of enzymes as many other digestive aids, the large number of capsules provides a dose markedly greater than that normally prescribed for maldigestion. In addition, the capsules are enterically coated, which may result in greater enzyme uptake.

The product information supplied by the manufacturer (MUCOS Pharma GmbH & Co, undated) indicates that the product may act by one or more of three mechanisms:

1) It may directly cause tumor necrosis through enzymatic action.

2) It may inhibit metastasis through stimulation of fibrinolytic activity.

3) It may facilitate an immune response. The product reportedly alters the protein configuration on the plasma membrane of tumor cells and digests the fibrin coating that surrounds tumors, either of which may expose tumor antigens to the immune system.

According to the manufacturer's literature (MUCOS Pharma GmbH & Co, undated), Wobe-Mugos appears to be somewhat effective in treating patients with pancreatic cancer. Over 30 patients with pancreatic cancer, treated solely with Wobe-Mugos and vitamin A, were still alive after 2 years. A number of these patients have survived at least five to nine years. Historically, the expected mean survival for patients with pancreatic cancer is seven months. If Wobe-Mugos is particularly effective in treating pancreatic cancer, it may be related to the enteropancreatic recycling of proteolytic digestive enzymes (Beynon and Kay, 1976; Gotze and Rothman, 1975; Leibow and Rothman, 1975). This system is thought to

---

[10] A number of herbal agents, such as *Artemisia capillaris (yin chen hao),* also dilate the bile duct and promote the excretion of bile (Zhou, 1985).

[11] The product that Wolf and Ransberger used prior to 1972 may not have been as concentrated as the current product. It contained 100 mg pancreatin, 40 mg bromelain, 60 mg papain, 10 mg lipase, 10 mg amylase, 24 mg trypsin, 1 mg alpha-chymotrypsin, and 50 mg rutin. The concentration of the pancreatin was not given, but it would need to have been 18X USP to be equivalent to the current strength.

spare digestive enzymes and, theoretically, may result in elevated pancreatic tissue concentrations after oral dosing.

Again, according to the manufacturer, Wobe-Mugos has shown some effectiveness in treating patients with breast cancer. Five-year survival rates for stage I and III postsurgical breast cancer patients who received Wobe-Mugos were 91% and 58% respectively, as compared to 78% and 42% for controls. Further studies are needed to verify these results.

Independent investigators have reported immune-enhancing effects. Administration of Wobenzyme, a similar multienzyme product, to healthy volunteers increased the secretion of interleukin-1-beta, interleukin-6, and tumor necrosis factor-alpha by peripheral blood mononuclear cells ex vivo (Desser et al., 1993). The increase in IL-1 may explain, in part, the fever and other symptoms that patients have exhibited after taking high doses of the enzymes.

15.3.3 Bromelain

Bromelain, a cysteine proteolytic enzyme derived from pineapple, has been used to treat various inflammatory diseases and maldigestion (reviewed by Murray, 1992:181-7). It consists of five closely related proteolytic enzymes and is capable of digesting collagen, globulins, and muscle fiber. Its main component is a glycoprotein proteolytic enzyme, but it also contains acid phosphatase, a peroxidase, several proteolytic inhibitors, and organically bound calcium (Taussig, 1980). Upon oral administration, a substantial percentage of bromelain appears to be absorbed into the blood. Up to 40% is absorbed unchanged in animal models (Lotz-Winter, 1990). However, bromelain's proteolytic activity is inhibited by serum factors (Leung, 1980:74-6).

Some authors suggest that the active ingredient in bromelain may not be the proteolytic enzyme, but a minor enzymatic component that is responsible for the release of an unidentified PGE_1-like compound (Felton, 1977). In fact, many of the in-vitro and in-vivo biologic activities of bromelain resemble those of PGE_1, such as the following:

- Stimulation of intestinal muscle contractions
- Smooth muscle relaxation
- Inhibition of platelet aggregation
- Enhanced antibiotic absorption and increased capillary permeability
- Increased cAMP levels
- Anti-inflammatory activities

- Antiulcer activities and appetite inhibition. Appetite inhibition and starvation are the major causes of death in animals fed high doses of bromelain. Rats fed 2 grams/kg per day essentially stopped eating and starved.
- Shortening of labor

Unrelated to PGE_1, bromelain acts similar to the protease plasmin and, like plasmin, has a high affinity for fibrin (Lotz-Winter, 1990). It increases the proteolytic and fibrinolytic activity of the blood in rats (Taussig and Batkin, 1988). The production of plasmin may be responsible for a number of the biologic activities discussed above, such as inhibition of platelet aggregation.

Bromelain in Cancer Treatment

A number of investigators have suggested that bromelain may be useful in treating cancer patients. Gerard (1972) was the first to use oral bromelain as an anticancer agent. In 12 patients with various tumors who were administered 600 mg bromelain daily, resolution of masses were reported in patients with ovarian carcinoma and breast cancer. Nieper (1976) experimented with high doses of bromelain in combination with standard chemotherapy and also reported some success. These physicians have suggested that the optimum dose of bromelain may be 1.0 to 2.4 grams daily.

Bromelain may produce anticancer effects through a number of mechanisms, including kinin degradation, fibrinolysis, globulin degradation, inhibition of platelet aggregation, induction of differentiation, peroxidase action, immune stimulation, and modification of cell surface proteins. Each of these are discussed briefly below.

Kinin Degradation

The anti-inflammatory effects of bromelain are due, in part, to its ability to deplete plasma kininogen, the precursor of inflammatory kinins, and prekallikrein, the precursor to the enzyme that activates kininogens (Kumakura et al., 1988; Fujiyoshi et al., 1989; Uchida and Katori, 1986).[12] Recall from Chapter 3 that the kinins bradykinin and substance P induce angiogenesis. Degrading kininogen limits kinin production. In addition, proteolytic degradation of kininogens produces some fragments that are powerful inhibitors of cysteine proteases such as papain, and human cathepsin (Vogel et al., 1988; Karlsrud et al., 1991). As protease inhibitors, these fragments may inhibit tumor invasion.

---

[12] Bromelain may also reduce inflammation by interfering with arachidonic acid metabolism.

Fibrinolysis

As a fibrinolytic agent, bromelain may degrade the fibrin gel that surrounds solid tumors, thereby depriving tumors of their structural stroma and unmasking blocked tumor surface antigens, which may expose the antigens to increased immune recognition.

Globulin Degradation

As a proteolytic enzyme that degrades globulins (including antibodies), bromelain may lyse tumor antigen-antibody complexes that block immune response (Maurer et al., 1988). In addition, bromelain has shown some effectiveness in degrading paraproteins (abnormal plasma proteins) and reducing hyperviscosity symptoms in patients with hematological neoplasms (Sakalova et al., 1992).

Inhibition of Platelet Aggregation

Platelet aggregation appears to facilitate metastasis, and bromelain inhibits platelet aggregation in vitro and in vivo (Taussig and Batkin, 1988; Felton, 1980).

Induction of Differentiation

Proteases may stimulate tumor cell differentiation and, paradoxically, may also stimulate cell proliferation in some cell lines. Bromelain induced differentiation in one animal and two human leukemic cell lines in vitro. In human leukemia K562 cells, bromelain caused a parallel dose-response increase in both cell proliferation and cell differentiation. Cell growth in human HL-60 and a mouse leukemia cell line was inhibited in a dose-dependent fashion. Heat treatment of bromelain, which destroys the proteolytic activity, reduced its ability to cause cell differentiation (Maurer et al., 1988). Trypsin and chymotrypsin also induce differentiation in human leukemia cell lines in vivo and ex vivo. Papain, plasmin, and other proteases have no effect (Fibach et al., 1985). In contrast to the above, mild concentrations of proteases, including bromelain, accelerated the growth of Ehrlich ascites tumor cells in vitro (Adamietz et al., 1989). The stimulation of growth was reversible and lasted for approximately two days.

Peroxidase Action

The peroxidase component of bromelain strongly inhibits the growth of Lewis lung carcinoma, YC-8 lymphoma, and MCA-1 ascitic cells in vitro in a dose-dependent fashion (Taussig et al., 1985). Growth inhibition was observed, even after heating bromelain past 70 °C. Temperatures above 70 °C (and less than 100 °C)

inactivate its proteolytic activity and its ability to inhibit platelet aggregation, but not its peroxidase activity. Heating past 100 °C eliminated its growth-inhibiting effects. In another study, bromelain decreased lung metastasis by 90% in mice implanted with Lewis lung cells (Batkin et al., 1988). Again, the effects were observed even when the protease component was inactivated by heat. However, in this study, the peroxidase component by itself was not able to inhibit cell growth in vitro, and previous studies by the authors indicated that in-vitro activity was necessary for in-vivo antimetastatic activity. Therefore, the authors suggest that components other than proteases or peroxidases may be responsible for the antimetastatic effects.

Immune Stimulation

Wobenzyme, as well as bromelain and papain, at 40 μg/ml stimulated the production of tumor necrosis factor-alpha in human peripheral blood mononuclear cells cultures. The activities of bromelain and Wobenzyme were similar at 16 hours of incubation, although bromelain was far more potent at every other time period from 4 to 24 hours. Papain was the least effective (Desser and Rehberger, 1990).

Modification of Cell Surface Proteins

The manufactures of Wobe-Mugos have applied for an international patent for the use of bromelain to reduce the metastatic potential of cancer cells by altering surface glycoproteins responsible for metastasis. The effect is enhanced by the addition of papain, trypsin, amylase, chymotrypsin, and pancreatin (Ransberger, abstract undated).

Bromelain and Tumor Invasion

Both proteolytic enzymes and their inhibitors have been proposed as anti-invasion drugs. Earlier, it was mentioned that bromelain may inhibit tumor invasion by degrading kininogens, thereby producing protease inhibitors. On the other hand, bromelain also stimulates the production of the proteolytic enzyme plasmin, an enzyme involved in tumor invasion. By stimulating plasmin, does bromelain stimulate invasion? It probably does not. It is likely that a number of proteolytic enzymes, including metalloproteinases and cathepsins, must act in concert with plasmin to degrade the basement membrane (Tannock and Hill, 1992:183; Thorgeirsson et al., 1985). This opinion is reinforced by William Stetler-Stevenson, M.D., Ph.D., an expert on matrix degradation and tumor invasion. He states that since invasion depends on a cascade of substrate-specific proteases, the use of oral digestive enzymes probably would not enhance invasion. However, he also states that invasion may possibly be enhanced in nonspecific ways, such as through damage to the endothelial lining of blood vessels (Stetler-Stevenson, 1994, personal communication). Damage of the endothelial lining may facilitate the attachment of migrating tumor cells.

15.4 UREA

The use of oral urea in the treatment of liver and skin cancers was first investigated by the Greek physicians Evangelos Danopoulos and Iphigenia Danopoulou (1974a,, 1974b, 1975, 1979, 1983). Urea apparently destabilizes the fibrin stroma of solid tumors, and, as discussed in Section 3.4, inhibits angiogenesis.[13] Urea inhibits HeLa cells in vitro, by undefined mechanisms (reviewed by Danopoulos et al., 1982).

Complete responses were reported in 15 of 22 patients with hepatic metastasis from primary adenocarcinomas (Danopoulos and Danopoulou, 1981). The dose was 12 to 15 grams/day divided into 6 portions. Treatment was well tolerated. Patients were eligible for study if metastatic disease was confined to the liver, but did not exceed one-third of the liver parenchyma; estimated survival was at least 6 weeks; the patients did not have ascites; and bilirubin counts were below 75 mg/dl.

The therapy was also administered locally, in combination with curettage, to 28 patients with extensive lip cancer. The response rate was 100%. Recurrences occurred in four patients, three of which responded to further treatment (Danopoulos et al., 1982).

The authors suggest that this therapy will not be effective against cancers other than liver (unless applied locally) since urea is rapidly excreted by the kidneys and the liver is the only organ that exhibits high concentrations after oral administration.

Other investigators have attempted to replicate these results without success. Using the same inclusion criteria and similar doses of urea, no response was seen in 15 patients with liver metastasis from colorectal adenocarcinoma (Levin et al., 1987). No response was seen in 10 patients with liver metastasis from colorectal carcinoma (Hooper et al., 1984). No response was seen in 20 patients with secondary liver tumors, predominantly from colorectal primary cancers (Clark et al., 1988). In this study urea was administered four times daily instead of six—a criticism made by Danopoulos and Danopoulou (1981) of earlier negative studies. Based upon these negative studies, urea does not appear to be effective against liver metastasis from colorectal cancers. Further clinical studies are warranted if improvements in protocol or application are developed, or if further in vitro or animal studies suggest a positive effect.

15.5 SUMMARY

Four dietary supplements that have a reported effect on cancer are DMSO, bovine or shark cartilage, bromelain and multienzyme formulas, and urea. DMSO may be useful as a free radical scavenger and as a solvent to carry other anticancer agents into tumor cells. Bovine and shark cartilage may be useful as antiangiogenic agents in treating solid tumors, as immune stimulants, or as collagenase inhibitors. Bromelain and other proteases may inhibit cancer growth through a number of mechanisms, including immune stimulation, globulin degradation, inhibition of inflammation, and inhibition of platelet aggregation. Urea may adversely affect the fibrin matrix of tumors and inhibit angiogenesis.

---

[13] The inhibitory effects of urea and glutathione on liver tumors may be due, in part, to similar antiangeogenic, free radical scavenging mechanisms. See sections 3.4 and 12.4.5.

16

PHYSICAL AND PSYCHOLOGICAL THERAPIES

The previous chapters have discussed natural agents that have potential anticancer activity that are administered by oral or intravenous routes. Other treatment modalities may also benefit the chancer patient. This chapter discusses two of these: physical and psychological therapies.

16.1 PHYSICAL THERAPIES

16.1.1 Acupuncture

Acupuncture is the insertion of fine needles into the skin at specific locations to affect the flow of *qi* in the *channels.* Although not soley a physical therapy, acupuncture is discussed under this heading as a matter of convienience. Acupuncture is used in many countries to treat a wide variety of disease patterns, especially superficial disease patterns that involve the *channels* (such as musculoskeletal disorders). In China, herbs are used much more frequently than acupuncture in treating cancer patients. In fact, there is a paucity of international studies on the use of acupuncture in cancer treatment. However, acupuncture may still be useful in treating cancer patients, especially for secondary, superficial symptoms and for inducing relaxation. Acupuncture may also be useful in normalizing immune indices in patients with mild myleosuppression. Studies conducted on acupuncture in cancer treatment are summarized below.

In a study on 376 medium- and advanced-stage cancer patients with chemotherapy-induced leukocytopenia, acupuncture and moxibustion (a type of local heat therapy) raised the leukocyte count in 38% of the patients. Patients with higher starting levels of leukocytes exhibited a greater response than did patients with lower starting levels. The authors suggest that acupuncture and moxibustion influence leukocyte counts only to the extent that the bone marrow is intact and functioning (Chen and Huang, 1991).

In a study on 122 patients with late-onset edema due to radiotherapy, acupuncture effectively relieved edema and reduced pain. Best results were achieved in patients with low-grade edema (Bardychev et al., 1988). In a study on 36 breast cancer patients with radiation-induced edema, acupuncture and laser acupuncture, in combination with routine drug therapy, massage, and application of DMSO, reduced edema by 22 to 37%. Treatment normalized immunological indices, especially lymphocyte counts (Kuzmina and Degtiareva, 1987a, 1987b).

In a study of 130 patients with chemotherapy-induced nausea and vomiting, electroacupuncture (on the point Pericardium 6 *(nei guan)*) resulted in improvement in approximately 96% of the patients. A limited cross-over study using a sham acupuncture point demonstrated that the effects were specific to Pericardium 6. However, relief lasted only about eight hours, and each treatment required a significant amount of staff time. Therefore, the authors recommend an alternative approach before it is adopted clinically (Dundee et al., 1989).

16.1.2 Electrotherapy

Numerous investigators have reported that locally applied direct current destroys a variety of human and animal tumors in vitro and in vivo. Highly reproducible destruction of subcutaneous mouse mammary tumors has been observed in vivo (Griffin et al., 1994). Destruction was greater when the tumor electrode was anodic rather than cathodic, and destruction increased with increasing charge. An anodic charge greater than 10.6 coulombs resulted in 100% mortality of the mice within 72 hours, while lower charges did not influence mortality. Mortality was associated with serum electrolyte imbalanccs and appeared to be due to an excessive metabolic load of tumor breakdown products. The authors state that this lysis syndrome should not present a problem in the treatment of humans, where the ratio of tumor mass to total body mass is normally much smaller.

Many other investigations have been conducted. Percutaneous electrical treatment (20 mA for 15 minutes) of mice with Lewis lung carcinoma resulted in smaller tumors at death and longer survival times than controls or mice treated with sham electrical therapy. The treatment reduced local tumor mass, but did not affect the degree of metastasis (Morris et al., 1992). Treatment of nude mice bearing subcutaneous human colon cancer with varying percutaneous electrical charges resulted in varying inhibition rates. Direct currents of 7.5 volts and 35 coulombs/cm^3 of tumor provided the greatest antitumor response (Heiberg et al., 1991). In a case study, one woman with breast cancer was treated with apparent success by two hours of percutaneous electrotherapy (Azavedo et al., 1991)

Researchers in China have also investigated electrotherapy. Results indicate that, in addition to superficial cancers, such as skin, thyroid, breast, and mouth cancers, electrotherapy can also treat deeper cancers such as liver, adrenal, lung, and cervical cancers. Of 216 patients with malignant tumors, the overall response rate was 78%. Very advanced lesions and patients with generalized metastasis responded poorly (Xin, 1992). In 211 patients with middle- and late-stage lung cancer, electrical treatment, combined with herbal medicine, resulted in a short-term response rate of 85% (based upon international standards). The response rate for electricity or herbs alone was 69% and 53% respectively. Four-year survival rates were 54% for the combined treatment, 46% for the group receiving electricity, and 40% for the group receiving herbs. The amount of electricity applied was approximately 100 coulombs/cm^3 of tumor. Needles were inserted into the tumors to act as electrodes (Xin, 1993).

Electrical currents may retard tumor growth by normalizing cell proliferation rates (Vodovnik et al., 1992). Nondividing cells (such as mature neurons) exhibit a high transmembrane potential (TMP). The TMP is the difference in electrical charge between the inside and outside of the plasma membrane. In contrast, cells with a high proliferation rate, such as some cancer cells, tend to have a low TMP. When exposed to direct current, one side of the cell becomes hyperpolarized, while the other becomes depolarized. In nondividing cells, direct current lowers the TMP, whereas the opposite is true in cells with a high division rate. The authors speculate that direct current may normalize tumor cell proliferation rates by normalizing the TMP.

A variation of electrotherapy under investigation is a combination of chemotherapy and electrotherapy, called electrical impulse chemotherapy (EIC) or electrochemotherapy (ECT). Electrochemotherapy markedly increases the uptake of a variety of drugs by tumor cells both in vitro and in vivo.[1] This effect may be due to an increase in membrane fluidity (and drug transport) secondary to an increase in transmembrane potential. In patients with squamous cell carcinomas of the head and neck, the use

of ECT resulted in partial responses and complete cures without any damaging side effects. The combination of ECT and interleukin-2 injections provided a maximum response, and the authors suggested that electrical treatment initiates an aggressive antitumor immune response (Dev and Hofmann, 1994; Belehradek et al., 1993). (Note that in Xin's study mentioned above, a maximum response was observed with a combination of electrotherapy and herbs. Quite likely the herbs included immunostimulants.) In further support of an immune effect, electrotherapy, in combination with interleukin-2, resulted in higher tumor inhibition in two mouse models than that observed for either treatment alone (Sersa et al., 1992; Mir et al., 1992).

Eighteen additional papers on electrotherapy and electrochemotherapy can be found in the *European Journal of Surgery* 1994, issue 574.

16.2 PSYCHOLOGICAL THERAPIES

It is becoming increasingly apparent to medical professionals that the mind and the body are interconnected and affect one another. Recent studies suggest that emotions may alter immune function and that repression of emotions may adversely affect cancer survival rates. Some investigators suggest that meditation and similar Eastern spiritual practices may benefit the immune system and increase cancer survival rates. Pertinent aspects of Western psychology and Eastern psychology are discussed below.

16.2.1 Western Psychology

As discussed elsewhere in this book, the immune and endocrine systems may have a significant impact on carcinogenesis and tumor growth. Each of these systems may be heavily influenced by stress or other emotional states. The study of the effects of the emotions on the nervous, immune, and endocrine systems is called psychoneuroimmunology or psychoneuroendocrinology.

The Effects of the Endocrine System on Immune Function

The reaction of the endocrine system to stress is complex and poorly understood. The hypothalamus appears to play a central role, as emotions can affect the release of hypothalamus-pituitary hormones such as adrenal corticotropic hormone (ACTH), thyroid-stimulating

---

[1] In experiments on rats injected with bleomycin, the experimental voltages were high, ranging from 0 to 5 kv (Okino et al., 1992). However, significant tumor inhibition can also be produced at low voltages. Tumor inhibition was observed with a single treatment (0.6 mA DC for 60 minutes) in mice bearing fibrosarcoma. Electrotherapy in combination with bleomycin further improved responses (Sersa et al., 1993).

hormone (TSH), gonadotrophins, prolactin, and growth hormone (GH). In turn, these hormones can affect the production of estrogens, androgens, glucocorticoids, and other hormones and hormone-like substances. Hormone interactions are very complicated, and altering any one hormone can affect the production of many others.

It has been known for many years that certain endogenous hormones, such as glucocorticoids (e.g., cortisol), suppress immune responses and are necessary to check the progression of inflammation or otherwise prevent excessive immune reactions. More recently, researchers have discovered that other hormones affect immune function. Neuroendocrine processes that affect the immune system may include the following (reviewed by O'Leary, 1990):

- Some catecholamines mobilize lymphocytes while reducing their functional activity.[2]
- Norepinephrine stimulates NK cell activity.
- Sympathetic innervation of lymphoid organs has been reported in the mouse.[3]
- Opioids suppress lymphocyte response to mitogens, enhance NK cell activity, and enhance monocyte migration.[4]
- Receptors for most hormones and neurotransmitters have been found on the surfaces of lymphocytes.
- Growth hormone and prolactin stimulate macrophage function (Plotnikoff, 1991).

It has now become apparent that not only does the endocrine system affect the immune system, but that the opposite is also true: the immune system affects the endocrine system. Evidence supporting a bidirectional communication between the immune and endocrine systems includes the following (reviewed by Plotnikoff et al., 1991):

- Lymphocytes and macrophages synthesize and appear to secrete several pituitary hormones.
- Lymphoid and myeloid cells secrete hormone-like molecules that act locally (cytokines), and act at distant sites, such as the brain, to affect the neuroendocrine system.
- Some cytokines affect hormonal response. For example, interleukin-2 has been shown to increase ACTH levels (Bovbjerg, 1991).

The Effects of Stress on Endocrine Function

Various stressors such as noise, light, movement, and electric shock can alter immune response in animals,

either positively or negatively (Vessey, 1964; Solomon, 1969; Monjan and Collector, 1977). Stress-induced alteration in immune function may occur via the sympathetic-adrenal-medullary (SAM) system, the hypothalamus-pituitary-adrenocortical (HPAC) system, or other endocrine systems (reviewed by O'Leary, 1990). The SAM system is sometimes referred to as the "fight or flight" system, and the HPAC system as the "distress" or "conservation-withdrawal" system. SAM activation is associated with the release of epinephrine, norepinephrine, and other catecholamines, and HPAC activation is associated with the release of ATCH and corticosteroids. During a stressful event, SAM activation usually occurs first, followed later by HPAC activation if the stress continues. However, both systems are often active to some degree. The release of glucocorticoids appears to be responsible for most of the immunosuppressive effects of stress. The cardinal sign of chronic stress is thymus involution caused by an increase in glucocorticoids.

The Effect of Stress on Immune Function

Studies on acute stress have demonstrated variable effects on the immune system, possibly due to differences in activation of the HPAC and SAM systems. The few available studies on chronic stress indicate that prolonged stress (such as loneliness and social disruption) may result in prolonged immunosuppression. Repressive coping, a coping style that involves repression of threatening material, has been associated with decreased monocyte counts and reduced lymphocyte response to mitogens (reviewed by O'Leary, 1990). Chronic clinical depression or the death of a spouse have been associated with a prolonged suppression of T-lymphocyte function (Holmes and Masuda, 1974; Schleifer et al., 1983; Kronfol et al., 1983; O'Leary, 1990). Prolonged psychological stress can reduce T-lymphocyte and NK cell activity (reviewed by Plotnikoff, 1991:78).

Even the anticipation of a stressful event, such as chemotherapy treatment, may initiate immune suppression and other reactions. Preliminary studies provide evidence of anticipatory immune suppression, nausea, and vomiting prior to repeat chemotherapy treatment in patients with ovarian cancer (Bovbjerg et al., 1990). Similarly, reductions in monocyte and NK cell activity have been reported in high-anxiety breast cancer patients immediately prior to repeat chemotherapy treatments (Fredrikson et al., 1993).

---

[2] Catecholamines (epinephrine and norepinephrine) affect metabolic rate, muscle contraction, and a host of other processes.

[3] The sympathetic division of the autonomic nervous system stimulates muscles and organs for physical action, whereas the parasympathetic division induces a rest-repose response.

[4] Opioids are endogenous morphine-like peptides that affect the nervous system. They are present in the brain, certain endocrine glands, and the gastrointestinal system. Endorphins are a type of opioid that decrease pain sensation.

TABLE 16.1. EFFECT OF EMOTIONAL STATES ON CANCER	
EFFECT	**REFERENCE**
Patients with melanoma who reported higher distress and a problem-solving orientation exhibited higher NK cell activity and lower nine-month relapse rates.	Rogentine et al., 1979
In a ten-year follow-up on breast cancer patients, those who were rated as being stoic or helpless exhibited lower survival rates then patients who were rated as having a fighting spirit.	Greer et al., 1979
Breast cancer patients who reported little psychiatric stress at the beginning of their treatment for recurrent disease, and who were rated as "well-adjusted," were more likely to die within one year as compared to patients who reported higher levels of psychiatric disturbance and who were rated as "disturbed."	Levy, 1985
In a seven-year follow-up of 36 patients with recurrent malignant disease, survival time was predicted by only one psychological factor: the level of joy at baseline testing.	Levy et al., 1988
In a study of 204 patients with advanced cancers of the breast, cervix, or lung, the longest survival times were found among patients who displayed "strong hostile drives without loss of emotional control."	Stavraky, 1968
Cancer patients who lived longer than expected tended to have less emotional stress and closer personal relationships, whereas those who lived shorter periods tended to display passivity and a stoic acceptance.	Weisman and Worden, 1975
Patients with melanoma who were defined as cooperative, unassertive, compliant, and had difficulty expressing anger exhibited increased tumor thickness and degree of invasion as compared to more assertive patients.	Temoshok, 1985
Poor prognosis in early-stage breast cancer was associated with low NK cell activity, and 51% of the NK cell activity variance could be accounted for by three factors: adjustment to illness, family support, and fatigue-depression.	Levy et al., 1985

On the other hand, social support may reduce stress and have a positive effect on the immune system. In a study of 23 spouses of cancer patients, those who reported higher levels of social support exhibited enhanced NK cell function as compared to those with lower levels of social support (Baron et al., 1990).

The Effects of Stress on Cancer

Stress may facilitate tumor growth by suppressing immune response and by increasing estrogen, androgen, or other hormone levels. In addition, stress may also reduce the level of some hormones that may prevent tumor growth. For example, melatonin can decrease the number of breast tumors in DMBA-treated rats and alter the growth of human breast cancer cells in vitro. Melatonin release may be dependent on sympathetic stimulation of the pineal gland by norepinephrine. In animal models, norepinephrine levels in the brain were depleted in response to helplessness in the face of stress (Seligman and Beagley, 1975). Studies at NCI have shown that breast cancer patients with estrogen receptor-positive tumors may have altered melatonin release curves. These patients exhibited decreased melatonin levels overall, and decreased amplitude of nighttime secretion (reviewed by Levy, 1985). Lastly, stress may facilitate carcinogenesis by adversely affecting DNA repair, a condition associated with increased cancer risk (Takabe et al., 1983; Kiecolt-Glaser et al., 1985).

The effects of acute stress may not always be destructive. Glucocorticoids inhibit the proliferation of leukemia and lymphoma cells by affecting glucocorticoid receptors sites on their plasma membranes. The cortisol levels required to saturate leukemia cell receptors are only minimally above normal circulating values and may be achievable by an acute stress response. This may account for many spontaneous remissions of these cancers (reviewed by Levy, 1985).

Coping Mechanisms and Cancer

Psychological stress is very common in patients with cancer. In a study of 215 cancer patients undergoing treatment, 47% could be diagnosed as having a DSM-III psychiatric disorder, with the most frequent disorder being reactive depression and anxiety (Derogatis et al., 1983). The method of coping with this stress may be more important than its occurrence. Helplessness, passivity, stoicism, and suppression of anger appear to be the most detrimental coping mechanisms. A number of studies have reported unfavorable prognosis in passive cancer patients. These are summarized in Table 16.1.

In spite of the above studies, the effects of coping skills on cancer survival are not widely agreed upon.

The experimental design used in Greer and Rogentine's studies (see Table 16.1) have been criticized for using too small a sample size, lack of adjustment for age differences, and for the fact that a healthier patient has more energy available for psychological disturbance (Greenwald, 1992:108). A study of 204 patients with late-stage cancer found no relationship between coping style and survival (Cassileth et al., 1985). However, the author recognized that psychology may be a factor in patients with a more favorable prognosis. Critics of Cassileth's study argue that the 32-question survey used was not adequate to fully characterize a patient's psychology (Vitaliano et al., 1985). A larger and more complex study of 536 cancer patients reported no relationship between tension, depression, or anger and survival (Seattle Longitudinal Assessment of Cancer Survival).

In addition to possible effects on patients with established cancers, coping mechanisms may also affect who develops cancer. In a study of 71 women awaiting breast biopsy, patients subsequently diagnosed as having cancer reported experiencing anger and "losing control in anger" less frequently than those with benign disease (Morris et al., 1981). A similar study with 56 women also found that women diagnosed with cancer had difficulty expressing anger, tended to avoid conflict, were more self-sacrificing, and were more optimistic (Wirsching et al., 1982). Other investigators have reported similar results (Cheang and Cooper, 1985; Jansen and Muenz, 1984). However, still other studies have been contradictory and investigators have not reached a consensus on these observations.

Psychotherapy in Cancer Treatment

A number of investigators have reported that psychological intervention may increase the life expectancy of patients with cancer. In a study on 225 patients with advanced cancer who received comprehensive psychotherapy in addition to conventional treatment, median patient survival time was approximately double that of national averages (Simonton et al., 1980). However, comparison of treatment results with historical data is often not statistically valid. In a study of 86 women with metastatic breast cancer who received conventional treatment, those receiving a one-year intervention with psychotherapy (weekly supportive group therapy) lived twice as long as those not receiving psychotherapy (19 months vs. 37 months). Survival differences became apparent eight months after the intervention ended (Spiegel et al., 1989).

In addition to affecting patient survival, relaxation techniques may also positively affect quality-of-life parameters. In a study on 67 cancer patients, a relaxation technique involving deep breathing, muscle relaxation, and imagery effectively reduced subjective pain ratings and analgesic intake as compared to controls (Sloman et al., 1994). In a study of 60 cancer patients receiving chemotherapy, those who received instruction in relaxation techniques exhibited less nausea prior to chemotherapy and lower blood pressure after chemotherapy as compared to controls (Vasterling et al., 1993). Relaxation techniques may also affect immune parameters. In a study of 13 patients with stage I breast cancer, those trained in relaxation, guided imagery, and biofeedback exhibited increased NK cell activity, increased mixed lymphocyte response, and an increased number of peripheral blood lymphocytes as compared to controls who received no training (Gruber et al., 1993).

16.2.2 Eastern Psychology

Eastern medical traditions such as Traditional Chinese Medicine and Ayurvedic medicine have long held that the mind directly affect the body and that therapy for any mental or emotional imbalance improves the treatment outcome for many physical diseases. TCM views emotional imbalance as a common cause of disease, and views various diseases as affecting the mind and emotions. China is now a world leader in integrating meditation exercises into modern clinical settings. Meditation is one of the primary tools used in Eastern traditions to correct imbalances of the mind.

Physiologic Aspects of Meditation

Studies on the biochemical effects of meditation have produced conflicting results. Although some investigators have reported mixed or no effects, others have reported that meditation may:

- increase serum DHEA-S (Glaser et al., 1992)[5]
- reduce serum cortisol
- increase serum total protein
- reduce blood pressure
- reduce pulse rate
- reduce lung vital capacity and tidal volume
- reduce reaction rates (Sudsuang et al., 1991)
- increase plasma norepinephrine levels (Morrell and Hollandsworth, 1986)
- decrease serum TSH, growth hormone, and prolactin levels (Werner et al., 1986)
- increase plasma free fatty acids (Cooper et al., 1985)

---

[5] Dehydroepiandrosterone sulfate (DHEA-S) is a hormone produced by the adrenal cortex and is a tissue percussor of androgen and estrogen. DHEA is protective against some forms of cancer.

Some of these physiologic changes may inhibit tumor growth or metastasis. For example, glucocorticoids may increase metastasis of solid tumors, probably through their immunosuppressive effects. Human studies demonstrate that glucocorticoids may produce extrapulmonary metastasis in tumors that would otherwise only metastasize to the lung (reviewed by DeVita, 1985). Meditation may reduce serum glucocorticoid levels, which in turn, may inhibit metastasis.

Few studies have been conducted on the effects of meditation on diseases. Those that have been conducted suggest that meditation may provide a positive benefit in many circumstances. In a five-year comparison study of medical insurance utilization by approximately 2,000 regular meditation practitioners and nonmeditating controls, the meditating group had 53% fewer inpatient admissions, 44% fewer outpatient visits, 55% fewer admissions for benign and malignant tumors, 87% fewer admissions for heart disease, and 87% fewer admissions for diseases of the nervous system. However, these results may have been confounded by patient self-selection (Orme-Johnson, 1987). That is, people who meditate may be inclined to do other activities that promote health, and may not be representative of the population at large. In a study on the residents of 73 homes for the elderly, those who were instructed in meditation exhibited a significant increase in life expectancy (Alexander et al., 1989).

Meditation and Qi Gong

For over two thousand years, Daoist monks have practiced meditation exercises to help ensure a long, healthy life and to reach a state of harmony with the *Dao,* the "way" of the universe. One of the central tenents of Daoism, *wu wei,* or "no active intervention" implies a way of living and acting that is completely natural to the given moment. Classic Daoist works include the *Dao De Ching* written by Lao Tzu , and *Chuang Tzu* written by Lao Tzu's contemporary Chuang Chou (369-286 B.C.).

Daoist, Buddhist, and other Eastern spiritual teachings contend that we experience misery (and stress) because our minds spin wildly and unceasingly. We are caught in a continual spasm of thoughts, a spasm that robs us of our peace. Through meditation, the mind is calmed and peace returns naturally. A calm mind also allows us to feel who we are, and we begin to experience that who we are is not just our mind, but something much greater and much deeper. This revelation, or even just a glimpse of it, can be of enormous value to cancer patients, who may be facing the ultimate loss of mind: their death. Eastern spiritual teachings hold that through the practice of meditation, we gain an understanding that

allows us to accept the natural flow from life to death. Because of these benefits, meditation increasingly is being used in clinical psychotherapy. For example, in a literature review of meditation in psychotherapy, Bogart (1991) states that "Meditation may be of great value ... through its capacity to awaken altered states of consciousness that may profoundly reorient an individual's identity, emotional attitude, and sense of well-being and purpose in life."

Meditation in Cancer Treatment

The late Ainslie Meares, an Australian psychiatrist, treated a number of cancer patients using meditation techniques. Based on his experience in treating 73 patients with advanced cancer, who attended at least 20 sessions of intensive meditation, Meares (1980) claimed that nearly all patients received a significant reduction in anxiety, depression, and pain. In addition, inhibition of tumor growth occurred in about 10%, and tumor regression occurred in about 10%. For those patients who later died, Meares claimed that intensive meditation improved the quality of life in 50% of the patients, and facilitated death with dignity in 90%. As patients deepened their meditation, they naturally developed a greater nonverbal understanding of life and death.

Meares (1982) published case reports of nine patients with tumor regression in the absence of conventional treatment. These included patients with breast cancer, sarcoma, rectal cancer, oat-cell lung cancer, Hodgkin's disease, lymphosarcoma, and melanoma. In a study of 17 cancer patients who were taught meditation exercises, all were reported to have survived several months longer than expected, and six (35%) improved dramatically (Meares, 1979). Patients receiving chemotherapy did not respond to intensive meditation as well as patients who relied solely on meditation. Two possible reasons for this may be that a reliance on chemotherapy reduces the motivation to meditate, and that chemotherapy reduces the competence of the immune system (Meares, 1983b).

Meares (1983a) characterized the meditation technique he used as an "effortless stilling of the mind." In this respect, it is similar to various Buddhist and Daoist meditation techniques. He discouraged active visualization, contemplation, mantra repetition, or concentration on the breath in favor of natural quietness. Patients attended a meditation session each weekday morning for a month, and then attended later sessions less frequently. The patients were also required to practice at home, anywhere from 30 minutes to 3 hours or more daily. The meditation experience of those patients who achieved remission generally had three attributes: their meditation was profound and prolonged, there was little or no conscious mental activity during meditation, and they carried the meditation experience into their daily lives.

In discussing the possible mechanisms for cancer regression, Meares (1983b) suggested the following:

- *Psychological activation of the immune system:* Stress stimulates the secretion of cortisone, and cortisone inhibits the immune system. Meditation, by reducing stress, may enable the immune system to function more optimally.
- *Psychologically induced changes in blood supply:* Meditation and relaxation are known to increase circulation in the peripheral and visceral blood vessels. With increased circulation, numerous physiological changes may occur.
- *Psychologically induced changes in endocrine functions:* Numerous cancers are hormone-sensitive. Meditation has been known to affect the production or release of a variety of hormones.
- *Changes in sympathetic and parasympathetic activity:* The reduction of anxiety induced by meditation can reduce sympathetic nervous activity. This may in turn positively affect the immune system.

Meditation may also help the cancer patient to change those negative coping responses to stress that may reduce survival expectancy. As discussed previously, a passive or stoic emotional response may be associated with poor survival. Patterned emotional responses are learned responses that may be altered through deep meditation. By stilling the mind, meditation brings a direct experience of the moment and allows reactions that are in direct response to the moment, rather than reactions that arise from habitual thought patterns.

Tibetan Medicine

A number of traditional medical systems other than TCM incorporate meditation and other spiritual practices in the treatment of disease. For example, Tibetan medicine views emotions (or mental attitudes) as both causes for disease and conditions under which diseases can ripen. In Tibetan medicine, 84,000 different types of afflictive emotions (such as desire or hatred) produce 84,000 different types of disorders. These are condensed into 404 types of disorders (Donden 1986:15-18):[6]

1) 101 disorders are under the strong influence of actions (karma) from previous lifetimes. When karma ripens and causes a disease to manifest, it is very powerful and generally fatal. Patients with these types of diseases are often compelled to renounce worldly activities and engage in spiritual practices. However, few survive.

2) 101 disorders are due to the actions of this life. These disorders will usually prove to be fatal unless treated. Sometimes medication is not sufficient, and spiritual practices such as confession of wrongdoing, engaging in virtuous practice, or altering harmful behavior are required.

3) 101 disorders involve spirits (unseen forces that can harm an individual). Medication cannot help patients with these disorders and spiritual methods must be used.

4) 101 disorders are superficial, and proper diet and behavior patterns can correct them.

In Tibetan medicine, any one of the four types of disorders can cause cancer. Cancer caused from past karma cannot be treated successfully and is usually fatal. Cancer caused by actions of this life can be cured if treated. Cancer caused by spirits is difficult to treat, and generally is fatal unless spiritual methods are employed. Cancer caused by a superficial factor can be cured by dietary and behavioral changes (Donden 1986:15-18).

These concepts from Tibetan medicine offer interesting suggestions on ways in which cancer treatment could be studied in the West. In conventional medicine, spiritual practice as a form of treatment is rarely considered for cancer or any other disease. Yet, it is possible that some physical diseases, including some cases of cancer, may originate and be sustained from a nonphysical driving force. To rely solely on physical treatment may deprive some patients of therapy that is essential to their healing process. In view of the positive effects that meditation may have on a patient's survival, sense of peace, and acceptance of death, and considering that meditation is low-cost and completely nontoxic, it is conceivable that instruction in meditation could be useful to a large number of patients. Further studies are warrented to confirm any benefits.

16.3 SUMMARY

Two physical therapies, acupuncture and electrotherapy, may be beneficial to the cancer patient. Acupuncture may be best suited to treating mild leukopenia or secondary, superficial symptoms. Electrotherapy may be best suited to treating superficial cancers, especially in conjunction with immunostimulating agents. Psychological therapies that may be beneficial include psychotherapy and meditation. These therapies may alter the neurological, endocrine, and immune system of the cancer patient and may improve their quality of life, if not their survival.

---

[6] Ayurvedic medicine, a traditional medicine from India, likewise recognizes some of these same causes of disease (Frawley, 1989:xvii-xx).

17
CONDUCTING RESEARCH ON NATURAL AGENTS

17.1 RESEARCH DESIGN

Nearly two hundred natural agents with potential anticancer activity have been mentioned in this book. Some of these may have little or no effect, while others may be quite effective. Further research is needed to determine the clinical value of these agents. Although the word "research" may inspire images of large and expensive clinical trials, a multitude of research designs exist that are less complicated and less expensive. Volumes have been written on the subject of research design and it is beyond the scope of this book to describe their intricacies. However, an overview of common research designs is provided in Appendix I.

One research design that may be particularly suited to the practitioner is case studies. Although the results of a case study or case series do not prove the efficacy of a given treatment, they can suggest directions for further research. Case studies can be valuable contributions to the body of knowledge on a subject. The Office of Alternative Medicine (OAM) at the National Institutes of Health has suggested the *best case series* as a means to determine whether a complementary anticancer therapy demonstrates potential efficacy and whether clinical development of the therapy should continue. The best case series is a retrospective analysis of clinical data that a practitioner has collected. The essential elements of a best case series are (OAM, 1994):

- A confirmation of the patient's diagnosis by tissue biopsy.
- A description of the measures used to define the extent of tumor reduction.
- A definition of the objective response criteria used. This must be consistent with the criteria used by NCI.
- A description of how patient's records will be maintained, and a schedule for follow-up examinations.
- A record of any cancer treatments the patients received concurrent with the trial.
- A record of any cancer treatments the patients received previous to the trial.
- A record of each patient's disease status at the onset of therapy and during treatment.
- An identification of the primary tumor site, and a record of dates when the cancer metastasized and the sites of metastasis.
- A description of each patient's overall clinical status and medical condition.
- The criteria used to modify treatment from that proposed in the original protocol due to clinical observations or treatment-associated toxicities.

The Office of Alternative Medicine should be contacted for additional information on the best case series.

In addition to case series design, other research designs can and should be utilized. Many of these require funding. Small amounts of grant money are available through OAM programs. Grants may also be available from other governmental agencies or private foundations.

In all cases, the ethical aspects of using unproven therapies must be thoroughly considered. Standard ethical guidelines for clinical and animal research have been developed and should be adhered to. Federal regulations for human subjects assurances and informed consent are provided in 45 CFR 46 and 21 CFR 50 and 56. For additional information regarding protocol development and implementation, see the *Investigators Handbook,* printed by the National Cancer Institute (NCI, 1993).

17.2 SUMMARY OF PROMISING AGENTS

A summary of what may be the most promising of those agents discussed in this text is provided in Table 17.1. Where appropriate, the active constituents are listed (in brackets). The reader should keep in mind that, in many cases, the accuracy of the listed actions may be uncertain and must be verified by further study. Also, for some plant products, hot water extracts may not contain adequate concentrations of active ingredients, and purified fractions may be required clinically. Appropriate references for the stated actions are provided in the preceding 16 chapters.

Agents that are not considered by this author to be among the most promising are listed in Appendix J. Since little data are available for most of the agents, the distinction between promising and less-promising is admittedly subjective. In general, agents that had only minor mention in this book were placed into Appendix J.

TABLE 17.1. SUMMARY OF THE MOST PROMISING AGENTS		
AGENT	**REPORTED ACTIONS**	**COMMENT**
Acanthopanax sp. (*wu jia pi, ci wu jia*)	○ stimulates immune cells in vitro ○ inhibits histamine release in vitro ○ antitumor activity	
Aesculus hippocastanum (horse chestnut) [escin]	○ inhibits collagenase activity in vitro ○ inhibits increased vascular permeability in humans	
Allium sativum (garlic, *da suan*) [thiol and other compounds]	○ fibrinolytic in humans ○ inhibits platelet aggregation in humans ○ inhibits production of angiogenic factors by macrophages ○ inhibits endothelial cell proliferation in vitro ○ scavenges free radicals	○ increases tPA
Aloe vera gel	○ reduces PGE_2 production in vitro ○ inhibits platelet aggregation in vitro ○ inhibits kinins in vitro ○ inhibits histamine release in vitro ○ antitumor activity ○ stimulates immune system in vivo ○ inhibits angiogenesis in vivo	
Angelica sinensis (dang gui)	○ stimulates immune cells in vivo ○ antitumor activity ○ inhibits platelet aggregation in humans ○ inhibits increased vascular permeability in vitro	
Arctium lappa (niu bang zi) [lignans]	○ induces differentiation in vitro ○ reduces sex hormone bioavailability ○ inhibits tumor cell proliferation in vitro ○ antitumor activity (*A. lappa* root, burdock root)	
Astragalus membranaceus (huang qi)	○ stimulates immune system in vivo ○ inhibits chemotherapy-induced immunosuppression in humans ○ antitumor activity ○ inhibits platelet aggregation in humans	
(Table continues)		

	TABLE 17.1. *(continued)*	
AGENT	**REPORTED ACTIONS**	**COMMENT**
Atractylodes macrocephala (bai zhu)	○ fibrinolytic/antithrombotic in humans ○ antitumor activity ○ increases leukocyte count in humans	
Berberine	○ induces differentiation in vitro ○ antitumor activity ○ inhibits tumor cell proliferation in vitro ○ stimulates immune cells in vitro	○ antibacterial effects may alter gut flora
Bromelain	○ stimulates plasmin production ○ fibrinolytic in animals ○ inhibits kinins in vitro ○ stimulates immune cells in vitro ○ induces differentiation in vitro ○ inhibits platelet aggregation in humans ○ stimulates globulin degradation in humans ○ modifies cell surface proteins in vitro ○ anticancer activity (ovarian carcinoma and breast cancer)	
Bufo bufo gargarizans (chan su)	○ induces differentiation in vitro ○ anticancer activity (acute and chronic leukemia)	
Bupleurum chinense (chai hu)	○ inhibits PAF production in vitro ○ inhibits increased vascular permeability ○ stimulates immune system in vivo ○ antitumor activity ○ induces apoptosis in vitro	
Camellia sinensis [green tea polyphenols]	○ stimulates immune system in vivo ○ inhibits platelet aggregation in vitro ○ inhibits tumor cell proliferation in vitro ○ blocks estrogen/growth factor binding in vitro ○ scavenges free radicals ○ inhibits metastasis in vivo ○ inhibits collagenase activity ○ source of (+)-catechin and EGCG	
Carthamus tinctorius (hong hua)	○ inhibits thrombin in humans ○ fibrinolytic in humans	
Cartilage, bovine and shark	○ inhibits angiogenesis in vivo ○ stimulates immune system in humans ○ anticancer activity (multiple cancers) ○ antitumor activity ○ inhibits collagenase activity in vitro	
Coenzyme Q10	○ induces remission in human cancer patients	
Crataegus oxyacantha (shan zha) [anthocyanins]	○ promotes collagen cross-linking in vitro ○ inhibits collagenase activity ○ source of (+)-catechin	
Cysteine (or N-acetyl cysteine)	○ reduces excess copper levels ○ increases insulin degradation ○ scavenges free radicals ○ inhibits endothelial cell proliferation in vitro ○ inhibits production of angiogenic factors by macrophages ○ precursor for glutathione	
	(Table continues)	

AGENT	REPORTED ACTIONS	COMMENT
	**TABLE 17.1.** *(continued)*	
DMSO	○ inhibits metalloproteinase production in vitro ○ inhibits invasion in vitro ○ induces apoptosis in vitro ○ induces differentiation in vitro ○ increases survival of humans with stomach and colon cancer ○ increases drug uptake by cancer cells in vivo ○ anticancer activity (with hematoxylin) ○ scavenges free radicals	
Echinacea purpurea	○ stimulates immune cells in vitro	
Eicosapentaenoic acid (EPA)	○ inhibits collagenase activity in vitro ○ induces differentiation in vitro ○ inhibits PAF production in vitro ○ inhibits platelet aggregation in humans ○ antitumor activity ○ decreases PGE_2 production ○ increases PGE_3 production ○ increases membrane fluidity and drug uptake ○ inhibits metastasis in vivo ○ inhibits cachexia in vivo	○ inhibits immune cells in vivo
Electrotherapy	○ normalizes transmembrane potential ○ increases membrane fluidity and drug uptake in vitro ○ antitumor activity ○ anticancer activity (multiple cancers) ○ stimulates immune system in vivo	
Ganoderma lucidum (ling zhi)	○ antitumor activity ○ induces differentiation ○ inhibits histamine release ○ stimulates immune system in vivo	
Genistein	○ induces apoptosis in vitro ○ increases SHBG production in humans ○ inhibits platelet aggregation in vitro ○ inhibits tumor cell proliferation in vitro ○ inhibits leukotriene production in vitro ○ inhibits angiogenesis in vitro ○ induces differentiation in vitro	
Glutathione	○ facilitates drug metabolism ○ scavenges free radicals ○ facilitates repair of DNA ○ required for optimal activation of T lymphocytes ○ antitumor activity ○ inhibits endothelial cell proliferation in vitro ○ inhibits production of angiogenic factors by macrophages ○ increases insulin degradation	
Glycyrrhiza uralensis (gan cao)	○ inhibits PAF production ○ stimulates immune system in vivo ○ inhibits histamine release in vitro ○ antitumor activity ○ may increase absorption of hydrophobic compounds	
Gynostemma pentaphyllum (jiao gu lan)	○ inhibits platelet aggregation in vivo ○ stimulates immune system in humans	
Indirubin (from *Isatis tinctoria, qing dai*)	○ antitumor activity ○ anticancer activity (leukemia) ○ stimulates immune system in vivo	
	*(Table continues)*	

	TABLE 17.1. *(continued)*	
AGENT	**REPORTED ACTIONS**	**COMMENT**
Ligusticum chuanxiong (chuan xiong)	○ inhibits platelet aggregation in humans ○ stimulates immune cells in vivo	
Ligustrum lucidum (nu zhen zi)	○ inhibits increased vascular permeability in vivo ○ inhibits PGE_2 production in vivo ○ stimulates immune system in humans ○ antitumor activity	
Limonene and perillyl alcohol	○ antitumor activity ○ anticarcinogenic activity ○ induces differentiation in vitro	
Linum usitatissimum (flax seed) [fiber, lignans]	○ antitumor activity ○ reduces sex hormone bioavailability ○ precursor for butyric acid ○ reduces risk for breast and colon cancer	
Low-fat diet	○ reduces sex hormone bioavailability in humans ○ reduces cancer incidence in humans ○ improves immune functioning in humans	
Low-sugar diet	○ inhibits tumor growth in vivo ○ reduces insulin production ○ reduces blood glucose levels	
Lycium barbarum (gou qi zi)	○ stimulates immune cells in vitro	
Meditation	○ increases survival of humans with various cancers ○ increases peace of mind ○ inhibits stress-induced immunosuppression	
Melatonin	○ stimulates immune system ○ antiestrogen activity in vitro ○ anticancer, especially in combination with IL-2	
Modified citrus pectin	○ inhibits metastasis in vivo	
Multienzymes	○ increases survival of humans with various cancers ○ inhibits metastasis in humans ○ stimulates immune cells in vitro	
Paeonia lactiflora (chi shao and bai shao)	○ fibrinolytic in vitro ○ inhibits fibrin production in vitro	
Panax ginseng (ren shen)	○ antitumor activity ○ inhibits platelet aggregation in humans ○ stimulates immune system in humans ○ inhibits chemotherapy-induced immune suppression in humans	○ increases plasminogen activator production in vitro
Picrorrhiza kurroa (hu huang lian)	○ inhibits histamine release ○ stimulates immune system in vivo	
Proanthocyanidins	○ inhibits collagenase and elastinase activity in vitro ○ induces collagen cross-linking in vitro ○ inhibits histamine release ○ scavenges free radicals ○ inhibits increased vascular permeability	○ promotes collagen synthesis in vitro
Pseudostellaria heterophylla (tai zi shen)	○ antitumor activity ○ stimulates immune cells in vitro	
PSP and PSK	○ stimulates immune system in humans ○ increases survival of humans with various cancers ○ PSK inhibits heparanase activity	
Psychotherapy	○ inhibits stress-induced immunosuppression ○ increases survival of humans with various cancers	
	(Table continues)	

TABLE 17.1. *(continued)*		
AGENT	**REPORTED ACTIONS**	**COMMENT**
Quercetin	○ induces apoptosis in vitro ○ inhibits histamine release in vitro ○ inhibits tumor cell proliferation in vitro ○ competes for type II estrogen binding sites in vitro ○ stimulates TGF-β_1 production in vitro ○ inhibits expression of multidrug resistance genes in vitro ○ inhibits heat shock resistance in vitro ○ scavenges free radicals	○ soluble form required for oral administration
Realgar (arsenic sulfide, *xiong huang*)	○ anticancer activity (acute and chronic leukemia)	
Rhein and emodin	○ anti-inflammatory ○ antitumor activity	○ laxative properties ○ may be immunosuppressive
Salvia miltiorrhiza (dan shen)	○ fibrinolytic/antithrombic in humans ○ inhibits collagen synthesis in vitro ○ anticancer activity (lymphoma) in combination with chemotherapy ○ stimulates plasmin production in vitro ○ some success in treating DIC	
Scutellaria baicalensis (huang qin)	○ antitumor activity ○ inhibits platelet aggregation in vitro ○ inhibits histamine release in vitro ○ baicalein inhibits tumor cell proliferation in vitro ○ induces apoptosis in vitro ○ stimulates immune system in vivo	○ antibacterial effects may alter gut flora
Soy foods [protease inhibitors, equol, and daidzein]	○ equol reduces estrogen bioavailability ○ antitumor activity ○ anticarcinogenic activity	
Tanacetum parthenium (feverfew)	○ fibrinolytic/antithrombotic in vitro ○ inhibits histamine release in vitro	
Vaccinium myrtillus (bilberry) [anthocyanins]	○ inhibits collagenase activity in vitro ○ scavenges free radicals ○ promotes collagen cross-linking in vitro	○ stimulates collagen synthesis in vitro
Viscum album (sang ji sheng)	○ antitumor activity ○ stimulates immune system in vivo ○ inhibits angiogenesis in vivo ○ induces apoptosis in vivo ○ cytotoxic	
Vitamin A (retinoic acid)	○ inhibits endothelial cell proliferation in vitro ○ inhibits angiogenesis in vitro ○ inhibits collagen synthesis ○ induces differentiation in vitro ○ induces apoptosis in vitro ○ increases production of metalloproteinase inhibitors by capillary cells in vitro	
Vitamin C	○ increases survival of humans with various cancers ○ facilitates immune function ○ scavenges free radicals ○ inhibits histamine release in vitro	○ facilitates collagen synthesis in vitro ○ enhance angiogenesis in vitro
Vitamin D_3 metabolites	○ may up-regulate vitamin A receptors ○ inhibits angiogenesis in vitro, synergistic with retinoic acid ○ antitumor activity ○ induces differentiation in vitro ○ induce apoptosis in vitro	○ may be best reserved for patients with low vitamin D levels

As an aid to the reader, the agents listed in Table 17.1 are listed again in Table 17.2, grouped according to the primary anticancer mechanism by which they have been shown to act or may theoretically act. For example, agents that scavenge free radicals are listed as inhibiting invasion, and agents that inhibit platelet aggregation are listed as inhibiting metastasis. Only major anticancer mechanisms are listed. Since little data are available on most of these agents, the accuracy of the information may be uncertain, and the discrimination between primary and secondary mechanisms is somewhat subjective.

TABLE 17.2. SUMMARY OF PROMISING AGENTS LISTED BY POSSIBLE MECHANISMS			
PRIMARY MECHANISM	**AGENT**	**SECONDARY MECHANISMS**	**POTENTIAL INDICATIONS**
Inhibit angiogenesis	*Aesculus hippocastanum* (horse chestnut)	inhibit invasion	most solid cancers
	Allium sativum (da suan)	inhibit metastasis	
	cartilage, bovine and shark	stimulate immune system, inhibit invasion	breast, prostate, primary brain, and ovarian cancers
	Picrorrhiza kurroa (*hu huang lian*)	stimulate immune system	most solid cancers; its hepatoprotective properties (reviewed by Bone, 1995) may make it particularly suitable for treating liver cancer
	glutathione and NAC	inhibit invasion, stimulate immune system	most cancers
Induce apoptosis	*Bupleurum chinense (chai hu)*	stimulate immune system, inhibit angiogenesis	most cancers, especially liver
Cytotoxic mechanisms	electrotherapy	stimulate immune system	superficial and localized cancers
	Isatis tinctoria (qing dai)	stimulate immune system	chronic myelogenous leukemia
	limonene and perillyl alcohol	induce differentiation	most cancers
	realgar (arsenic sulfide, *xiong huang*)	none known	chronic and acute leukemias
	rhein/emodin	inhibit angiogenesis	most cancers
Induce differentiation	*Arctium lappa (niu bang zi)*	cytotoxic	cancers known to differentiate: leukemia, melanoma, colon carcinoma, bladder carcinoma, brain cancer (glioblastoma multiforme), choriocarcinoma, hepatoma, ovarian adenocarcinoma, and neuroblastoma
	vitamin A	induce apoptosis, inhibit angiogenesis, inhibit invasion	
	berberine	cytotoxic, stimulate immune system	
	Bufo bufo gargarizans (*chan su*, toad skin)	none known	
Reduce sex hormone bioavailability	*Linum usitatissimum* (flax seed)	none known	estrogen and androgen sensitive tumors
	low-fat diet	facilitate immune function	
	soy foods	inhibit invasion	
Stimulate the immune system	*Acanthopanax sp.* (*wu jia pi, ci wu jia*)	inhibit angiogenesis	cancers known to respond to immunotherapy: melanoma and renal cell carcinoma; and possibly lymphoma, leukemia, osteosarcoma, and colorectal, lung, bladder, ovarian, and breast cancers
	Aloe vera gel	inhibit metastasis, inhibit angiogenesis	
(column continues)	*Astragalus membranaceus* (*huang qi*)	inhibit metastasis	
(Table continues)			

PRIMARY MECHANISM	AGENT	SECONDARY MECHANISMS	POTENTIAL INDICATIONS
Stimulate the immune system *(continued)*	*Atractylodes macrocephala (bai zhu)*	inhibit metastasis	cancers known to respond to immunotherapy: melanoma and renal cell carcinoma; and possibly lymphoma, leukemia, osteosarcoma, and colorectal, lung, bladder, ovarian, and breast cancers
	Echinacea purpurea	none known	
	Ganoderma lucidum (ling zhi)	induce differentiation, inhibit angiogenesis	
	Glycyrrhiza uralensis (gan cao)	inhibit angiogenesis	
	Gynostemma pentaphyllum (jiao gu lan)	inhibit metastasis	
	Ligustrum lucidum (nu zhen zi)	inhibit angiogenesis	
	Lycium barbarum (gou qi zi)	none known	
	meditation and pychotherapy	improve *qi* and *blood* circulation, provide peace of mind	
	melatonin	reduce sex hormone bioavailability, stimulate immune system	
	Panax ginseng (ren shen)	inhibit metastasis	
	Pseudostellaria heterophylla (tai zi shen)	none known	
	PSP and PSK	inhibit metastasis	
	vitamin C	inhibit angiogenesis	
Inhibit invasion	*Crataegus oxyacantha (shan zha)*	none known	most solid cancers
	DMSO	induce apoptosis and differentiation	
	proanthocyanidins	inhibit angiogenesis	
	Vaccinium myrtillus (bilberry)	none known	
Inhibit metastasis	*Angelica sinensis (dang gui)*	stimulate immune system, inhibit angiogenesis	most solid cancers except brain
	Carthamus tinctorius (hong hua)	none known	
	Ligusticum chuanxiong (chuan xiong)	stimulate immune system	
	modified citrus pectin	none known	
	Paeonia lactiflora (chi shao and *bai shao)*	none known	
	Salvia miltiorrhiza (dan shen)	inhibit angiogenesis	
	Tanacetum parthenium (feverfew)	inhibit angiogenesis	
Agents that act by four or more mechanisms	bromelain	inhibit metastasis, stimulate immune system, inhibit angiogenesis, induce differentiation	most cancers
	Camellia sinensis (EGCG)	inhibit invasion, inhibit metastasis, cytotoxic, stimulate immune system	
(column continues)	eicosapentaenoic acid (EPA)	inhibit invasion, inhibit angiogenesis, induce differentiation, inhibit metastasis	

(Table continues)

183

		TABLE 17.2. *(continued)*	
PRIMARY MECHANISM	**AGENT**	**SECONDARY MECHANISMS**	**POTENTIAL INDICATIONS**
Agents that act by four or more mechanisms *(continued)*	genistein	cytotoxic, reduce sex hormone bioavailability, induce apoptosis, inhibit metastasis, inhibit angiogenesis, induce differentiation	most cancers
	multienzymes	stimulate immune system, induce differentiation, inhibit angiogenesis, inhibit metastasis	
	quercetin	cytotoxic, reduce estrogen bioavailability, induce apoptosis, inhibit angiogenesis	
	Scutellaria baicalensis (huang qin)	induce apoptosis, inhibit metastasis, inhibit angiogenesis, stimulate immune system	
	Viscum album (sang ji sheng)	cytotoxic, stimulate immune system, inhibit angiogenesis, induce apoptosis	
	vitamin D_3	induce differentiation, inhibit angiogenesis, stimulate immune system, inhibit apoptosis	

17.3 DISCUSSIONS ON INDIVIDUAL AGENTS

Discussions on the pharmacokinetics and clinical use of selected agents are provided below. If a promising agent is not discussed below, it is because no additional information has been collected beyond what has already been presented in this text or in standard reference books. The following discussions are not intended to be used as a sole resource for developing research protocols. Before using any of these therapies, a thorough literature search, and consultation with appropriate experts, is advised. It may not be appropriate to use some of these therapies on human patients until additional laboratory data can be generated.

In general, there is a lack of pharmacokinetic data on the natural agents discussed in this book. The estimates that follow are often based on gross assumptions and may not reflect actual conditions in humans. The dosage calculations are not intended to be a final pronouncement, but are intended only to provide rough figures as a starting point for further research, and to suggest research data that must be gathered. As with all aspects of this book, the author welcomes corrections and additional information that may improve the accuracy of the information presented.

The discussions below are based on a number of assumptions. These include the following:

- Mice are assumed to weigh 20 grams, rats 200 grams, guinea pigs 300 grams, and rabbits 2 kg unless stated otherwise. Humans are assumed to weigh 70 kg.
- The ratio between the equivalent dose for mice and humans is assumed to be 12.5 to 1, and the ratio for rats and humans is assumed to be 4.3 to 1. These ratios are based upon differences in metabolic weight using a K factor of 0.75 (see Section 11.3.1).
- When compounds are administered every half-life, the average plasma concentration is assumed to be double that of the maximum plasma concentration achieved after a single dose. See Gibaldi (1991:11) for further information on this subject.

Lastly, information on the traditional use and the common dosage of individual herbs was obtained from Bensky and Gamble (1993) and Hsu et al. (1986) unless stated otherwise.

17.3.1 *Aesculus Hippocastanum* (Horse Chestnut)

Aesculus extracts may inhibit angiogenesis (by inhibiting increased vascular permeability) and may inhibit invasion (by inhibiting collagenase activity). The fruits of the *Aesculus sp.* have been used in both Chinese and

Western herbal medicine. In Chinese herbal medicine *A. chinensis (suo luo zi)* is used to *rectify the qi* (for example, to treat *qi stagnation*), and is used at a dose of 3 to 9 grams in decoction. In Germany, preparations of *A. hippocastanum* are used to treat diseases of the venous system, such as thrombophlebitis, varicose veins, and many types of edema. Aesculus extracts are the second most prescribed herbal monopreparation in Germany, with retail sales of $103 million (U.S.) (Grunwald, 1995).[1]

The primary active constituent is escin, an acidic saponin. There are two forms known: alpha- and beta-escin. Beta-escin is the natural form and can be converted to alpha-escin. Beta-escin is practically insoluble in water, whereas alpha-escin is quite soluble (Budavari et al., 1989:3647). Esculin, a coumarin derivative, is also somewhat active (reviewed by Weiss, 1991:188).

Escin appears to reduce capillary permeability and increase uptake of edemic fluids into capillaries. In animal experiments, escin was 600 times more potent than the flavonoid rutin in reducing edema (reviewed by Weiss, 1991:188). As discussed in Table 3.4, horse chestnut extract is effective against many forms of edema, including brain edema. This suggests that it could be useful in reducing angiogenesis-associated increases in capillary permeability in numerous tumors, including brain tumors.

The bioavailability of the beta-escin is low. Weiss (1991:188-9) reports that escin, in its natural state, is not absorbed and that the alpha form, such as Reparil (Madaus, Germany), should be used. However, other studies suggest that oral escin (100 mg), as contained in crude chestnut extracts (Venostasin), is effective in reducing capillary permeability in humans (Hitzenberger, 1989; Bisler et al., 1986). This effect may be due to the escin, or may be due to other agents in the extract. It may also be due to interactions between agents. For example, the addition of the crude flavonoids to escin (10:1 ratio) increases escin bioavailability by as much as 50% in mice (Obolentseva and Khadzhai, 1969). As discussed in Table 3.4, oral administration of the crude extract is effective in animals. Pretreatment with 10 to 40 mg/kg of alpha-escin inhibited increased capillary permeability caused by carbon tetrachloride in rabbits (Hampel et al., 1970). This corresponds to a human dose of approximately 280 to 1120 mg, which is somewhat greater than that for Venostasin, as mentioned above.

The toxicity of escin is of some concern. The oral LD50 of alpha-escin in mice, rats, and guinea pigs is 320, 720, and 475 mg/kg respectively. That of sodium beta-escin is 134, 400 and 188 mg/kg respectively. These correspond to human doses of 1.8 to 11 grams of alpha-escin, and 0.75 to 6.2 grams of beta-escin. The manufacture's recommended dose should not be exceeded.

17.3.2 Anthocyanins and Proanthocyanidins

Anthocyanins

Anthocyanins may inhibit invasion by inhibiting collagenase activity. However, they may also facilitate angiogenesis by promoting collagen cross-linking. Until more information is available, agents that stimulate collagen synthesis or cross-linking should be used with caution in patients with cancer, and it may be prudent to combine them with antiangiogenic agents. However, as discussed in Sections and 3.2.3 and 4.3, vitamin C also stimulates collagen synthesis and enhances angiogenesis in CAM assays, but is widely used by cancer patients and some investigators have reported beneficial effects.

Two potential sources of anthocyanins are *Vaccinium myrtillus* (bilberry) and *Crataegus oxyacantha (shan zha)*. For arthritic conditions and reducing capillary permeability, bilberry is commonly used at doses of 20 to 40 mg (calculated as pure anthocyanidins) 3 times per day (reviewed by Pizzorno and Murray, 1987). Crataegus is used in Chinese medicine to treat maldigestion, and is used in both western herbology and Chinese medicine to treat heart disease. It contains both (+)-catechin and anthocyanins. The normal dose in Chinese medicine is 9 to 15 grams/day of the whole fruit.

Proanthocyanidins

Similar to anthocyanins, proanthocyanidins inhibit collagenase activity in vitro and promote collagen cross-linking and synthesis in vitro. In addition, they scavenge free radicals and inhibit increased vascular permeability, two qualities that are also likely shared by anthocyanins. Due to their effect on collagen synthesis, similar cautions apply to both anthocyanidins and proanthocyanidins.

Proanthocyanidins are readily absorbed after oral administration, with peak serum concentrations occurring in 45 minutes. The half-life is approximately five hours (Schwitters and Masquelier, 1993:24-7). Maximal uptake occurs in connective tissue, especially the aorta. They appear to be clinically useful in reducing capillary fragility (Schwitters and Masquelier, 1993:57-8). Proanthocyanidin extracts are commercially available and are commonly used in divided doses of 50 to 100 mg/day.

---

[1] *Ginkgo biloba* extracts are the most prescribed herbal monopreparation, with annual sales of $280 million (U.S.). The extracts are used to enhance circulation.

17.3.3 *Bufo Bufo Gargarizans (Chan Su, Toad Skin)*

Bufo bufo gargarizans has been used with apparent success in treating acute leukemia. This substance is toxic, and must be used cautiously. The traditional dose for the venom of bufo is 0.015 to 0.03 grams/day in pill form. When the entire skin is used, the dose is 9 to 15 grams/day (Zhang, 1989:158). As discussed in Section 11.5.3, the alcohol extract has been used in leukemia studies at a dose of 15 to 30 ml, 3 times per day until improvement, followed by a resting period. Unfortunately, the amount of bufo in the alcohol extract was not specified. If the extract was prepared at a 1:5 weight/volume ratio, then each 5 ml of extract contains 1 gram of bufo skin, which would put the daily dose at 9 to 18 grams. However, this is only speculative.

17.3.4 *Bupleurum Chinense (Chai Hu)*

Bupleurum may induce apoptosis, inhibit angiogenesis (by inhibiting PAF production), and stimulate the immune system. In Chinese herbal medicine, bupleurum is classified as a cool herb and is used to treat *liver qi stagnation* and certain types of fever. Bupleurum is generally prescribed at a dose of 3 to 12 grams/day in decoction.

Bupleurum saponins (saikosaponins) exhibit anti-inflammatory activity equivalent to prednisolone in animal studies. An oral dose of 100 to 400 mg was effective in mice, which was approximately 10 times the effective intravenous dose. Therefore the bioavailability is approximately 10%. The content of total saponins in bupleurum *(B. falcatum)* is approximately 2.8% (reviewed by Chang and But, 1987:967). A dose of 100 to 400 mg of total saponins would, therefore, require approximately 4 to 14 grams of the raw herb, which is similar to the standard dosage. The saponins exhibit low toxicity in animal studies, the oral LD50 in mice being 4.7 g/kg (reviewed by Chang and But, 1987:967).

As discussed in Table 2.4, saikosaponin-a induces apoptosis in human hepatoma cells in vitro at concentrations of 50 μg/ml. The pharmacokinetics of bupleurum saponins are not known at this time and, therefore, the dose of bupleurum required to produce a 50 μg/ml plasma level cannot be calculated. Since the studies on bupleurum and apoptosis were originally conducted on human hepatoma cells, and since bupleurum is traditionally used against liver diseases, continued research on liver cancer lines may be warranted.

17.3.5 *Camellia Sinensis*

Camellia (green tea) contains two compounds that are of particular interest. These are (+)-catechin, and epigallocatechin gallate (EGCG). Each is discussed separately below.

Epigallocatechin Gallate

As discussed in Table 14.2, the concentration of epigallocatechin gallate that inhibits tumor cell proliferation in vitro varies from 10 to 1,000 μg/ml. For the purposes of our discussion, we will use a target concentration of 500 μg/ml. If we assume that EGCG possesses similar pharmacokinetic properties as (+)-catechin (see below—a 2-gram oral dose produced a peak plasma level of 1.5 μg/ml in humans; the half-life was 3 hours), than the oral dose of EGCG required to produce a plasma level of 500 μg/ml is 330 grams, when administered every 3 hours. Obviously, this is a prohibitively high dose. Even if we assume that a concentration of 50 μg/ml is effective, this would still require a dose of 33 grams every 3 hours. Since one cup of tea contains approximately 10 to 30 mg of EGCG (Lea et al., 1993a), this is the equivalent of approximately 3,000 cups of tea every 3 hours.

It may be more reasonable to use a lower dose, similar to the doses used in animal experiments. Oral doses of 500 mg/kg per day of green tea extract inhibited the proliferation of EA carcinoma by 32% in mice (Yan, 1992). Assuming that green tea extract is 49% EGCG (Wang et al., 1992c), this corresponds to a human dose of 1.4 grams of EGCG. In another study, 130 mg/kg per day of EGCG (85% pure) inhibited lung metastasis of melanoma in mice. This would correspond to a human dose of 850 mg/day. Due to the low plasma concentrations that these doses would be expected to produce, it is possible that the antitumor effects seen in the animal experiments were due to immune stimulation rather than cytotoxicity. Since human tumors may respond differently to immunotherapy than experimental animal tumors, it is not known if similar anticancer effects would be produced in humans. Alternatively, the antitumor effect seen in the animal studies could be due to free radical scavenging effects.

(+)-Catechin

As discussed in Section 14.4.4, (+)-catechin inhibits invasion in vitro at concentrations of 0.5 μM (0.15 μg/ml). In humans, an oral dose of 2 grams has produced a maximum (+)-catechin plasma level of 5.2 μM (1.5 μg/ml) at 3 hours (Smillie et al., 1987). The half-life was 2.7 hours. This would suggest that the dose necessary to produce 0.5 µM may be 100 mg every 3 hours. Recall that (+)-catechin stimulates the production of IL-1 by lymphocytes in vitro at concentrations less than 64 µg/ml. Therefore, this dose is likely to stimulate immune activity, including IL-1 production.

Adverse effects of (+)-catechin may be significant. The pure compound has been used clinically for the treatment of hepatitis in several countries at oral doses of approximately two grams/day. Its use has been associated with life-threatening episodes of intravascular hemolysis in some patients (Gandolfo et al., 1992). (+)-Catechin binds tightly with RBC membranes and may facilitate antibody reactions against blood cells (Salama and Mueller-Eckhardt, 1987). Drug-induced acute renal failure secondary to hemolytic anemia has been reported in humans after doses of 500 mg (Imbasciati et al., 1987). Drug-induced fever has also been widely reported, and may be due to increased IL-1 secretion by lymphocytes (Daniel et al., 1988). Increased IL-1 production may also facilitate angiogenesis, since IL-1 is angiogenic.

Depending upon the manufacturing process, the concentration of (+)-catechin in green tea polyphenol solids may be approximately 2% (Wang et al., 1992c). Therefore, a dose of 5 grams of solid green tea polyphenols contains approximately 100 mg of (+)-catechin. This same dose of green tea polyphenols contains approximately 2.5 grams of EGCG.

In light of the above discussion, it does not appear that green tea compounds are promising anticancer agents. However, green tea also has two other activities that are of interest: its ability to inhibit platelet aggregation and its ability to scavenge free radicals. Green tea extract may be useful in lower doses for these actions. At low doses it may also be useful as an anticarcinogenic agent. (+)-Catechin also inhibits ulcers by inhibiting hydrochloric acid secretion (Murakami et al., 1992), and reduces cholesterol absorption (Ikeda et al., 1992). It is moderately lipophilic (Ring et al., 1976) and of low molecular weight (MW 290). Therefore, it may be capable of crossing the blood-brain barrier.

17.3.6 DMSO

DMSO is attractive as an anticancer agent for a number of reasons. It inhibits metalloproteinase production in vitro; inhibits invasion in vitro; induces apoptosis in vitro; induces differentiation in vitro; may increase the survival of humans with stomach and colon cancer; increases drug uptake by cancer cells in vivo; and scavenges free radicals. However, not all of the in-vitro activity can be easily produced in vivo. Maximum blood levels of DMSO cannot exceed 0.1% without producing toxic effects (Jacob, 1995, personal communication).

This is significantly lower than the 1 to 2% concentration that causes differentiation in vitro. However, it may be possible to use lower doses of DMSO by administering it in combination with other differentiating agents. As discussed in Section 2.2.2, vitamin A reduces the effective in-vitro concentration of DMSO by 400%. To reduce it still further, vitamin D_3, EPA/DHA, berberine, bromelain, or ganoderma could also be employed. Even in combination with other differentiating agents, intravenous administration is likely to be necessary to produce adequate plasma concentrations.

A more accessible use of DMSO may be as a free radical scavenger. As discussed in Section 15.1.2, DMSO apparently increased survival in postoperative gastric and colon cancer patients. This may have been due to a free radical scavenging effect. The oral dose of DMSO used in these studies was 200 mg/day (500 mg of a 10% DMSO solution 4 times per day).

It should be noted that 200 mg/day of DMSO is a very low dose. In human studies measuring the synergistic effects of DMSO and chemotherapy drugs, dosages have been as high as 80 grams/day (Fuks et al., 1981). In one case study (of lipoid proteinosis) an oral dose of 2.8 to 4.2 grams/day for 3 years did not produce adverse effects (Wong and Lin, 1988). Oral solutions of 2 to 10% have been given to humans (Egorin et al., 1982; Aisner and Wiernik, 1978). Solutions exceeding 50% should not be administered orally. Intravenous dosages of 50 to 100 grams/day are not uncommon (Walker, 1993:46).

DMSO may also be of use as a drug carrier. It carries compounds of low molecular weight (<1,000 grams/mole) through a variety of human membranes (Jacobs, 1995, personal communication). However, systemic therapy may not be practical for at least two reasons. First, many drug-DMSO complexes will split in the gastrointestinal tract and drug absorption will not be increased (Jacob, 1995, personal communication). Second, it may be difficult to systemically obtain the concentrations of DMSO required to produce a solvent effect. Therefore, to act as a drug carrier, localized treatments may be more practical. For example, a 10% DMSO solution synergistically increased the cytotoxicity of a variety of antineoplastic agents against human ovarian tumors ex vivo, suggesting that intraperitoneal administration to humans with ovarian cancer may be useful (Pommier et al., 1988).

DMSO should not be used topically at concentrations exceeding 50 to 80%. The face and neck may be more sensitive than other areas. The redness that often occurs after application may be controlled with *Aloe vera* gel. Due to possible contaminants, only pharmaceutical grade DMSO should be used on humans. Pharmaceutical grade

DMSO is available from various suppliers, at least one of which carries a deodorized product.

17.3.7 Eicosapentaenoic Acid (EPA)

EPA may induce differentiation, inhibit invasion (by inhibiting collagenase activity), and inhibit angiogenesis (by inhibiting PAF production, inhibiting platelet aggregation, and decreasing PGE_2 production). It may also increase drug uptake and inhibit proliferation by increasing membrane fluidity. Lastly, it may be useful in treating cachexia.

Theoretically, increases in membrane fluidity could be maximized by using EPA in combination with other agents that increase membrane fluidity, such as rhein, indirubin, or electrotherapy. Likewise, differentiation could be maximized by using EPA in combination with other agents that induce differentiation, such as DMSO and vitamins A and D_3. The optimal dose of EPA and its efficacy in treating cancer has not been determined. As discussed in Section 12.3.6, an estimated dose for treating cachexia is 6.4 to 25.6 grams of pure EPA per day. For inhibiting platelet aggregation, 2 to 4 grams/day may be adequate. Effects may become apparent four weeks after beginning therapy.

DHA and EPA occur together in fish oil, and appear to have some of the same actions. In contrast to EPA, DHA actually stimulated tumor growth in mice in some cases (see Section 12.3.6). Therefore, fish oil products that contain a high ratio of EPA to DHA may be most appropriate. Commercial products are available with a EPA/DHA ratio of at least 5:2.

17.3.8 Genistein

Genistein may induce apoptosis; decrease estrogen bioavailability (by increasing SHBG production), inhibit metastasis (by inhibiting platelet aggregation), inhibit cell proliferation, inhibit angiogenesis, and induce differentiation. Unfortunately, the majority of studies on genistein have been in vitro, and little animal or human data are available.

As discussed in Table 14.4, genistein is active in vitro at concentrations of approximately 5 to 100 µM. For our purposes, we will assume that the target concentration may be 40 µM, or 11 µg/ml. Limited pharmacokinetic data are available on genistein. In one study, oral administration of 2.0 mg/kg of genistein to healthy volunteers resulted in a maximum plasma concentration of 2.15 µM (Xu et al., 1994). The half-life of genistein is quite likely on the order of a few hours. Based upon this data, plasma concentration of 40 µM would require a

dose of 18 mg/kg of genistein every 3 hours. This is 10 grams/day of genistein—a very large dose.

Limited data are available concerning the amount of genistein in foods and herbs. The content of genistein in soy is quite low (0.0014-0.0044%) (Eldridge and Kwolek, 1983; Coward et al., 1993). The soy food with the highest concentration of genistein is soy miso, at 0.0497%. For the dose specified above, 20,000 grams of miso would be required on a daily basis. Obviously, this is an unmanageable dose, and new sources of genistein need to be explored.

Most common foods probably contain an insufficient amount of genistein to act as anticancer agents. The plasma genistein concentration of 14 healthy Japanese men consuming a high-soy diet was 0.28 µM (Adlercreutz et al., 1993)—over 1,000 times lower than our target concentration of 40 µM.

A study is currently under way at the University of Michigan to assess the genistein and daidzein content in a wide range of plant products, including some Chinese herbs. Preliminary results of that study suggest that *Psoralea corylifolia (bu gu zhi)* may contain over 2.1 grams/kilogram of genistein (0.21%), more than 80 times that of most other herbs and seeds tested (Kaufman et al., in progress). Further research will examine methods to improve yields from psoralea and/or other sources.

17.3.9 Glutathione and Cysteine

As a source of thiol, glutathione and cysteine may inhibit angiogenesis and scavenge free radicals. In addition, glutathione has demonstrated antitumor activity.

Glutathione

As discussed in Section 12.4.5, oral glutathione caused partial or complete regression in 81% of established aflatoxin-induced liver tumors in rats. The dose used was 330 mg/kg per day. This corresponds to a human dose of 5.9 grams/day.[2] However, the bioavailability of oral glutathione in humans is uncertain. Oral administration of approximately 3 grams did not increase plasma glutathione or cysteine concentrations in 7 healthy subjects (Witschi et al., 1992). In contrast, other investigators reported that oral administration does increase plasma levels in humans, and that administration of the seperate amino acids is not effective (Jones et al., 1989; reviewed by Jones et al., 1992). An oral dose of approximately 1 gram increased plasma glutathione levels by 1.5 to 10-fold over baseline levels in 4 out of 5 healthy subjects. Maximum plasma concentrations occurred after one hour. Oral administration produced a

---

[2] The rats in this experiment weighed approximately 300 grams.

prolonged increase in plasma glutathione levels in rats, in large part due to absorption of intact glutathione molecules. Maximum concentrations occurred after 90 to 120 minutes and remained high for approximately 2 hours. Doses of 375 mg/kg produced optimal increases in plasma concentrations, whereas higher or lower doses produced substantially lower plasma concentrations. Administration of the constituent amino acids did not increase plasma glutathione levels (Hagen et al., 1990). Note that the dose producing an antitumor effect in rats was 330 mg/kg—nearly the optimum dose for glutathione absorption.

The narrow optimal dose window does not explain why administration of one gram increased plasma glutathione levels in humans, but administration of three grams did not. The human dose equivalent to 375 mg/kg, the optimal dose in rats, is approximately 6.1 grams. Extrapolating from the rat data, neither one nor three grams would be expected to increase glutathione levels in humans.

A recent epidemiological study lends further support to the theory that glutathione is absorbed by humans. In a study on 1,830 subjects, ingestion of glutathione derived from raw fruits and vegetables reduced the risk of oral and pharyngeal cancer (Flagg et al., 1994).

Increases in the plasma concentration of glutathione can be expected to produce increases in intercellular levels, at least in some cells. Endogenous glutathione is taken up by lung, kidney, and small intestine epithelial cells in rats in vitro (reviewed by Hagen et al., 1990).

Dietary intake of glutathione may vary between 2.9 to 131 mg/day in Americans. Common supplemental dosages are approximately one to three grams daily (Chaitow, 1988:104).[3] [4]

Cysteine

Although glutathione is synthesized from cysteine, glycine, and glutamic acid, only cysteine is usually in limited supply. The ability of N-acetyl cysteine to increase glutathione levels in humans is uncertain. Oral NAC (400 mg/day) did not statistically change intracellular glutathione levels in healthy, exercise-stressed volunteers, although it did increase helper T-cell count in glutathione-deficient individuals (Kinscherf et al., 1994). However, the timing of the assessment may not have been optimal to detect increases in glutathione. A single oral dose of approximately two grams of NAC increased intercellular cysteine in humans, but not glutathione levels (De Quay et al., 1992). In addition, intravenous administration of NAC in humans did not

significantly increase plasma glutathione concentrations (Ammon et al., 1992). Cysteine itself may be a better choice for increasing glutathione levels since NAC is a relatively poor glutathione precursor in endothelial cells as compared to cysteine (Cotgreave et al., 1991). However, as discussed above (Hagen et al., 1990), administration of cysteine to humans did not increase plasma glutathione levels.

When treating acetaminophen overdose, high loading doses of oral NAC are used (~140 mg/kg). At this dose, side effects may include nausea, vomiting, and diarrhea. Anaphylactic reactions may occur in up to 10% of patients after intravenous administration. Fatalities have occurred with overdose (Flanagan and Meredith, 1991). Both cysteine and glutathione may be contraindicated in insulin-dependent diabetes, since glutathione acts as a coenzyme for degrading insulin in the liver and kidney (Chaitow, 1988:82; Bionostics, 1986).

The terminal half-life of oral NAC is 6.25 hours in humans, which suggests that NAC should be administered in four divided doses per day (Holdiness, 1991). Other investigators reported that the terminal half-life is closer to 2.3 hours, and that no NAC is found in human plasma 12 hours after an oral dose of 600 mg (Borgstrom et al., 1986). As a dietary supplement, NAC is commonly prescribed at 1.5 grams/day in divided doses.

17.3.10 Glycyrrhiza Uralensis (Gan Cao)

As discussed in Box 8.1, licorice stimulates natural killer cell activity, induces interferon production, and inhibits suppressor T-lymphocyte activity. Intraperitoneal administration of glycyrrhizin (20 mg/kg every 3 days) caused either a complete remission or delayed tumor growth in 60% of Meth A tumor-bearing mice (Suzuki et al., 1992), apparently by modulating immune function. The equivalent human dose is approximately 1.6 mg/kg, or 112 mg, every 3 days.

After oral administration intestinal flora metabolize glycyrrhizin to glycyrrhetinic acid, the primary active form. In 6 geographically diverse samples of licorice root, the glycyrrhizin content was 2.22 to 3.23% (Spinks and Fenwick, 1990). The half-life of glycyrrhetinic acid in humans is 11 to 39 hours (Krahenbuhl et al., 1994). If we assume that licorice root contains 2.7% glycyrrhizin and that all glycyrrhizin is metabolized to glycyrrhetinic acid, then the dose of licorice required to provide 112 mg of glycyrrhizin every half-life (~24 hours) is 4.1 grams. This is within the traditional dose of 2 to 12 grams. This dose of glycyrrhizin is not expected to produce severe adverse aldosterone-like effects. The lowest observed

---

[3] Glutathione is an expensive amino acid. However, prices may vary greatly between suppliers.
[4] All doses for this part of the study were mixed in food and ingested over one hour or less.

adverse effect level in humans is 100 mg/day of glycyr-rhizic acid (Stormer et al., 1993). Most humans experience adverse effects at 400 mg/day.

Theoretically, the intestinal absorption of some hydrophobic compounds can be increased by mixing them with licorice saponins. This may be one reason that glycyrrhiza is used in such a high percentage of herbal formulas in Chinese medicine.

17.3.11 Isatis Tinctoria (Qing Dai)

The active agent of interest in *Isatis tinctoria* is indirubin. As discussed in Section 11.3.3 , indirubin shows possible antileukemic activity in humans, particularly against chronic myelocytic leukemia. Pure indirubin has a higher antileukemic activity than *Qing dai,* a traditional product made by processing the raw herb. *Qing dai* contains 0.1% indirubin (Chang and But, 1986:694).

Indirubin is soluble in acetic acid, but insoluble in alcohol and water (Ma and Yao, 1983). It is slowly and poorly absorbed from gastrointestinal tract, and high concentrations appear in the bile, stomach, intestines, liver, marrow, and brain in mice. Bioavailability in mice is 47% after intragastric administration. The terminal half-life is 17 to 20 hours. Indirubin is chiefly excreted in feces (Ma and Yao, 1983). Due to its poor absorption, adverse effects are primarily located in the intestinal tract.

In treating CML, the oral dose of indirubin in Chinese studies has been 150 to 200 mg/day, which may be reduced after remission. This dose requires 150 to 200 grams of *qing dai* per day, an amount that greatly exceeds the normal daily dose of 3 grams. However, some investigators have reported success with markedly lower dosages. In one study, a 36% response rate was seen in 22 patients treated with 6 to 12 grams of *qing dai* daily (Chang, 1985). The reason for the inconsistency in the reported effective doses is not clear. Patients are treated for 26 to 172 days (an average of 72 days) before maximal effects are observed (Ma and Yao, 1983).

Two natural agents may be useful in optimizing indirubin treatment. Indirubin may act by altering the fluidity of leukocyte membranes, in which case, EPA and rhein may potentiate treatment. Second, agents that increase indirubin absorption may reduce its adverse effects in the intestines and allow a reduction in dosage. Theoretically, glycyrrhiza saponins could be useful in this regard.

17.3.12 Limonene and Perillyl Alcohol

As discussed in Section 11.3.4, limonene, the primary constituent in orange oil, induces regression of stomach, lung, skin, breast, and liver cancers in rodent models. The dose expected to be effective in humans is a rather massive 90 to 100 grams/day, based upon rat studies. Phase I trials of limonene are now being conducted in London by R.C. Coombes M.D., Ph.D.

In contacts with Mr. Tom Moore of Tallahassee, Florida (see below), Dr. Coombes unofficially reported that 29 patients have received approximately 14 grams/day of limonene during 18 months of study. In spite of the fact that this is a very low dose, one patient did exhibit a partial response. Mild nausea and diarrhea were reported, which Dr. Coombes noted was possibly due to the drug carrier. No other adverse effects were reported. Further study of limonene at higher dosage levels is anticipated.

Perillyl alcohol, a common chemical used in the perfume industry, is a limonene analog that may be more potent than limonene in inducing tumor regression. The estimated effective dose in humans is 10 grams/day. In addition to its effects on cancer, perillyl alcohol has also been investigated as an antibacterial and antifungal agent for use in humans (Chastain, 1992).

Tom Moore is a Florida lawyer whose wife, Maria, suffered a recurrence of breast cancer in 1994. Maria's cancer did not respond to other conventional or experimental chemotherapy agents and, after researching the issue, Maria decided that she would like to try perillyl alcohol. Mr. Moore worked with University of Wisconsin researchers and NCI and FDA officials to enable Maria to become the first known cancer patient to take perillyl alcohol. Mr. Moore was instrumental in obtaining FDA approval of an emergency investigational new drug (EIND) application for perillyl alcohol, even though human studies at the University of Wisconsin had not yet begun.

Maria began taking perillyl alcohol in mid-February 1995, at the low dose of 0.75 grams per day, and progressively increased her dosage in accordance with the approved protocol. By early April her dose had increased to six grams per day. Maria's cancer was advanced by the time she started treatment with perillyl alcohol, but by the end of April she was starting to show symptomatic improvement (normalized liver enzymes and elimination of the need for supplemental oxygen). In early May, Maria required palliative radiotherapy for tumors in her spine, and, unfortunately, her EIND protocol required that treatment with perillyl alcohol cease when other treatment is provided. Radiotherapy-induced nausea also interfered with perillyl alcohol treatment. She resumed perillyl alcohol in June and was authorized to take 12 grams per day. Sadly, by this time the cancer had

TABLE 17.3. TRADITIONAL DOSES FOR IMMUNOSTIMULATING AGENTS		
AGENT	**MAXIMUM TRADITIONAL DOSE (g/day)**	**ACTIVE POLYSACCHARIDES**
Acanthopanax sp. (wu jia pi, ci wu jia)	15	yes
Aloe vera gel	***	yes
Astragalus membranaceus (huang qi)	60	yes
Atractylodes macrocephala (bai zhu)	9	
Echinacea purpurea	9 *	yes
Ganoderma lucidum (ling zhi)	15	yes
Glycyrrhiza uralensis (gan cao)	12	
Gynostemma pentaphyllum (jiao gu lan)	60 **	yes
Lentinus edodes (shiitake mushroom)	food item	yes
Ligustrum lucidum (nu zhen zi)	18	
Lycium barbarum (gou qi zi)	15	yes
Panax ginseng (ren shen)	9	
Pseudostellaria heterophylla (tai zi shen)	30	yes
Ziziphus jujuba (da zao)	30	

   * Source: Tierra, 1988
  ** Unreferenced.
*** Has been used at doses of up to one gallon per day (Dharmananda, 1995, personal communication).

returned with a vengeance, and Maria died June 20th (Tom Moore, 1995, personal communication).[5]

Maria never experienced any acute adverse effects from perillyl alcohol. Just prior to her death, and reportedly in direct response to Maria's "favorable" reaction to the drug, FDA authorized University of Wisconsin researchers to double the dosage level (to approximately 4.0 grams per day) for the first group of subjects in the upcoming Phase I trials.

Limonene and perillyl alcohol are not expected to produce severe adverse reactions at the effective dose. However, irritation to gastrointestinal and kidney tissues may occur. To reduce irritation, the terpenes could be mixed with an oil carrier and placed in gelatin capsules. They could also be taken with meals. Agents such a plantain, which are protective of the stomach mucosa, may also be of use. Due to their rapid metabolism, the daily dose of limonene and perillyl alcohol should be divided into four or more equal portions.

17.3.13 Polysaccharide-containing Agents

High molecular weight polysaccharides (HMWPs) are active ingredients in a number of herbs that stimulate the immune system. From the few reports available, it appears that large doses of HMWPs are necessary to produce immunostimulating effects. A HMWP dose of 50 to 500 mg/kg appears to provide optimal results in humans (Dharmananda, 1995, personal communication).[6] This corresponds to 3.5 to 35 grams/day for a 70-kg adult. In studies on mice, optimal antitumor effects were observed at doses of 100 to 250 mg/kg i.p. Assuming a 10% bioavailability (Ronca and Conte, 1993), this corresponds to an oral human dose of 5.6 to 14 grams/day for a 70-kg human (Boik, paper in progress). In China, it is common to prescribe decoctions containing 30 to 90 grams/day of HMWP-rich herbs to cancer patients. The HMWP content of these herbs is approximately 7%. For example, the amount of HMWP in lycium fruit is about 5 to 8% (Wang et al., 1991). Therefore, patients may be receiving approximately 2.1 to 6.3 grams/day of HMWPs. Some of the major immunostimulating agents, and their traditional dosages, are listed in Table 17.3. Those that are high in HMWPs are marked as such. The majority of these herbs are used in Chinese medicine to *supplement the qi.*

To achieve significant levels of HMWPs without using excessive amounts of any single herb, herbs can be combined. For example, the following combination

---

[5] Mr. Moore welcomes inquires regarding Maria's experience with perillyl alcohol and the prospects of obtaining EIND approval for other cancer patients. He can be reached at (904) 893-6015.

[6] Subhuti Dharmananda, Ph.D. is director of the Institute of Traditional Medicine in Portland, Oregon, and is the author of numerous books on Chinese herbal medicine.

contains a dose of 6.1 grams of HMWPs per day, assuming that each herb contains 7% HMWPs: 12 grams of lycium, 30 grams of astragalus, 15 grams of acanthopanax, and 30 grams of gynostemma. A model formula for this type of approach is *Bu Zhong Yi Qi Tang*.

A number of purified polysaccharides and proteoglycans have been isolated from HMWP-rich herbs. Some of these, such as PSP, PSK, and lentinan (from *Lentinus edodes*) may prolong the life-span of tumor-bearing animals and humans (reviewed by Chihara, 1992; Chihara et al., 1987; and Yang and Kwok, 1993). Oral doses are normally about three grams per day. Lower doses are used when the agents are administered intravenously.

It may be worthwhile to combine melatonin and glutathione (or NAC or cysteine) with herbal immunostimulants, since these may all act together to increase interleukin-2 activity. Oral melatonin is well absorbed. A dose of 50 mg every 4 hours can produce plasma peaks up to 80 times higher than endogenous peak levels (Kane et al., 1994). As discussed in Section 8.4.2, the dosage used in most studies was 1 to 50 mg/day. The dose used to treat insomnia is commonly 3 to 9 mg/day. Acute adverse side effects or addiction are not expected.

17.3.14 Quercetin

Quercetin may induce apoptosis, scavenge free radicals, inhibit angiogenesis (by inhibiting histamine release), inhibit proliferation, and reduce estrogen bioavailability (by competing for type II estrogen binding sites). It may also inhibit expression of multidrug resistance genes, and in this respect may be useful with cytotoxic agents.

Quercetin (and many other flavonoids discussed in this book) are metabolized relatively quickly. An intravenous injection of 100 mg quercetin produced a plasma concentration of 3.7 µg/ml in humans after 5 minutes. The terminal half-life was 2.4 hours (Gugler et al., 1975). No toxic effects were observed. An oral dose of four grams produced a zero plasma concentration, suggesting that quercetin is not absorbed in humans. Absorption is severely limited by its low solubility in water and lipids.

The 10 µM (4.4 µg/ml) concentration used in many of the in-vitro studies would require an intravenous dose of 59 mg every 2.4 hours. Although this concentration can be achieved in vivo, an injectable form of quercetin is not commercially available. One U.S. company is producing a soluble form of quercetin, which may eliminate the need for intravenous administration.

Pharmacokinetic data on this product are not yet available.

In studies on radiolabeled quercetin in rats, quercetin or its metabolic byproducts was concentrated primarily in the kidneys and liver, and to a lesser extent, in the blood, lungs, and ribs (Ueno et al., 1983). Negligible concentrations of quercetin were observed in the tissues after 48 hours.

17.3.15 Rhein and Emodin

The primary constituents of interest in *Cassia tora (jue ming zi)*, *Polygonum cuspidatum (hu chang)*, *Polygonum multiflorum (he shou wu)*, and *rheum palmatum (da huang)* are the anthraquinones rhein and emodin. Each is discussed separately below.[7]

Rhein and emodin are likely among the most active compounds in the Hoxsey and Essiac herbal formulas (see Box 14.1). Due to continued strong interest in these formulas by patients and practitioners, the pharmacokinetics of these anthraquinones are discussed at length here. The methods and data used to derive the concentration-time curves are discussed in Appendix K. These curves are based upon data obtained by administering ^{14}C-labeled emodin and rhein to rats. Since this data reflects the total amount of anthraquinones, which includes unknown anthraquinone metabolites, the actual amount of rhein and emodin present may be overestimated. For example, more than 40% of emodin may undergo break-down to non-anthraquinone fragments, most of which are excreted in the feces (Bachmann and Schlatter, 1981). However, plasma ^{14}C activity may reflect mostly the anthraquinone, as has been shown for rhein (Lang, 1988).

Rhein

The total rhein content in 24 samples of *da huang* obtained from various Asian markets was approximately 2.6% of the dry weight (pure rhein anthraquinone is present at approximately 0.3%) (Kashiwada et al., 1989, Oshio and Kawamura, 1985).[8] The bioavailability of orally administered rhein anthraquinone is approximately 30% in rats (Lang, 1988). Both rhein and emodin appear to undergo enterohepatic recycling at a rate of 20 to 30% (Lang, 1988; Bachmann and Schlatter, 1981).

As discussed in Section 11.3.7, the daily intraperitoneal dosage of rhein required for antitumor activity in mice appears to be approximately 40 mg/kg. The calculated plasma concentration-time curve for oral

---

[7] The author is currently preparing a paper containing refined data on rhein, emodin, and the Essiac formula.
[8] Total rhein includes rhein anthraquinone and rhein sennosides and glycosides. In addition, it includes approximately 50% of chrysophanol and chrysophanol glycosides, since these are converted in the body to rhein and aloe-emodin.

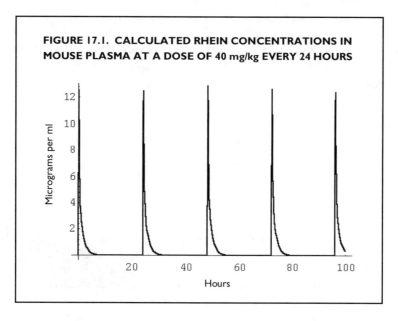

FIGURE 17.1. CALCULATED RHEIN CONCENTRATIONS IN MOUSE PLASMA AT A DOSE OF 40 mg/kg EVERY 24 HOURS

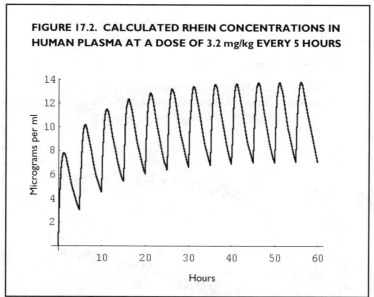

FIGURE 17.2. CALCULATED RHEIN CONCENTRATIONS IN HUMAN PLASMA AT A DOSE OF 3.2 mg/kg EVERY 5 HOURS

administration of this dose in mice is shown in Figure 17.1. Although the curve for intraperitoneal administration is likely to show greater retention than that for oral administration, due to the short half-life both curves are likely to display periods of low concentration between dosages. Therefore, it may be possible to optimize treatment by using a more frequent dosage schedule. In-vitro studies suggest that a maximum cytotoxic effect occurs when cells are continually exposed to rhein, and that rhein is cytotoxic at concentrations of 6 to 18 µg/ml (20 to 65 µM). For the purposes of this discussion, this is assumed to be equal to 6 to 18 µg/gram in wet tissue.

Based on the data and model presented in Appendix K, a calculated oral dose that may maintain a consistent plasma concentration within this range in humans is 3.2 mg/kg every 5 hours. The concentration-time curve for this dose is shown in Figure 17.2. This is equal to a daily dose of 1.1 grams of pure rhein (15 mg/kg). Assuming a 12% extraction efficiency in hot water (such as for emodin, see below), and a 10% conversion of sennosides to rhein anthraquinone in the intestines, the daily dose of rhubarb required for decoction is approximately 1.5 kilograms, or 250 times the normal dose for this herb. It would appear that purified rhein in capsule form may be more appropriate. If provided in this form, the required dose may not produce severe purgation. The dose of rhein that causes a purgative action in mice is 98 mg/kg (Oshio and Kawamura, 1985). If we divide this by 2 to account for administration every half-life, the purgative dose becomes 49 mg/kg. The equivalent human dose is 3.8 mg/kg every 5 hours, which is just above the target dose of 3.2 mg/kg.

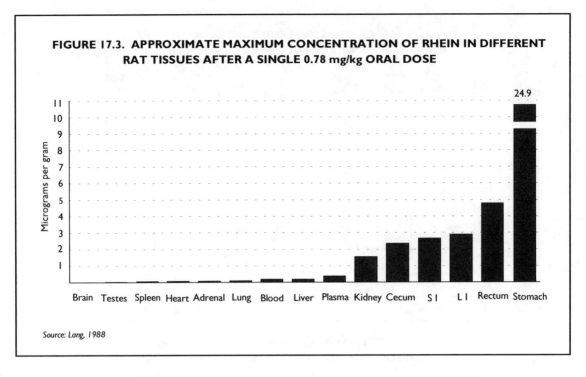

FIGURE 17.3. APPROXIMATE MAXIMUM CONCENTRATION OF RHEIN IN DIFFERENT RAT TISSUES AFTER A SINGLE 0.78 mg/kg ORAL DOSE

Source: Lang, 1988

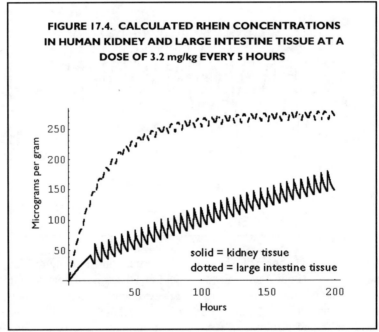

FIGURE 17.4. CALCULATED RHEIN CONCENTRATIONS IN HUMAN KIDNEY AND LARGE INTESTINE TISSUE AT A DOSE OF 3.2 mg/kg EVERY 5 HOURS

solid = kidney tissue
dotted = large intestine tissue

Concentrations of rhein are higher in kidney and intestinal tissue than in plasma (De Witte and Lemli, 1988a; Lang, 1988), and toxicity in these organs may limit the dosage.[9] Concentrations in various rat organs are shown in Figure 17.3. The concentration of rhein that is toxic to healthy tissue has not been determined, although rhein has demonstrated some cytotoxic specificity to neoplastic cells. As discussed in Section 11.3.7, concentrations of 100 µg/ml were only minimally toxic to

human bronchial epithelial cells in vitro. For our purposes we will assume that the concentration in kidney tissue should be maintained within 10 times the concentration cytotoxic to neoplastic cells in vitro, or approximately 100 µg/ml (~100 µg/gram wet weight).

The calculated concentration-time curve for human kidney and large intestine tissue for an oral dose of 3.2 mg/kg administered every 5 hours is shown in Figure 17.4. Concentrations in the stomach and rectum are

[9] The use of rhubarb in Chinese folk medicine for treating kidney cancer may reflect its uptake by that organ.

194

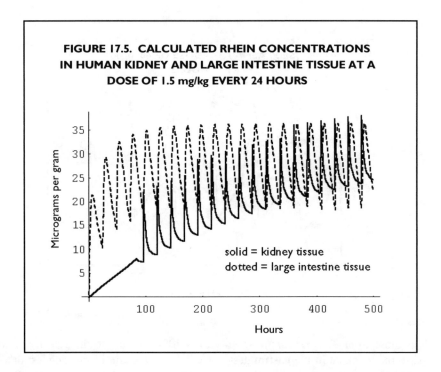

FIGURE 17.5. CALCULATED RHEIN CONCENTRATIONS IN HUMAN KIDNEY AND LARGE INTESTINE TISSUE AT A DOSE OF 1.5 mg/kg EVERY 24 HOURS

likely to be even greater. As can be seen, concentrations may exceed 100 µg/gram and, in the case of kidney tissue, continue to rise with time.

Two methods may be used to prevent toxicity to the kidneys. The first is to suspend administration of rhein for 48 hours after every 100 hours of treatment. This may limit rhein concentrations in the kidney to approximately 100 µg/gram, although the concentration in the large intestine may reach 250 µg/gram. It is not known if intestinal tissue is less sensitive than kidney tissue to rhein, although this is likely to be the case.

Second, the required dose could be significantly reduced by limiting treatment to cancers of the kidney and gastrointestinal system. A dose that produces an average concentration of approximately 30 µg/gram in the kidney and large intestine is 1.5 mg/kg every 24 hours. The concentration-time curves for this dose are shown in Figure 17.5. The maximum and minimum swings can be drawn tighter by dosing at 0.75 mg/kg every 12 hours. This dose will produce an average plasma concentration of approximately 1.5 µg/ml, well below the cytotoxic range.

A daily dose of 1.5 mg/kg requires 105 mg of rhein for a 70-kg human. This amount of rhein is contained in a decoction made from approximately 150 grams of rhubarb (again, assuming a 12% extraction efficiency in hot water and a 10% conversion of sennosides to rhein anthraquinone in the intestines). This is approximately 25 times the common dose for this herb. As can be seen, a number of technical difficulties arise when rhubarb is used as a source for rhein. First, rhein is not soluble in water and is only slightly soluble in alcohol. This requires extraction in other solvents. Second, a large percentage of the rhein contained in rhubarb is in the form of rhein glycosides and sennosides (see Figure 11.2). These must be converted to rhein anthraquinone prior to administration or a strong purgative effect and low rhein absorption will occur.

A number of strategies may increase the cytotoxic effect of rhein. One strategy is to administer rhein with agents that increase drug uptake in cancer cells, such as EPA/DHA, DMSO, or electrotherapy. DMSO and electrotherapy may be more appropriate for localized treatment, and EPA/DHA may be more appropriate for systemic use. As discussed in Section 12.3.2, DHA can increase the number of unsaturated double bonds in the plasma membrane of certain tumor cells in vitro by 31%. This may increase membrane fluidity and drug uptake. Incorporation of DHA into L1210 leukemia cells produced a 10-fold decrease in survival after doxorubicin treatment in vitro. Reduced survival was primarily due to increased intracellular concentrations of doxorubicin (Burns and Spector, 1990). It may prove optimal to administer EPA/DHA for one month prior to administration of rhein to allow cells to increase their omega-3 fatty acid content. Monitoring RBC fatty acids may provide a guide to treatment. A second advantage of administering EPA/DHA is that it inhibits the production of PGE_2, which is thought to be partially responsible for the purgative action of anthraquinones.

Another strategy that may theoretically increase plasma concentrations and decrease intestinal concentrations is to mix rhein with saponins prior to

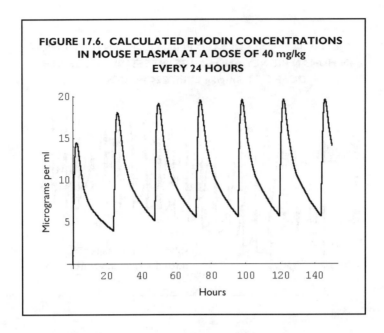

FIGURE 17.6. CALCULATED EMODIN CONCENTRATIONS IN MOUSE PLASMA AT A DOSE OF 40 mg/kg EVERY 24 HOURS

administration, such as those from *Glycyrrhiza sp. (gan cao)*. This may increase rhein uptake in the gastrointestinal system, potentially reducing the risk of toxicity in gastrointestinal organs. As mentioned above, approximately 30% of orally administered rhein is absorbed in rats, much of which undergoes enterohepatic recycling. Data are required to model this strategy.

Rhein does not appear to be carcinogenic. Sennosides and rhein have not produced genotoxic effects in vitro or in vivo (reviewed by Heidemann et al., 1993). However, rhein has been shown to act as a tumor-promoting agent in rat livers in vivo (Wolfle et al., 1990).

Emodin

As discussed in Section 11.3.7, emodin shows antitumor activity and has been reported to increase the leukocyte count in chemotherapy patients. Studies in mice suggest that emodin may produce an antitumor effect at a daily intraperitoneal dose of 5 to 75 mg/kg. The midpoint of this range (40 mg/kg) corresponds to a human dose of 3.2 mg/kg. The active in-vitro concentration ranges from 4 to 20 μg/ml (~4 to 20 μg/gram).

The average free emodin content in 23 *Rheum palmatum (da huang)* samples obtained from different markets in Asia was 0.16%. It was as low as 0.029% in some samples (Kashiwada et al., 1989). The concentration of emodin in *Polygonum cuspidatum (hu chang)*, *Polygonum multiflorum (he shou wu)*, and *Cassia tora (jue ming zi)* is approximately 1.1%, 0.006%, and 0.005% respectively (Liang et al., 1995). Studies on rabbit blood using HPLC suggest that the bioavailability of emodin after oral administration is very low (likely less

than 10%) (Liang et al., 1995). In contrast, studies on ^{14}C-labeled emodin in rats suggest that the bioavailability is closer to 50% (data in Appendix K). This higher value may be due to a higher absorption rate in rodents, or may be due to the detection of high levels of emodin metabolites in plasma or the calculation of bioavailability by excretion rather than by comparison of oral and intravenous responses. For example, the bioavailability of rhein in rats is approximately 50% when computed from excretion rates and 30% when computed from comparison of oral and intravenous responses (Lang, 1988). Due to its low water solubility, less then 12% of the emodin contained in plants is extracted by hot water (Liang et al., 1995).

Based on data presented in Appendix K, the calculated plasma concentration-time curve for a daily oral dose of 40 mg/kg in mice is shown in Figure 17.6. Although the curve for intraperitoneal administration is likely to vary from the curve for oral administration, both curves may display some similar characteristics. Figure 17.6 suggests that this dose produces an average plasma concentration of approximately 12 μg/ml, which is within the range of in-vitro cytotoxic activity.

The data and model presented in Appendix K do not allow the accurate extrapolation of emodin data from rats to humans. This is due to the difference in dose between that given to rats and the human dose of interest (see Appendix K). For those interested, the model predicts that the oral dose required to produce an average plasma concentration of 20 μg/ml in humans is 1.5 mg/kg every 24 hours. The time concentration curve for this dose is shown in Figure 17.7. This is equal to 100 mg/day for a 70-kg human, or the emodin contained in 79 grams of *Polygonum cuspidatum (hu chang)* (assuming a 12%

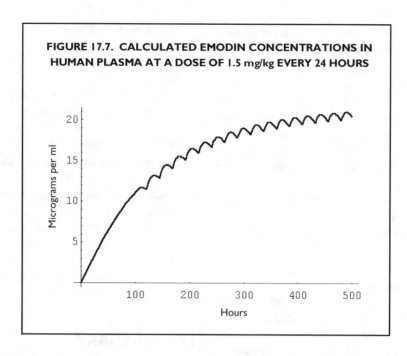

FIGURE 17.7. CALCULATED EMODIN CONCENTRATIONS IN HUMAN PLASMA AT A DOSE OF 1.5 mg/kg EVERY 24 HOURS

extraction efficiency in hot water). This is almost three times the normal dose of this herb.

A dose of 100 mg/day of pure emodin is not expected to produce purgation. The purgative dose in mice is greater than 500 mg/kg for a single administration (Natori et al., 1981:424). The equivalent human dose would be approximately 2.8 grams (40 mg/kg). A slight purgative action was caused by a single dose of 50 mg/kg in rats (Bachmann and Schlatter, 1981). The equivalent human dose is 770 mg (11 mg/kg).

Like rhein, emodin appears to concentrate in kidney and intestinal tissue in rats. In addition, emodin accumulates in adipose tissue (Bachmann and Schlater, 1981). Unfortunately, insufficient data are available to generate concentration-time curves for emodin in these tissues. If emodin possesses similar properties as rhein, quite likely the dose of emodin must be reduced below the 1.5 mg/kg per day calculated above to prevent the accumulation of toxic levels in these tissues. However, the amount of reduction required is unknown. Emodin appears to be markedly more persistent in the plasma than rhein, and if it is persistent in other tissues, a toxic dose could easily accumulate over time. When additional pharmacokinetic data are available, it may be possible to exploit these characteristics for clinical use. For example, its ability to accumulate in adipose tissue may allow its use against breast cancer and other cancers that are surrounded by large amounts of adipose tissue.

17.4 MULTIAGENT APPROACH TO TREATMENT

As suggested throughout this chapter, in theory it may be possible to obtain optimal clinical results by judiciously combining therapeutic agents. There are two ways in which this can be done:

- *Agents can be combined to reinforce one another.* For example, EPA could be combined with rhein to increase the cell uptake of rhein and reduce rhein's purgative effect. To inhibit invasion and metastasis, PSK could be combined with cartilage to inhibit both the heparanases and metalloproteinases that degrade the ECM. Other examples include the combination of glutathione, melatonin, and astragalus for their effects on IL-2, and the combination of limonene and quercetin for their effects on the secretion of transforming growth factor-beta. Many possibilities exist for these types of combinations. Natural agents can also be combined with traditional chemotherapy drugs to increase their efficacy. For example, quercetin could be combined with cytotoxic drugs to inhibit the development of drug resistance.

- *Agents can be combined to address multiple targets of a cancer.* For example, agents that may be effective against breast cancer include angiogenesis inhibitors, cytotoxic agents, agents that reduce estrogen bioavailability, immunostimulants, agents that inhibit invasion, and agents that inhibit metastasis (see Table 17.2). Agents that perform more than one of these actions, such as genistein or EPA, could be combined with other appropriate agents.

Individual agents can be chosen to address patient-specific conditions. For example:

- Immunostimulants could be used in patients who are immunosuppressed or are diagnosed with *qi vacuity*.

- Agents that inhibit platelet aggregation or induce fibrinolysis could be used in patients diagnosed with *blood stagnation* or coagulation disorders.

- Melatonin could be used in patients who have low plasma melatonin concentrations, especially if their tumors are estrogen-responsive.

- EPA could be used in patients with low tissue levels of omega-3 fatty acids.

- Vitamin D_3 could be used in patients with low plasma D_3 levels.

- Agents can be chosen to address the TCM diagnosis of the patient. This is particularly true of herbal agents. For example, appropriate immunostimulants for patients who are diagnosed with *yin vacuity* might be *Ligustrum lucidum (nu zhen zi)* and *Lycium barbarum (gou qi zi)*, which *supplement the yin and blood*, rather than *Astragalus membranaceus (huang qi)* and *Atractylodes macrocephala (bai zhu)*, which are contraindicated in patients with *yin vacuity*.

The above list is not inclusive, but suggests the general dual approach of tailoring the treatment to each patient and attempting to direct treatment using laboratory data wherever possible.

17.5 LABORATORY ANALYSIS

As mentioned above, laboratory assays can help to direct treatment. Obviously, laboratory assays are also important in many types of research. In addition to common laboratory assays (such as tumor-marker concentrations), other lab analyses may be useful for assessing the health of the cancer patient and monitoring the success of treatment. Where appropriate, these may include:

- **Digestive function assays:** These include comprehensive stool and digestive analysis (CSDA), intestinal permeability, and serum IgE/IgG4 food allergy panels. Chronic digestive malfunction is common in patients with chronic disease, but treatment can also impair digestive function. For example, chemotherapy may increase intestinal permeability to microorganisms and their endotoxins (O'Dwer et al., 1988), or otherwise compromise digestive function.

- **Liver function assays:** Liver enzyme assays detect the presence of gross liver damage. However, these tests are not designed to detect functional abnormalities. Functional assays, in particular, detoxification assays, may be useful. Various nutritional programs can be devised to support or stimulate P_{450} metabolism and conjugation reactions if necessary (Bland and Bralley, 1992).

- **Nutrient assays:** These include assays for amino acids, minerals, antioxidants, vitamins, fatty acids, and organic acids. Wherever possible, a program of nutritional supplementation should be based upon assay results and should be monitored periodically to evaluate the effectiveness of therapy.

- **Immune function assays:** These include natural killer cell function and population, macrophage function, and secretory IgA levels.

- **Other assays to direct treatment:** This book discusses numerous plasma factors which may affect the progression of cancer. Analysis for any of these may be appropriate to direct treatment. For example, sex hormone binding globulin levels could be monitored to direct treatment with certain antiestrogen agents.

17.6 SUMMARY

A large number of natural agents may be useful in treating cancer. Some of these may be beneficial when used singularly, but many may produce optimal results when combined judiciously with other agents and when selected to meet the specific conditions of the individual patient in question. Unfortunately, this approach of combined and patient-specific therapies is not easily transferred to the arena of research. This makes it all the more imperative that practitioners who are familiar with these treatment concepts and with the traditional uses of natural agents become involved in research. The possibilities for combining the resources of both conventional and traditional medicines within the same research project are greater today then they ever have been. This is truly an exciting time. Which of the agents discussed in this book will be recognized in the not-to-distant future as components of a successful anticancer therapy?

APPENDIX A: LIST OF CHINESE HERBS

This appendix lists the majority of Chinese herbs mentioned in the text or in other appendices. It is not intended to be a definitive listing of herbal agents, and the reference sources should be consulted when additional information is needed. Note that a number of mandarin and pharmaceutical names may refer to one or more genus and/or species names in addition to those listed. For example, *wang bu liu xing* (Semen Vaccariae) refers to *Vaccaria segetalis*, as listed, but may also refer to the seed of *Ficus pumila*, *Hypericum sampsoni*, or *Vicia sativa*, depending on what part of China the herb comes from. See the references for these additional listings. Obviously, the lack of exclusive nomenclature is problematic. Also note that the maximum dose listed in the table generally refers to that for hot water decoctions or infusions. However, in some cases, the dose refers to powders. See the references for additional information.

BOTANICAL/ ZOOLOGICAL NAME	MANDARIN NAME	PHARMACEUTICAL NAME	MAX. DOSE gram/d	CATEGORY	COMMON NAME
Acanthopanax senticoccus	*ci wu jia*	Radix Acanthopanacis Senticosi	15	*Dispel wind dampness*	
Achyranthes bidentata	*huai niu xi, niu xi*	Radix Achyranthis Bidentatae	15	*Regulate the blood*	
Aconitum carmichaelii	*chuan wu, wu tou*	Radix Aconiti Carmichaeli	9	*Warm the interior*	Sichuan aconite
Acorus ramineus	*shi chuang pu, chuang pu*	Rhizoma Acori Graminei	9	*Open the portals*	Sweetflag rhizome
Actinidia chinensis	*teng li*	Fructus Actinidiae Chinensis	60	*Clear heat*	
Adenophorae stricta	*nan sha shen*	Radix Adenophorae	15	*Supplement the yin*	Ladybell root, southern sand root
Adina rubella	*shui yang mei*	Herba Adinae	15	*Clear heat toxins*	
Aesculus hippocastanum	*so lo tzu*	Aesculi Fructus	9	*Supplement the qi*	Horse chestnut
Agkistrodon acutus	*bai hua she*	Agkistrodon seu Bungarus	10	*Dispel wind dampness*	Agkistrodon snake
Agrimonia pilosa	*xian he cao*	Herba Agrimoniae Pilosae	15	*Stop bleeding*	
Ailanthus altissima	*chun pai pi, chuen gen bi*	Cortex Ailanthi	9	*Astringent*	Tree of heaven bark
Akebia trifoliata	*mu tong*	Caulis Mutong	9	*Percolate damp*	
Alisma plantago-aquatica	*ze xie*	Rhizoma Alismatis Plantago-Aquaticae	15	*Percolate damp*	Water plantain rhizome
Allium bakeri	*xie bai*	Allii Chinensis Bulbus	18	*Rectify the qi*	Chinese chive
Allium sativum	*da suan*	Allii Bulbus	15	*Expel parasites*	Garlic
Allium tuberosum	*jiu zi*	Semen Allii Tuberosi	9	*Supplement the yang*	Chinese leek seeds
Alpinia oxyphllya	*yi zhi ren*	Fructus Alpiniae Oxyphyllae	9	*Supplement the yang*	Wild cardamon seed
Alum	*ming fan, bai fan*	Alumen	3	*Topical application*	
Amorphophallus rivieri	*ju ruo*	Rhizoma Amorphophalli	15	*Transform cold phlegm*	
Amyda rinensis	*bie jia*	Carpax Amydae Sinensis	30	*Supplement the yin*	Chinese soft-shell turtle shell
Andrographitis paniculatae	*chuan xin lian*	Herba Andrographitis Paniculatae	15	*Clear heat toxins*	
Angelica dahurica	*bai zhi*	Radix Angelicae	9	*Warm and resolve the exterior*	Chinese angelica root
(Table continues)					

199

TABLE A.1. (continued)					
BOTANICAL/ ZOOLOGICAL NAME	**MANDARIN NAME**	**PHARMACEUTICAL NAME**	**MAX. DOSE gram/d**	**CATEGORY**	**COMMON NAME**
Angelica sinensis or A. acutiloba	*dang gui*	Radix Angelicae Sinensis	15	*Supplement the blood*	
Arca inflata	*wa leng zi*	Concha Arcae	30	*Regulate the blood*	Cockle/ark shell
Arctium lappa	*niu bang zi*	Fructus Arctii Lappae	9	*Cool and resolve the exterior*	Burdock fruit
Ardisia japonica	*zi jin niu*	Herba Ardisiae	12	*Regulate blood*	
Ardisia japonica	*jin niu cao*	Herba Ardisiae	12	*Clear heat*	
Areca catchu	*bing lang*	Semen Arecae Catechu	12	*Expel parasites*	
Arisaema consanguineum	*tian nan xing*	Rhizoma Arisaematis	9	*Transform cold phlegm*	Jack-in-the-pulpit rhizome
Aristolchia debilis	*ma dou ling*	Fructus Aristolochiae	9	*Stop coughing*	Birthwort fruit
Aristolochia mollissima	*xun gu feng*	Herba Aristolochiae	15	*Dispel wind dampness*	Hairy birthwort
Artemesia annua	*qing hao*	Herba Artemesiae Annuae	9	*Clear heat*	Sweet wormwood
Artemisia anomala	*liu ji nu*	Herba Artemisiae Anomalae	9	*Regulate the blood*	
Artemisia argyi	*ai ye*	Folium Artemisiae	9	*Stop bleeding*	Mugwort leaf
Asclepius curassavica	*ma li jin*	Asclepiadis Herba		*Clear heat*	
Asparagus cochinchinensis	*tian men dong*	Tuber Asparagi Cochinchinensis	15	*Supplement the yin*	Asparagus tuber
Astragalus complanatus	*sha yuan ji li*	Semen Astragali	15	*Supplement the yang*	Flattened milk-vetch seed
Astragalus membranaceus	*huang qi*	Radix Astragali	30	*Supplement the qi*	Yellow milk vetch root
Atractylodes macrocephala	*bai zhu*	Rhizoma Atractylodis Macrophalae	9	*Supplement the qi*	
Atractylodis lancea	*cang zhu*	Atractylodes Lanceae Rhizoma	9	*Transform damp*	Red atractylodes
Baphicacanthus cusia	*ban lan gen*	Radix Isatidis sue Baphicacanthi	30	*Clear heat toxins*	Woad root
Belamcanda chinensis	*she gan*	Rhizoma Belamcandae Chinensis	9	*Clear heat toxins*	Blackberry lily rhizome
Benincasa cerifera	*dong gua zi*	Benincasae Semen	30	*Clear Heat and Phlegm*	Wax gourd seed, wintermelon seed
Bletilla striata	*bai ji*	Rhizoma Bletillae Striatae	15	*Stop bleeding*	
Bombyx mori	*jiang can*	Bombyx Batryticatus	9	*Extinguish wind*	Silkworm
Bos taurus domesticus	*niu huang*	Calculus Bovis	15	*Open the portals*	Ox or water buffalo gallstone
Boswellia carterii	*ru xiang*	Gummi Olibanum	9	*Regulate the blood*	Frankincense
Brucea javanica	*ya dan zi*	Fructus Brucae Javanicae	1	*Expel parasites*	Java brucea fruit
Bufo bufo gargarizans	*chan su*	Secretio Bufonis	0.03	*Topical application*	Toad venom
Bufo bufo gargarizans	*chan su*	Pericarpium Bufonis	15	*Topical application*	Toad skin
Bupleurum chinense	*chai hu*	Radix Bupleuri	12	*Cool and resolve the exterior*	
Buthus martensi	*quan xie*	Buthus Martensi	6	*Extinguish wind*	Scorpion
Camelliae folium	*cha ye*	Camelliae Folium	9	*Percolate damp*	
Camptotheca acuminata	*xi shu*	Fructus Camptothecae	9	*Regulate the blood*	
Canarium album	*gan lan*	Fructus Canarii	9	*Clear heat toxins*	Chinese olive
Cannabis sativa	*huo ma ren*	Semen Cannabis Sativae	15	*Drain precipitation*	Hemp seed, marihuana seed
(Table continues)					

		TABLE A.1. *(continued)*			
BOTANICAL/ ZOOLOGICAL NAME	**MANDARIN NAME**	**PHARMACEUTICAL NAME**	**MAX. DOSE gram/d**	**CATEGORY**	**COMMON NAME**
Carthamus tinctorius	*hong hua*	Flos Carthami Tinctorii	9	*Regulate the blood*	Safflower flower
Cassia acutifolia	*fan xie ye*	Sennae Folium	9	*Drain precipitation*	
Cassia obtusifolia, C. tora	*jue ming zi*	Cassiae Torae Semen	15	*Quell fire*	
Catharanthus roseus	*chang chun hua*	Catharanthi Herba	15	*Calm Spirit*	Madagscar periwinkle
Centipeda minima	*shi hu sui*	Herba Centipedae	9	*Transform cold phlegm*	
Cephalanoplos segetum	*xiao ji*	Herba Cephalanoplos	18	*Stop bleeding*	Small thistle. field thistle
Cervus nippon, C. temmiinck	*lu rong*	Cornu Cervi Parvum	2.4	*Supplement the yang*	Velvet of young deer antler
Chaenomeles lagenaria	*mu gua*	Fructus Chaenomelis Lagenariae	12	*Dispel wind dampness*	Chinese quince
Chinemys reevesii	*gui ban*	Plastrum Testudinis	30	*Supplement the yin*	Fresh-water turtle shell
Chrysanthemum indicum	*ye ju hua*	Flos Chrysanthemi Indici	12	*Cool and resolve the exterior*	Wild chrysanthemum flower
Cibotium barometz	*gou ji*	Rhizoma Cibotii Barometz	9	*Supplement the yang*	Chain fern rhizome
Cinnamomum cassia	*rou gui*	Cortex Cinnamomi Cassiae	4.5	*Warm the interior*	Cinnamon bark
Cinnamomum cassia	*gui zhi*	Ramulus Cinnamomi Cassiae	9	*Warm and resolve the exterior*	Cinnamon twig
Cirsium japonicum	*da xiao ji, da ji*	Herba Cirsii Japonici	15	*Stop bleeding*	Japanese thistle
Cistanchesalsa	*rou cong rong*	Herba Cistanches	18	*Supplement the yang*	Stem of broomrape
Citrus reticulata	*chen pi, ju pi*	Pericarpium Citri Reticulatae	9	*Rectify the qi*	Tangerine peel
Clematis chinensis	*wei ling xian*	Radix Clemetidis Chinensis	12	*Dispel wind dampness*	
Cnidium monnieri	*she chuang zi*	Fructus Cnidii Monnieri	9	*Topical application*	Snake's bed seeds
Codonopsis pilosula	*dang shen*	Radix Codonopsis Pilosulae	9	*Supplement the qi*	Asiabell root
Coix lalchryma-jobi	*yi yi ren*	Semen Coicis Lachryma-Jobi	30	*Percolate damp*	Job's tears seeds
Commiphora myrrha	*mo yao*	Resinae Myrrhae	12	*Regulate the blood*	Myrrh gum-resin
Coptis chinensis	*huang lian*	Rhizoma Coptidis	9	*Clear damp heat*	
Cordyceps sinensis	*dong chong xia cao*	Cordyceps Sinensis	15	*Supplement the yang*	Chinese caterpillar fungus
Cornus officinalis	*shan zhu yu*	Fructus Corni Officinalis	12	*Astringent*	
Corydalis yanhusuo	*yan hu suo*	Rhizoma Corydalis Yanhusuo	12	*Regulate the blood*	
Crataegus oxyacantha	*shan zha*	Crataegi Fructus	12	*Relieve food accumulation*	
Cremastra variabilis	*shan ci gu*	Tuber Shancigu	15	*Topical application*	
Crocus sativa	*fan hong hua*	Crocus (Croci Stigma)	3	*Regulate the blood*	Saffron
Crotalaria sessiliflora	*ye bai he*	Herba Crotalariae Sessiliflorae	30	*Clear heat toxins*	Narrow-leaved rattlebox
Cryptotympana atrata	*chan tui*	Cicidae Periostracum	30	*Cool and resolve the exterior*	Cicada
Cucurbita maxima	*nan gua zi*	Cucurbitae Semen	120	*Expel parasites*	Pumpkin seed
		(Table continues)			

201

TABLE A.1. *(continued)*					
BOTANICAL/ ZOOLOGICAL NAME	**MANDARIN NAME**	**PHARMACEUTICAL NAME**	**MAX. DOSE gram/d**	**CATEGORY**	**COMMON NAME**
Cudrania tricuspidata	*da ding huang*	Lignum Cudraniae	60	*Dispel wind dampness*	
Curculigo orchioiodes	*xian mao*	Rhizoma Curculiginis Orchioidis	9	*Supplement the yang*	
Curcuma zedoaria	*e zhu*	Rhizoma Curcumae Zedoariae	9	*Regulate the blood*	
Curcuma longa	*yu jin*	Tuber Curcumae	9	*Regulate the blood*	Tumeric tuber
Cuscuta chinensis, C. australis	*tu si zi*	Semen Cuscutae	15	*Supplement the yang*	Dodder seed
Cycas revoluta	*tieh shu*	Folium Cycadis	15	*Clear heat*	
Cynomorium songaricum	*suo yang*	Herba Cynomorii Songarici	15	*Supplement the yang*	
Daemonorops draco	*xue jie*	Sanguis Draconis	1.5	*Regulate the blood*	Dragon's blood
Daphne genkwa	*yuan hua*	Flos Daphnes Genkwa	3	*Drain precipitation*	
Dendrobium nobile	*shi hu*	Herba Dendrobii	12	*Supplement the yin*	
Desmodium styracifolium	*jin qian cao*	Herba Desmodii	60	*Clear heat*	
Dianthus superbus	*qu mai*	Herba Dianthi	12	*Percolate damp*	
Dichondra repens	*xiao jin qian cao*	Herba Dichondra	60	*Percolate damp*	
Dichroa febrifuga	*chang shan*	Radix Dichroae Febrifuga	9	*Expel parasites*	
Dictamnus dasycarpus	*bai xian pi*	Cortex Dictamni Dasycarpi Radicis	9	*Clear heat toxins*	Dittany root bark
Dioscorea opposita	*shan yao*	Radix Dioscoreae Oppositae	30	*Supplement the qi*	Wild Chinese yam
Dioscorea bulbifera	*huang yao zi*	Tuber Dioscoreae Bulbiferae	15	*Transform hot phlegm*	
Diospyros kaki	*shi di*	Calyx Diospyri Kaki	12	*Regulate the qi*	
Dipsacus japonica	*xu duan*	Radix Dipsaci	12	*Supplement the yang*	Teasel root
Duchesnea indica	*she mei*	Herba Duchesneae	15	*Clear heat toxins*	Snake strawberry
Eclipta prostrata	*han lian cao*	Herba Ecliptae Prostratae	30	*Supplement the yin*	
Ephedra sinica	*ma huang*	Herba Euphedrae	9	*Warm and resolve the exterior*	Hemp yellow
Epimedium grandiflorum	*yin yang huo, xian ling pi*	Herba Epimedii	12	*Supplement the yang*	
Epimedium sagittatum	*yin yang huo*	Herba Epimedii	15	*Supplement the yang*	Licentious goat wort
Equus asinus	*e jiao*	Gelatinum Corii Asini	15	*Supplement the blood*	Donkey hide gelatin
Eriobotrya japonica	*pi pa ye*	Folium Eriobotryae Japonicae	12	*Stop coughing*	Loquat leaf
Eucommia ulmoides	*du zhong*	Cortex Eucommiae Ulmoidis	15	*Supplement the yang*	
Eugenia caryophyllata	*ding xiang*	Carophylli Flos	5	*Warm the interior*	Cloves
Eupatorium fortunei, E. japonicum	*pei lan*	Herba Eupatorii Fortunei	9	*Transform dampness*	Boneset, feverwort
Euphoria longan	*long yan rou, gui yuan rou*	Arillus Euphoriae Longanae	15	*Supplement the blood*	Logan fruit
Eupolyphaga sinensis	*tu bie chong*	Eupolyphagae seu Opisthoplatiae	6	*Regulate the blood*	Wingless cockroach
Ficus carica	*wu hua guo*	Fici Caricae Flos	60	*Clear heat*	Fig flower
(Table continues)					

TABLE A.1. (continued)					
BOTANICAL/ ZOOLOGICAL NAME	**MANDARIN NAME**	**PHARMACEUTICAL NAME**	**MAX. DOSE gram/d**	**CATEGORY**	**COMMON NAME**
Ficus pumila	*xue li shi*	Fructus Fici Pumilae	15	*Supplement the yang*	Fig
Foeniculum vulgare	*xiao hui xiang*	Foeniculi Fructus	5	*Warm the interior*	Fennel
Forsythia suspensa	*lian qiao*	Fructus Forsythiae Suspensae	15	*Clear heat toxins*	Forsythia fruit
Fritillaria thunbrergii	*zhe bei mu*	Bulbus Fritillariae Thungergii	9	*Transform hot phlegm*	
Galium aparine	*zhu yang yang*	Herba Galii Aparines	60	*Clear heat*	
Gallus gallus domesticus	*ji nei jin*	Endithelium Corneum Gigeraiae Galli	9	*Relieve food accumulation*	Chicken gizzard internal lining
Ganoderma lucidum	*ling zhi*	Ganoderma	9	*Quiet the spirit*	Reishi
Gardenia jasminoides	*zhi zi*	Fructus Gardenia Jasminoidis	12	*Quell fire*	
Gekko chinensis	*tian long, ge jie*	Gekko gecko	15	*Supplement the yang*	
Gentiana scabra	*long dan cao*	Radix Gentianae Scabrae	9	*Clear damp heat*	
Geranium wilfordii	*gennoshiouko* (Japanese)	Herba Geranii	15	*Extinguish wind*	Japanese geranium
Ginkgo biloba	*yin xing*	Ginkgo Semen	15	*Astringent*	
Gleditsia sinensis	*zao jiao ci*	Spina Gleditsiae Sinensis	1.5	*Transform cold phlegm*	Honeylocust fruit, soap bean
Glehnia littoralis	*bei sha shen*	Radix Glehiae Littoralis	15	*Supplement the yin*	Northern sand root
Glycyrrhiza uralensis	*gan cao*	Radix Glycyrrhizae Uralensis	12	*Supplement the qi*	Licorice root
Gossypium herbaceum	*mian hua gen*	Radix Gossypii	60	*Stop coughing*	Cotton root
Grifola umbellata	*zhu ling*	Polyporus	15	*Percolate damp*	
Gynostemma pentaphyllum	*jiao gu lan*	Herba Gynostemma Pentaphyllum	20	*Supplement the qi*	
Heliotropium indicum	*er gou cao*	Herba Heliotropii	12	*Clear heat*	
Hibiscus mutabilis	*fu rong ye*	Folium Hibisci Mutabilis	18	*Clear heat*	
Hirudo nipponia	*shui zhi*	Hirudo seu Whitmaniae	3	*Regulate the blood*	Leech
Homo sapien	*zi he che, tai yi*	Placenta Hominis	9	*Supplement the yang*	Human placenta
Houttuynia cordata	*yu xing cao*	Herba Houttuyniae Cordatae	60	*Clear heat toxins*	Fish smell plant
Hypericum japonicum	*tian ji huang*	Hyperici Herba	60	*Clear heat*	
Impatiens balsamina	*ji xing zi*	Semen Impatientis	60	*Regulate the blood*	Touch-me-not seed
Impatiens balsamina	*tou gu cao*	Herba Impatiens	15	*Warm and resolve the exterior*	Touch-me-not
Imperata cylindrica	*mao gen*	Rhizoma Imperatae Cylindricae	30	*Stop bleeding*	
Inula helerium	*mu xiang*	Saussureae Radix	9	*Rectify the qi*	
Iris pallasii	*ma lin zi*	Iridis Semen	9	*Clear heat*	Iris seed
Isatis tinctoria	*qing dai*	Indigo pulverata pevis	4	*Clear heat toxins*	Indigo
Isatis tinctoria	*da qing ye*	Folium Daqingye	30	*Clear heat toxins*	Woad leaf
Juglans regia	*hu tao ren*	Semen Juglandis Regiae	30	*Supplement the yang*	Walnut
Laminaria japonica	*kun bu*	Thallus Algae	15	*Transform hot phlegm*	Kelp kombu
Lasiosphaera nipponica	*ma bo*	Frucificatio Lasiosphaerae	4.5	*Clear heat toxins*	Puffball
(Table continues)					

BOTANICAL/ ZOOLOGICAL NAME	MANDARIN NAME	PHARMACEUTICAL NAME	MAX. DOSE gram/d	CATEGORY	COMMON NAME
Ledebouriella divaricata, L. sesoloides	*fang feng*	Radix Ledebouriellae	9	*Warm and resolve the exterior*	Guard against wind
Leonurus heterophyllus	*yi mu cao*	Herba Leonuri Heterophylii	30	*Regulate the blood*	Motherwort
Lepidium apetalum	*ting li zi*	Semen Tinglizi	9	*Drain precipitation*	Tansy mustard seed
Lespedeza cuneata	*ye guan men*	Herba Lespedezae	30	*Regulate the blood*	
Ligusticum wallichii	*chuan xiong*	Radix Ligustici Wallichii	6	*Regulate the blood*	Szechuan lovage root
Ligustrum lucidum	*nu zhen zi*	Fructus Ligustri Lucidi	15	*Supplement the yin*	Privet fruit
Lindera strychnifolia	*wu yao*	Radix Linderae Strychnifoliae	9	*Regulate the qi*	
Liquidambar orientalis	*su he xiang*	Styrax	1	*Open the portals*	Sweet gum
Lithospermum erythrorhizon	*zi cao*	Radix Lithospermi seu Arnebiae	9	*Cool blood*	Groomwell fruit
Livistona chinensis	*kui shu zi*	Semen Livistonae	30	*Clear heat*	Fan palm seed
Lobelia chinensis	*ban bian lian*	Herba Lobeliae Chinensis cum Radice	30	*Percolate damp*	
Lonicera japonica	*jin yin hua*	Flos Lonicerae Japonicae	15	*Clear heat toxins*	Honeysuckle flower
Lopthatherum gracile	*dan zhu ye*	Herba Lophatheri Gracilis	9	*Quell fire*	Bamboo leaf and stem
Loranthus parasiticus	*sang ji sheng*	Ramus Loranthi seu Visci	16	*Supplement the yin*	Mulberry mistletoe
Luffa cylindrica	*si gua luo*	Fasciculus Vascularis Luffae	12	*Regulate the blood*	Luffa sponge
Lycium chinense	*gou qi zi*	Fructus Lycii Chinensis	15	*Supplement the blood*	Wolfberry fruit
Lycopus lucidus	*ze lan*	Herba Lycopi Lucidi	9	*Regulate the blood*	Bugleweed
Lygodii japonici	*hai jin sha*	Spora Lygodii Japonici	15	*Clear heat toxins*	Climbing fern spore
Lysimachia christinae	*jin qian cao*	Herba Lysimachiae	60	*Percolate damp*	
Magnolia liliflora, M. salicifolia	*xin ye hua*	Magnolia Flos	6	*Cool and resolve the exterior*	Magnolia flower
Magnolia officinalis	*hou po*	Cortex Magnoliae Officinalis	9	*Transform dampness*	
(Mammal bones)	*long gu*	Os Draconis	30	*Quiet the spirit*	
Manis pentadactyla	*chuan shan jia*	Squama Manitis Pentadactylae	9	*Regulate the blood*	Anteater scales, pagolin scales
Melia toosendan	*chuan lian zi*	Fructus Meliae Toosendan	9	*Rectify the qi*	Chinaberry fruit, pagoda tree fruit
Millettia dielsiana	*ji xue teng*	Radix et Caulis Jixueteng	15	*Regulate the blood*	Chicken blood vine
Momordica grosvenori	*luo han guo*	Fructus Momordicae Grosvenori	15	*Supplement the yin*	
Mori alba	*sang shen*	Fructus Morialbae	15	*Supplement the blood*	White mulberry fruit bud
Morinda officinalis	*ba ji tian, ba ji*	Radix Morindae Officinalis	15	*Supplement the yang*	
Moschus moschiferus	*she xiang*	Secretio Moschus Moschiferi	0.15	*Open the portals*	Musk
Mylabris phalerata	*ban mao*	Mylabris	0.06	*Topical application*	Chinese blistering beetle
Myrica rubra	*yang mei pi*	Myricae Cortex	21	*Rectify the qi*	
Nelumbo nucifera	*ou jie*	Nodus Nelumbinis Nuciferae	15	*Stop bleeding*	Lotus node

(Table continues)

204

	TABLE A.1. *(continued)*				
BOTANICAL/ ZOOLOGICAL NAME	**MANDARIN NAME**	**PHARMACEUTICAL NAME**	**MAX. DOSE gram/d**	**CATEGORY**	**COMMON NAME**
Oldenlandia diffusa (Heydyotis diffusa)	*bai hua she she cao*	Herba Oldenlandiae Diffusae	60	*Clear heat toxins*	
Ophiopogon japonicus	*mai men dong*	Tuber Ophiopogonis Japonici	15	*Supplement the yin*	Creeping lily-turf tuber
Ostrea gigas	*mu li*	Concha Ostreae	30	*Quiet the spirit*	Oyster shell
Paeonia lactiflora	*bai shao yao, bai shao*	Radix Paeoniae Lactiflorae	15	*Supplement the blood*	White peony root
Paeonia obovata	*chi shao yao, chi shao*	Radix Paeoniae Ruba	9	*Regulate the blood*	Red peony root
Paeonia moutan	*mu dan pi*	Moutan Radicis Cortex	9	*Cool the blood*	Moutan
Panax ginseng	*ren shen*	Radix Ginseng	9	*Supplement the qi*	
Panax pseudoginseng	*tian san qi, san qi*	Radix Pseudoginseng	3	*Stop bleeding*	Notoginseng root
Panax quinquefolium	*xi yang shen*	Radix Panacis Quinquefolii	9	*Supplement the yin*	American ginseng root
Paridis polyphyllae, P. formosana	*cao he che*	Rhizoma Paridis Polyphyllae	30	*Clear heat*	Snakeweed rhizome
Patrina villosa	*bai jiang cao*	Thlaspi Herba	30	*Clear heat toxins*	Penny-cress, Snow-thistle
Patrinia scabiosaefolia, Paridis formosana	*bai jiang cao*	Herba Baijiangcao	15	*Clear heat*	Patrinia
Perilla frutescens	*su zi*	Fructus Perillae Frutescentis	9	*Stop coughing*	
Peucedanum praeruptorum	*qian hu*	Radix Peucedani	9	*Transform hot phlegm*	
Peucedanum praeruptorum	*qian hu*	Radix Peucedani	9	*Transform hot phlegm*	
Phellodendron amurense	*huang bai, huang bo*	Cortex Phellodendri	12	*Clear damp heat*	
Pheretima aspergillum	*di long*	Lumbricus	12	*Extinguish wind*	Earthworm
Picrorrhiza kurroa	*hu huang lian*	Rhizoma Picrorhizae	9	*Clear heat*	
Pinellia ternata	*ban xia*	Rhizoma Pinelliae Ternatae	12	*Transform cold phlegm*	
Pinus tabulaeformis	*song jie*	Lignum Pini Nodi	15	*Dispel wind damp*	
Piper kadsure	*pi bo*	Piperis Longi Fructus	5	*Warm the interior*	Long pepper
Piper wallichii	*shi nan teng*	Piperis Wallichi Caulis et Folium	15	*Dispel wind damp*	Wild pepper
Plantago asiatica	*che qian cao*	Herba Plantaginis	30	*Percolate damp*	Plantain
Platycodon grandiflorum	*jie geng, ku jie geng*	Radix Platycodi Grandiflori	9	*Transform cold phlegm*	Balloonflower root
Podohyyllum pleianthum [=Dysosma pleianthum]	*ba jiao lian*	Rhizome Podophylli	12	*Clear heat*	
Polistes mandarinus	*lu feng fang*	Nidus Vespae	12	*Topical application*	Hornet's nest, wasp's nest
Polygonatum odoratum	*yu zhu*	Rhizoma Polygonati Odorati	15	*Supplement the yin*	Fragrant Solomon's seal
Polygonatum Sibiricum	*huang jing*	Rhizoma Polygonati	18	*Supplement the qi*	Siberian Solomon's seal
Polygoni salicifolii	*shui hong hua zi*	Fructus Polygoni Salicifolii	9	*Clear heat toxins*	Water pepper
Polygonum perfoliatum	*gang ban gui*	Herba Polygoni Perfoliati	15	*Percolate damp*	Prickly polygonum
Polygonum multiflorum	*he shou wu, shou wu*	Radix Polygoni Multiflori	30	*Supplement the blood*	Fleeceflower root, fo-ti root
	(Table continues)				

205

		TABLE A.1. (continued)			
BOTANICAL/ ZOOLOGICAL NAME	MANDARIN NAME	PHARMACEUTICAL NAME	MAX. DOSE gram/d	CATEGORY	COMMON NAME
Polygonum multiflorum	ye jiao teng	Caulis Polygoni Multiflori	30	Quiet the spirit	Fleeceflower stem, fo-ti stem
Polygonum cuspidatum	hu zhang	Radix et Rhizoma Polygoni Cuspidati	30	Regulate the blood	Giant knotweed rhizome
Polyporus umbellatus	zhu ling	Sclerotium Polypori Umbellati	15	Percolate damp	
Poria cocos	fu ling	Sclerotium Poriae Cocos	15	Percolate damp	Hoelen, tuckahoe
Portulaca oleracea	ma chi xian	Herba Portulacae Oleraceae	60	Clear heat toxins	Purslane
Prunella vulgaris	xia ku cao	Spica Prunellae Vulgaris	15	Quell fire	Selfheal spike,
Prunus persicae	tao ren	Semen Persicae	9	Regulate the blood	Peach seed kernal
Pseudostellaria heterophylla	hai er shen, tai zi shen	Radix Pseudostellariae Heterophyllae	15	Supplement the qi	Prince ginseng root
Psoralea corylifolia	bu gu zhi	Fructus Psoralae Corylifoliae	9	Supplement the yang	
Pueraria lobata	ge gen	Radix Puerariae	12	Cool and resolve the exterior	
Pulsatilla chinensis	bai tou weng	Radix Pulsatillae Chinensis	15	Clear heat toxins	Anemone root
(Pyritum)	zi ran tong	Pyritum	9	Regulate the blood	Pyrite
Pyrrosia lingua	shi wei	Folium Pyrrosiae	9	Percolate damp	
Rabdosia rubescens	dong ling cao	Herba Rabdosiae Rubescens	6		
Ranunculus teratus	mao zhua cao	Radix Ranunculi Ternati	15	Clear heat toxins	
(Realgar)	xiong huang	Realgar	0.3	Topical application	Arsenic disulfide
Rehmannia glutinosa	sheng di huang	Radix Rehmanniae Glutinosae	30	Cool blood	Fresh Chinese foxglove root
Rehmannia glutinosa	shu di huang, shu di	Radix Rehmanniae Glutinosae Conquitae	30	Supplement the blood	Prepared Chinese foxglove root
Rhaponticum uniflorum	lou lu	Radix Rhapontici seu Echinops	12	Clear heat toxins	Echinops root
Rheum tanguticum	da huang	Rhizoma Rhei	6	Drain precipitation	Rhubarb root
Rhus chinensis / Melaphis chinensis	wu bei zi	Galla Rhi Chinensis	6	Astringent	Gallnut of Chinese sumac
Rubia cordifolia	qian cao gen	Radix Rubiae Cordifoliae	9	Stop bleeding	Madder root
Rumex japonicus	yang ti	Radix Rumecis	15	Stop bleeding	
Salvia chinensis	shi jian chuan	Herba Salviae Chinensis	30	Regulate the blood	
Salvia miltiorrhiza	dan shen	Radix Salvia Miltiorrhizae	15	Regulate the blood	Red sage root
Sargassum fusiforme	hai zao	Herba Sargassii	15	Transform hot phlegm	Sargassum seaweed
Sargentodoxa cuneata	hong teng	Caulis Sargentodoxae	15	Clear heat toxins	
Saururus chinensis	san bai cao	Herba Saururi	15	Percolate damp	
Schisandra chinensis	wu wei zi	Fructus Schisandrae Chinensis	9	Astringent	Northern schisandra fruit
Scolopendra subspinipes	wu gong	Scolopendra Subspinipes	4.5	Extinguish wind	Centipede
Scrophularia ningpoensis	xuan shen	Radix Scrophulariae Ningpoensis	30	Cool blood	Figwort root
Scutellaria baicalensis	huang qin	Radix Scutellariae Baicalensis	15	Clear damp heat	
Scutellariae barbatae	ban zhi lian	Herba Scutellariae Barbatae	30	Clear heat toxins	
Selaginella doederleinii	shi shang bai	Herba Selaginellae Doederleinii	60	Clear heat toxins	
Semiaquilegia adoxoides	tian kui zi	Radix Semiaquilegia	9	Clear heat toxins	
		(Table continues)			

TABLE A.1. *(continued)*

BOTANICAL/ ZOOLOGICAL NAME	MANDARIN NAME	PHARMACEUTICAL NAME	MAX. DOSE gram/d	CATEGORY	COMMON NAME
Senecio integrifolius	*kou she cao*	Herba Senecionis Integrifolii	15	*Clear heat toxins*	Dog tongue grass
Sesamum indicum	*hei zhi ma*	Semen Sesami Indici	30	*Supplement the yin*	Black sesame seed
Smilax glabra	*tu fu ling*	Rhizoma Smilacis Glabrae	30	*Clear heat toxins*	
Solanum nigrum	*long kui*	Herba Solani	30	*Clear heat toxins*	
Solanum indicum	*huang shui qie*	Solani Xanthocarpi Herba	15	*Percolate damp*	
Solanum lyratum	*shu yang quan*	Herba Solani Lyrati	15	*Clear heat toxins*	Climbing nightshade
Sophora japonica	*huai hua*	Flos Sophorae Japonicae	15	*Regulate the blood*	Pagoda tree flower
Sophora flavescens	*ku shen*	Radix Sophorae Flavescentis	15	*Clear damp heat*	Bitter ginseng root
Sophora subprostrata	*shan dou gen*	Radix Sophorae Subprostratae	9	*Clear heat toxins*	Pigeon pea
Sparganium simplex	*san leng*	Rhizoma Sparganii	9	*Regulate the blood*	Bur-reed rhizome
Stephania tetranda	*han fang ji*	Radix Stephaniae Tetrandrae	9	*Percolate damp*	Stephania root
Strychnos nux-vomica	*ma qian zi*	Semen Strychnotis	1.2	*Topical application*	Nux-vomica seed
Taraxacum mongolicum	*pu gong ying*	Herba Taraxaci Mongolici cum Radice	30	*Clear heat toxins*	Dandelion
Terminalia chebula	*he zi*	Fructus Terminaliae Chebulae	9	*Astringent*	Myrobalan fruit
Trachelospermum jasminoides	*luo shi teng*	Trachelospermi Caulis	15	*Dispel Wind Damp*	Star jasmine stem
Tremella fuciformis	*bai mu er*	Fructificatio Tremellae Fuciformis	9	*Supplement the yin*	Wood ear fungus
Trichosanthes kirilowii	*tian hua fen*	Radix Trichosanthis	15	*Transform hot phlegm*	Snakegourd root
Trichosanthes kirilowii	*gua lou*	Fructus Trichosanthis	12	*Transform hot phlegm*	Snakegourd fruit
Trigonella foenum-graecum	*hu lu ba*	Semen Trigonellae Foeni-Graeci	9	*Supplement the yang*	Fennugreek seed
Trogopterus xanthipes	*wu ling zhi*	Excrementum Trogopterori seu Pteromi	9	*Regulate the blood*	Flying squirrel feces
Typha augustifolia	*pu huang*	Pollen typhae	12	*Stop bleeding*	
Typhonium giganteum	*bai fu zi, yu bai fu*	Rhizoma Typhonii Gigantei seu Radix Aconiti Coreani	6	*Transform cold phlegm*	
Uncaria gambir	*a xian yao*	Gambir		*Topical application*	Black catechu
Uncaria rhynchophylla	*gou teng*	Ramulus cum Uncis Uncariae	15	*Extinguish wind*	Hook vine
Vaccaria segetalis	*wang bu liu xing*	Semen Vaccariae Segetalis	30	*Regulate the blood*	Cow soap wort seed
Veratrum nigrum	*li lu*	Radix et Rhizoma Veratri	0.9	*Induce vomiting*	
Verbena officinalis	*ma pian cao*	Herba Verbenae	30	*Regulate the blood*	Vervain
Vitex negundo	*pu jiang gen*	Victis Qinatae Radix	9	*Stop coughing*	
Wikstroemia indica	*pu yin gen*	Radix Wikstroemiae	9	*Clear heat toxins*	
Wisteria sinensis, W. floribunda	*fugikobu* (Japanese)	Galla Wisteriae	10		
Xanthium sibiricum	*cang er zi*	Fructus Xanthii	9	*Dispel wind dampness*	Cocklebur fruit
Zanthoxylum nitidum	*liang mian zhen*	Zanthoxyli Nitidi Folium et Radix	9	*Dispel wind damp*	Shiny bramble
Ziziphus jujuba	*da zao, hong zao*	Fructus Ziziphi Jujubae	20	*Supplement the qi*	Chinese date

Sources: Hsu et al., 1986; Bensky and Gamble, 1993; Foster and Yue, 1992:73

APPENDIX B: HERBAL FORMULAS MENTIONED IN TEXT

This appendix lists the ingredients of the herbal formulas mentioned in the text. Indications and additional information on most of these formulas can be found in Bensky and Barolet (1990) and Huang and Wang (1993). Where available, daily dosages (for decoctions) are provided for unusual formulas. See the above references for further dosage information.

TABLE B.1 HERBAL FORMULAS MENTIONED IN TEXT	
FORMULA	**INGREDIENTS**
Ba Wei Di Huang Wan	*Rehmannia glutinosa (sheng di huang)* 24g, *Cornus officinalis (shan zhu yu)* 24g, *Dioscorea opposita (shan yao)* 24g, *Alisma plantago (ze xie)* 15g, *Poria cocos (fu ling)* 24g, *Paeonia suffruticosa (mu dan pi)* 24g, *Schisandra chinensis (wu wei zi)* 15g, *Astragalus membranaceus (zhi huang qi)* 30g
Bu Yang Huan Wu Tang	*Astragalus membranaceus (huang qi)*, *Angelica sinensis (dang gui)*, *Ligusticum chuanxiong (chuan xiong)*, *Paeonia lactiflora (chi shao)*, *Prunus persica (tao ren)*, *Carthamus tinctorius (hong hua)*, *Pheretima aspergillum (di long)*
Bu Zhong Yi Qi Tang	*Astragalus membranaceus (huang qi)*, *Panax ginseng (ren shen)*, *Atractylodes macrocephala (bai zhu)*, *Glycyrrhiza uralensis (zhi gan cao)*, *Angelica sinensis (dang gui)*, *Cimicifuga foetida (sheng ma)*, *Bupleurum chinense (chai hu)*, *Citrus reticulata (chen pi)*
CML pills	*Ranunculi ternati (mao zhua cao)*, *Sophora flavescens (ku shen)*, *Scutellaria baicalensis (huang qin)*, *Phellodendron chinense (huang bai)*, *Realgar (xiong huang)*, *Angelica sinensis (dang gui)*, *Terminalia chebula (he zi)*, *Isatis tinctoria (qing dai)*, *Hirudo nipponia (shui zhi)*, *Eupolyphaga sinensis (tu bie chong)*
Da Chai Hu Tang	*Bupleurum chinense (chai hu)*, *Scutellaria baicalensis (huang qin)*, *Citrus aurantium (zhi shi)*, *Rheum officinale (da huang)*, *Pinellia ternata (ban xia)*, *Paeonia lactiflora (bai shao)*, *Zingiber officinale (sheng jiang)*, *Ziziphus jujuba (da zao)*
Dang Gui Shao Yao San	*Angelica sinensis (dang gui)*, *Paeonia lactiflora (shao yao)*, *Poria cocos (fu ling)*, *Atractylodes macrocephala (bai zhu)*, *Alisma plantago-aquatica (ze xie)*, *Ligusticum chuanxiong (chuan xiong)*
Er Chen Tang	*Pinellia ternata (ban xia)*, *Citrus reticulata (ju hong)*, *Poria cocos (fu ling)*, *Glycyrrhiza uralensis (zhi gan cao)*
Er Xian Tang	*Curculigo orchioides (xian mao)* 6 to 15g, *Epimedium grandiflorum (yin yang huo)* 9 to 15g, *Morinda officinalis (ba ji tian)* 9g, *Angelica sinensis (dang gui)* 9g, *Phellodendron chinense (huang bai)* 4.5 to 9g, *Anemarrhena asphodeloides (zhi mu)* 4.5 to 9g
Fei Liu Ping	*Astragalus membranaceus (huang qi)*, *Codonopsis pilosula (dang shen)*, *Oldenlandia diffusa (bai hua she ye cao)*, *Prunus armeniaca (xing ren)*, *Paris polyphylla (cao he che)*, *Houttuynia cordata (yu xing cao)*, *Patrina villosa (bai jian cao)*, *Glehnia littoralis (bei sha shen)*
Formula #1	*Paeonia lactiflora (chi shao)*, *Ligusticum chuanxiong (chuan xiong)*, *Angelica sinensis (dang gui)*, *Prunus persica (tao ren)*, *Carthamus tinctorius (hong hua)*, *Millettia reticulata (ji xue teng)*, *Pueraria lobata (ge gen)*, *Citrus reticulata (chen pi)*, *Salvia miltiorrhiza (dan shen)*, *Astragalus membranaceus (huang qi)*
Formula #2	*Codonopsis pilosula (dang shen)*, *Astragalus membranaceus (huang qi)*, *Atractylodes macrocephala (bai zhu)*, *Solanum lyrati (shu yang quan)*, *Hedyosis diffusae (bai hua she she cao)*, *Salvia chinesis (shi jian chuan)*
Formula #3	*Astragalus membranaceus (huang qi)*, *Acanthopanax gracilistylus (wu jia pi)*
Fu Zheng Sheng Jin Decoction	*Ophiopogon japonicus (mai dong)*, *Asparagus cochinchinensis (tian dong)*, *Scrophularia ningpoensis (yuan shen)*, *Rehmannia glutinosa (sheng di huang)*, *Imperata cylindrica (bai mao gen)*, *Polygonatum odoratum (yu zhu)*, *Lonicera japonica (yin hua)*, *Oldenlandia diffusa (bai hua she she cao)*, *Solanum lyratum (bai mao teng)*, *Codonopsis pilosula (dang shen)*, *Poria cocos (fu ling)*, *Atractylodes macrocephala (bai zhu)*, *Glycyrrhiza uralensis (gan cao)*, *Salvia miltiorrhiza (dan shen)*
Gui Zhi Fu Ling Wan	*Cinnamomum cassia (gui zhi)*, *Poria cocos (fu ling)*, *Paeonia lactiflora (shao yao)*, *Paeonia suffruticosa (mu dan pi)*, *Prunus persica (tao ren)*
(Table continues)	

TABLE B.1 *(continued)*

FORMULA	INGREDIENTS
Gui Zhi Tang	*Cinnamomum cassia (gui zhi), Paeonia lactiflora (shao yao), Zingiber officinalis (sheng jiang), Ziziphus jujuba (da zao), Glycyrrhiza uralensis (zhi gan cao)*
Jian Pi Jin Dan	Components not specified
Jin Gui Shen Qi	*Aconitum carmichaeli (fu zi)* 3g, *Cinnamomum cassia (gui zhi)* 3g, *Rehmannia glutinosa (sheng di huang)* 24g, *Cornus officinalis (shan zhu yu)* 12g, *Dioscorea opposita (shan yao)* 12g, *Alisma plantago (ze xie)* 9g, *Poria cocos (fu ling)* 9g, *Paeonia suffruticosa (mu dan pi)* 9g
Kang Fu Xin	Components not specified
Kang Shuai Sen Fang	Components not specified
Kanzo Shashin To	Similar to Chinese formula *Gan Cao Xie Xin Tang*
Li Wei Hua Jie Decoction	*Codonopsis pilosula (dang shen), Atractylodes macrocephala (bai zhu), Poria cocos (fu ling), Glycyrrhiza uralensis (gan cao), Astragalus membranaceus (sheng huang qi), Rehmannia glutinosa (shu di huang), Polygonatum sibricum (huang jing), Solanum lyratum (bai mao teng), Oldenlandia diffusa (bai hua she she cao), Euryale ferox (qian shi), Nelumbo nucifera (lian rou), Panax notoginseng (tian san qi), Ziziphus jujuba (da zao), Adenophora tetraphylla (sha shen), Ovine calculi (yang du zao), Lycium barbarum (gou qi zi)*
Liu Wei Di Huang Tang	*Rehmannia glutinosa (shu di huang), Cornus officinalis (shan zhu yu), Dioscorea opposita (shan yao), Alisma plantago (ze xie), Paeonia suffruticosa (mu dan pi), Poria cocos (fu ling)*
Manli Pill	*Ranunculus ternatus (mao zhao cao), Sophora flavescens (ku shen), Scutellaria baicalensis (huang qin), Phellodendron amurense (huang bai), Realgar (xiong huang), Angelica sinensis (dang gui), Terminalia chebula (he zi rou), Baphicacanthus cusia (qing dai san), Eupolyphaga sinensis (tu bie zi), Hirudo nipponia (shui zhi)*
Mieai Decoction	*Hirudo nipponia (shui zhi), Salammonite and Halite (nao sha), Prunella vulgaris (xia ku cao), Codonopsis pilosula (dang shen), Saussurea lappa (mu xiang), Alum (bai fan), Borax (peng sha), Erosaria caputserpentis (zi bei chi), Areca catechu (bing lang), Scrophularia ningpoensis (xuan shen), Hematite (zhe shi), Rheum palmatum (chuan jun), Salvia miltiorrhiza (dan shen), Citrus reticulata (chen pi)*
Mieai Powder	*Rheum palmatum (sheng jun), Alum (bai fan), Daemonorops draco (xue jie), Moschus moschiferus (she xiang), Human urine sediment (ren zhong bei), Panax ginseng (ren shen)*
Pishen Fang	*Codonopsis pilosula (dang shen), Atractylodes macrocephala (bai zhu), Cuscuta chinensis (tu si zi), Psoralen corylifolia (bu gu zhi), Ligusticum lucidum (nu zhen zi), Lycium chinense (gou qi zi)*
Ren Shen Tang	Major known ingredient: *Panax ginseng (ren shen)*
Ren Shen Yang Rong Tang	*Panax ginseng (ren shen), Rehmannia glutinosa (shu di huang), Atractylodes macrocephala (bai zhu), Angelica sinensis (Dang gui), Paeonia lactiflora (bai shao yao), Poria cocos (fu ling), Astragalus membranaceus (huang qi), Cinnamomum cassia (rou gui), Schisandra chinensis (wu wei zi), Polygala tenuifolia (yuan zhi), Citrus reticulata (chen pi), Glycyrrhiza uralensis (zhi gan cao), Zingiber officinale (sheng jiang), Ziziphus jujuba (da zao)*
Saiboku To	*Perilla frutescens (zi su zi), Panax ginseng (ren shen), Ziziphus jujuba (da zao), Glycyrrhiza uralensis (gan cao), Magnolia officinalis (hou po), Poria cocos (fu ling), Pinellia, Scutellaria baicalensis (huang qin), Bupleurum chinense (chai hu)*
San Zhuang Wan	Components not specified
Shen Cao Fu Zheng Kangai	*Panax ginseng (ren shen), Astragalus membranaceus (huang qi), Atractylodes macrocephala (bai zhu), Poria cocos (fu ling), Solanum nigra (long kui), Oldenlandia diffusa (bai hua she she cao), Scutellaria barbata (ban zhi lian), Ligustrum lucidum (nu zhen zi)*
Shen Xue Tang	*Astragalus membranaceus (huang qi), Pseudostellaria heterophylla (tai zi shen), Atractylodes macrocephala (bai zhu), Poria cocos (fu ling), Ligustrum lucidum (nu zhen zi), Cuscuta chinensis (tu si zi), Lycium chinensis (gou qi zi), Millettia reticulata (ji xue teng)*
Sheng Mai San	*Panax ginseng (ren shen), Ophiopogon japonicus (mai men dong), Schisandra chinensis (wu wei zi)*

(Table continues)

TABLE B.1 *(continued)*	
FORMULA	**INGREDIENTS**
Shi Quan Da Bu Tang	*Astragalus membranaceus (huang qi), Cinnamomum cassia (rou gui), Panax ginseng (ren shen), Rehmannia glutinosa (shu di huang), Atractylodes macrocephala (bai zhu), Angelica sinensis (dang gui), Paeonia lactiflora (bai shao yao), Ligusticum chuanxiong (chuan xiong), Poria cocos (fu ling), Glycyrrhiza uralensis (zhi gan cao), Zingiber officinale (sheng jiang), Ziziphus jujuba (da zao)*
Si Jun Zi Tang	*Panax ginseng (ren shen), Atractylodes macrocephala (bai zhu), Poria cocos (fu ling), Glycyrrhiza uralensis (zhi gan cao)*
Wu Zi Yan Zong	Components not specified
Xiao Chai Hu Tang	*Bupleurum chinense (chai hu), Scutellaria baicalensis (huang qin), Pinellia ternata (ban xia), Zingiber officinale (sheng jiang), Panax ginseng (ren shen), Glycyrrhiza uralensis (gan cao), Ziziphus jujuba (da zao)*
Xiao Yao San	*Bupleurum chinense (chai hu), Angelica sinensis (dang gui), Paeonia lactiflora (bai shao), Atractylodes macrocephala (bai zhu), Poria cocos (fu ling), Mentha haplocalyx (bo he), Zingiber officinale (sheng jiang), Glycyrrhiza uralensis (zhi gan cao)*
Ye Qi Sheng Xue Tang	*Astragalus membranaceus (huang qi), Angelica sinensis (dang gui), Equus asinus (e jiao), Spatholobi sp., Pyrrosia lingua (shi wei), Ziziphus jujuba (da zao), Hordeum vulgare (mai ya), Citrus reticulata (chen pi), Glycyrrhiza uralensis (gan cao)*
Yi Kang Ling	Components not specified
Yi Qi Jian Pi	Components not specified
Yi Qi Yang Yin	*Pseudostellaria heterophylla (tai zi shen), Scrophularia ningpoensis (xuan shen), Ophiopogon japonicus (mai men dong), Rehmannia glutinosa (shu di huang), Ligusticum lucidum (nu zhen zi), Dendrobium officinale (shi hu), Trichosanthes kirilowii (gua lou), Hedyosis diffusa (bai hua she she cao), Scutellaria barbata (ban zhi lian), Glycyrrhiza uralensis (gan cao)*
You Gui Yin	*Rehmannia glutinosa (shu di huang), Aconitum carmichaeli (fu zi), Cinnamomum cassia (rou gui), Cornus officinalis (shan zhu yu), Lycium chinense (gou qi zi), Dioscorea opposita (shan yao), Eucommia ulmoides (du zhong), Glycyrrhiza uralensis (zhi gan cao)*
Zhu Ling Tang	*Polyporus umbellatus (zhu ling), Poria cocos (fu ling), Alisma plantago-aquatica (ze xie), Equus asinus (e jiao), Talc (hua shi)*

APPENDIX C: CANCER INCIDENCE AND SURVIVAL DATA

TABLE C.1. UNITED STATES CANCER STATISTICS, ALL RACES				
PRIMARY CANCER SITE	**INCIDENCE (1985-89)**	**MORTALITY (1985-89)**	**5-YEAR RELATIVE SURVIVAL (%) (1983-88)**	**MEDIAN AGE AT DIAGNOSIS (1985-89)**	**MEDIAN AGE AT DEATH (1985-89)**
All Sites	377.8	172	52	67	70
Oral Cavity and Pharynx:	11	3.1	51.3	63	66
— Lip	1.2	0	93.1	68	75
— Tongue	2.2	0.7	46.3	63	66
— Salivary gland	1	0.2	70.9	63	70
— Floor of mouth	1.2	0.1	55	63	66
— Gum and other oral cavity	1.9	0.5	53.1	63	69
— Nasopharynx	0.6	0.3	46.6	57	63
— Tonsil	1.1	0.2	37.1	62	64
— Oropharynx	0.3	0.2	24.1	64	66
— Hypopharynx	1.1	0.2	23	64	65
— Other oral cavity and pharynx	0.4	0.6	26	64	66
Digestive system:	79.2	41.3	40.8	71	72
— Esophagus	3.9	3.4	8.1	67	67
— Stomach	8.1	4.9	16.9	71	72
— Small intestine	1.2	0.3	46.6	67	70
— Colon and rectum	50.1	19.8	57.5	71	73
— — colon	35.7	—	58.1	72	73
— — rectum	14.4	—	56	69	72
— — anus	0.8	0.1	60.1	65	67
— Liver and Intrahepatic	2.8	2.6	5.7	67	70
— — liver	2.5	2.2		67	70
— — gallbladder	1.1	0.8	13.9	73	74
— — other biliary	1.1	0.7	14.2	72	74
— Pancreas	9.3	8.4	3.2	71	72
— Retroperitoneum	0.4	0.1	41.9	59	69
— Peritoneum, and mesentery	0.2	0.1	23.4	65	69
— Other digestive system	0.3	0.2	3.2	75	77
Respiratory system:	63.7	49.8	17.4	67	68
— Nose, nasal cavity and middle ear	0.7	0.2	54.2	64	68
(Table continues)					

PRIMARY CANCER SITE	INCIDENCE (1985-89)	MORTALITY (1985-89)	5-YEAR RELATIVE SURVIVAL (%) (1983-88)	MEDIAN AGE AT DIAGNOSIS (1985-89)	MEDIAN AGE AT DEATH (1985-89)
— Larynx	4.6	1.4	65.5	64	67
— Lung and bronchus	57.5	48	13	67	68
— Pleura	0.7	0.1	4.4	69	70
— Trachea and other respiratory	0.3	0.1	42	47	66
Bones and Joints	0.8	0.4	55.1	34	60
Soft Tissue (including heart)	2.1	1.1	60.1	57	64
Skin (excluding basal and squamous cell):	14	2.9	69.8	48	65
— Melanoma	10.7	2.2	82.5	54	63
— Other nonepithelial	3.4	0.8	32.6	38	69
Breast	58.9	15.4	78	64	66
Female genital system:	25.6	8.5	65.8	63	69
— Cervix uteri	4.6	1.7	65.6	48	61
— Corpus uteri	11.5	1.1	83.2	66	71
— Uterus, NOS	0.2	1	27.6	71	73
— Ovary	7.7	4.4	39.5	63	68
— Vagina	0.4	0.1	39.8	69	75
— Vulva	0.9	0.2	73.3	71	77
— Other female genital system	0.3	0.1	50.2	61	69
Male genital system:	43.3	9.5	76.9	72	76
— Prostate	40.8	9.3	75.9	72	77
— Testis	2.1	0.1	92.4	32	34
— Penis	0.3	0.1	71.3	67	71
— Other male genital system	0.1	0	70.4	68	71
Urinary system:	26	6.8	70.2	69	73
— Bladder	17	3.3	78.3	70	76
— Kidney and renal pelvis	8.3	3.4	54.8	66	69
— Ureter	0.5	0.1	60.9	72	75
— Other urinary system	0.3	0.1	48.6	69	72.5
Eye and orbit	0.6	0.1	76.2	61	70
Brain and nervous system:	6.2	4.1	25.9	56	63
— Brain	5.9	4	23.9	57	63

(Table continues)

PRIMARY CANCER SITE	INCIDENCE (1985-89)	MORTALITY (1985-89)	5-YEAR RELATIVE SURVIVAL (%) (1983-88)	MEDIAN AGE AT DIAGNOSIS (1985-89)	MEDIAN AGE AT DEATH (1985-89)
— Cranial nerves and other	0.3	0.1	63	43	62
Endocrine system:	5	0.7	89.2	44	66
— Thyroid	4.4	0.3	93.9	44	72
— Other endocrine and Thymus	0.6	0.3	50.4	51	53
Lymphomas:	16.3	6.5	56.8	62	70
— Hodgkin's disease	2.8	0.6	77.3	33	54
— Non-Hodgkin's lymphomas	13.5	5.9	51.3	65	70
Multiple myeloma	4.2	2.9	26.8	70	72
Leukemias:	10.1	6.3	36.5	67	71
— Lymphocytic:	4.5	1.8	59.9	66	72
— — acute	1.5	0.6	51.1	11	40
— — chronic	2.9	1.1	66.2	71	75
— — other	0.1	0.1	29.9	71	76
Myeloid:	3.9	2.6	14.3	67	69
— — acute	2.3	1.7	9.7	67	69
— — chronic	1.4	0.8	21.7	67	67
— — other	0.3	0.1	16.5	67	76
Monocytic:	0.3	0.1	9.5	66	72
— — acute	0.2	0.1	8.5	64	71
— — chronic	0	0	—	64	76
— — other	0	0	11.9	79	78
— Other:	1.4	1.8	28	70	71
— — other acute	0.6	1	7.7	71	70
— — other chronic	0	0.1	44.9	78	77
— — NOS	0.7	0.7	43.7	69	73
Ill-defined and unspecified	10.7	12.6	9.7	71	71

Note: Incidence and mortality rates are per 100,000 people, and age-adjusted to the 1970 U.S. standard population.
Adapted from: Miller et al., 1992

APPENDIX D: STUDIES ON PLATELET AGGREGATION AND FIBRINOLYSIS

When reading this appendix, recall that agents that reduce thromboxane A_2 (TXA_2) or increase prostacyclin (PGI_2) will inhibit platelet aggregation.

- Administration of *Ligusticum chuanxiong (chuan xiong)* to rabbits with experimentally induced acute renal failure reduced elevated levels of plasma thromboxane B_2 (TXB_2), elevated levels of 6-keto-$PGF_{1\text{-alpha}}$, and inhibited platelet aggregation (Hu and Ma, 1993).[1] Similarly, administration of *Ligusticum chuanxiong* to rats with experimentally induced glomerulonephritis resulted in a reduction of elevated levels of TXA_2 and elevated depressed levels of 6-keto-PGF_1 (Yuan, 1993). In humans with acute cerebral infarction, administration of *Ligusticum chuanxiong* reduced elevated levels of TXB_2, increased depressed levels of 6-keto-$PGF_{1\text{-alpha}}$, and inhibited platelet aggregation (Liu, 1991). Similar results were obtained in rabbits with experimentally induced cerebral ischemia (Liu, 1990).

- In a study on the effects of 18 Chinese herbs on TXA_2 and PGI_2 production in vitro, *Glehnia littoralis (sha shen)* inhibited synthesis of TXA_2 and stimulated synthesis of PGI_2 (Wang et al., 1993b). *Codonopsis pilosula (dang shen)*, *Astragalus membranaceus (huang qi)*, *Angelica sinensis (dang gui)*, ginsenosides (from *Panax ginseng, ren shen*), and baicalin (from *Scutellaria baicalensis, huang qin*) markedly inhibited synthesis of TXA_2 and mildly increased PGI_2. *Rheum palmatum (da huang)* inhibited synthesis of TXA_2 but had no effect on PGI_2.

- In a placebo-controlled study on 14 patients with exercise induced angina pectoris, administration of a formula consisting of *Panax ginseng (ren shen)*, *Astragalus membranaceus (huang qi)*, and *Angelica sinensis (dang gui)* resulted in a 59% reduction in platelet aggregation, and a 91% reduction in the frequency and severity of angina episodes. No adverse side effects of the formula were observed (Liao et al., 1989).

- Administration of *Codonopsis pilosula (dang shen)* and *Astragalus membranaceus (huang qi)* to 22 patients with arteriosclerosis resulted in a significant inhibition of platelet aggregation. In-vitro studies produced similar results (Li et al., 1986).

- In a study on 24 patients with angina pectoris, administration of *Codonopsis pilosula (dang shen)* reduced plasma TXB_2. Similar results were obtained in vitro (Wang and Zhu, 1990).

- *Rheum palmatum (da huang)* blocked the synthesis of TXB_2 in rabbit kidneys (Guo et al., 1989).

- Saponins obtained from *Gynostemma pentaphyllum (jiao gu lan)* inhibited platelet aggregation and TXA_2 release in rabbits (Li and Jin, 1989).

- Scoparone, a coumarin found in *Artemisia capillaris (yin chen hao)* and *Angelica dahurica (bai zhi)*, dilated rat aorta rings and scavenged free radicals. Vasodilation appeared to be mediated by enhanced PGI_2 release (Huang, 1992b).

- The bulb of *Allium bakeri* effectively inhibited platelet aggregation in vitro (Shibata, 1985).

- In a study of 308 patients with abnormal blood lipid values, the essential oil of *Allium sativum* (garlic, *da suan*) reduced blood lipids, reduced platelet aggregation rates, and reduced blood pressure (CGEOG, 1986). Allitridi, a component of *Allium sativum*, inhibited platelet aggregation in vitro (Yue et al., 1984). In a placebo-controlled double-blind study, administration of 800 mg of garlic powder for 4 weeks eliminated spontaneous platelet aggregation, increased microcirculation in the skin, decreased plasma viscosity, and decreased blood glucose in humans (Kiesewetter et al., 1991).

- In a study on 112 extracts prepared from 37 different animal crude drugs, water extracts of *Bombyx mori (jiang can)* demonstrated potent anticoagulant effects (Wang, et al., 1989).

- Components of *Typha latifolia (pu huang)* increased PGI_2 production, inhibited smooth muscle cell proliferation, and inhibited platelet aggregation in vitro (Zhao et al., 1990, 1989).[2]

- Extracts of *Andrographis paniculata (chuan xin lian)* promoted the synthesis of PGI_2, inhibited production of TXA_2, and inhibited platelet aggregation in dogs with mechanical coronary artery injury or dogs with experimental myocardial infarction (Zhao and Fang, 1990, 1991). In a study on dogs with induced myocardial infarction, flavones from *Andrographis paniculata* increased plasma 6-keto-PGF1-alpha production, decreased TXB_2 production, decreased

---

[1] Thromboxane B_2 is a metabolite of thromboxane A_2. 6-keto-$PGF_{1\text{-alpha}}$ is a stable metabolite of PGI_2 and therefore can be used to measure PGI_2 levels. Many prostaglandins are difficult to measure directly in vivo since they are rapidly metabolized in the body.

[2] Smooth muscle cells surround blood vessels larger than capillaries.

platelet aggregation, and inhibited thrombus formation (Zhao and Fang, 1991).

- An extract of *Tanacetum parthenium* (feverfew, also known as *Chrysanthemum parthenium*) demonstrated antithrombotic activities in vitro. The extract inhibited the deposition of platelets on human collagen, inhibited platelet aggregation, and protected endothelial cells from salt-induced injury (Loesche et al., 1988).

- An extract of *Ginkgo biloba* administered intravenously or orally to rabbits reduced experimentally induced thrombus formation (Borzeix et al., 1980).

- *Aloe vera* decreased thromboxane A_2 and B_2 production in vitro (Klein et al., 1988).

- Capsaicin (from cayenne pepper, *Capsicum frutescens*) is a potent inhibitor of platelet aggregation in vitro (Wang et al., 1984a).

- Extracts of *Paeonia lactiflora (bai shao)* prolonged prothrombin time, inhibited thrombin, stimulated plasminogen, and inhibited urokinase activity in vitro (Wang and Ma, 1990).

APPENDIX E: NATURAL AGENTS THAT AFFECT cAMP LEVELS

TABLE E.1. NATURAL AGENTS THAT AFFECT cAMP LEVELS		
AGENT	**EFFECT**	**REFERENCE**
AGENTS THAT INCREASE cAMP		
Aconitum carmichaeli (fu zi), and *Cinnamomum cassia* (*rou gui*)	Administration of the herbs to rats with excess thyroid or adrenocortical hormone increased the elevated plasma cAMP levels in the kidneys.	Yi et al., 1987
Actinidia chinensis (*teng li gen*)	A polysaccharide compound isolated from the root and administered intraperitoneally to tumor-bearing mice markedly increased spleen cell cAMP levels, nearly to the level of healthy mice.	Lin, 1988
Andrographis paniculata (*chuan xin lian*)	Stimulated synthesis of cAMP by platelets in vitro.	Zhao and Fang, 1991, 1990
Caffeine	Caffeine inhibits phosphodiesterases and, therefore, raises cAMP levels.	Reviewed by Tannock and Hill, 1992:215
Cnidium monnieri (*she chuang zi*)	In rats with hydrocortisone-induced adrenal damage, plasma PGE_2 and cAMP levels are significantly reduced compared to levels in normal rats. Administration of the total coumarins or a water extract of *Cnidium monnieri* increased these levels to normal. The essential oil of *Cnidium monnieri* had no effect.	Qin et al., 1993
Kanzo Shashin To (formula)	In a study of 59 formulas, this formula showed the highest inhibitory effect on cAMP phosphodiesterase.	Suzuki et al., 1991
Li Wei Di Huang Tang (formula)	Increased intercellular cAMP in mice bearing U-14 tumor.	Pan, 1992:35
Polyporus umbellatus (*zhu ling*)	Stimulated synthesis of cAMP by platelets in vitro. Increased intracellular cAMP in mice bearing sarcoma-180.	Zhao and Fang, 1991, 1990; Pan, 1992:35
Saiboku To (formula)	Increased intracellular cAMP levels in cultured tracheal epithelium cells from dogs.	Tamaoki et al., 1992
Salvia miltiorrhiza (*dan shen*)	Inhibited human platelet aggregation in vitro. The mechanism is likely due to an inhibition of cAMP phosphodiesterase and an associated increase in cAMP.	Wang et al., 1982b
Yi Qi Jian Pi (formula)	Elevated depressed spleen cell and plasma cAMP levels in mice with rhubarb-induced diarrhea.	Zhang SL, 1990
You Gui Yin (formula)	Elevated depressed plasma cAMP and cortisol levels in mice with hydrocortisone-induced adrenal damage.	Li et al., 1990
Ziziphus jujuba (da zao)	The herb contains 100 to 600 nM/g of cAMP. Cyclic AMP inhibits histamine release, and the cAMP content of *Ziziphus jujuba* may explain, in part, the reason this herb is traditionally used to treat allergies and depression (some evidence suggests that histamine may have neurotransmitter-like properties).	Hsu et al., 1985:752
AGENTS THAT DECREASE cAMP		
Rehmannia glutinosa (shu di huang) and *Chinemys reevesii* (*gui ban*)	Administration of the herbs to rats with excess thyroid or adrenocortical hormone reduced the elevated plasma cAMP levels in the kidneys.	Yi et al., 1987
Qing Wen Bai Dou Yin (formula)	Reduced the fever and reduced elevated levels of plasma cAMP in rabbits with experimentally induced fevers. This formula is traditionally used to treat fevers and other heat conditions.	Xie, 1993

APPENDIX F: COMPOUNDS SHOWING CYTOTOXIC OR ANTITUMOR ACTIVITY IN CHINESE STUDIES

This appendix lists some botanical compounds that have shown cytotoxic or antitumor activity. The review sources used to construct this appendix often did not cite the original sources of their data or provide details of the study designs. If cited, the original data were not verified by this author. Therefore, the accuracy of the information contained in Table F.1 is uncertain. See Table 11.2 for a list of cell line codes.

TABLE F.1. COMPOUNDS SHOWING CYTOTOXIC OR ANTITUMOR ACTIVITY IN CHINESE STUDIES			
CHEMICAL GROUP	**COMPOUND**	**PLANT SOURCE**	**PHARMACOLOGIC ACTIVITY**
1. Aliphatic Compounds[1]			
Alcohols	podophyllotoxin	*Dysosma pleiantha* *Podophyllum versipelle* *P. pleianthum*	○ Inhibits TLX-5 cells and nasopharyngeal carcinoma.[2] ○ Antileukemic.[4]
	deoxypodophyllotoxin	*Dysosma pleintha* *Podophyllum versipelle* *P. pleianthum* *Hernandia ovigera*	○ Inhibits TLX-5 cells and nasopharyngeal carcinoma.[2] ○ Antileukemic and cytotoxic.[4]
Acids, Esters, Lactones	coixenolide	*Coix lacryma-jobi*	○ Inhibits cervical cancer U14 and HCA solid tumor (mice).[3]
2. Aromatic Compounds			
Naphthoquinones	irisquinone	*Iris pollasii*	○ Inhibits cervical carcinoma U14, hepatoma, lymphatic sarcoma, and Ehrlich ascites carcinoma (mice).[2]
Anthraquinones	rhein, emodin	*Rheum palmatum* *R. tanguticum* *R. coreanum* *Cassia obtusifolia* *C. tora* *C. fistula* *C. angustifolia* *C. acutifolia*	○ Inhibits melanoma, EA, and breast carcinoma (mice).[3]
Benzo-a-Pyrone derivitives	psoralen	*Psoralea corylifolia* *Glehnia littoralis* *Angelica pubescens* *A. dahurica* *A. japonica* *Ledebouriella seseloides* *Ficus carica*	○ Inhibits SA, EA (mice), bone sarcoma, and lung cancer.[2]
Flavonoids (flavones, flavonols, flavanones, flavanonols, etc.)	liquiritin	*Glycyrrhiza uralensis*	○ Inhibits ascitic liver carcinoma (rats), and Ehrlich ascites carcinoma (mice). Inhibits Jitian sarcoma, prevents induced liver carcinoma.[3]
	trifolirhizin	*Trifolium pratense* *Sophora subprostrata* *S. flavescens*	○ Inhibits SA (mice).[3]
(column continues)	maackiain	*Trifolium pratense* *Sophora subprostrata*	○ Inhibits SA (mice).[3]
(Table continues)			

TABLE F.1. *(continued)*			
CHEMICAL GROUP	**COMPOUND**	**PLANT SOURCE**	**PHARMACOLOGIC ACTIVITY**
Flavonoids *(continued)*	sophoraponicin	*Sophora subprostrata*	○ Inhibits SA (mice).[3]
	bavachinin	*Psoralea corylifolia*	○ Inhibits SA, Ehrlich ascites (mice), bone sarcoma, and lung cancer.[2]
	corylifolinin	*Psoralea corylifolia*	○ Inhibits SA, Ehrlich ascites cells (mice), bone sarcoma, and lung cancer.[2]
4. Alicyclic Compounds			
Monoterpenoids	Asperuloside	*Oldenlandia diffusa* *Galium verum* *Heydotis corymbosa* *Paederia scandens* *Asperula odorata* *Daphniphyllum macropodum*	○ Stimulates reticuloendothelial system.[2]
Sesquiterpenoids	curcumenol, curcumol	*Curcuma zedoria*	○ Inhibits cervical carcinoma (humans), SA, ascites cells, cervical U14 cells (mice). May stimulate immune system.[2] ○ Inhibits early stage cervical cancer. Inhibits S-37, cervical cancer U14, and Ehrlich ascites carcinoma (mice). Increases fibroblasts around tumor, lymphocytes within tumor, and macrophage engulfment of tumor cells.[3]
	curdione	*Curcuma zedoria*	○ Inhibits SA, ascities carcinoma, and cervical U-14 (mouse). Enhances immunity.[5] ○ Inhibits S-37, cervical cancer U14, and Ehrlich ascites carcinoma (mice). Increases fibroblasts around tumor, lymphocytes within tumor, macrophage engulfment of tumor cells.[3]
	molephantinin	*Elephantopus elatus* *E. mollis*	○ Inhibits P-388 lymphocytic tumor and ascites cells.[2] ○ Antileukemic and cytotoxic.[4]
	elephantopin	*Elephantopus elatus* *E. mollis*	○ Inhibits P-388 lymphocytic tumor and ascites cells.[2] ○ Antitumor and cytotoxic.[4]
Diterpenoids	triptolide A	*Tripterygium wilfordii*	○ Inhibits L-615 leukemia cells (mice).[2]
	triptolide	*Tripterygium wilfordii*	○ Inhibits S-37 (mice), L-615 (mice), hepatoma, and solid Walker-256 (rats).[3] ○ Antileukemic.[4]
	tripdiolide	*Tripterygium wilfordii*	○ Inhibits L-615 (mice).[3]
	triptonide	*Tripterygium wilfordii*	○ Inhibits human nasopharyngeal KB cells in vitro.[3]
	quassin	*Ailanthus altissima* *Picrasma quassioides*	○ Inhibits SA (mice).[2]
Triterpenoids	glycyrrhetinic acid and derivatives	*Glycyrrhiza uralensis*	○ Inhibits Oberling-Guerin myeloma (rats). Antileukemic (mice).[3] ○ Inhibits melanoma, cancer-preventive, stimulates immunity.[4]
	glycyrrhizin	*Glycyrrhiza uralensis*	○ Inhibits ascitic liver carcinoma (rats) and Ehrlich ascites carcinoma (mice). Inhibits Jitian sarcoma, prevents induced liver carcinoma.[3]
(Table continues)			

218

TABLE F.1. *(continued)*			
CHEMICAL GROUP	**COMPOUND**	**PLANT SOURCE**	**PHARMACOLOGIC ACTIVITY**
Steroids	beta-sitosterol and analogs	many plant species	○ Inhibits SA (mice), Yoshida sarcoma, and Ehrlich ascites cells.[2] Antitumor in various animal studies, inhibits Hela cells.[3] ○ Antileukemic.[4]

5. Alkaloids

Alkaloids	tetrandrine	*Stephania tetrandra* *Sinomenium acutum* *Sophora flavescens*	○ Inhibits Walker carcinoma 256.[2] Inhibits Ehrlich ascites carcinoma and SA in vitro. Inhibits KB, Hela, various liver carcinoma strains, Ehrlich ascites carcinoma, and rat Walker carcinoma 256 in vitro.[3] Analgesic, inhibits lung tumor.[4]
	celacemine	*Tripterygium wilfordii*	○ Antileukemic.[3]
	beta-dichroine/ febrifugine	*Dichroa febrifuga*	○ Iinhibits Ehrlich ascites carcinoma, SA, melanoma (mice), ascitic hepatoma, S-45, and Walker carcinoma (rats).[3]
	matrine	*Sophora flavescens* *S. subprostrata* *S. alopecuroides*	○ Inhibits SA (mice), leukemia, and hepatoma.[2] Inhibits SA, Ehrlich ascites carcinoma (mice).[3]
	oxymatrine	*Sophora flavescens* *S. subprostrata*	○ Inhibits SA (mice).[3]
	fangchinoline	*Stephania tetrandra*	○ Inhibits Walker carcinoma 256.[2]
	nitidine chloride	*Zanthoxylum nitidum* *Z. ailanthoides* *Z. avicennae* *Z. cuspidatum*	○ Inhibits leukemia, L-1210 and P-388 lung carcinoma (mice).[2]
	dauricine	*Sophora subprostrata* *Menispermum dauricum*	○ Inhibits SA (mice), leukemia, hepatoma.[2]
	anagyrine	*Sophora subprostrata* *Thermopsis lanceolata*	○ Inhibits SA (mice), leukemia, hepatoma.[2]
	trigonelline	*Trigonella foenum-graecum* *Abrus precatorius* *Coffea arabica* *Strophanthus sp.* *Cannabis sativa* *Quisqualis indica* *Arabacia pustulosa* *Velella spirans*	○ Inhibits liver carcinoma (mice).[3] Inhibits cervical and liver cancer.[4]
	rubescensine B	*Rabdosia rubescens*	○ Inhibits hepatoma cells. May stimulate immune system in cancer bearing animals.[2]
	pterocarpine	*Sophora subprostrata*	○ Inhibits SA (mice).[3]
	maytansine	*Maytenus serrata*	○ Antileukemic and antimelanotic.[4]

[1] Chemical outline adapted from Hsu et al., 1982
[2] Huang KC, 1993
[3] Chang and Butt, 1986, 1987
[4] Duke, 1992
[5] Chang, 1992

APPENDIX G: HERBAL PRODUCTS WITH REPORTED ANTITUMOR OR ANTICANCER EFFECTS

This appendix lists the antitumor effects of some crude herbal agents. The review sources used to construct this appendix often did not cite the original sources of their data or provide details of the study designs. If cited, the original data were not verified by this author. Therefore, the accuracy of the information contained in Table G.1 is uncertain. Although it was not always clearly specified in the sources, it is assumed that the activities listed in Table G.1 are in vivo. When specified in the source, the testing animal is listed. Note that, in some cases, clinical trials may have used the crude drug externally. Also note that some of these extracts may act by mechanisms other than cytoxicity. Lastly, in some cases, the botanical name was estimated based on the mandarin name, or the mandarin name was estimated based on the botanical or pharmaceutical name. See Table 11.2 for a list of cell line codes.

TABLE G.1. HERBAL AGENTS WITH REPORTED ANTITUMOR OR ANTICANCER EFFECTS	
HERB	**ANTITUMOR OR ANTICANCER ACTIVITY**
Actinidia chinensis (teng li)	Inhibits SA.[2]
Ailanthus altissima (feng yen cao)	Inhibits SA, sarcoma-37, and leukemia-16 (mice).[1] Inhibits SA.[2]
Amorphophallus rivieri (ju ruo)	Inhibits SA.[1]
Arisaema consanguineum (tian nan xing)	Inhibits SA.[2] Inhibits SA, HCA solid type, and carcinoma of cervix U14 (mice). Out of 105 cases, 78% effective rate against human carcinoma of cervix.[3]
Aristolochia mollissima (xun gu feng)	Inhibits sarcoma-37, EA, and subcutaneous Ehrlich's cancer.[1]
Asparagus cochinchinensis (tian men dong)	Inhibits SA.[2]
Atractylodes macrocephala (bai zhu)	Inhibits SA.[1] Inhibits EA.[3]
Bombyx mori (jiang can)	Inhibits SA.[1,3]
Bos tarus domesticus (niu huang)	Inhibits SA, S-37, solid EA, and WA.[1]
Brucea javanica (ya dan zi)	Strongly inhibits EA. Inhibits S37, SA, and B16.[1,2] Inhibits EA, WA, PS, and human esophageal cancer. Marked effects and short term remission with no relapse in 2 to 5 years were observed in treatment of squamous carcinoma of the cervix in humans.[1,3]
Bufo bufo gargarizans (chuan su)	Inhibits SA, B and P tumors (rabbits). Strengthens tumor-inhibitory effect of some antineoplastic drugs. Short term inhibition of skin cancer, basal cell carcinoma, lung cancer, liver cancer, breast cancer, lymphosarcoma, and nasopharyngeal cancer in humans.[1,3]
Camptotheca acuminata (xi shu)	Decoction of the fruit and the alcohol extract inhibits ascites and stomach cancer in mice. The ethanol extract of the bark inhibits CA.[1] Strongly inhibits many animal tumors in vivo and in vitro (PS, LE, EA, WA and others).[2]
Carthamus tinctorius (hong hua)	Inhibits SA.[1]
Catharanthus roseus (chang chun hua)	Inhibits breast tumor, CA, LE, AKR-leukemia, SA, EA, ascitic hepatoma, and P-4 in mice. Inhibits WA, IRC 741/1398 leukemia, and ascitic Jitian sarcoma (rats).[3]
Chaenomeles lagenaria (mu gua)	Inhibits LE, PS, and EA.
Coix Lachryma-jobi (yi yi ren)	Inhibits ascites cancer and Yoshida's sarcoma.[1] Inhibits SA and Yoshida sarcoma.[2] Inhibits EA, cervical cancer U14, and HCA solid tumor (mice).
Cordyceps sinensis (dong chong xia cao)	Increases survival period of mice with EA. Shows significant anticancer effect on terminal carcinoma of lung in humans.[3] This herb is thought to act, in part, as an immunostimulant.
Cremastra variabilis (shan ci gu)	Inhibits WA.[3]
(Table continues)	

TABLE G.1. *(continued)*	
HERB	**ANTITUMOR OR ANTICANCER ACTIVITY**
Crotalaria sessiliflora (ye bai he)	Inhibits SA, L-615 leukemia, and EA. In humans inhibits skin carcinoma, cervical cancer, rectal cancer.[2] Inhibitits WA by 70 to 100%, and SA by 59 to 70% . Inhibits S-37, lymphosarcoma ascitic type L1, EA, metastatic LL, B16, reticulocytic leukemia L615, and LE. Inhibits plasma cell tumor and adenoma 755 (hamsters). Shrinkage of tumor and symptomatic improvement obtained by local application and injection into base of tumor in human skin and cervical cancers.[3]
Curcuma zedoaria (e zhu)	Inhibits SA, ascites cells, and cervical U-14 cells (mice). Protects leukocyte counts after radiation.[2] Inhibits SA, S-37, cervical cancer U14, and EA. Enhances specific immunity of host. Inhibits human cervical cancer with an effective rate of 70 to 71%.[3]
Dianthus superbus (qu mai)	Inhibits SA, human cardiac cancer, cystocancer.[1]
Dichroa febrifuga (chang shan)	Inhibits EA by 50 to 100%, EA solid type by 45%, SA by 45%, and melanoma by 75% (mice). Inhibits ascitic hepatoma by 55%, sarcoma-45 by 30%, and WA by 45% (rats).[3]
Duchesnea indica (she mei)	Inhibits EA and SA (mice).[1,2]
Eclipta prostrata (han lian cao)	Inhibits oncocytoplasia (in vitro and in vivo).[1]
Ficus pumila (xue li shi)	Inhibits ascites, subcutaneous lymphosarcoma-1, and WA.[1]
Ganoderma lucidum (ling zhi)	Inhibits SA.[2] Note: this herb is thought to act as an immunostimulant.
Gardenia jasminoides (zhi zi)	Inhibits SA.[1]
Gentiana scabra (long dan cao)	Inhibits SA.[1]
Gleditsia sinensis (zao jiao)	Inhibits sarcoma (rats).[1] Inhibits SA.[2]
Glycyrrhiza uralensis (gan cao)	Inhibits Oberling-Guerin myeloma (rats), leukemia (mice), and Jitian sarcomas. Inhibits ascitic carcinoma of liver (rats) and EA (mice). Prevents induced liver carcinoma in mice.[3]
Gossypium herbaceum (mian hua gen)	Inhibits S-37, SA, and WA.[1,2] Inhibits Jitian sarcoma, EA, WA, and breast cancer (mice). Applied locally dissolves melanoma (animals).[3]
Hirudo nipponia (shui zhi)	Inhibits liver cancer (mice).[1]
Houttuynia cordata (yu xing cao)	Inhibits stomach cancer. Used in the treatment of lung cancer and related infections.[1]
Impatiens balsamina (ji xing zi)	Inhibits S-37 (mice).
Isatis tinctoria (qing dai)	Inhibits WA (increases survival period by 43%). Inhibits LL and breast carcinoma (mice). Complete and partial remission of chronic granulocytic leukemia in humans.[3]
Iris pallasii (ma lin zi)	Inhibits mouse U-14 cancer, hepatoma, lymphatic sarcoma, EA, and carcinoma of cervix.[2]
Juglans regia (hu tao ren)	Inhibits various ascites cancer, SA, S-37, and spontaneous mammary cancer (mice). Inhibits S-37 cells (mice) and solid tumors.[2]
Ligustrum lucidum (nu zhen zi)	Inhibits carcinoma of cervix U14 (rats) by 49%.[3] This herb is thought to act, in part, as an immunostimulant.
Lobelia chinensis (bab bian lian)	Inhibits S-37.[1] Inhibits SA.[2]
Manis pentadactyla (chuan shan jia)	Anti-leukemia action in humans.[1]
Moschus moschiferus (she xinag)	Shows short-term therapeutic effect on early and middle stages of alimentary tract cancers in humans.[3]
Mylabris phalerata (ban mao)	Inhibits SA and inhibits cellular metabolism of other cancers.[1] Shrinks and inhibits solid tumors.[2] Inhibits ascitic malignant hepatoma and reticulosarcoma ARS (mice).[3]
Oldenlandia diffusa (bai hua she she cao)	Inhibits acute lymphatic, granulocytic, and monocytic leukemias; Yoshida's sarcoma; EA; uterine cancer-14; SA; and ascitic lymphosarcoma-1 (mice).[1] Inhibits SA by 57.4%. Short-term therapeutic effects in treatment of human lymphosarcoma, fibrosarcoma, carcimomas of cervix, breast, and rectum.[3] Note: this herb is thought to act, in part, as an immunostimulant.
(Table continues)	

221

HERB	ANTITUMOR OR ANTICANCER ACTIVITY
Ostrea gigas (mu li)	Inhibits SA and Kreb's tumor-2. Immunostimulant.[1]
Paeonia obovata (chai shao)	Inhibits solid and ascitic SA.[1]
Panax ginseng (ren shen)	Inhibits EA.[3] Inhibits SA (mice), adenocarcinoma-755 (mice), and human cervical cancer-26. Injection into leukemic guinea pigs results in 99% remission and doubling of lifespan.[1] Note: this herb is thought to act in part as an immunostimulant.
Patrinia scabiosaefolia (bai jiang cao)	Inhibits human cervical cancer cells.[2]
Phellodendron amurense (huang bai)	Inhibits SA.[1]
Pinellia ternata (ban xia)	Inhibits cervical cancer-14, SA, and solid liver cancer.[1] Inhibits SA, liver carcinoma (HCA), cervix carcinoma U14, Hela cells (animals). Inhibits cervical carcinoma (short term), and skin carcinoma in humans.[3]
Polistes mandarinus (lu feng fang)	Inhibits liver and gastric cancer.[1]
Polyporus umbellatus (zhu ling)	Inhibits SA and stimulates immunity.[2] Inhibits SA by 62% and hepatoma (mice) by 37 to 54%. Stimulates specific and nonspecific immunity. In humans with esophageal cancer may protect bone marrow during chemotherapy.[3]
Prunella vulgaris (xia ku cao)	Inhibits SA and cervical cancer-14 (mice).[2] Inhibits EA and SA.[3]
Psoralea corylifolia (bu gu zhi)	Inhibits SA, and EA cells.[2]
Rabdosia rubescens	Inhibits Hela cells, EA cells, SA cells, and hepatoma cells. Analgesic.[2] Inhibits Ehrlich ascites carcinoma, SA, cervical carcinoma U14 (mice), WA, hepatoma, and reticular cell sarcoma. Prolongs the survival period of animals. Iincreases survival period and reduces side effects when used with other anti-neoplastic drugs in humans with esophageal carcinoma. Improvement of liver pain and anorexia in patients with human liver carcinoma.[3]
Ranunculus teratus (mao zhua cao)	Inhibits SA, S-37, and EA.[2]
Realgar *(xiong huang)*	Inhibits human carcinoma cell JTC-26, effective rate 90%. Inhibits S-27.[1]
Rheum tanguticum (da huang)	Inhibits melanoma, EA, breast carcinoma, and S-37 in mice.[3] Inhibits S-27 (mice), melanoma (mice), and SA.[1]
Rubia cordifolia (qian cao gen)	Inhibits PS, LE, LL, human carcinoma cell JTC-26, and ascites SA.[1]
Salvia chinensis (shi jian chuan)	Inhibits SA.[1,2]
Salvia miltiorrhiza (dan shen)	Inhibits EA, and increases survival period.[3]
Scutellaria baicalensis (huang qin)	Inhibits SA, sarcoma-37, and cervical cancer-14.[1]
Scutellariae barbatae (ban zhi lian)	Inhibits SA and EA.[1,2]
Senecio integrifolius (kou she cao)	Inhibits leukemia (animals).[1]
Smilax chinensis (tu fu ling)	Inhibits SA.[1]
Solanum nigrum (long kui)	Inhibits SA, WA, ascites cancer (mice), and cervical cancer.[1] Inhibits transplanted animal tumors, effective rate 40 to 50%. Suppresses growth of meningeal tumor cells, inhibits Hela cells and ascitic SA (mice). Reduces signs and symptoms of carcinomas of cervix, esophagus, breast, lung, liver and ovary, chorioepithelioma, hepatoma, and sarcoma in humans.[3]
Solanum lyratum (shu yang quan)	Inhibits EA, SA, sarcoma-37, and lymphatic leukemia-615 (rats).[1]
Sophora subprostrata (shan dou gen)	Inhibits SA.[2] Inhibits carcinoma of cervix-U14 (mice), EA, and SA. Inhibits ascitic Jitian sarcoma. Inhibits solid ascitic carcinoma of liver (rats) by 60%.[3]
Sophora flavescens (ku shen)	Inhibits SA.[3]

(Table continues)

TABLE G.1. *(continued)*	
HERB	**ANTITUMOR OR ANTICANCER ACTIVITY**
Stephania tetranda (han fang ji)	Inhibits ascites cells (mice).[1] Inhibits WA.[2] Inhibits EA, liver carcinoma (mice), and WA.[3]
Trichosanthes kirilowii (gua lou or *gua lou ren)*	Is clinically effective on trophoblastic cell tumor of placenta. Reduces ascites and prolongs survival period of mice with ascitic carcinoma of liver. Inhibits carcinoma of cervix-U14 in mice. Cured 42 out 43 cases of malignant hydatidiform mole in humans. Cured 50% of chorioepithelioma.[3]
Tripterygium wilfordii	Inhibits L-615 leukemia cells, increases suvival time (mice).[2] Inhibits LE, PS, L615, sarcoma 37, hepatoma, and WA. Significantly prolonged survival period of animals with leukemia L615.[3]
Vaccaria segetalis (wang bu liu xing)	V. pyramidata inhibits EA.[2]
Xanthium sibiricum (cang er zi)	Inhibits EA and SA.[1]
Zanthoxylum nitidum (liang mian zhen)	Inhibits LE and PS.[2]
[1] Chang, 1992 [2] Huang KC, 1993 [3] Chang and Butt, 1986, 1987	

APPENDIX H: OVERVIEW OF SELECTED CANCERS

This appendix provides information on the pathophysiology, etiology, presentation, treatment, and patient survival for selected cancers. Unless otherwise specified, pathophysiology, etiology, and presentation data were obtained from Calabresi and Schein (1993), treatment data were obtained from Tierney et al. (1993), and survival data were obtained from Miller et al. (1992).

HODGKIN'S DISEASE

Hodgkin's disease is a little-understood neoplasm of the lymphoid tissue, most commonly affecting prepubescent and advanced-age males. Its etiology is unknown, although it has been associated with familial clustering, altered response to Epstein-Barr virus, tonsillectomy, appendectomy, and infectious mononucleosis. In spite of its infectious-disease-like symptoms, no specific pathogenetic organisms have been identified. It is frequently associated with defects in cell-mediated immunity, including T-cell lymphocytopenia and T-lymphocyte dysfunction. B-lymphocyte function tends to be normal. As such, serious infections are a common complication of the disease.

Altered cytokine production may be responsible for the characteristic inflammation. The bulk of the lymphoid swelling may be attributed to inflammatory cells rather than neoplastic cells, and many investigators question whether this disease should even be considered a true neoplasm.

The clinical course can be quite variable and treatment may result in complications that are difficult to separate from the disease itself. Patients usually experience swelling of the involved lymph nodes and may also experience pruritus, anemia, and involvement of the spleen, liver, lung, and bone marrow. In advanced cases, high fever, drenching sweats, fatigue, anorexia, and weight loss may occur. Elevations of serum fibrinogen, copper, and zinc are common. A moderate to marked neutrophilic leukocytosis and thrombocytosis are characteristic of the active phase.

Patients in early stages of the disease (stages IA or IIA) have a 90% probability of a cure with radiotherapy. In patients with more advanced disease combination chemotherapy is commonly used, sometimes in conjunction with additional radiotherapy. The current treatment of choice for patients with stage III and IV disease is combination chemotherapy with doxorubicin (Adriamycin), bleomycin, vinblastine, dacarbazine (ABVD); or mechlorethamine, vincristine, prednisone, procarbazine (MOPP); or combinations of MOPP and ABVD. The associated five-year survival rate is 25 to 80%. Relative survival rates are illustrated in Figure H.1.

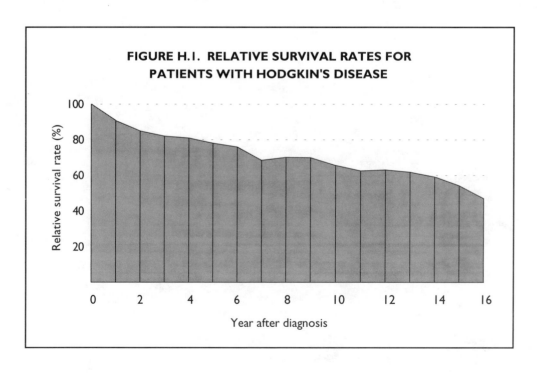

FIGURE H.1. RELATIVE SURVIVAL RATES FOR PATIENTS WITH HODGKIN'S DISEASE

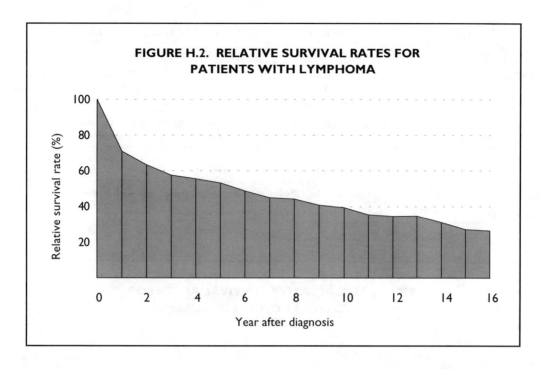

FIGURE H.2. RELATIVE SURVIVAL RATES FOR PATIENTS WITH LYMPHOMA

LYMPHOMAS

Lymphomas (non-Hodgkin's lymphomas, NHL) are a very diverse group of immune cell neoplasms. At least ten major subtypes exist. They occur in lymphoid tissues such as the lymph nodes, spleen, and bone marrow, and are similar in many respects to Hodgkin's disease and lymphatic leukemias. Some subtypes of NHL are very aggressive, and others are mildly aggressive. The etiology NHL is unknown, although various subtypes have been associated with immunodeficiency states, autoimmune diseases, and viral infections (EBV and HTLV).

Unlike Hodgkin's disease, NHL is often systemic in nature rather than localized. Signs may vary considerably between subtypes. Characteristic signs include lymph node enlargement, fever, night sweats, weight loss, and fatigue. Gastrointestinal involvement may include obstruction, ulceration, perforation, and hemorrhage. Lymphocytosis may be present.

Survival ranges from a few months to 10 years or more, depending upon the subtype and stage. In general, aggressive types of NHL are responsive to chemotherapy. Patients with advanced stages of low-grade lymphomas generally respond poorly to treatment, and a palliative program is usually employed. In early stages of low-grade lymphomas, many patients are best managed with no initial therapy. In all subtypes, radiotherapy is seldom used because of the diffuse nature of the disease. Survival data are illustrated in Figure H.2.

Current conventional treatments of choice include combination chemotherapy, usually including cyclophosphamide, vincristine, doxorubicin, and prednisone.

LEUKEMIAS

Leukemias are a diverse group of neoplasms of the blood and bone marrow. They are divided into two main subtypes, acute and chronic. Each of these are further divided into the classifications of myeloid (nonlymphocytic) and lymphoid. Like lymphoma, they are systemic in nature.

Although the etiology of leukemia is often unknown, heredity, viruses, radiation, antineoplastic drugs, and chemical exposures have all been implicated. The virus associated with leukemia is adult T-cell leukemia/lymphoma virus (ATLV).

Clinical signs and lab abnormalities of acute leukemia commonly include anemia, leukocytosis, leukopenia or leukocyte dysfunction, thrombocytopenia, fatigue, anorexia and weight loss, fever, hemorrhage, splenomegaly, hepatomegaly, infection, lymphadenopathy, and sternal tenderness.

Lab abnormalities in chronic leukemia commonly include increased production or sensitivity to hematopoietic growth factors such as GM-CSF, or decreased production or sensitivity to inhibitors of myelopoiesis such as PGE_2. During the chronic phase there is increased production of normal functioning granulocytes, monocytes, and platelets. During the acute phase, these cells exhibit a loss of differentiation, and fail to mature. Interferons, which have antiproliferative properties, have been tested for use in the chronic phase of chronic leukemia.

The clinical course ranges from rapidly fatal to slowly growing, depending upon the subtype and stage.

TABLE H.1. CURRENT CONVENTIONAL TREATMENTS OF CHOICE FOR LEUKEMIAS	
TYPE	**TREATMENT OF CHOICE**
Acute lymphatic leukemia	**Initial**: Combination chemotherapy. Adults: vincristine, prednisone, and daunorubicin, with or without asparaginase. Children: vincristine, prednisone, and asparaginase. **Remission maintenance:** Methotrexate and mercaptopurine.
Acute myelocytic and myelomonocytic leukemia	**Initial**: Combination chemotherapy including cytarabine and daunorubicin. **Consolidation:** Autologous or allogenic bone marrow transplantation, chemotherapy.
Chronic myelocytic leukemia	Hydroxyurea with or without interferon-alpha. Allogenic bone marrow transplantation in young patients.
Chronic lymphocytic leukemia	If treatment is indicated, chlorambucil and prednisone or fludarabine.
Hairy cell leukemia	Interferon-alpha or 2-chlorodeoxyadenosine

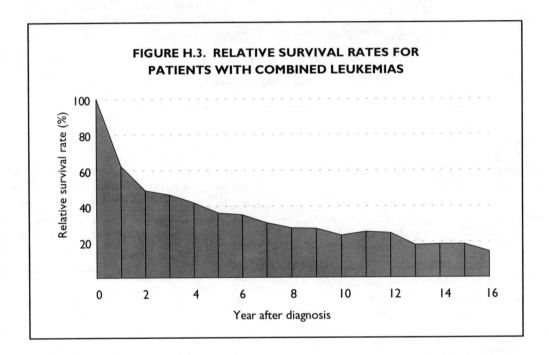

FIGURE H.3. RELATIVE SURVIVAL RATES FOR PATIENTS WITH COMBINED LEUKEMIAS

A complete remission rate of 90% is commonly seen in children with acute lymphocytic leukemia. Of these, 55 to 70% may enjoy long-term survival. Adults generally do not respond as well, with remission periods being considerably shorter. Survival data are illustrated in Figure H.3. Treatments of choice are listed in Table H.1.

MELANOMA

Sunlight plays a major etiological role in melanoma. Incidence and mortality rates are inversely related to the distance a person lives from the equator. There has been a dramatic eightfold increase in the incidence of melanoma in the last 40 years, which may be related to cyclic changes in sunspot activity or other factors. The incidence rate continues to increase, in some locations doubling every 10 to 17 years.

Dysplastic nevi is both a risk factor and precursor for melanoma. A large number of common acquired nevi (common moles) may increase melanoma risk by up to 10 to 50 times, although these lesions are usually not melanoma precursors.[1]

Melanoma may be associated with immunosuppression as evidenced by increased incidence among patients with Hodgkin's disease, other lymphoproliferative malignancies, and bone and renal transplants. Sun exposure may be a factor due to sunlight's immunosuppressive effects.

Melanomas may have a latency period of over 25 years between the time of resection of the primary lesion and metastatic disease, although commonly the latency period is less than 5 years. Five-year survival is 100% for patients whose lesions are surgically removed during

---

[1] It is possible that the increased risk is due to immune suppression as evidenced by an increased number of virally-induced moles.

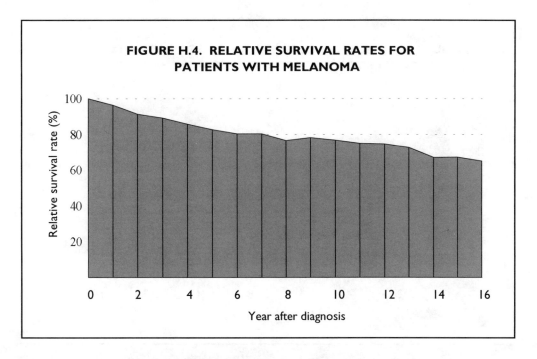

FIGURE H.4. RELATIVE SURVIVAL RATES FOR PATIENTS WITH MELANOMA

TABLE H.2. DISTRIBUTION AND SURVIVAL RATES FOR PATIENTS WITH MELANOMA

STAGE AT DIAGNOSIS	STAGE DISTRIBUTION (%) (all races, males and females)	FIVE-YEAR RELATIVE SURVIVAL (%) 1983-87
All stages	100	82.5
Localized	81	90.7
Regional	8	53.6
Distant	4	12.8
Unstaged	7	58.6

stage I. Once the disease has spread, long term survival is poor. The 10-year survival for stage II disease is 13%, and is less than 2% for stage III disease. Survival data for patients with melanoma are provided in Table H.2 and Figure H.4.

Since the immune system appears to play a role in the initiation and progression of melanoma, immunotherapy drugs have been tested. Although uncommon, immunotherapy has produced complete remissions. Of all the cytokines, interferons have received the most extensive testing. The overall response rate to rIFN-alpha is 17%, with a complete response rate of 5%. IFN-gamma and IFN-beta have also been tested. Response to high doses of IL-2 is 20%, with a complete response rate of 8%. Drugs that interrupt melanin synthesis are also being studied.

Tumors are generally managed initially with surgery, with or without adjuvant chemotherapy and radiotherapy. Palliative chemotherapy and radiotherapy are commonly used in patients with metastatic disease. The chemotherapy agent of choice is dacarbazine, along with the adjuvants interferon-alpha, and interleukin-2 with or without LAK cells.

Receptors for a number of hormones and growth factors have been identified on certain melanomas. Estrogen receptors have been identified, and both estrogens and antiestrogens have been reported to have an inhibitory effect on tumor growth in a small percentage (<10%) of patients. Insulin, transforming growth factor-alpha (TGF-alpha), epidermal growth factor (EGF), nerve growth factor (NGF), and basic fibroblast growth factor (bFGF) have all been shown to stimulate the growth of certain melanoma cells.

To prevent the initiation of melanoma, excessive sun exposure should be minimized. Sunscreens with a sun protection factor of 15 or higher may be useful. Early detection is crucial to successful treatment. As summarized by the mnemonic ABCD, a patient with any pigmented lesions that are *a*symmetric, have an irregular *b*order, have multiple *c*olors, and a *d*iameter greater than a pencil eraser (6 mm) should be referred to an appropriate physician.

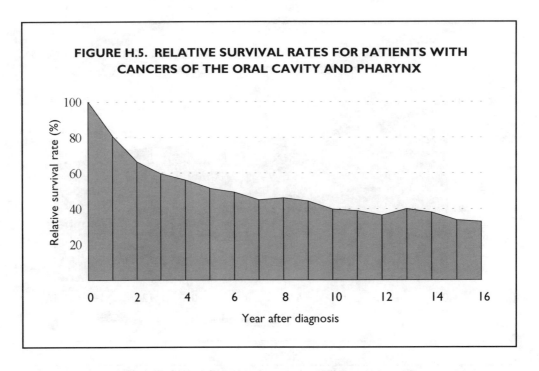

FIGURE H.5. RELATIVE SURVIVAL RATES FOR PATIENTS WITH CANCERS OF THE ORAL CAVITY AND PHARYNX

TABLE H.3. DISTRIBUTION AND SURVIVAL RATES FOR PATIENTS WITH CANCERS OF THE ORAL CAVITY AND PHARYNX

STAGE AT DIAGNOSIS	STAGE DISTRIBUTION (%) (all races, males and females)	FIVE-YEAR RELATIVE SURVIVAL (%) 1983-87
All stages	100	51.5
Localized	37	76.2
Regional	43	40.9
Distant	10	18.9
Unstaged	10	41.7

NEOPLASMS OF THE HEAD AND NECK

Neoplasms of the head and neck include cancers of the lip, oral cavity, tongue, oropharynx, nasal cavity and paranasal sinuses, nasopharynx, hypopharynx, larynx, and salivary glands. Exposure to environmental factors, such as sunlight, tobacco, alcohol, vitamin deficiencies, and wood dust and other occupational exposures, have all been associated with or are suspected of causing head and neck cancers. Squamous cell carcinomas are the most common malignant tumors within this category.

Symptoms of head and neck neoplasms may include ulcerations, leukoplakia, symptoms due to local obstruction, infection, pressure, dysphagia, and sore throat.

Localized lesions may be cured with radiotherapy and/or surgery. Chemotherapy is used to treat metastatic disease, although the survival of responders is only about three to five months from the start of therapy. Survival data are presented in Table H.3 and Figure H.5.

The chemotherapy agent of choice is combination chemotherapy using cisplatin and fluorouracil. Palliative radiotherapy may be used to treat metastatic disease.

LUNG CANCER

Lung cancer is the most common cause of cancer death in United States men over 35 years old, and its incidence is increasing faster than that of any other cancer except melanoma. The most significant causal factor is cigarette smoking.

Cancers arising from the endobronchial epithelium (bronchogenic cancers) constitute 90% of all lung cancers. They are commonly classified into five types: squamous cell, adenocarcinoma, large cell, small cell, and broncho-alveolar.

Symptoms generally include cough, sputum production, hemoptysis, stridor, infection, and paraneoplastic syndromes (ACTH and HGH irregularities, etc.). Regional and distant spread is common. The course is

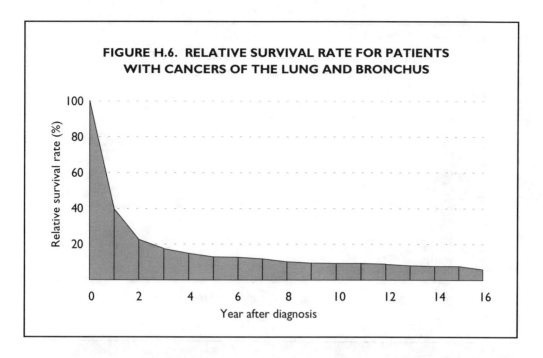

FIGURE H.6. RELATIVE SURVIVAL RATE FOR PATIENTS WITH CANCERS OF THE LUNG AND BRONCHUS

TABLE H.4. DISTRIBUTION AND SURVIVAL RATES FOR PATIENTS WITH CANCER OF THE LUNG AND BRONCHUS		
STAGE AT DIAGNOSIS	**STAGE DISTRIBUTION (%)** (all races, males and females)	**FIVE-YEAR RELATIVE SURVIVAL (%) 1983-87**
All stages	100	13.1
Localized	16	45.6
Regional	32	13.1
Distant	37	1.3
Unstaged	15	7.8

rapid, and more than half of the patients with bronchogenic cancers die within the first year of diagnosis (nearly half of the patients have widely disseminated disease at the time of diagnosis). Surgery, radiotherapy, and chemotherapy have been largely unsuccessful, and there has been little change in five-year survival rates since the 1950s. Survival data are presented in Table H.4 and Figure H.6.

Tumors are generally managed initially with surgery, with or without adjuvant chemotherapy and radiotherapy. Palliative chemotherapy and radiotherapy are commonly used in patients with metastatic disease. The chemotherapy of choice for small cell carcinoma is a combination of cisplatin and etoposide. Chemotherapy of choice for non-small cell carcinoma is a combination of cisplatin, mitomycin, and vinblastine.

ESOPHAGEAL CANCER

Although the etiological factors of esophageal cancer are largely unknown, incidence is associated with the use of tobacco and alcohol, deficiencies of vitamins and minerals, genetic factors, fungal contamination of foodstuffs, consumption of pickled and preserved foods, and a history of head, neck, and lung cancer. Common signs and symptoms include dysphagia, substernal pain, anemia, hoarseness, coughing after eating or drinking, and hemorrhage.

Esophageal carcinomas tend to metastasize early, often to the lungs, liver, bones, and kidneys. At diagnosis, the majority of patients have disseminated disease. However, death may be caused by lateral invasion. Therapy has not been very successful, and the median survival of patients receiving surgery, radiation, and chemotherapy is between 12 and 29 months. Survival data are provided in Table H.5 and Figure H.7.

Tumors are generally managed initially with surgery, with or without adjuvant chemotherapy and

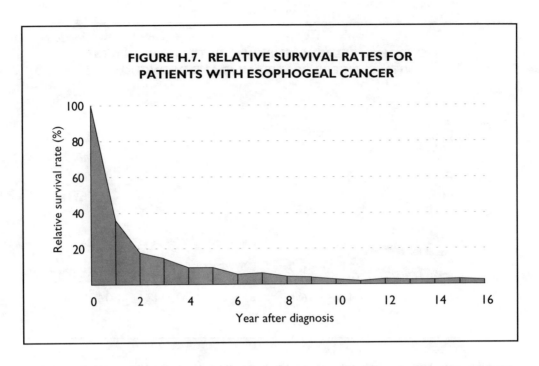

FIGURE H.7. RELATIVE SURVIVAL RATES FOR
PATIENTS WITH ESOPHOGEAL CANCER

TABLE H.5. DISTRIBUTION AND SURVIVAL RATES FOR
PATIENTS WITH ESOPHAGEAL CANCER

STAGE AT DIAGNOSIS	STAGE DISTRIBUTION (%) (All races, males and females)	FIVE-YEAR RELATIVE SURVIVAL (%) 1983-87
All stages	100	8
Localized	25	18.5
Regional	22	5.2
Distant	28	1.8
Unstaged	26	7.6

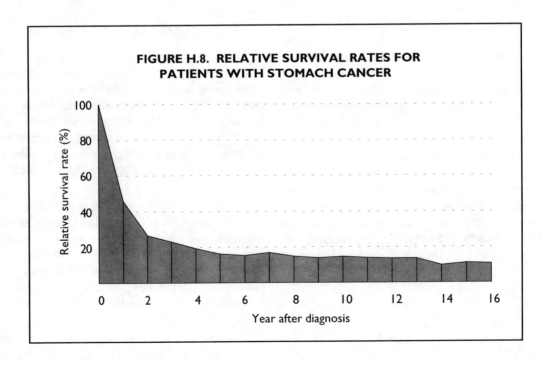

FIGURE H.8. RELATIVE SURVIVAL RATES FOR
PATIENTS WITH STOMACH CANCER

TABLE H.6. DISTRIBUTION AND SURVIVAL RATES FOR PATIENTS WITH STOMACH CANCER		
STAGE AT DIAGNOSIS	STAGE DISTRIBUTION (%) (all races, males and females)	FIVE-YEAR RELATIVE SURVIVAL (%) 1983-87
All stages	100	16.8
Localized	16	55.4
Regional	34	17.3
Distant	36	2.1
Unstaged	13	9.6

radiotherapy. Palliative chemotherapy and radiotherapy are commonly used in patients with metastatic disease. The chemotherapy agents of choice is combination chemotherapy using fluorouracil, cisplatin, and mitomycin.

STOMACH CANCER

Epidemiological evidence suggests that dietary and environmental factors play a significant role in the incidence of stomach cancer. Dietary intake of nitrites (found in high amounts in processed or "cured" meats) is suspected as a causative factor. Predisposing factors include pernicious anemia, atrophic gastritis, adenomas, familial stomach cancer, high intake of pickled or preserved foods, and gastric ulcer. The majority (95%) of all stomach cancers are adenocarcinomas.

Signs and symptoms include mild epigastric discomfort similar to a typical peptic ulcer, anorexia, early satiety, distortions of taste and smell, weight loss, nausea, vomiting, palpable abdominal masses, anemia, and disseminated intravascular coagulation (DIC).

If detected at an early stage, surgery may be curative. However, the majority of patients have disseminated advanced disease at the time of diagnosis. Surgery, chemotherapy, and radiotherapy are largely ineffective for these patients, and five-year survival rates are low. Survival data are presented in Table H.6 and Figure H.8.

Tumors are generally managed initially with surgery, with or without adjuvant chemotherapy and radiotherapy. Palliative chemotherapy and radiotherapy are commonly used in patients with metastatic disease. The chemotherapy agent of choice is combination chemotherapy using fluorouracil, doxorubicin, methotrexate; or using doxorubicin, etoposide, and cisplatin.

PANCREATIC CANCER

The etiology of pancreatic cancer is unknown, and reports of associated factors have been contradictory. The prognosis of patients with pancreatic cancer is very poor, the average survival being less than two years even in patients with local tumors. Chemotherapy, radiotherapy, and surgery are of very limited efficacy. Survival data are presented in Table H.7 and Figure H.9.

Signs and symptoms are often vague and insidious. They include weight loss, jaundice, back pain, depression, hepatomegaly, anorexia, dark urine, and light stools. In part due to the vague nature of the presentation, experienced physicians misdiagnose the disease 50% of the time. By the time of diagnosis, the disease has usually metastasized.

Tumors are generally managed initially with surgery, with or without adjuvant chemotherapy and radiotherapy. Palliative chemotherapy and radiotherapy are commonly used in patients with metastatic disease. The chemotherapy agent of choice is fluorouracil.

LIVER CANCER

Numerous etiological factors have been associated with liver cancer. These include viruses (hepatitis-B and hepatitis-C), hepatic cirrhosis, alcohol consumption, chemical carcinogens, aflatoxin, oral contraceptives, and anabolic steroid use. Hepatocellular cancer accounts for 90% of primary hepatic malignancies.

Signs and symptoms include weight loss, abdominal pain, anorexia, fatigue, hepatomegaly, ascites, splenomegaly, jaundice, and elevated liver enzymes. Hormonal syndromes and paraneoplastic phenomena are common. Generally, the disease is confined locally, although there are cases of distant malignant spread. Although not specific for hepatoma, serum alpha-fetoprotein (AFP) is normally elevated and may provide a useful tumor marker during treatment.

Surgery, radiotherapy and chemotherapy are all of limited value in the treatment of this disease, and five-year survival rates are relatively low. The most effective chemotherapy agent appears to be doxorubicin. Survival data are provided in Table H.8 and Figure H.10.

TABLE H.7. DISTRIBUTION AND SURVIVAL RATES FOR PATIENTS WITH PANCREATIC CANCER		
STAGE AT DIAGNOSIS	**STAGE DISTRIBUTION (%)** (all races, males and females)	**FIVE-YEAR RELATIVE SURVIVAL (%) 1983-87**
All stages	100	3.2
Localized	9	8.1
Regional	21	3.7
Distant	50	1.4
Unstaged	19	5.2

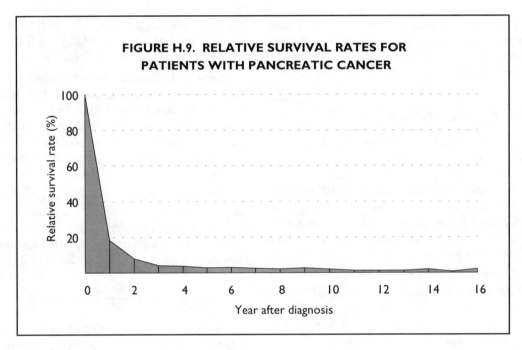

FIGURE H.9. RELATIVE SURVIVAL RATES FOR PATIENTS WITH PANCREATIC CANCER

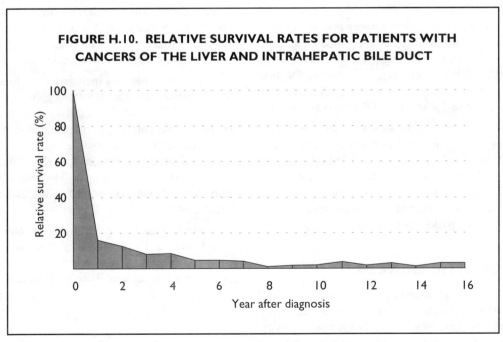

FIGURE H.10. RELATIVE SURVIVAL RATES FOR PATIENTS WITH CANCERS OF THE LIVER AND INTRAHEPATIC BILE DUCT

TABLE H.8. DISTRIBUTION AND SURVIVAL RATES FOR PATIENTS WITH CANCER OF THE LIVER AND INTRAHEPATIC BILE DUCT		
STAGE AT DIAGNOSIS	STAGE DISTRIBUTION (%) (All races, males and females)	FIVE-YEAR RELATIVE SURVIVAL (%) 1983-87
All stages	100	6
Localized	21	15.1
Regional	23	5.8
Distant	26	1.9
Unstaged	30	2.9

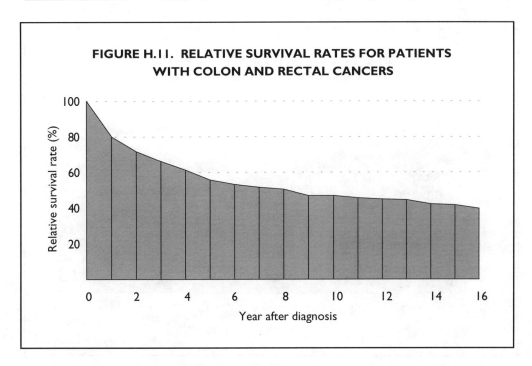

FIGURE H.11. RELATIVE SURVIVAL RATES FOR PATIENTS WITH COLON AND RECTAL CANCERS

COLORECTAL CARCINOMA

Risk factors for colorectal carcinoma includes familial polyposis syndromes; inflammatory bowel disease; a past history of colorectal, breast, or endometrial cancer; decreased physical activity; a high-fat and low-fiber diet; and low intake of vitamin C, calcium, selenium, flavones and indoles.

Signs and symptoms include vague abdominal pain, peptic-ulcer-like symptoms, low-grade chronic blood loss in stool, alterations in bowel habits, and tenesmus. Poor prognosis is associated with low serum protein level and high carcinoembryonic antigen (CEA) levels.

Responses to chemotherapy are generally low (less than about 30%). Biological response modifiers such as interferons, and interleukins have been studied, although success has been limited. Survival data are presented in Table H.9 and Figure H.11.

Tumors are generally managed initially with surgery, with or without adjuvant chemotherapy and radiotherapy. Palliative chemotherapy and radiotherapy are commonly used in patients with metastatic disease. The chemotherapy agent of choice is fluorouracil, in combination with the adjuvant agents levamisole or leucovorin.

BREAST CANCER

Risk factors for breast cancer include a family history of breast cancer, radiation exposure, and obesity (postmenopausal women). Early menarche, late menopause, and late or no childbearing may increase risk due to increased life time exposure to estrogen. Hormonal replacement therapy may also increase risk. Lymph node involvement and menstrual status are two of the most useful parameters to determine prognosis. Low serum cholesterol and low body weight may double five-year disease free survival rates compared to patients with high cholesterol and high body weight. Breast cancer is often

TABLE H.9. DISTRIBUTION AND SURVIVAL OF PATIENTS WITH COLON AND RECTAL CANCER		
STAGE AT DIAGNOSIS	**STAGE DISTRIBUTION (%)** (all races, males and females)	**FIVE-YEAR RELATIVE SURVIVAL (%) 1983-87**
All stages	100	77.9
Localized	53	92.7
Regional	37	71.1
Distant	7	17.8
Unstaged	4	50.1

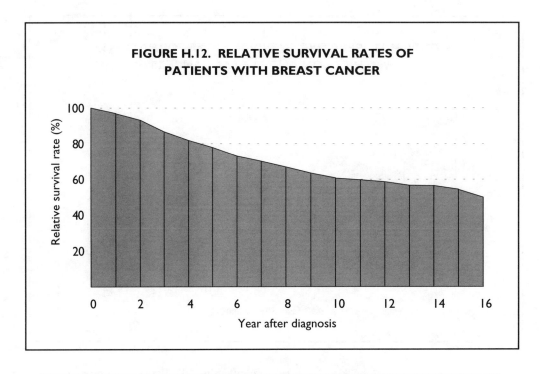

FIGURE H.12. RELATIVE SURVIVAL RATES OF PATIENTS WITH BREAST CANCER

TABLE H.10. DISTRIBUTION AND SURVIVAL OF PATIENTS WITH BREAST CANCER		
STAGE AT DIAGNOSIS	**STAGE DISTRIBUTION (%)** (all races, females)	**FIVE-YEAR RELATIVE SURVIVAL (%) 1983-87**
All stages	100	77.9
Localized	53	92.7
Regional	37	71.1
Distant	7	17.8
Unstaged	4	50.1

a chronic disease, and patients with stage I and II cancer may live for 20 years or more.

Signs and symptoms include a lump or thickening in the breast, pain in the breast, and nipple discharge. Local and regional treatments alone generally fail to lengthen survival times, and the majority of deaths are due to disseminated disease. Radical mastectomy has been found to be no more effective than lumpectomy or other more conservative procedures when the tumor is small (<3 cm).

The antiestrogen tamoxifen is commonly used if the disease is not advanced, and if the tumor is ER-positive. If the tumor is also progesterone sensitive, response rates may be as high as 80%. The median duration of response exceeds six months. Tamoxifen appears to be more effective in postmenopausal women, and less

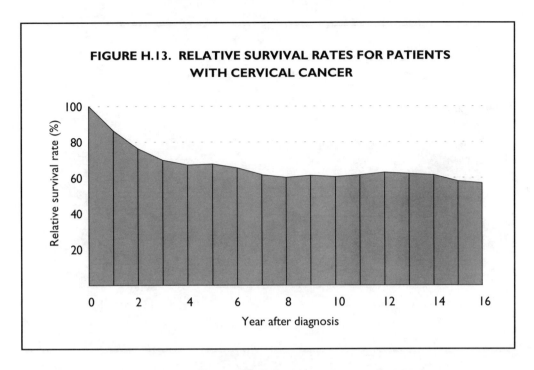

FIGURE H.13. RELATIVE SURVIVAL RATES FOR PATIENTS WITH CERVICAL CANCER

TABLE H.11. DISTRIBUTION AND SURVIVAL RATES OF PATIENTS WITH CERVICAL CANCER

STAGE AT DIAGNOSIS	STAGE DISTRIBUTION (%) (all races, females)	FIVE-YEAR RELATIVE SURVIVAL (%) 1983-87
All stages	100	65.9
Localized	48	89.2
Regional	34	51.5
Distant	10	13.5
Unstaged	7	54.5

effective in premenopausal women. Combination chemotherapy used against aggressive cancers results in response rates ranging from 50 to 75%, with complete response rates generally below 20%. The median duration of complete and partial responses is six to eight months. The median survival is one to two years after the start of chemotherapy. The optimal duration of treatment appears to be 4 to 6 months, with longer durations resulting in negligible additional improvement. Chemotherapy appears to be more effective in premenopausal women. Survival data are provided in Table H.10 and Figure H.12.

Tumors are generally managed initially with surgery, with or without adjuvant chemotherapy and radiotherapy. Palliative chemotherapy and radiotherapy are commonly used in patients with metastatic disease. The chemotherapy agent of choice is combination chemotherapy using cyclophosphamide, doxorubicin, and fluorouracil.

CANCER OF THE CERVIX

Death rates from cancer of the cervix have been falling since 1935. This decline is often attributed to screening with the PAP smear. Cancer of the cervix acts epidemiologically like a sexually transmitted disease. It is associated with increased sexual exposure and poor economic status. A low incidence exists in groups with reduced sexual exposure, such as Roman catholic nuns. The causative factor appears to be human papilloma virus (HPV), the virus responsible for genital warts. A subtype of HPV has been identified in 95% of squamous cell cancers of the cervix. Other unknown etiologic factors are likely.

Signs and symptoms include abnormal vaginal bleeding, foul smelling discharge, pelvic or low-back pain, and ulceration.

Prognosis is closely related to the stage of the disease at diagnosis. Surgery is curative if the disease is identified at an early stage. Cure at a late stage is rare.

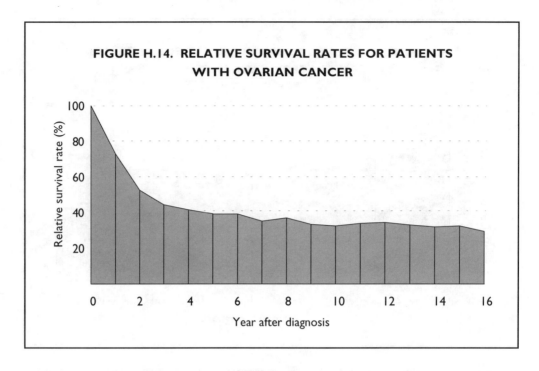

FIGURE H.14. RELATIVE SURVIVAL RATES FOR PATIENTS WITH OVARIAN CANCER

TABLE H.12. DISTRIBUTION AND SURVIVAL RATES OF PATIENTS WITH OVARIAN CANCER

STAGE AT DIAGNOSIS	STAGE DISTRIBUTION (%) (all races, females)	FIVE-YEAR RELATIVE SURVIVAL (%) 1983-87
All stages	100	39.1
Localized	23	88.5
Regional	26	36.6
Distant	46	17.6
Unstaged	5	20.8

Survival data are presented in Table H.11 and Figure H.13.

Palliative chemotherapy and radiotherapy are commonly used in patients with metastatic disease. The chemotherapy agents of choice are combinations of methotrexate, doxorubicin, cisplatin, and vinblastine; or mitomycin, bleomycin, vincristine, and cisplatin.

OVARIAN CANCER

Etiologic factors associated with ovarian cancer include breast cancer, no children, family history of ovarian cancer, and obesity. The cause of ovarian cancer is unknown.

Ovarian cancer is often an occult disease, as symptoms are nonspecific. Therefore, ovarian cancers are commonly diagnosed at an advanced stage. Signs and symptoms may include vague pelvic or abdominal discomfort, indigestion, urinary frequency, abnormal vaginal bleeding, abdominal swelling, and palpable abdominal masses.

Surgery is rarely curative in early stage disease, since metastasis into the abdominal cavity is common even with small tumors. Chemotherapy is used for disseminated disease. Chemotherapy may provide remissions in about 50% of the patients, and median survival rates are generally 3 years or less. Survival data are presented in Table H.12 and Figure H.14.

The chemotherapy of choice is combinations that include cyclophosphamide, and cisplatin or carboplatin. Immunotherapy with interferon-alpha has shown modest effects. Treatment with interleukin-2 has also been studied. The use of radiotherapy is controversial since the entire abdomen and pelvis must be treated.

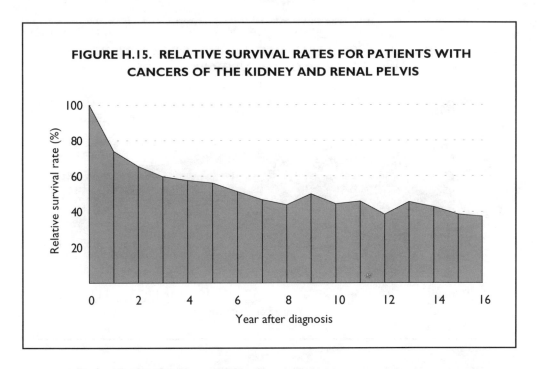

FIGURE H.15. RELATIVE SURVIVAL RATES FOR PATIENTS WITH CANCERS OF THE KIDNEY AND RENAL PELVIS

STAGE AT DIAGNOSIS	STAGE DISTRIBUTION (%) (all races, males and females)	FIVE-YEAR RELATIVE SURVIVAL (%) 1983-87
All stages	100	54.9
Localized	43	85.4
Regional	25	56.3
Distant	27	9
Unstaged	6	30.3

TABLE H.13. DISTRIBUTION AND SURVIVAL RATES OF PATIENTS WITH CANCERS OF THE KIDNEY AND RENAL PELVIS

NEOPLASM OF THE KIDNEY

The etiology of renal tumors is unknown, although associated factors include tobacco use, obesity, and diets rich in animal fats and cholesterol. Hormonal imbalance has been suggested as a possible cause.

Early tumor growth is commonly asymptomatic, and patients usually present with later stage diseases at diagnosis. At the time of diagnosis, approximately 20 to 40% of the patients have metastasis. Without surgery, the disease is normally fatal within one year. Nephrectomy can increase five-year survival in stage I, II, and III diseases to 59 to 60%, 51 to 64%, and 34 to 48% respectively. Radiotherapy has not been shown to be useful in increasing survival. Renal cell carcinoma is resistant to chemotherapy and hormonal therapy, with response rates generally less than 10%. Vinblastine is the most common chemotherapy agent used. Due to reports of spontaneous regression of renal cell carcinoma, immunotherapy has been investigated. Trials with alpha- and gamma-

interferon have resulted in response rates of approximately 15% and 9 to 28% respectively. Trials with tumor necrosis factor have been more disappointing. Use of interleukin-2 has resulted in response rates of 22%. Survival data are provided in Table H.13 and Figure H.15.

BLADDER CANCER

Smoking may be responsible for approximately 37 to 45% of deaths due to bladder cancer. Occupational exposure may also be a causative factor. Bladder cancer may develop through the two-stage process of initiation, possibly through a single exposure to a low-dose carcinogen, and promotion through contact with a noncarcinogenic agent.

Diagnosis is commonly made when the disease is still localized. Signs and symptoms may include hematuria, urinary frequency, urinary urgency, and dysuria. Bladder cancer can be an aggressive disease. Early-stage

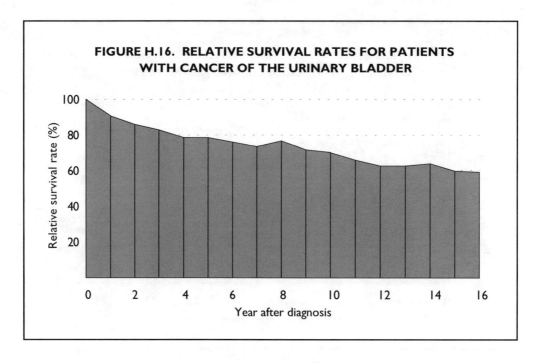

FIGURE H.16. RELATIVE SURVIVAL RATES FOR PATIENTS WITH CANCER OF THE URINARY BLADDER

TABLE H.14. DISTRIBUTION AND SURVIVAL RATES OF PATIENTS WITH URINARY BLADDER CANCER

STAGE AT DIAGNOSIS	STAGE DISTRIBUTION (%) (all races, males and females)	FIVE-YEAR RELATIVE SURVIVAL (%) 1983-87
All stages	100	78.1
Localized	74	90
Regional	19	46
Distant	3	9.1
Unstaged	4	55.6

diseases are commonly treated with transurethral resection and fulguration of the bladder (TURB). Using this method, reported five-year survival rates for stage I, II, and II diseases is 62 to 77%, 57 to 59%, and 2 to 23% respectively. Stage III disease may be treated with radiotherapy and total cystectomy. The associated five-year survival rate is 40 to 50%. Survival of patients with stage IV disease is generally less than one year. If chemotherapy is used, the agents of choice are combinations of methotrexate, vinblastine, doxorubicin and cisplatin. Intravesical BCG (a bacteria which stimulates the immune system) or thiotepa may also be used. Survival data are presented in Table H.14 and Figure H.16.

PROSTATE CANCER

The etiology of prostate cancer is unknown, but appears to be related to a high-fat diet. Epidemiologic studies have failed to consistently identify associated factors. The disease is hormonally related since regression may follow estrogen therapy or castration. A relationship between prostate cancer and benign prostatic hyperplasia (BPH) has not been confirmed.

Prostate cancer grows very slowly. However, the progression is highly unpredictable and a focal tumor can rapidly progress to widespread metastasis rather than to a localized disease. Symptoms usually do not appear until the disease progresses to the point of impinging on surrounding tissue. Signs and symptoms may include urinary hesitancy, frequency, nocturia, and dysuria.

Treatment for prostate cancer varies according to the patient's specific condition and the physicians preference. Commonly, no specific treatment is warranted in stage A disease, as survival is similar to age-matched controls. Surgery or radiotherapy may be used in stage B disease. Potentially, these may be curative. Surgery may also be used in stage C. Treatment in stage D often includes palliative measures and hormonal manipulation (androgen deprivation), usually by bilateral orchiectomy, antagonists of the release of luteinizing hormone (such as

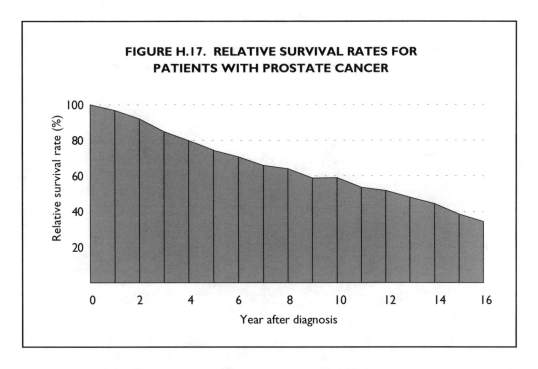

FIGURE H.17. RELATIVE SURVIVAL RATES FOR PATIENTS WITH PROSTATE CANCER

TABLE H.15. DISTRIBUTION AND SURVIVAL RATES OF PATIENTS WITH PROSTATE CANCER

STAGE AT DIAGNOSIS	STAGE DISTRIBUTION (%) (all races, males)	FIVE-YEAR RELATIVE SURVIVAL (%) 1983-87
All stages	100	75.6
Localized	58	91
Regional	14	80.4
Distant	18	28
Unstaged	9	67.5

leuprolide), or antiandrogens (such as flutamide). Serial measurements of prostate-specific antigen (PSA) may provide a useful marker for detecting early relapse and for following treatment response. In stage C disease, serial PSA measurements have a 50 to 80% accuracy for documenting treatment response. Trials with chemotherapy agents have resulted in response rates less than 10%. Survival data are presented in Table H.15 and Figure H.17.

TUMORS OF THE CENTRAL NERVOUS SYSTEM (BRAIN CANCERS)

The World Health Organization has classified over 34 different types of primary brain tumors, many of which have diverse characteristics. In addition to primary development, brain tumors can also arise from metastatic spread from distant sites. Brain tumors are unique for a number of reasons:

- Due to the confinement of the skull, tumors may cause symptoms and signs by increasing intracranial pressure.
- Small lesions may cause extensive damage since central nervous system tissue does not regenerate, adjacent healthy tissue will not compensate for damaged tissue, and function is precisely located. For these same reasons, surgery is sometimes highly restricted.
- Brain tumors spread by invading adjacent tissue but rarely metastasize.
- Due to the blood-brain barrier, many chemotherapy drugs are not able to reach target sites in the brain and spinal cord, and are thus of limited value. Agents of small molecular size (less than 450 daltons) and high lipid solubility have shown the most promise (Edward et al., 1980).

The etiology of brain cancer is unknown. Heredity, chemical exposure, viral exposure, and exposure to radiation have shown minor associations. A number of brain

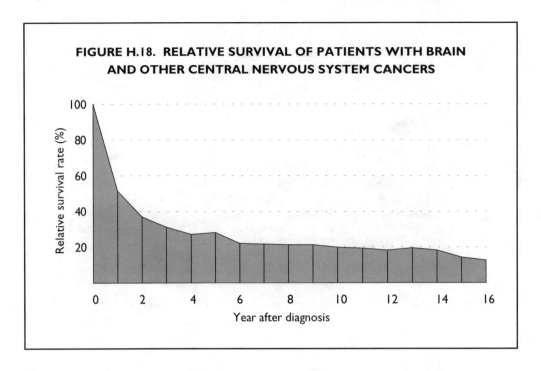

FIGURE H.18. RELATIVE SURVIVAL OF PATIENTS WITH BRAIN AND OTHER CENTRAL NERVOUS SYSTEM CANCERS

TABLE H.16. DISTRIBUTION AND SURVIVAL OF PATIENTS WITH BRAIN CANCER AND OTHER NERVOUS SYSTEM CANCERS		
STAGE AT DIAGNOSIS	**STAGE DISTRIBUTION (%) (all races, males and females)**	**FIVE-YEAR RELATIVE SURVIVAL (%) 1983-87**
All stages	100	25.9
Localized	66	26
Regional	22	27.9
Distant	2	23.6
Unstaged	10	21.7

tumors may be affected by hormonal factors. In addition, overexpression of receptors for platelet-derived growth factor and epidermal growth factor have been identified in cell lines derived from primary brain tumors. Signs and symptoms vary widely, but may include headache, seizures, mental symptoms, and neurologic defects.

Therapy may include surgery, radiotherapy, and chemotherapy. Treatments vary depending upon the type and location of the tumor. Survival data are presented in Table H.16 and Figure H.18.

APPENDIX I: OVERVIEW OF COMMON RESEARCH DESIGNS

Why should practitioners of conventional or complementary medicine get involved in research? First, because practitioners tend to be interested in unique research questions. If you are interested in the effects of a particular herb on macrophage activity, you may have to wait a long time before university or government researchers become interested in the same question. Research on complementary medicine can progress much faster if practitioners are working to push it forward.

Second, practitioners may be more familiar with a natural agent. This may allow the practitioner to create a design that optimally reflects the theory or application of the therapy being tested.

Third, practitioners of both conventional and complementary medicine tend to look at research questions from a clinical, rather than an academic, viewpoint. When research is left solely to academia, there is a greater risk that the results of the research will have less clinical relevance.

There are other good reasons to get involved with research, not the least of which is to expand your own knowledge on a given topic and improve your clinical effectiveness.

A wide variety of research designs can be used to gather information on anticancer agents. These range from simple information-gathering surveys to large clinical trials (see Tables I.1 to I.4). Designs can be ordered in terms of their ability to establish cause and effect. The designs listed in the tables below are presented in order from weakest to strongest (i.e., descriptive designs, correlational designs, quasi-experimental designs, and experimental designs).

The descriptive and correlational designs are weakest because they lack a comparison group. To establish that a particular therapy is beneficial, one must show that its effects are superior to an alternative therapy. The alternative therapy can be "no therapy" or "placebo".

Most quasi-experimental designs explicitly include a comparison group. The primary weakness of quasi-experimental designs is that they do not rule out alternative hypotheses that may explain differences between the experimental and control groups. That is, quasi-experimental designs do not control for confounding variables. For example, consider the post-test only with nonequivalent groups design. Observed differences between the treatment and control group could be due to the therapy or could be due to pre-existing characteristics of the two groups (e.g., patients in the treatment group have

greater motivation to get well; are less severely ill; or have healthier lifestyles).

Experimental designs overcome the problem of confounding through random assignment of patients to treatment groups. Random selection of patients is not required. Random assignment assures the investigator that, on the average, patients in treatment and control groups are comparable with respect to all possible confounding variables (even those that the investigator hasn't thought of). Confounding variables that the investigator knows to be important also can be controlled by blocking (stratification, matching). To block on a confounding variable (for example, severity or stage of disease), patients are grouped into homogeneous subsets (blocks) with respect to the confounding variable. Within each block, treatments are randomly assigned to patients. The overall strategy in experimental designs is to block on variables that are known to be potential confounding factors and to use randomization to control for all others.

The outline of research design presented in these tables is adapted from Burns and Grove (1987) with minor changes. Other authors may refer to these designs by different titles, but the contents are generally similar. The reader is referred to Payton (1988) for a slightly different presentation. For further information concerning the nuts and bolts of designing and conducting research, see Burns and Grove (1987), Payton (1988), and Lewith and Aldridge (1993).

The following considerations may be of use when developing a research project:

- Data for all patients and all trials should be reported, not just the successful ones. Data for failures are just as important as data for successes.

- Toxicity and quality of life data should be reported wherever appropriate. Standard forms for assessing toxicity reactions are contained in the *Investigators Handbook* (NCI, 1993). One instrument that may be particularly suited for assessing quality of life parameters is the Sickness Impact Profile. See Lewith and Aldridge (1993), and Deyo et al. (1982, 1983) for more information on this instrument.

- Tissue biopsies must be included in all human studies to verify the diagnosis of cancer.

TABLE I.1. DESCRIPTIVE DESIGNS

DESCRIPTIVE DESIGN: The purpose of descriptive studies is to describe a phenomena. They are used to gain information in a field of study for the purpose of developing theories, identifying problems with current therapies, or determining the therapies that other practitioners are using in similar situations. In general, the researcher in descriptive study does not manipulate variables (such as providing a treatment). Rather, the researcher describes what is naturally occurring. An exception to this is case study design, where the researcher may describe the effects of treatment on an individual or group.

SUBTYPE	EXAMPLE
Nominal Descriptive Designs. The purpose of nominal (or exploratory) design is to explore and describe a phenomena that is poorly understood.	An interview of 50 licensed acupuncturists to identify the types of biomedical diseases that they commonly treat.
Typical Descriptive Design. This is the most common type of descriptive design. It is used to examine the characteristics of a single sample group.	An interview with 50 acupuncturists to determine how they treat patients with *heart blood vacuity*.
Comparative Descriptive Design. This design identifies and describes differences in variables between two or more groups.	An comparison between how 50 acupuncturists and 50 TCM herbalists treat *heart blood vacuity*.
Case Study Designs. The case study is an intensive exploration of a single subject or group of subjects (the later is referred to as a case series). Case studies are used as evidence supporting or negating theories, for demonstrating the effectiveness of a technique (in a particular subject or group), and for generating new hypotheses for later testing in experimental studies. Case studies can not be used to generalize the effect of an action to the population at large. Case study designs often contain elements of one of the time dimensional descriptive designs discussed below.	An examination of the quality of life of 15 patients with breast cancer that were treated with a particular method. Treatment could be altered over time to suit the patients, or could be provided and then withheld in cycles.
Surveys. Surveys are questionnaires or interviews of randomly sampled individuals within a population of interest to describe their characteristics.	A survey of the eating habits of 50 patients diagnosed with *stomach fire*.

PRIMARY SUBTYPE	SECONDARY SUBTYPE	EXAMPLE
Time Dimensional Descriptive Design. This is also called a cohort design (a cohort is a group of subjects born in a particular period and traced through life). Cohort designs can be retrospective (based upon past medical records) or prospective (based upon current and future medical records).	**Longitudinal Descriptive Design.** Longitudinal designs follow a cohort for an extended period of time.	A prospective longitudinal study may follow 500 female patients diagnosed with *spleen qi vacuity* for 20 years to determine which patients, if any, develop breast cancer.
	Trend Design. This type of design examines changes in a sample population over time in order to predict further changes.	An examination of the diagnostic skills of 10 first-year naturopathic students, and examination of the same 10 students one year later, to predict their skills in the third year of school.
	Event Partitioning Designs. This type of design is a cross between cross-sectional or longitudinal and trend studies. It allows for merged data between time-separated subject groups.	An examination of the changes in TCM diagnosis over time after initial and concurrent diagnosis of liver cancer and *liver qi* stagnation. Patients would be enrolled in the study as they are diagnosed, and examination would occur 3 times yearly for 10 years.

TABLE I.2. CORRELATIONAL DESIGNS

CORRELATIONAL DESIGN: The purpose of a correlational design is to describe whether a correlation exists between two or more variables. It is used to examine relationships. Correlational designs do not establish cause and effect.

SUBTYPE	EXAMPLE
Descriptive Correlational Design. This type of design describes and examines the correlation between two variables. This is also called a Cross-sectional design.	Interviewing 1,000 people from the general public to determine if a correlation exists between smoking cigarettes and a diagnosis of *lung yin vacuity.*
Case-Control Design. This design is widely used in medical literature to measure the change in risk of disease (or health) due to exposure to some agent. Unlike other correlational designs, subjects are intentionally selected to have certain scores on one variable (case vs. control). Scores on the second variable are free to vary.	Interviewing 500 people who have a diagnosis of *lung yin vacuity* (cases) and 500 people who do not (controls) to identify if a correlation exists between a diagnosis of *lung yin vacuity* and smoking cigarettes. Controls are selected to be as similar as possible to cases (i.e., gender, age, etc.).
Predictive Correlational Design. This type of design is used to predict a the value of a variable based upon the value of another variable.	Interviewing 1,000 people from the general public to determine the accuracy of a mathematical formula that predicts that 10% of patients with a diagnosis of *lung yin vacuity* also smoke cigarettes.
Theory Testing Correlational Design. This type of design can include adjustments of a correlation based upon an intervening variable.	Interviewing 1,000 people from the general public to determine if a correlation exists between smoking cigarettes and a diagnosis of *lung yin vacuity,* after accounting for any previous exposure to asbestos.

TABLE I.3. QUASI-EXPERIMENTAL STUDY DESIGNS

QUASI-EXPERIMENTAL STUDY DESIGNS: The purpose of a quasi-experimental design is to examine cause-and-effect relationships. It is used when an experimental design (see below) is not ethical or possible, such as when random assignment is not possible. Subjects in a quasi-experimental design are rarely randomly selected.

PRIMARY SUBTYPE	SECONDARY SUBTYPE	EXAMPLE
Nonequivalent Control Group Design. This type of design is used when treatments can not be randomly assigned to patients (or patients cannot be randomly assigned to a treatment).	**One-Group Post-Test-Only Design.** In this design, no control group is used, and no pretest is given. This is the weakest of the quasi-experimental designs, since there is no direct way to measure change.	The leukocyte count is measured in 10 post-chemotherapy patients 5 days after treatment with an herbal formula that is expected to increase the leukocyte count.
	Post-Test-Only Design with Nonequivalent Groups. This is a slight improvement on the previous design, in that a nonequivalent control group is used.	The leukocyte count is measured in 10 post-chemotherapy patients 5 days after treatment with an herbal formula that is expected to raise the leukocyte count. In addition, identical tests are conducted in 10 similar patients that self-selected not to receive the herbal formula (i.e., they were not equivalent to the experimental group).
(column continues)	**One-Group Pretest-Post-Test Design.** This design uses no control group but uses a pretest and post-test. This design has serious weaknesses, and the findings are often uninterpretable.	The leukocyte count is measured in 10 post-chemotherapy patients just before and 5 days after treatment with an herbal formula that is expected to raise the leukocyte count.

(Table continues)

	Table I.3. *(continued)*	
PRIMARY SUBTYPE	**SECONDARY SUBTYPE**	**EXAMPLE**
Nonequivalent Control Group Design *(continued)*	**Untreated Control Group Design with Pretest and Post-Test.** This design is frequently used in social science research. This is the first quasi-experimental study discussed so far that is generally interpretable.	The leukocyte count is measured in 10 post-chemotherapy patients just before and 5 days after treatment with an herbal formula that is expected to raise the leukocyte count. In addition, identical tests are conducted on 10 similar patients that self-selected not to receive the herbal formula.
	Nonequivalent Dependent Variables Design. This design uses the same group both as controls (with a variable that should not be affected by treatment), and as the experimental group (with a variable that is expected to be altered by treatment). It is mostly used to test theories.	The leukocyte count is measured in 10 post-chemotherapy patients just before and 5 days after treatment with an herbal formula that is expected to raise the leukocyte count but not affect blood pressure. Blood pressure is also monitored just before and five days after treatment.
	Removed-Treatment Design with Pretest and Post-Test. This design is similar to the one-group pretest-post-test design except that measurements are carried out on a regular time interval before, after, shortly after, and long after treatment. Results are difficult to interpret, and there may be ethical problems in withdrawing an effective treatment.	The leukocyte count is measured in 10 post-chemotherapy patients just before, and 5, 10, and 15 days after treatment with an herbal formula that is expected to raise the leukocyte count.
	Repeated-Treatment Design. This is similar to the previous design, except that a treatment is introduced, withdrawn, and then reintroduced. Outcomes of this design are difficult to interpret.	The leukocyte count is measured in 10 post-chemotherapy patients just before and 5 days after treatment with an herbal formula. After 5 more days the leukocyte count is measured again and the formula is readministered. Five days after the second treatment the leukocyte count is measured a last time.
	Reversed-Treatment Nonequivalent Control Group Design with Pretest and Post-Test. In this design, two experimental groups are used. One receives a proposed positive treatment and one receives a proposed negative treatment. Pretests and post-tests are used. There may be ethical problems in providing a treatment that causes a negative effect. This design is more useful for theory testing then the no-treatment control group design.	The leukocyte count is measured in 10 post-chemotherapy patients just before and 5 days after treatment with an herbal formula that is expected to raise the count. Identical measurements are made on a second group of 10 similar patients who receive an herbal formula that is expected to lower the count.
Interrupted Time-Series Designs. These are similar to descriptive designs except that a treatment is given at some point in the observations. Repeated pretests can be used to assess trends in test scores beforetreatment. *(column continues)*	**Simple Interrupted Time Series**	The leukocyte count is measured in 10 post-chemotherapy patients every 5 days for 50 days. On day 25 the patients are given an herbal formula that is expected to raise the leukocyte count.
	(Table continues)	

244

	Table I.3. *(continued)*	
PRIMARY SUBTYPE	**SECONDARY SUBTYPE**	**EXAMPLE**
Interrupted Time-Series Designs. *(continued)*	**Interrupted Time Series with a Nonequivalent No-Treatment Control Group**	The leukocyte count is measured in 10 post-chemotherapy patients every 5 days for 50 days. On day 25 the patients are given an herbal formula that is expected to raise the leukocyte count. In addition, identical measurements are made in 10 similar patients that self-selected not to receive the herbal formula.
	Interrupted Time Series with Nonequivalent Dependent Variables. This design is used mainly to test theories. A variable not expected to be changed by treatment is measured in conjunction with a variable that is expected to change. No control group is used.	The leukocyte count and blood pressure is measured in 10 post-chemotherapy patients every 5 days for 50 days. On day 25 the patients are given an herbal formula that is expected to raise the leukocyte count but not affect the blood pressure.
	Interrupted Time Series with Removed Treatment. This design is an interrupted time series with an elongated treatment time.	The leukocyte count is measured in 10 post-chemotherapy patients every 5 days for 60 days. On days 20 to 40 the patients are given an herbal formula that is expected to raise the leukocyte count.
	Interrupted Time Series with Multiple Replications. This is a powerful design for determining cause-and-effect. It consists of a series of interrupted time series. To be interpretable, pretest and post-test values must show differing trends. Treatments can be modified in this type of design.	The leukocyte count is measured in 10 post-chemotherapy patients every 5 days for 50 days. On day 25 the patients are given an herbal formula that is expected to raise the leukocyte count. The exact same series is repeated on days 55 to 105 and 110 to 160. The formula is modified in this last series by removing three herbs.
	Interrupted Time Series with Switching Replications. This powerful design includes two similar experimental groups who initially receive the treatment at different times.	The leukocyte count is measured in 10 post-chemotherapy patients every 5 days for 50 days. On day 25 the patients are given an herbal formula that is expected to raise the leukocyte count. Identical measurements are made in a second group of 10 similar patients, only this group receives the formula on day 35.

TABLE I.4. EXPERIMENTAL STUDY DESIGNS	
EXPERIMENTAL STUDY DESIGNS: The purpose is to study cause-and-effect relationships between variables in a highly controlled environment. Experimental study designs provide the greatest accuracy in describing cause and effect, and for this reason are considered the "gold standard" in clinical research. However, experimental study designs are rarely the first type of design used when testing a new clinical activity. Commonly an experimental study will be preceded by a series of descriptive, correlational, and quasi-experimental trials, often in that order. In experimental designs, treatments are randomly assigned to patients.	
SUBTYPE	**EXAMPLE**
Pretest-Post-Test Control Group Design. This type of design provides treatment to the experimental group, and pretest and post-test to both experimental and control groups. It is the most commonly used type of experimental design.	Twenty post-chemotherapy patients are randomly assigned to one of two treatments. Each treatment group consists of 10 patients. Patients in the first group are treated with an herbal formula that is expected to raise their leukocyte count. Patients in the second group serve as a control and receive no treatment. Leukocyte count is measured in all patients at the start of the experiment and again five days later (after the experimental group receives the herbal treatment).
(Table continues)	

Table I.4. *(continued)*	
PRIMARY SUBTYPE	**EXAMPLE**
Post-Test-Only Control Group Design. This type of design is used when pretesting is not practical or possible (for example, when measuring length of survival). Fewer statistical tools can be used with this type of design.	Same patients and treatment as in the first example. The leukocyte count is measured in all patients five days after the start of the experiment.
Solomon Four-Group Design. This rather involved design is used to determine the effects of pretesting on post-test scores. Two experimental and two control groups are used. One of each these groups receives a pretest and post-test, while the other two receive only a post-test.	Same patients, treatment, and measurements as in the first example. In addition, in a second pair of experimental and control groups, identical treatments and measurements are made, except that no pretest is given.
Randomized Block Design. This design is the same as the pretest-post-test control group design or the post-test-only control group design, except that subjects are ranked according to a variable that is expected to confound the study findings. The effects of confounding factors can also be evaluated statistically using the Analysis of Covariance method without conducting the ranking procedure, but care must be taken not to violate the assumptions of the statistical method.	The degree of immunosuppression may influence the ability of an herbal formula to elevate the leukocyte count. Using the same patients, treatment, and measurements in the first example, the patients are ranked according to the level of their leukocyte count on the pretest, and appropriate statistical evaluations are performed.
Factorial Design. In this type of design two or more variables are independently varied within the study. This allows analysis of multiple causality. Commonly, two levels of two treatments will be varied. This is referred to as a 2 x 2 factorial design. This design produces four groups of subjects.	Same patients and measurements as in the first example. However, all 20 patients receive the herbal formula and 10 of these are randomly assigned to receive identical acupuncture treatments. Identical measurements are made in new group of 10 patients that are randomly assigned to a control group that does not receive the formula or acupuncture. Identical measurements are also made in a second new group of 10 patients that are randomly assigned to receive acupuncture but no formula. A 4 X 4 factorial design would have 16 groups and could allow for different doses of the formula and different retention times of the acupuncture needles.
Nested Designs. This type of design is used when there are variables that may be "nested" within the independent variable. For example, race, gender, or state of birth may be a nested variable.	A nested variable may be the clinic in which a treatment is provided. In a six-clinic study on two different acupuncture treatments for back pain, three clinics are randomly assigned to perform treatment #1 on 20 patients, and three are randomly assigned to perform treatment #2. The responses from the 20 patients in each of the six clinics are examined to determine differences in outcome between treatments. In this example, clinics are nested within treatments.
Multivariate Design. This type of design involves multiple variables. Any type of experimental design can be altered to include multiple variables. the design is used to examine complex relationships between variables.	Same patients, treatment, and measurements as in the first example. In addition, measurements are made for body weight and platelet count in each group. These last two variables are analyzed in relationship to changes in leukocyte count.
Repeated Measures Designs with Counterbalancing. This design includes aspects of the interrupted time series with multiple replications design. Treatment order is varied between experimental groups to counterbalance carryover effects.	The leukocyte count is measured in 30 post-chemotherapy patients every 5 days for 50 days. Of these, ten patients are randomly assigned as controls and receive no treatment. Ten are randomly assigned to receive an herbal formula on day 10 and an acupuncture treatment on day 25. And 10 are randomly assigned to receive acupuncture on day 10 and an herbal formula on day 25.
Randomized Clinical Trials. These are similar to the controlled trials discussed above, except that the control group may be receiving an alternate treatment. Clinical trials tend to involve large numbers of patients and, therefore, are frequently conducted at multiple locations. They have been in use since 1945.	Length of survival is measured in 500 patients diagnosed with advanced liver cancer and *liver qi* stagnation. Half of these are treated with palliative chemotherapy, and half are treated with an herbal formula and glutathione supplements. The trial is conducted at ten different institutions. Within each institution, treatments are randomly assigned to patients.

In addition to the designs mentioned in the tables above, other designs are possible. These include primary prevention and health promotion studies (which measure an event that does not occur after intervention), secondary analysis designs (which involve analysis of data previously collected in another study), meta-analysis designs (which involve analysis of data from multiple independent studies), and methodological designs (which involve analysis of the validity and reliability of research instruments, such as a questionnaire).

APPENDIX J: LESS-PROMISING NATURAL AGENTS

TABLE J.1. SUMMARY OF LESS-PROMISING NATURAL AGENTS		
AGENT	**REPORTED ACTIONS**	**COMMENT**
Achyranthes bidentata (niu xi)	o stimulates immune system	
Actinidia chinensis (teng li)	o antitumor activity	
Acupuncture	o increases leukocyte count in humans o reduces edema of extremities in humans o reduces stress o normalizes flow of *qi* in *channels*	o may be best reserved for *channel* disorders
Agkistrodon acutus (bai hua she)	o fibrinolytic/antithrombotic action in vitro	
Agrimonia pilosa (xian he cao)	o antitumor activity	
Allium bakeri (xie bai)	o inhibits platelet aggregation	
Altheae officinalis (marsh mallow)	o stimulates immune system	
Andrographis paniculata (chuan xin lian)	o inhibits platelet aggregation	
Angelica dahurica (bai zhi)	o inhibits platelet aggregation	
Aristolochia debilis (mu xiang or tian xian teng, or ma dou ling)	o stimulates immune system	
Artemisia argyi (ai ye)	o inhibits thrombin in vitro o inhibits plasmin in vitro o fibrinolytic/antithrombotic activity in vitro	o induces bFGF production in vitro o stimulates endothelial cell proliferation in vitro
Artemisia capillaris (yin chen hao)	o inhibits platelet aggregation in vitro o antitumor activity	o may have same disadvantages as *Artemisia argyi*
Berberis aquifolium (Oregon grape)	o source of berberine	o concentrated berberine may be more effective
Bombyx mori (jiang can)	o inhibits platelet aggregation	
Brinase, a proteolytic enzyme from *Aspergillus oryzae*	o inhibits platelet aggregation o fibrinolytic/antithrombotic in humans	o not readily available
Bu Yang Huan Wu Tang (formula)	o inhibits fibrin production in vitro o fibrinolytic/antithrombotic activity in vitro	o see *Astragalus membranaceus, Angelica sinensis, Ligusticum chuanxiong, Paeonia lactiflora,* and *Carthamus tinctorius* in Table 17.1
Bu Zhong Yi Qi Tang (formula)	o antitumor activity	o see *Astragalus membranaceus, Panax ginseng, Atractylodes macrocephala, Glycyrrhiza uralensis, Angelica sinensis,* and *Bupleurum chinense* in Table 17.1
Buthus martensi (quan xie)	o fibrinolytic/antithrombotic in vitro	
Butyric acid	o induces differentiation in vitro o induces apoptosis in vitro	o see *Linum usitatissimum* in Table 17.1
Caffeine	o induces apoptosis	o adverse side effects
Calcium	o inhibits initiation of colon cancer	o may be best reserved for patients with low calcium levels
Cannabis sativa (marijuana)	o decreases testosterone bioavailability in vivo	o illegal
Capsicum annuum (cayenne pepper)	o fibrinolytic in humans o inhibits platelet aggregation in vitro	o normally used in low doses
(Table continues)		

	TABLE J.1. *(continued)*	
AGENT	**REPORTED ACTIONS**	**COMMENT**
Cassia angustifolia and *Cassia acutifolia* (*fan xie ye,* senna)	○ source of rhein/emodin	○ strong purgative
Cassia tora and *Cassia obtusifolia* (*jue ming zi*)	○ source of rhein/emodin	○ low emodin content
(+)-Catechin	○ binds tPA and inhibits invasion in vitro ○ inhibits elastinase activity	○ may induce intravascular hemolysis
Centipeda minima (*shi hu sui*)	○ inhibits histamine release	
Cesium	○ anticancer activity ○ antitumor activity	○ stimulates growth of some tumors in vivo
Cinnamomum cassia (*rou gui*)	○ stimulates immune system in vivo ○ antitumor activity ○ source of (+)-catechin	○ normally used in low dosages
Codonopsis pilosula (*dang shen*)	○ inhibits platelet aggregation in humans ○ stimulates immune system in humans	○ reduces leukocyte count in vivo
Copper	○ required for cross-linking of collagen	○ increase angiogenesis in some tumors
Coptis chinensis (*huang lian*)	○ source of berberine	○ concentrated berberine may be more effective
Cordyceps sinensis (*dong chong xia cao*)	○ antitumor activity ○ stimulates immune system in vivo	○ inhibits immune system in vivo ○ expensive
Corydalis turtschaninovii (*yan hu suo*)	○ inhibits increased vascular permeability	
Crocus sativa (saffron)	○ antitumor activity	
Curcuma aromatica (*yu jin* or *e zhu*)	○ antitumor activity	
Curcuma longa (*jiang huang*)	○ fibrinolytic in vitro	
Cuscuta australis (*tu si zi*)	○ stimulates immune system	
Daidzein (isoflavone)	○ induces differentiation in vitro	○ see soy in Table 17.1 for source
Dang Gui Shao Yao San (formula)	○ reduces estrogen production in vitro	○ conflicting reports of individual ingredients
Docosahexaenoic acid (DHA)	○ induces differentiation in vitro ○ inhibits PAF production in vitro ○ inhibits platelet aggregation in humans ○ antitumor activity ○ decreases PGE_2 production ○ increases PGE_3 production ○ increases membrane fluidity	○ inhibits immune cells in vivo ○ stimulates tumor growth in vivo ○ see EPA in Table 17.1
Eclipta prostrata (*han lian cao*)	○ stimulates immune system	
Epimedium sagittatum (*yin yang huo*)	○ inhibits fibrin and fibronectin deposition in vitro	
Er Xiang Tang (formula)	○ stimulates immune system	○ see *Angelica sinensis* in Table 17.1
Eugenia caryophyllata (*ding xiang*)	○ induces differentiation	○ must be used at low dosages
Eupatorium cannabinum (hemp agrimony)	○ stimulates immune system	
Eupatorium perfoliatum (boneset)	○ stimulates immune system	
Fei Liu Ping (formula)	○ increases survival of humans with lung cancer	○ see *Astragalus membranaceus* in Table 17.1
	(Table continues)	

	TABLE J.1. *(continued)*	
AGENT	**REPORTED ACTIONS**	**COMMENT**
Formula #1	○ increases survival of humans with nasopharyngeal cancer in combination with radiotherapy	○ see *Paeonia lactiflora, Ligusticum chuanxiong, Angelica sinensis, Carthamus tinctorius,* and *Astragalus membranaceus* in Table 17.1
Formula #2	○ increases survival of humans with stomach cancer in combination with chemotherapy	○ see *Astragalus membranaceus* and *Atractylodes macrocephala* in Table 17.1
Formula #3	○ increases leukocyte count in radiotherapy patients	○ see *Astragalus membranaceus* and *Acanthopanax sp.* in Table 17.1
Fu Zheng Jie Du Tang (formula)	○ stimulates immune system in vivo	○ unspecified ingredients
Fu Zheng Sheng Jin decoction (formula)	○ increases survival of humans with nasopharyngeal cancer in combination with radiotherapy	○ see *Salvia miltiorrhiza, Glycyrrhiza uralensis,* and *Atractylodes macrocephala* in Table 17.1
Ginkgo biloba	○ inhibits PAF production ○ inhibits histamine release in vitro ○ scavenges free radicals ○ stimulates immune system in humans ○ fibrinolytic/antithrombotic activity in vivo	○ Gingko dilates peripheral blood vessels and increases cerebral blood flow. These actions have unknown effects on cancer in vivo.
Glehnia littoralis (bei sha shen)	○ inhibits platelet aggregation in vitro	
Glucosamine	○ may protect GI lining during chemotherapy	○ stimulates collagen synthesis
Gui Zhi Fu Ling Wan (formula)	○ inhibits estrogen synthesis in vivo	○ conflicting studies on individual components
Hirudo nipponia (shui zhi)	○ inhibits platelet aggregation	○ contains heparin
Humulus lupulus (hops)	○ reduces estrogen production in vivo	
Hydrastis canadensis (goldenseal)	○ source of berberine	○ concentrated berberine may be more effective
Jian Pi Jin Dan (formula)	○ stimulates immune system	○ unspecified components
Jin Gui Shen Qi (formula)	○ increases survival of humans with small cell lung cancer in combination with chemotherapy	○ component herbs not otherwise discussed
Kang Fu Xin (formula)	○ stimulates immune system	○ unspecified components
Kang Shuai Sen Fang (formula)	○ stimulates immune system	○ unspecified components
Laminaria sp. (kun bu), Sargassum sp. (hai zao) and other brown algae	○ inactivates thrombin	
Leonurus heterophyllus (yi mu cao)	○ inhibits PAF production in vitro	
Li Wei Hua Jie Tang (formula)	○ increases survival of humans with stomach cancer in combination with conventional therapy	○ see *Glycyrrhiza uralensis, Astragalus membranaceus, Ziziphus jujuba, Lycium barbarum,* and *Atractylodes macrocephala* in Table 17.1
Liu Wei Di Huang Tang (formula)	○ antitumor activity ○ increases survival of humans with small cell lung cancer in combination with chemotherapy	○ component herbs not otherwise discussed
Magnolia salicifolia (xin yi hua)	○ inhibits histamine release in vitro ○ inhibits angiogenesis in vitro ○ inhibits endothelial cell proliferation in vitro	○ the amount of the active ingredient magnosalin in magnolia flowers, and its pharmacokinetic properties in humans or animals is unknown
	(Table continues)	

AGENT	REPORTED ACTIONS	COMMENT
Manli pill	○ anticancer (CML)	○ see *Scutellaria baicalensis*, *realgar*, and *Angelica sinensis* in Table 17.1
Matrine and oxymatrine	○ antitumor activity ○ increases leukocyte counts in chemotherapy patients	○ numerous studies, but inconclusive results
Methionine	○ reduces excess copper levels ○ inhibits proliferation of some cancers in vitro	○ stimulates proliferation of some cancers in vitro
Mieai powder and *Mieai* decoction (formulas)	○ increases survival of humans with esophageal cancer ○ increases survival of humans with stomach cancer	○ see *Rheum palmatum* and *Salvia miltiorrhiza* in Table 17.1 and J.1
Organic foods	○ may reduce exposure to xenoestrogens ○ may be nutritionally superior to conventionally grown foods	○ long-term effects only will be evident
Panax pseudoginseng (san qi)	○ stimulates immune system in vivo	○ expensive
Panax quinquefolium (American ginseng, *xi yang shen*)	○ stimulates immune system in vivo	○ expensive
Paris formosana (quan shen)	○ stimulates immune system	
Peucedanum praeruptorum (qian hu)	○ inhibits histamine release in vitro	
Pheretima aspergillum (di long)	fibrinolytic/antithrombic in vitro	
Pinshen Fang (formula)	○ increases survival of humans with stomach cancer in combination with chemotherapy	○ see *Atractylodes macrocephala*, *Lycium barbarum*, and *Ligustrum lucidum* in Table 17.1
Piper kadsura (hai feng tang) and *Piper wallichii (shi nan teng)*	○ inhibits PAF production in-vitro	○ normally used in small doses
Plantago sp. (i.e., psyllium seed)	○ stimulates immune cells in vitro ○ source of fiber	○ flax seed may be more active
Polygonatum odoratum (yu zhu)	○ stimulates immune system in vivo	
Polygonum cuspidatum (hu chang)	○ source of emodin ○ increases WBC count in chemotherapy patients	○ purifed emodin may be more useful
Polygonum multiflorum (he shou wu)	○ source of emodin ○ source of (+)-catechin	○ low emodin content
Proline, Glycine, and Arginine	○ promotes collagen synthesis	○ arginine stimulates proliferation of some tumors
Psoralea corylifolia (bu gu zhi)	○ source of psoralen	○ see psoralen
Psoralen	○ antitumor activity	○ carcinogenic
Ren Shen Tang (formula)	○ antitumor activity ○ stimulates immune system in vivo	○ unspecified components
Ren Shen Yang Rong Tang (formula)	○ stimulates immune cells in vitro	○ see *Paeonia lactiflora*, *Angelic sinensis*, *Astragalus membranaceus*, *Cinnamomum cassia*, *Panax ginseng*, *Atractylodes macrocephala*, and *Glycyrrhiza uralensis* in Table 17.1
Rhamnus frangula (alder buckthorn)	○ source of rhein/emodin	○ strong purgative

(Table continues)

	TABLE J.1. *(continued)*	
AGENT	**REPORTED ACTIONS**	**COMMENT**
Rhamnus purshiana (cascara sagrada)	∘ source of rhein/emodin	∘ strong purgative
Rheum palmatum (da huang)	∘ inhibits platelet aggregation in vivo ∘ stimulates immune system in vivo ∘ increases leukocyte count in chemotherapy patients ∘ source of (+)-catechin ∘ source of rhein/emodin	∘ purifed rhein/emodin may be more useful
Rubia cordifolia (qian cao gen)	∘ antitumor activity	
Rumex crispus (yellow dock)	∘ source of rhein/emodin	∘ purifed rhein/emodin may be more useful
Ruscus aculeatus (butcher's broom)	∘ inhibits increased vascular permeability in vitro	
Saiboku To (formula)	∘ inhibits histamine release in vitro	∘ see *Panax ginseng, Ziziphus jujuba, Glycyrrhiza uralensis, Scutellaria baicalensis,* and *Bupleurum chinense* in Table 17.1
San Zhuang Wan (formula)	∘ decreases testosterone bioavailability in vivo	∘ unspecified components
Schisandra chinensis (wu wei zi)	∘ antitumor activity	
Scolopendra subspinipes mutilans (wu gong)	∘ fibrinolytic/antithrombic in vitro	
Serenoa repens (saw palmetto)	∘ decrease testosterone bioavailability in vivo ∘ inhibits eicosanoid production	∘ may be best reserved for BPH
Shen Cao Fu Zheng Kangai (formula)	∘ stimulates immune system in vivo	∘ see *Panax ginseng, Astragalus membranaceus, Atractylodes macrocephala,* and *Ligusticum lucidum* in Table 17.1
Shen Xue Tang (formula)	∘ reduces chemotherapy side effects in humans ∘ stimulates immune system in humans ∘ increases survival of humans with stomach cancer in combination with chemotherapy	∘ see *Astragalus membranaceus, Atractylodes macrocephala, Ligustrum lucidum,* and *Lycium barbarum* in Table 17.1
Sheng Mai San (formula)	∘ stimulates immune system	∘ see *Panax ginseng* in Table 17.1
Shi Quan Da Bu Tang (formula)	∘ antitumor activity ∘ stimulates immune system in vivo	∘ see *Angelica sinensis, Atractylodes macrocephala, Astragalus membranaceus, Ligusticum chuanxiong, Panax ginseng,* and *Glycyrrhiza uralensis* in Table 17.1
Si Jun Zi Tang (formula)	∘ increases survival of humans with liver cancer in combination with radiotherapy	∘ see *Panax ginseng, Atractylodes macrocephala,* and *Glycyrrhiza uralensis* in Table 17.1
Silicon	∘ may facilitate collagen cross-linking	∘ may be best reserved for patients with low silicon levels ∘ facilitates collagen synthesis
Selenium	∘ required for glutathione peroxidase production	∘ may be best reserved for patients with low selenium levels
Solanum indicum (huang shui qie)	∘ antitumor action	
Sophora flavescens (ku shen)	∘ source of matrine and oxymatrine	∘ see matrine
	(Table continues)	

252

TABLE J.1. *(continued)*		
AGENT	**REPORTED ACTIONS**	**COMMENT**
Sophora subprostrata (shan dou gen)	○ source of matrine and oxymatrine	○ see matrine
Symphitum sp. (i.e., comfrey)	○ stimulates immune cells in vitro	○ alkaloids may be toxic
Thymus extracts	○ stimulates immune system in humans	○ crude extract may not be as active as purified fractions
Typha angustifolia and *Typha latifolia (pu huang)*	○ inhibits platelet aggregation in vitro ○ fibrinolytic/antithrombotic in vitro	○ stimulates tPA production in vitro
Urea	○ anticancer effects (liver cancer) ○ scavenges free radicals	○ numerous studies suggest little effect
Vitamin B6	○ may facilitate immune function	○ stimulates growth of some tumors in vivo
Vitamin E	○ scavenges free radicals ○ may inhibit platelet aggregation ○ may inhibit leukotriene production	○ may be best reserved for patients with low vitamin E levels
Vitex negundo (huang jing zi)	○ decrease testosterone production in vivo	
Xiao Chai Hu Tang (formula)	○ antitumor activity ○ induces apoptosis in vitro ○ stimulates immune system in vivo	○ see *Bupleurum chinense, Scutellaria baicalensis, Panax ginseng, Glycyrrhiza uralensis,* and *Ziziphus jujuba* in Table 17.1
Xiao Yao San and *Er Chen Tang* (formulas)	○ reduces estrogen levels in humans	○ conflicting studies on individual components
Ye Qi Sheng Xue Tang (formula)	○ increased leukocyte count in patients treated with chemotherapy	○ see *Astragalus membranaceus, Angelica sinensis,* and *Atractylodes macrocephala* in Table 17.1
Yi Kang Ling (formula)	○ antitumor activity	○ unspecified components
Yi Qi Yang Yin Tang (formula)	○ increases survival of humans with nasopharyngeal cancer in combination with radiotherapy	○ see *Pseudostellaria heterophylla, Ligusticum lucidum,* and *Glycyrrhiza uralensis* in Table 17.1
Zhu Ling Tang (formula)	○ antitumor activity ○ stimulates immune system in vivo	
Zinc	○ required for SOD production ○ required for optimal immune function	○ may be best reserved for patients with low zinc levels
Ziziphus jujuba (da zao)	○ stimulates immune system in vivo ○ source of cAMP	

APPENDIX K: DERIVATION OF CONCENTRATION-TIME CURVES FOR RHEIN AND EMODIN

RAW DATA

This appendix provides background information on the methods used to derive the concentration-time curves for emodin and rhein in human tissues, as displayed in Chapter 17. The data that forms the basis for these curves were obtained by administration of ^{14}C-labeled rhein and emodin to rats (see Table K.1). Although the recovery by this method is over 90%, recovery has been much lower in pharmacokinetic studies that did not use ^{14}C-labeled rhein and emodin. In these studies, recovery was closer to 20 to 40% (reviewed by De Witte and Lemli, 1988a, 1988b). Anthraquinone chemistry is complex, and the difference in recovery between these two methods is likely due to the production of unidentified anthraquinone metabolites. These metabolites would not be recovered as rhein or emodin, but would be recovered as ^{14}C-labeled anthraquinone. Therefore, calculations based on the data contained in Table K.1 are likely to overestimate actual rhein and emodin concentrations. However, the metabolites of these rhein and emodin may also possess some degree of biologic activity.

BLOOD CONCENTRATION CURVES FOR RHEIN IN RATS

The data for blood concentration as a function of time can be estimated by a formula in the form of Equation K.1. The first term governs the absorption rate, the second governs the initial decay period, and the third term governs the secondary decay period.

TIME (hours)	RHEIN			EMODIN
	BLOOD (µg/ml) 0.78 mg/kg dose	LARGE INTESTINE (µg/gram wet weight) 0.78 mg/kg dose	KIDNEY (µg/gram wet weight) 0.78 mg/kg dose	BLOOD (µg/ml) 50 mg/kg dose
0	0	0	0	0
0.25	0.221	0	1.5	—
0.33	0.245	0	—	—
0.5	0.235	0	—	—
0.75	0.152	0	—	—
1	0.124	0.04	0.733	7.7
2	0.08	—	—	14
3	0.057	2.75	0.353	—
4	—	—	—	13.7
6	0.027	—	—	12.7
8	0.0185	1.36	0.25	—
10	0.015	—	—	—
24	0.0061	0.322	0.21	4.1
28	0.0051	—	—	—
30	0.0039	—	—	—
48	0.0034	0.0715	0.128	2.1
72	—	—	—	0.8
96	—	0.0143	0.137	0.5
120	—	—	—	0.3
168	—	—	0.14	—

Table caption: **TABLE K.1 RHEIN ANTHRAQUINONE AND EMODIN CONCENTRATIONS IN RAT AFTER ^{14}C-LABELED ORAL DOSE**

Source: Lang (1988) and Bachmann and Schlatter (1981). All rhein concentrations were measured as ^{14}C activity equivalents and were converted using the factor 1×10^3 dpm = 0.0024 µg. Values for emodin and rhein were estimated from plotted points.

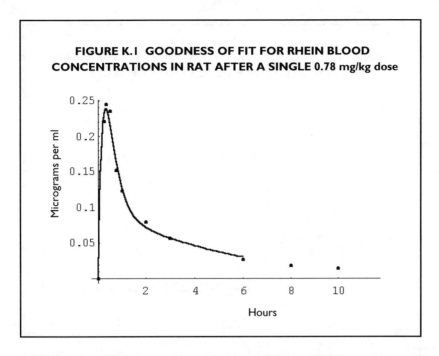

FIGURE K.1 GOODNESS OF FIT FOR RHEIN BLOOD CONCENTRATIONS IN RAT AFTER A SINGLE 0.78 mg/kg dose

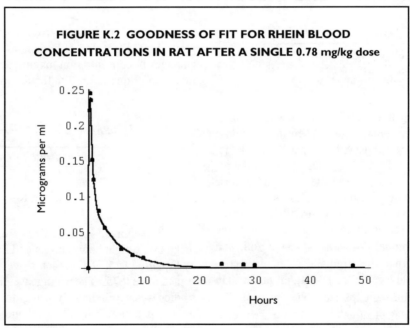

FIGURE K.2 GOODNESS OF FIT FOR RHEIN BLOOD CONCENTRATIONS IN RAT AFTER A SINGLE 0.78 mg/kg dose

$$-(A + B)e^{-kt} + Ae^{-\alpha t} + Be^{-\beta t}$$

Equation K.1

Data were fit to this equation using the software Mathematica, and the following values were determined for the constants:

$$-(7.274)\, e^{-3.81t} + 7.168\, e^{-3.57t} + 0.106\, e^{-0.207t}$$

Equation K.2

As shown in Figures K.1 and K.2, this formula provides a reasonable fit for the data at $t < 10$ hours, but slightly underestimates the concentration values beyond this point. However, a term for the tertiary decay period was not added since the equation is accurate to approximately $\pm\, 0.02$ µg/ml as is.

To account for changes in the concentration-time curve in response to changes in dosage, Equation K.2 can be multiplied by the term:

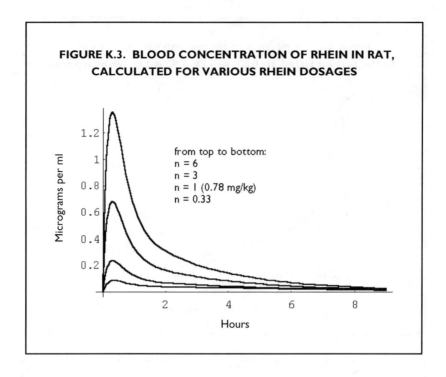

FIGURE K.3. BLOOD CONCENTRATION OF RHEIN IN RAT, CALCULATED FOR VARIOUS RHEIN DOSAGES

from top to bottom:
n = 6
n = 3
n = 1 (0.78 mg/kg)
n = 0.33

$$1 + \frac{NewDose - OriginalDose}{(e^{\beta t})(OriginalDose)}$$

Equation K.3

This term is equal to 1.0 when the new (hypothetical) dose equals the original dose. When the new dose does not equal the original dose, it is equal to a time dependent value between 1.0 and n, where n equals the ratio of the new dose to the original dose (NewDose/OriginalDose). Equation K.3 is necessary since simply multiplying the formula by n would artificially raise or lower the asymptote. For example, if the asymptote for the original dose was 0.0034 μg/ml, and the new dose is 100 times the original dose, the new concentration curve would level off at 0.34 μg/ml rather than 0.0034 μg/ml as would be expected. The factor $e^{\beta t}$ is used to match the decay of Equation K.3 with the secondary decay of Equation K.2. Therefore, the value of Equation K.3 slowly changes from n to 1.0. Using Equation K.3, concentration curves for various doses are shown in Figure K.3.

BLOOD CONCENTRATION CURVES FOR RHEIN IN HUMANS

In order to extrapolate rat data to human equivalents, additional adjustments must be made to Equations K.2 and K.3. The blood concentration for a given dose will be lower in a human than in a rat, and the rate of drug clearance will be slower. Therefore, the blood concentration curve for a given dose will be smaller and more spread out for a human as compared to a rat. Changes in concentration magnitude can be estimated by modifying Equation K.3 to the following:

$$1 + \frac{HumanDose - \dfrac{OriginalRatDose}{4.3}}{e^{\beta t} \dfrac{OriginalRatDose}{4.3}}$$

Equation K.4

The factor of 4.3 is derived from the differences in metabolic weight between rats and humans, as calculated by Equation K.5. The K factor (see Section 11.3.1) is assumed to be 0.75. The average weight of the rats in these studies was approximately 200 grams and the weight of a human is assumed to be 70 kilograms. (When extrapolating rat data to mice, the value of Equation K.5 was 0.56.).

$$\frac{\dfrac{weight_{rat}}{weight_{human}}}{\left(\dfrac{weight_{rat}}{weight_{human}}\right)^{0.75}} = 4.3$$

Equation K.5

To adjust for the differences in drug clearance between rats and humans, the time factor (t) in Equations

256

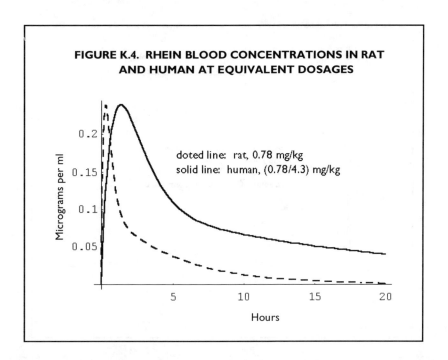

FIGURE K.4. RHEIN BLOOD CONCENTRATIONS IN RAT AND HUMAN AT EQUIVALENT DOSAGES

K.2 and K.4 was also divided by 4.3 (or 0.56 for mice). Using these modifications, Figure K.4 illustrates the differences in blood concentration between rats and humans at equivalent dosages.

VERIFICATION OF MODEL

The extrapolation rat pharmacokinetic data to humans would not be necessary if human pharmacokinetic studies on rhein and emodin had been conducted. Unfortunately only a limited amount of human data is available. Data from Krumbiegal and Schultz (1993) can be used to partially verify the equations derived above. In this study, two senna laxatives were administered to humans, and plasma levels of rhein were determined at various time periods. Unfortunately, the amount of rhein anthraquinone in the senna material was not established. In addition, only maximum plasma concentration levels were reported.

The first laxative product contained approximately 7.6 mg of potential rhein (rhein glycosides, sennosides, and anthraquinone), and the second contained 13.1 mg potential rhein. Maximum plasma concentrations were approximately 43.8 ng/ml and 65.1 ng/ml respectively. Both products produced plasma peaks at 3 to 5 and 10 to 11 hours. The maximum plasma peak for the first product was at 10 to 11 hours, and the maximum for the second was at 3 to 5 hours. The initial peak appears to correspond to absorption of free anthraquinone (in the small intestine) and the second peak to absorption of anthraquinone liberated by bacterial action (in the large intestine). Apparently, the second product contained a slightly greater percentage of free rhein. The ratio between the dose and plasma concentration for each product is roughly similar (0.17 vs. 0.20 mg/kg per μg/ml).

To use this data to verify our models, we must first estimate the amount of rhein anthraquinone that produced these peaks. It would appear that approximately half of the absorbed rhein was present as free anthraquinone, and the other half was liberated by bacterial action. Sennidins are readily converted to rhein in the intestinal tract, but recovery of rhein from intestinal contents is quite low. In rat intestines in vitro, recovery is on the order of 10%, suggesting that physical adsorption on solid fecal particles and chemical alteration takes place, which reduces the amount of rhein available for absorption (De Witte, 1993). If we assume that: 1) all potential rhein that reaches the large intestine is converted to rhein anthraquinone; 2) only 10% of the liberated rhein is absorbed; and 3) the absorbed amount is equal to the amount of free anthraquinone, then the amount of free anthraquinone in senna must be roughly 9% of the total potential rhein. This value roughly corresponds with data reported by Grimminger and Witthohn (1993), which suggests that the percentage of rhein anthraquinone in the total rhein content in a variety of senna products is approximately 3%. In rhubarb, 11% of the total rhein content is rhein anthraquinone (see page 192). Therefore, we will use the midpoint 3 and 9%, or 6%, and estimate that 13.1 mg x 6%, or 0.79 mg produced a rhein plasma concentration of 65 ng/ml. This dose is equal to 0.011 mg/kg in a 70-kilogram human.

According to our derived formulas, a dose of 0.011 mg/kg should produce a peak blood concentration of 34 ng/ml at 2.5 hours. Since rhein levels in rat plasma are

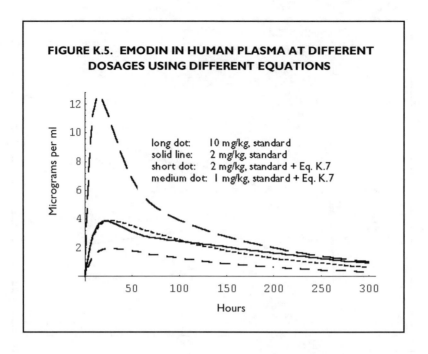

FIGURE K.5. EMODIN IN HUMAN PLASMA AT DIFFERENT DOSAGES USING DIFFERENT EQUATIONS

long dot: 10 mg/kg, standard
solid line: 2 mg/kg, standard
short dot: 2 mg/kg, standard + Eq. K.7
medium dot: 1 mg/kg, standard + Eq. K.7

approximately double the levels in rat blood (Lang, 1988), this must be multiplied by two.[1] With this adjustment, the calculated plasma level is 68 ng/ml, which is almost exactly the 65 ng/ml observed value. The calculated time of the peak concentration (2.5 hours) is just short of the observed peak at 3 to 5 hours. Therefore, this model provides a reasonable fit for this singular data point, given the stated assumptions.

PERIODIC DOSING

The last step in calculating rhein plasma concentrations in humans is to determine the effects of periodic, rather than singular, dosing. Plasma concentrations after periodic dosing can be calculated by the formula:

$$f(t)_{\text{periodic}} = f(t)_{\text{single}} + \sum_i \left[f(t - (i\,\tau))_{\text{single}} \right]$$
$$i = 0 \rightarrow \left(\frac{t}{\tau} \right)$$

Equation K.6

Where $f(t)_{\text{periodic}}$ is the plasma concentration after periodic dosing, $f(t)_{\text{single}}$ is the equation for plasma concentration after a single dose, and τ is the dosing rate in hours[-1].

CONCENTRATION-TIME CURVES FOR RHEIN AND EMODIN IN HUMAN TISSUE

Concentrations of rhein in kidney and large intestine tissues and emodin in plasma are calculated similar to that described above. The two differences are that 1) adjustments must be made for large intestine concentrations that initially remain at zero for a few hours, and 2) adjustments must be made to emodin concentrations when using a dose of emodin below approximately 2 mg/kg. The emodin concentration must be adjusted for low dosages because the standard equations developed above are not valid when the entire concentration-time curve is governed by the secondary decay term (the third term in Equation K.2). For doses reasonably below 2 mg/kg, Equation K.7 could be used to provide the adjusting factor. This factor is then multiplied to the value obtained using the standard equations. The value of 2.5 in Equation K.7 was derived empirically. However, even with this adjustment, the model is likely to be inaccurate at low doses. The concentration of emodin in human plasma at different dosages using the adjusted and nonadjusted standard equations (as appropriate) is shown in Figure K.5.

$$\frac{(-2.5)\,EmodinDose}{e^{\left(\frac{0.435\,t}{4.3} \right)}} + \frac{(2.5)\,EmodinDose}{e^{\left(\frac{0.0294\,t}{4.3} \right)}}$$

Equation K.7

---

[1] Concentration-time curves for emodin in Chapter 17 also assume that concentrations of emodin in the plasma are double that of the blood.

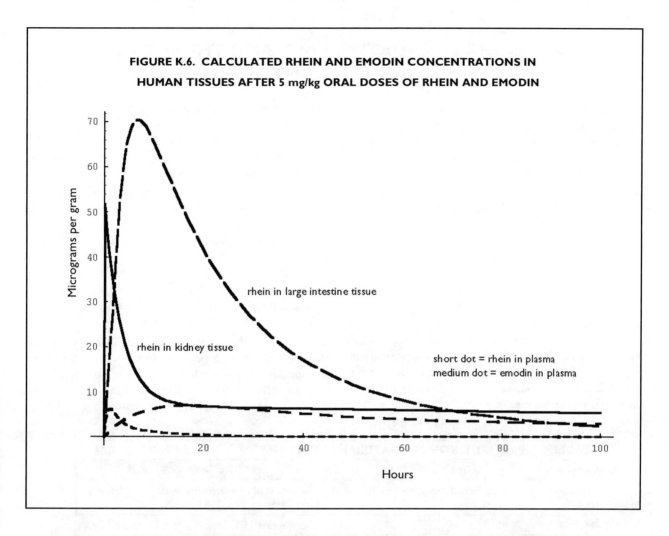

FIGURE K.6. CALCULATED RHEIN AND EMODIN CONCENTRATIONS IN HUMAN TISSUES AFTER 5 mg/kg ORAL DOSES OF RHEIN AND EMODIN

Graphs of estimated rhein and emodin concentrations in human tissues are provided in Figure K.6. Three important observations can be made from this figure:

1) The concentration peaks for rhein in the kidney and large intestine are of similar high magnitude, and the concentration peaks of rhein and emodin in the plasma are of similar low magnitude. Therefore, toxic levels of rhein and emodin may be reached in the kidney and large intestine before high plasma levels are achieved.

2) The concentration of rhein in the kidney remains elevated for an extended period of time. Toxic levels may be produced in this organ if frequent dosing schemes are employed.

3) The concentration peak for emodin in plasma is significantly later than that for rhein in plasma, and the concentration remains elevated for an extended time period. However, it should be kept in mind that the model used may not be produce accurate estimates at the applied dosage.

The accumulation of emodin in kidney and adipose tissue is of some concern and is not well defined. Based upon the limited data by Bachmann and Schlatter (1981), it would appear that emodin concentrations in kidney and adipose tissue in rats are similar to that of rhein concentrations in kidney tissue in rats (see Figure 17.3), at least at values of t greater than 72 hours. One difference is that emodin concentrations actually appear to increase slightly in these tissues between 72 and 120 hours. However, insufficient data is available to determine concentration-time curves for emodin in these tissues.

APPENDIX L: RADIOTHERAPY AND THE USE OF ANTIOXIDANTS

As discussed in Section 9.1.1, radiotherapy causes DNA damage to neoplastic (and normal) cells by inducing free radical production. Since a high percentage of the natural agents discussed in this book possess antioxidant activity (see Table L.1), there is some question as to the overall effect of administering these agents to patients undergoing radiotherapy. Agents that stimulate DNA repair mechanisms, such as *Panax ginseng (ren shen)* (Rhee et al., 1991) are also of concern.

One the one hand, studies on mice suggest that high doses of vitamin C protect normal tissue from radiation damage, but do not protect implanted tumor tissue (Okunieff, 1991). The reason for the differential effect between normal and neoplastic tissue appears to be due to differences in oxygen tension. Since radiotherapy is less capable of inducing free radical damage in hypoxic tissue than euoxic (oxygenated) tissue, hypoxic tissue is naturally more resistant to radiotherapy. Therefore, it follows that euoxic tissue, such as non-neoplastic tissue, is more readily protected from the acute effects of radiation by antioxidants than is hypoxic tissue. Hypoxic tissue is frequently found within solid tumors, and in fact, is the tissue that is most likely to survive radiotherapy and form the base for continued tumor growth.

That the body uses antioxidant stores to protect itself from radiotherapy damage is suggested by the reduced serum levels of antioxidants in leukemia patients receiving total body irradiation (Arterbery et al., 1994; Hunnisett et al., 1993; Clemens et al., 1989).[1] Similarly, the accumulation of lipid peroxidation products in irradiated rats and guinea pigs is diminished, but not completely normalized, by administration of vitamins E, C, and catechin (Baraboi et al., 1994a, 1994b).

Although the forgoing suggests that antioxidants may be beneficial to patients undergoing radiotherapy, the opposite is as likely to be true. A sizable percentage of most solid tumors is comprised of euoxic tissue (see Section 3.4). Therefore, this tissue may also be

TABLE L.1 PARTIAL LISTING OF NATURAL AGENTS THAT SCAVENGE FREE RADICALS	
AGENT	**REFERENCE**
Astragalus membranaceus and *Astragalus mongholicus (huang qi)*	Sugiura et al., 1993; Wang et al., 1994; Oleinik and Ovsiannikova, 1983
DMSO	See Section 15.1
Ligusticum chuanxiong (chuan xiong)	Ge and Zhang, 1994
Lycium barbarum (gou qi zi)	Zhang, 1993
Melatonin	See Section 8.4.2
Numerous phenol-containing agents, including numerous flavonoids	See Section 14.4
Numerous vitamins	See Section 13.1
Panax ginseng (ren shen)	Kim et al., 1992; Sun et al., 1989
Rhein *	Malterud et al., 1993
Salvia miltiorrhiza (dan shen)	Zhang et al., 1994; Huang and Zhang, 1992
Scutellaria baicalensis (huang qin)	Hamada et al., 1993
Thiol-continaing agents (for example, glutathione, cysteine, and garlic)	See Section 3.4
Urea	See Sections 15.4 and 3.4
Note: This table is only a partial listing. Numerous other natural agents scavenge free radicals. * Not all anthraquinones scavenge free radicals under all conditions. Some anthraquinones, such as emodin, stimulate free radical production. Free radical-induced DNA damage may account for the immunosuppressive effects of emodin (Huang et al., 1992a, 1991).	

---

[1] Free radicals may also be induced secondary to radiotherapy, such as from massive cellular lysis. This may also account for reduced antioxidant levels.

protected, to some degree, from radiation damage by antioxidants.

It is also possible that moderate doses of antioxidants may have little or no effect on radiotherapy-induced damage of normal or neoplastic cells. In Okunieff's study mentioned above, mice were administered a massive dose of vitamin C—up to 4.5 g/kg intravenously. Lower doses of vitamin C were not effective at providing radiation protection (Okunieff, 1995, personal communication).[2] The dose of antioxidants required to provide radiation protection is likely related to the degree of radiation exposure. NASA and other institutions have been studying thiol compounds for some time as agents to reduce the adverse effects of low-level radiation (Bogo, 1988; Aguilera et al., 1992). The high doses of radiation used during radiotherapy may require either very high doses, or moderate doses of very potent antioxidants, to produce significant protection.

The above discussion has concentrated on the use of antioxidants during radiation exposure. Based on available data, it is possible that antioxidants may interfere with the desired effects of radiotherapy, and their use may place the patient at unnecessary risk of tumor survival. More data on this issue is expected soon from trials using thiol compounds to protect patients with head and neck cancer from radiotherapy-induced damage to salivary glands (McDonald et al., 1994).

Potentially, antioxidants may be of more use in protecting patients from the late effects of radiation exposure, such as the development of alopecia, ulceration, and fibrosis. Preliminary data suggest that late effects of radiation may be due to inflammatory processes, and that antioxidants and other anti-inflammatory agents may inhibit these effects (Okunieff, 1995, personal communication). Tumor cell destruction continues for a prolonged period of time after radiotherapy ceases (possibly many months), and the optimum time to begin antioxidant treatment, and its efficacy, have not been established.

---

[2] Paul Okunieff, M.D., is the Branch Chief of the Radiation Oncology Branch, Division of Cancer Treatment, National Cancer Institute.

REFERENCES

Abdullaev FI, Frenkel GD: The effect of saffron on intracellular DNA, RNA and protein synthesis in malignant and non-malignant human cells. *Biofactors* 1992; 4(1):43-5.

Aburada M, Takeda S, Ito E, et al: Protective effects of juzen-taihoto, dried decoctum of 10 Chinese herbs mixture, upon the adverse effects of mitomycin C in mice. *J Pharmacobiodyn* 1983; 6(12):1000-4.

Achbarou A, Kaiser S, Tremblay G, et al: Urokinase overproduction results in increased skeletal metastasis by prostate cancer cells in vivo. *Cancer Res* 1994; 54(9):2372-7.

Aclimandos WA, Heinemann D, Kelly SB, et al: Erythrocyte stearic to oleic acid ratio in patients with ocular melanoma. *Eye* 1992 6(Pt4):416-9.

Adamietz IA, Kurfurst F, Muller U, et al: Growth acceleration of Ehrlich ascites tumor cells treated by proteinase in vitro. *Eur J Cancer Clin Oncol* 1989; 25(12):1837-41.

Adlercreutz H, Markkanen H, Watanabe S: Plasma concentrations of phyto-oestrogens in Japanese men. *Lancet* 1993 Nov 13; 342(8881):1209-10.

Adlercreutz H, Mousavi Y, Clark J, Hockerstedt K, et al: Dietary phytoestrogens and cancer: in vitro and in vivo studies. *J Steroid Biochem Mol Biol* 1992; 41(3-8):331-7.

Affany A, Salvayre R, Blazy L: Comparison of the protective effect of various flavonoids against lipid peroxidation of erythrocyte membranes induced by cumene hydroperoxide. *Fundamental and Clinical Pharmacology* 1987; 1:451-7.

Agarwal R, Katiyar SK, Zaidi SI, et al: Inhibition of skin tumor promoter-caused induction of epidermal ornithine decarboxylase in sencar mice by polyphenolic fraction isolated from green tea and its individual epicatechin derivatives. *Cancer Res* 1992; 52(13):3582-8.

Agrez MV, Bates RC: Colorectal cancer and the integrin family of cell adhesion receptors: current status and future directions. *Eur J Cancer* 1994; 30A(14):2166-70.

Aguilera JA, Newton GL, Fahey RC, Ward JF: Thiol uptake by Chinese hamster V79 cells and aerobic radioprotection as a function of the net charge on the thiol. *Radiat Res* 1992; 130(2):194-204.

Agullo G, Gamet L, Besson C: Quercetin exerts a preferential cytoxic effect on active dividing colon carcinoma HT29 and caco-2 cells. *Cancer Letters* 1994; 87:55-63.

Ahmed N, Weidemann MJ: Purine metabolism in promyelocytic HL60 and dimethylsulphoxide-differentiated HL60 cells. *Leuk Res* 1994 Jun; 18(6):441-51.

Aisner J, Wiernik PH: Thiotepa (NSC-6396) and dimethyl sulfoxide (NSC-763) in the treatment of renal cell carcinoma. *Cancer Clinical Trials* 1978; Spring:23-25.

Akiba S, Sato T, Fujii T: Enhancement of A23187-induced aracidonic acid liberation by vasopressin is sensitive to genistein in rabbit platelets. *Biochem Mol Biol Int* 1993 Sep; 31(1):135-42.

Al-Awadi F, Fatania H, Shamte U: The effect of a plants mixture extract on liver gluconeogenesis in streptozotocin induced diabetic rats. *Diabetes Res* 1991; 18(4):163-8.

Alba E, Visentin L, Farina C, et al: Prevention of infection and improvement of cenesthesia with thymostimulin during chemotherapy following mastectomy. *Minerva Ginecol* 1991; 43(12):585-7.

Albanes D: Energy balance, body size, and cancer. *Crit Rev Oncol Hematol* 1990; 10(3):283-303.

Albert-Puleo M: Fennel and anise as estrogenic agents. *J Ethnopharmacol* 1980 Dec; 2(4):337-44.

Aldeghi R, Lissoni P, Barni S, et al: Low-dose interleukin-2 subcutaneous immunotherapy in association with the pineal hormone melatonin as a first-line therapy in locally advanced or metastatic hepatocellular carcinoma. *Eur J Cancer* 1994; 30A(2):167-70.

Alexander CN, Langer EJ, Newman RI, et al: Transcendental meditation, mindfulness, and longevity: an experimental study with the elderly. *J Pers Soc Psychol* 1989; 57(6):950-64.

Alexander HC, Prudden JF: The causes of abdominal wound disruption. *Surg Gynecol Obstet* 1966 Jun; 122(6):1223-9.

Ali M, Afzal M, Gubler CJ, et al: A potent thromboxane formation inhibitor in green tea leaves. *Prostaglandins Leukot Essent Fatty Acids* 1990; 40:281-3.

Allen J, Prudden JF: Histologic response to a cartilage powder preparation in a controlled human study. *Am J Surg* 1966; 112(6):888-91.

Alpha-Tocopherol, Beta Carotene Cancer Prevention Study Group: The effect of vitamin E and beta carotene on the incidence of lung cancer and other cancers in male smokers. *The New England Journal of Medicine* 1994; 330(15):1029-35.

Ambrus JL, Stoll HL, Klein EA, et al: Increased prostaglandin E2 and cAMP phosphodiesterase levels in Kaposi's sarcoma-a virus against host defense mechanism. *Res Commun Chem Pathol Pharmacol* 1992; 78(2):249-52.

Amdur MO, Doull J, Klaassen CD, editors. *Casarett and Doull's Toxicology; The basic science of poisons* New York: Pergamon Press 1991.

Amellal M, Bronner C, Briancon F, et al: Inhibition of mast cell histamine release by flavonoids and bioflavonoids. *Planta Medica* 1985; 16-20.

Ames BN, Shigenaga MK, Hagen TM: Oxidants, antioxidants and the degenerative diseases of aging. *Proc Natl Acad Sci USA* 1993 Sep; 90:7915-22.

Ammon HP, Muller PH, Eggstein M, et al: Increase in glucose consumption by acetylcysteine during hyperglycemic clamp. A study with healthy volunteers. *Arzneimittelforschung* 1992 May; 42(5):642-5.

Anderson JA, Gow LA, Ogston D: Influence of cider on the fibrinolytic enzyme system. *Acta haemat* 1983; 69:344-48.

Anderson P, Yu SG, Kwon R, et al: A comparison of the anti-carcinogenic activities of two monoterpenes d-limonene and geraniol. *FASEB (Meeting Abstract)* 1993; 7(3):A70.

Andrade SP, Vieira LB, Bakhle YS, et al: Effects of platelet aggravating factor (PAF) and other vasoconstrictors on a model of angiogenesis in the mouse. *Int J Exp Pathol* 1992; 73(4):503-13.

Anton R, Haag-Berrurier M: Therapeutic use of natural an-thraquinone for other than laxative actions. *Pharmacology* 1980; 20(suppl 1):104-12.

Apitz-Castro R, Badimon JJ, Badimon L: Effect of ajoene, the major platelet compound from garlic, on platelet thrombus formation. *Thromb Res* 1992; 68(2):145-55.

Arcangeli A, Carla M, Del Bene MR, Becchetti A, et al: Polar/apolar compounds induce leukemia cell differentia-tion by modulating cell-surface potential. *Proc Natl Acad Sci USA* 1993 Jun 15; 90(12):5858-62.

Arlow, F: Presentation at the American College of Gastroen-terology meeting, 1989.

Armand JP, De Forni M, Recondo G, et al: "Flavonoids: A new class of anticancer agents? Preclinical and clinical data of flavone acetic acid." *Plant Flavonoids in Biology and Medicine II* Alan R. Liss, Inc., 1988; 235-41.

Arnold M, Przerwa M: Therapeutic effects on experimentally induced edemas. *Arzneim-Forsch* 1976; 26(3):402-9.

Arora RC, Arora S, Gupta RK: The long-term use of garlic in ischemic heart disease—an apraisal. *Atherosclerosis* 1981; 40(2):175-9.

Arterbery VE, Pryor WA, Jiang L, Sehnert, SS, Foster WM, Abrams RA, Williams JR, Wharam MD Jr, Risby TH: Breath ethane generation during clinical total body irradia-tion as a marker of oxygen-free-radical-mediated lipid per-oxidation: a case study. *Free Radical Biol Med* 1994; 17(6):569-76.

Asahi M, Yanagi S, Ohta S, Inazu T, et al: Thrombin-induced human platelet aggregation is inhibited by protein-tyrosine kinase inhibitors, ST638 and genistein. *FEBS Lett* 1992; 309(1):10-4.

Atal CK, Sharma ML, Kaul A, Khajuria A: Immunomodulating agents of plant origin. I: preliminary screening. *J Ethno-pharmacol* 1986; 18:133-41.

August L: Food & Hormones. *Townsend Letter* 1995 Apr:141:56-61.

Austin CA, Patel S, Ono K, et al: Site-specific DNA cleavage by mammalian DNA topoisomerase II induced by novel fla-vone and catechin derivatives. *Biochem J* 1992; 282 (Pt 3):883-9.

Avila MA, Velasco JA, Cansado J, Notario V: Quercetin medi-ates the down-regulation of mutant p53 in the human breast cancer cell line MDA-MB468. *Cancer Res* 1994; 54(9):2424-8.

Azavedo E, Svane G, Nordenstrom B: Radiological evidence of response to electrochemical treatment of breast cancer. *Clin Radiol* 1991; 43(2):84-7.

Azizi E, Brenner HJ, Shoham J: Postsurgical adjuvant treatment of malignant melanoma patients by the thymic factor thymostimulin. *Arzneimittelforschung* 1984; 34(9):1043-7.

Azuine MA, Kayal JJ, Bhide SV: Protective role of aqueous turmeric extract against mutagenicity of direct-acting car-cinogens as well as benzo [alpha] pyrene-induced genotox-icity and carcinogenicity. *J Cancer Res Clin Oncol* 1992; 118(6):447-52.

Bachman M, Schlatter C: Metabolism of [14C]emodin in rat. *Xenobiotica* 1981; 11(3):217-25.

Baggot JE, Ha T, Vaughn WH, et al: Effect of miso (Japanese soybean paste) and NaCl on DMBA-induced rat mammary tumors. *Nutr Cancer* 1990; 14:103-09.

Bailar JC, Smith EM: Progress against cancer? *The New Eng-land J of Med* 1986; 314(19):1226-32.

Bailey JM, Fletcher-Cieutat M: "Prostaglandins and Leuko-trienes in the T-Helper and T-Suppressor cell system." *Prostaglandins in Cancer Research.* E Garaci, R Paoletti, MG Santoro editors. Berlin: Springer-Verlag, 1987.

Baker ME: Licorice and enzymes other than 11B-hydroxysteroid dehydrogenase; An evolutionary per-spective. *Steroids* 1994 59(2):136-41.

Banda MJ, Howard EW, Herron GS, et al: Secreted inhibitors of metalloproteinases (IMPs) that are distinct from TIMP. *Matrix Suppl* 1992; 1:294-8.

Baraboi VA, Oleinik SA, Blium IA, Khmelevskii IuV: [Pro-oxidant and antioxidant homeostasis in guinea pigs follow-ing fractionated x-ray irradiation at low doses and the cor-rection of disorders with and antioxidant complex.] *Radiats Biol Radioecol* 1994b; 34(2):240-6.

Baraboi VA, Oliinyk SA, Blium IO, Korniichuk HM, Khmielievs'kyi IuV: [Dynamics of lipid peroxidation in blood and organs of rats after irradiation at low doses and the effect of antioxidants.] *Ukr Biokhim Zh* 1994a; 66(5):39-47.

Baranes J, Hellegouarch A, LeHegarat M, et al: The effects of PAF-acether on the cardiovascular system and their inhibi-tion by a new highly specific PAF-acether receptor antago-nist BN 52021. *Pharmacol Res Commun* 1986 Aug; 18(8):717-37.

Barbul A, Rettura G, Levenson SM, et al: Arginine: a thymo-tropic and wound-healing promoting agent. *Surgical Fo-rum* 1977 Oct; XVIII:101-3.

Bardychev MS, Guseva LI, Zubova ND: Acupuncture in edema of the extremities following radiation or combination ther-apy of cancer of the breast and uterus. *Vopr Onkol* 1988; 34(3):3 19-22.

Barnes S, Grubbs C, Setchell KDR, et al: "Soybeans inhibit mammary tumors in models of breast cancer." *Mutagens and Carcinogens in the Diet.* M. Pariza, ed. New York: Wiley-Liss, 1990, 239-53.

Barnett G, Chiang CW, Licko V: Effects of marijuana on tes-tosterone in male subjects. *J Theor Biol* 1983 Oct 21; 104(4):685-92.

Baron RS, Cutrona CE, Hicklin D, et al: Social support and immune function among spouses of cancer patients. *J of Personality and Social Psychology* 1990; 59(2):344-52.

Barone J, Hebert JR: Dietary fat and natural killer cell activity. *Med Hypotheses* 1988; 25:223-26.

Barone J, Hebert JR, Reddy MM: Dietary fat and natural-killer-cell activity. *Am J Clin Nutr* 1989 Oct; 50(4): 861-867.

Baruch J: Effects of endotelon in postoperative edema. Results of a doulbe-blind study with placebo on a group of thirty-two patients. *Ann Chir Plast Esthet* 1984(4).

Bashar H, Urano T, Fukuta K, et al: Plasminogen activators and plasminogen activator inhibitor 1 in urinary tract cancer. *Urol Int* 1994; 52(1):4-8.

Batkin S, Taussig SJ, Szekerezes J: Antimetastic effect of bromelain with or without its proteolytic and anticoagulant activity. *J Cancer Res Clin Oncol* 1988; 114:507-8.

Beard J: *The enzyme treatment of cancer and its scientific basis.* London: Chatto & Windus, 1911.

Beck SA, Smith KL, Tisdale MJ: Anticachectic and antitumor effect of eicosapentaenoic acid and its effect on protein turnover. *Cancer Res* 1991; 51(22):6089-93.

Begin ME, Ells G, Das UN, et al: Differential killing of human cacinoma cells supplemented with n-3 and n-6 polyunsaturated fatty acids. *JNCL* 1986 Nov; 77(5):1053-60.

Begin ME; Sircar S, Weber JM: Differential sensitivity of tumorigenic and genetically related non-tumorigenic cells to cytotoxic polyunsaturated fatty acids. *Anticancer Res* 1989; 9(4):1049-52.

Belehradek M, Domenge C, Luboinski B, Orlowski S et al: Electrochemotherapy, a new antitumor treatment. *Cancer* 1993; 72(12):3694-700.

Belman S, Garte SJ: "Proteases and cyclic nucleotides." *Arachidonic Acid Metabolism and Tumor Promotion*, SM Fischer and TJ Slaga editors. Boston: Martinus Nijhoff Publishing, 1985.

Benediktsson R, Edwards CR: Apparent mineralocorticoid excess. *J Hums Hypertens* 1994; 8(5)371-5.

Bennett SA, Leite LC, Birnboim HC: Platelet activating factor, an endogenous mediator of inflammation, induces phenotypic transformation of rat embryo cells. *Carcinogenesis* 1993; 14(7):1289-96.

Bensky D, Barolet R. *Chinese Herbal Medicine: Formulas & Strategies* Seattle, Washington: Eastland Press; 1990.

Bensky D, Gamble A: *Chinese Herbal Medicine Materia Medica.* Seattle: Eastland Press, 1993.

Beranek JT: Ingrowth of hypoplastic capillary sprouts into fibrin clots: Further evidence in favor of the angiogenic hypothesis of repair and fibrosis. *Med Hypotheses* 1989; 28(4):271-3.

Beretz A, Cazenave JP: "The effect of flavonoids on blood-vessel wall interactions." *Plant Flavonoids in Biology and Medicine II* Alan R. Liss, Inc., 1988; 187-200.

Berg P, Daniel PT: "Effects of flavonoid compounds on the immune response." *Plant Flavonoids in Biology and Medicine II* Alan R. Liss, Inc., 1988; 157-171.

Bergamaschi G, Rosti V, Danova M, Ponchio L, et al: Inhibitors of tyrosine phosphorylation induce apoptosis in human leukemic cell lines. *Leukemia* 1993 Dec; 7(12):20-8.

Bernardi P, Pace V: Correlations between folic acid, human papilloma virus (HPV) and cervix neoplasms. *Minerva Ginecol* 1994 May; 46(5):249-55.

Best R, et al: The anti-ulcerogenic activity of the unripe plantian banana (Musa species). *British Journal of Pharmacology* 1984; 82:107-16.

Beynon RJ, Kay J: Letter: Enteropancreatic circulation of digestive enzyme. *Nature* 1976 Mar 4; 260(5546):78-90.

Bhargava SK: Antiandrogenic effects of a flavanoid-rich fraction of Vitex negundo seeds: a histological and biochemical study in dogs. *J Ethnopharmacol* 1989 Dec; 27(3):327-39.

Bibby MC, Double JA: Flavone acetic acid—from laboratory to clinic and back. *Anticancer Drugs* 1993; 4(1):3-7.

Billings PC, Lognecker MP, Keary M, et al: Protease inhibitor content of human dietary samples. *Nutr Cancer* 1990; 14:85-93.

Bionostics, Inc.: Functions of Amino Acids. *Technical Memorandum 2*, 1986; 1-36.

Birchmeier W, Behrens J: Cadherin expression in carcinomas: role in the formation of cell junctions and the prevention in invasiveness. *Biochim Biophys Acta* 1994; 1 198(1):11-26.

Bisler H, Pfeifer R, Kluken, et al: Effects of horse-chestnut seed extract on transcapillary filtration in chronic venous insufficiency. *Dtsch Med Wochenschr* 1986 Aug 29; 111(35):1321-9.

Bland J, Bralley JA: Nutritional upregulation of hepatic detoxication enzymes. *Journal of Applied Nutrition* 1992; 44(3-4):1-18.

Bocci V: Mistletoe (viscum album) lectins as cytokine inducers and immunoadjuvant in tumor therapy. A review. *J Biol Regul Homeost Agents* 1993; 7(1):1-6.

Bockman RS, Hickok N, Rapuano B: "Prostaglandins and calcium metabolism in cancer." *Prostaglandins in Cancer Research*. E Garaci, R Paoletti, MG Santoro editors. Berlin: Springer-Verlag, 1987.

Bodor N, Brewster ME: Improved delivery through biological membranes; XV-Sustained brain delivery of berberine. *Eur J Med Chem* 1983; 18(3):235-40.

Bogart G: The use of meditation in psychotherapy: a review of the literature. *Am J Psychother* 1991; 45(3):383-412.

Bogo V: Radiation: behavioral implications in space. *Toxicology* 1988; 49(2-3):299-307.

Bonata IL, Ben-Efraim S: "Leukotrienes and Prostaglandins mutually govern the antitumor potential of macrophages." *Prostaglandins in Cancer Research*. Berlin: Springer-Verlag, 1987.

Bone K: Picrorrhiza important modulator of immune function. *Townsend Letter* 1995; 142:88-94.

Booyens J, Maguire: Dietary fats and cancer. *Med Hypotheses* 1985; 17:351-362.

Borgstrom L, Kagedal, Paulsen O: Pharmacokinetics of N-acetylcysteine in man. *Eur J Clin Pharmacol* 1986; 31:217-22.

Borovskaia TG, Udintsev SN, Zueva EP, et al: Dilution of the toxic action of 5-fluorouracil on the mucosa of the small intestine in mice using the sap of plantain. *Vopr Onkol* 1987; 33(7):60-64.

Borzeix MG, Labos M, Hartl C: Researches on the antiaggregative activity of Gingko biloba extract (author's translation). *Sem Hop* 1980; 56(7-8):393-8.

Bostick RM, Potter JD, Kushi LH, Sellers TA, et al: Sugar, meat, and fat intake and non-dietary risk factors for colon cancer incidence in Iowa women (United States). *Cancer Causes Control* 1994; 5(1):38-52.

Bouchet C, Spyratos F, Marin PM, et al: Prognostic value of urokinase-type plasminogen activator (uPA) and plasminogen activator inhibitors PAI-1 and PAI-2 in breast carcinomas. *Br J Cancer* 1994; 69(2):398-405.

Bourut C, Chenu E, Mathe G: Can neo-adjuvant chemotherapy prevent tumors? *J Surg Res* 1988; 45(6):513-22.

Bouskela E, Cyrino FZ, Marcelon G: Inhibitory effect of the Ruscus extract and of the flavonoid hesperidine methylchalcone on increased microvascular permeability induced by various agents in the hamster cheek pouch. *J Cardiovasc Pharmacol* 1993 Aug; 22(2):225-30.

Bovbjerg DH: Psychoneuroimmunology: Immplications of oncology? *Cancer Supp* 1991; 67:828-31.

Bovbjerg DH, Redd WH, Maier LA, et al: Anticapatory immune suppression and nausea in women receiving cyclic chemotherapy for ovarian cancer. *J Consult Clin Psychol* 1990 Apr; 58(2):153-7.

Boyar AP, Rose JR, Loughridge A, et al: Response to a diet low in total fat in women with postmenopausal breast cancer: a pilot study. *Cancer and Nutrition* 1988; 11:93-99.

Bracke M, Castronovo V, De Bruyne G, et al: Interactions of invasive cells with native and modified extracellular matrix in vitro. *Adv Exp Med Biol* 1988b; 233:171-178.

Bracke M, Van Cauwenberge R, Mareel M: Inhibitory effect of different flavanoids on the invasion of malignant MO4 calls into embryonic chick heart in vitro. *Treatment of Metastasis; Problems and Prospects* 1985; pp. 339-42.

Bracke M, Van Cauwenberge RML, Mareel MM, et al: "Flavonoids: Tools for the study of tumor invasion in vitro." *Plant Flavonoids in Biology and Medicine II* Alan R. Liss, Inc. 1986; 441-44.

Bracke M, Vyncke B, Opdenakker G, et al: Effect of catechins and citrus flavonoids on invasion in vitro. *Clin Exp Metastasis* 1991; 9(1):13-25.

Bracke ME, De Pestel G, Castronovo V, et al: "Flavonoids inhibit malignant tumor invasion in vitro." *Plant Flavonoids in Biology and Medicine II: Biochemical, Cellular, and Medicinal Properties* Alan R. Liss, Inc., 1988a; 2 19-33.

Bracke ME, Van Cauwenberge RM, Mareel MM: (+)-Catechin inhibits the invasion of malignant fibrosarcoma cells in chick heart in vitro. *Clin Exp Metastasis* 1984; 2(2):161-70.

Bradford PG, Autieri M: Increased expression of the inositol 1,4,5-trisphosphate receptor in human leukaemic (HL-60) cells differentiated with retinoic acid or dimethyl sulphoxide. *Biochem J* 1991 Nov 15; 280(Pt 1):205-10.

Braunhut, SJ, Palomares, M. *Microvasc Res* 1991; 41:47-62.

Braunhut SJ, Moses MA: Retinoids modulate endothelial cell production of matrix-degrading proteases and tissue inhibitors of metalloproteinases (TIMP). *J Biol Chem* 1994; 269(18):13472-9.

Bravard A, Beaumatin J, Dussaulx E, et al: Modifications of the anti-oxidant metabolism during proliferation and differentiation of colon tumor cell lines. *Int J Cancer* 1994 Dec 15; 59(6):843-7.

Braverman AS: Medical oncology in the 1990s. *The Lancet* 1991; 337:901-2.

Braverman ER, Pfieffer CC: *The Healing Nutrients Within.* New Canaan, CT: Keats Publishing, Inc; 1987.

Breitman TR: "The role of prostaglandins and other arachidonic acid metabolites in the differentiation of HL-60." *Prostaglandins in Cancer Research.* E Garaci, R Paoletti, and MG Santoro editors. Berlin: Springer-Verlag, 1987.

Breitman TR, He RY: Combinations of retinoic acid with either sodium butyrate, dimethyl sulfoxide, or hexamethylene bisacetamide synergistically induce differentiation of the human myeloid leukemia cell line HL60. *Cancer Res* 1990 Oct 1; 50(19):6268-73.

Brem SS, Zagzag D, Tsanaclis AM, Gately S, et al: Inhibition of angiogenesis and tumor growth in the brain. Suppression of endothelial cell turnover by penicillamine and the depletion of copper, an angiogenic cofactor. *Am J Pathol* 1990; 137(5):1121-42.

Breu W, Hagenlocher M, Redl K, Tittel G, et al: Anti-inflammatory activity of sabal fruit extracts prepared with supercritical carbon dioxide. In vitro antagonists of cyclooxygenase and 5-lipoxygenase metabolism. *Ger Arzneimittelforschung* 1992; 42(4):547-51.

Brewer AK: The high pH therapy for cancer tests on mice and humans. *Phar Biochem & Behavior* 1984; 21(1):1-5.

Brewer AK, Passwater RA: Physics of the cell membrane mechanism involved in cancer. *Am Lab* 1976; 8:37-45.

Brohult A, Brohult J, Brohult S, et al: Reduced mortality in cancer patients after administration of alkoxyglycerols. *Acta Obstst Gynecol Scand* 1986; 65:779-85.

Broitman SA, Cannizzo, Jr F: "A model system for studying nutritional interventions on colon tumor growth: effects of marine oil." *Exercise, Calories, Fat and Cancer.* MM. Jacobs, editor. New York: Plenum Press, 1992.

Brown DC, Purushotham AD, George WD: Inhibition of pulmonary tumor seeding by antiplatelet and fibrinolytic therapy in an animal experimental model. *J Surg Oncol* 1994; 55(3):154-9.

Brown LF, Dvorak AM, Dvorak HF, et al: Leaky vessels, fibrin deposition, and fibrosis: a sequence of events common to solid tumors and to many other types of disease. *Am Rev Respir Dis* 1989; 140(4):1104-7.

Bruseth S, Enge A: Mistletoe in the treatment of cancer. *Tidsskr Nor Laegeforen* 1993 30; 113(9):1058-60.

Bu L, Aasen AO, Karlsrud TS, et al: The role of proteases in the growth, invasion and spread of cancer cells. *Tidsskr Nor Laegeforen* 1990; 110(29):3753-6.

Buckley AR, Buckley DJ, Gout PW, Liang H, et al: Inhibition by genistein of prolactin-induced Nb2 lymphoma cell mitogenisis. *Mol Cell Endrocrinol* 1993 Dec; 98(1):17-25.

Budavari S, O'Neal MJ, Smith A, et al (ed.s): *The Merck Index*. 11th edition. New Jersey: Merck & Co, 1989.

Burns CP, Petersen ES, North JA, et al: Effect of docosahexaenoic acid on rate of differentiation of HL-60 human leukemia. *Cancer Research* 1989; 49:3252-58.

Burns N, Grove SK: *The practice of nursing research conduct, critique and utilization*. Philadelphia: WB Saunders Co, 1987.

Burns PC, Spector AA: Effects of lipids on cancer therapy. *Nutrition Reviews* 1990; 48(6):223-40.

Burton TS, Marsh MC: Therapy of spontaneous mouse cancer: failure of tuberculin, karkinolysin and some inorganic compounds therein. *Am Surg* 1931; 93:169-179.

Buset M, et al: Inhibition of human colonic epithelial cell proliferation in vivo and in vitro by calcium. *Cancer Res* 1986; 46(10):5426-30.

Butrum RR, Messina MJ: "Cancer." *Health effects of w-3 polyunsaturated fatty acids in seafoods*. *World Rev Nutr Diet* Simopoulos AP et al., editors. Basel, Karger, 1991; 66:48-50.

Butterworth CE Jr: Effect of folate on cervical cancer. Synergism among risk factors. *Ann NY Acad Sci* 1992 Sept 30; 669:293-9.

Caccamo DV, Keohane ME, McKeever PE: Plasminogen activators and inhibitors in gliomas: an immunohistochemical study. *Mod Pathol* 1994; 7(1):99-104.

Cahn J, Borzeix MG: Administration of procyanidolic oligomers in rats. Observed effects on changes in the permeability of the blood-brain barrier. *Sem Hop* 1983; 59:2031-4.

Cairns J: The treatment of disease and the war against cancer. *Scientific American* 1985; 253(5):51-59.

Calabresi P, Schein P. *Medical Oncology* Second Edition. New York: McGraw-Hill, Inc.; 1993.

Cameron E: Protocol for the use of vitamin C in the treatment of cancer. *Med Hypothesis* 1991; 36:190-94.

Cameron E, Campbell A: Innovation vs. quality control: an 'unpublishable' clinical trial of supplemental ascorbate in incurable cancer. *Medical Hypotheses* 1991; 36(3):185-9.

Cameron E, Pauling L: Supplemental ascorbate in the supportive treatment of cancer: prolongation of survival times in terminal human cancer. *Proc Natl Acad Sci USA* 1976 Oct; 73(10):3685-9.

Canovas FA, Alonso J, Gonzales de Zarate P, et al: The use of thymostimulin in lymphoma and myeloma patients. *An Med Interna* 1991; 8(2):69-73.

Cantrill RC, Ells G, Chisholm K, et al: Concentration-dependent effect of iron on gamma linolenic acid toxicity in ZR-75-1 human breast tumor cells in culture. *Cancer Lett* 1993; 72(1-2):99-102.

Carilla E, Briley M, Fauran F, Sultan C, Duvilliers C: Binding of Permixon, a new treatment for prostatic benign hyperplasia, to the cytosolic androgen receptor in the rat prostate. *J Steroid Biochem* 1984 Jan; 20(1):515-9.

Carroll KK: Dietary fats and cancer 1-3. *Am J Clin Nutr* 1991; 53:1064s-67s.

Carson DA, Ribeiro JM: Apoptosis and disease. *The Lancet* 1993; 341:1251-53.

Casarosa C, Cosci di Coscio M, Fratta M: Lack of effects of a lyposterolic extract of Serenoa repens on plasma levels of testosterone, follicle-stimulating hormone, and luteinizing hormone. *Clin Ther* 1988; 10(5):585-8.

Cascinu S, Catalano G: Intensive weekly chemotherapy for elderly gastric cancer patients, using 5-fluorouracil, ciplatin, epi-doxorubicin, 6S-leucovorin and glutathione withthe support of G-CSF. *Tumori* 1995 Jan-Feb; 81(1):32-5.

Cassady JM: Natural products as a source of potential cancer chemotherapeutic and chemopreventive agents. *Journal of Natural Products* 1990; 53(1):23-41.

Cassileth BR, et al: Psychosocial correlates of survival in advanced malignant disease? *New Engl J Med* 1985; 312:1551-5.

Cassileth BR, Lusk EJ, Guerry D, et al: Survival and quality of life among patients receiving unproven as compared with conventional cancer therapy. *The New England Journal of Medicine* 1991; 324(17):1180-85.

Castiglione S, Maurizio F, Bruno T, et al: Rhein inhibits glucose uptake in ehrlich ascites tumor cells by alteration of membrane-associated functions. *Anti-cancer* 1993; 4:407-14.

Castiglione S, Paggi MG, Delpino A, et al: Inhibition of protein synthesis in neoplastic cells by rhein. *Biochem Pharmacol* 1990; 40(5):967-73.

Castillo MH, Perkins E, Campbell JH, Doerr R, et al: The effects of the bioflavinoid quercetin on squamous cell carcinoma of head and neck origin. *Am J Surg* 1989; 158(4):351-5.

Cavallo F, et al: Zinc and copper in breast cancer: a joint study in northern Italy and southern France. *Cancer* 1991; 67:738-745.

CGEOG, Cooperative group for essential oil of garlic: The effect of essential oil of garlic on hyperlipidemia and platelet aggregation—an analysis of 308 cases. *J of Tradit Chinese Med* 1986; 6(2)-117-20.

266

Chaitow L: *Amino acids in therapy: A guide to the therapeutic application of protein constituents.* Rochester: Healing Arts Press, 1988.

Chan D, Lamande SR, Cole WG, et al: Regulation of procollagen synthesis and processing during ascorbate-induced extracellular matrix accumulation in vitro. *Biochem J* 1990; 269(1):175-81.

Chan TC, Chang CJ, Koonchak NM, et al: Selective inhibition of the growth of ras-transformed human bronchial epithelial cells by emodin, a protein-tyrosine kinase inhibitor. *Biochem Biophys Res Commun* 1993; 193(3):1152-8.

Chang CN: "Anti-leukemia Chinese herbs and the effective ingredients." *Advances in Chinese Medicinal Materials Research* Chang HM, Yeung HW, Tso W, Koo A. editors. Singapore: World Scientific, 1985. pp.369-76.

Chang HM, But PPH. *Pharamacology and Applications of Chinese Materia Medica* Vol. 2. Teaneck, NJ: World Scientific Publishing Company, 1987.

Chang HM, But PPH. *Pharmacology and Applications of Chinese Materia Medica* Vol. 1. Teaneck, NJ: World Scientific Publishing Company, 1986.

Chang KS: Down-regulation of c-Ki-ras2 gene expression associated with morphologic differentiation in human embryonal carcinoma cells treated with berberine. *Taiwan I Hsueh Hui Tsa Chih* 1991; 90(1):10-4.

Chang KSS, Gao C, Wang LC: Berberine-induced morphologic differentiation and down-regulation of c-Ki-ras2 protooncogene expression in human teratocarcinoma cells. *Cancer Letters* 1990; 55:103-08.

Chang M: *Anticancer Medicinal Herbs.* Hunan Changha, China: Hunan Science and Technology Press; 1992.

Chastain DE: Patent No. 5,110,832, issued May 5, 1992.

Cheang A, Cooper CL: Psychosocial factors in breast cancer. *Stress Med* 1985; 1:61-6.

Chen HL, Huang XM: Treatment of chemotherapy-induced leukocytopenia with acupuncture and moxibustion. *Chung Hsi I Chieh Ho Tsa Chih* 1991; 11(6):350-2.

Chen J, Wu Z, Yang H, et al: Cytokinetic effects of emodin on human lung cancer A-549 cell. *Zhongcaoyao* 1991; 22(12):543-6.

Chen MF, Chen LT, Boyce HW Jr: 5-fluorouracil cytoxicity in human colon HT-29 cells with moderatley increased or decreased cellular glutathione level. *Anticancer Res* 1995 Jan-Feb; 15(1):163-7.

Chen Q, Liu C, Qui C: Studies of chinese rhubarb: XII. Effect of anthraquinone derivatives on the respiration and glycolysis of ehrlich ascites carcinoma cell. *Yao Hsueh Hsueh Pao* 1980; 15(2):65-70.

Chen Y, Shen L, Yang Y: Determination of emodin in caulis polygoni multiflori and huangshen infusion by TLC-scanning. *Zhongguo Zhongyao Zazhi* 1994; 19(5):284-5.

Chen ZN, Yu PZ, Xu PJ: Anti-platelet activiating factor constituents, 2,5-diaryltetrahydrofuran type lignans, from Piper futokadsura Sied. et Zucc. *Chung Kuo Chung Yao Tsa Chih* 1993; 18(5):292-4.

Cheng JH, Zhang SL, Zhao DH, et al: Treatment of 20 patients with terminal primary bronchogenic carcinoma using feiliuping. *Jiangxi Journal of Traditional Chinese Medicine* 1991; 22(6):344-47.

Cheng Q: Effect of cordyceps sinensis on cellular immunity in rats with chronic renal insufficiency. *Chung Hua I Hsueh Tsa Chih* 1992; 72(1):27-9.

Cheng QL, Chen XM, Shi SZ: Effects of Epimedium sagittatum on immunopathology and extracellular matrices in rats with chronic renal insufficiency. *Chung Hua Nei Ko Tsa Chih* 1994 Feb; 33(2):83-6.

Chi CW, Chang YF, Chao TW, et al: Flowcytometric analysis of the effect of berberine on the expression of glucocorticoid receptors in human hepatoma Hep-g2 cells. *Life Sciences* 1994; 54(26):2099-2107.

Chiang HC, Tseng TH, Wang CJ, et al: Experimental antitumor agents from Solanum indicum. *Anticancer Res* 1991; 11(5):1911-7.

Chiang HC, Wang JJ, Wu RT: Immunomodulators from Paris formosana hayata. *Anticancer Res* 1992; 12(3):949-57.

Chu D, Sun Y, Lin J, et al: F3, a fractionated extract of Astragalus membranaceus, potentiates lymphokine-activated killer cell cytotoxicity generated by low-dose recombinant interleukin-2. *Chung Hsi I Chieh Ho Tsa Chih* 1990; 10(1):34-6.

Chu DT, Lepe-Zuniga J, Wong WL, et al: Fractionated extract of Astragalus membranaceus, a Chinese medicinal herb, potentiates LAK cell cytotoxicity generated by a low dose of recombinant interleukin-2. *J Clin Lab Immunol* 1988a; 26(4):183-7.

Chu DT, Sun Y, Lin JR: Immune restoration of local xenogeneic graft-versus-host reaction in cancer patients in vitro and reversal of cyclophosphamide induced immune suppression in the rat in vivo by fractionated astragalus membranaceus *Chung Hsi I Chieh Ho Tsa Chih* 1989; 9(6):351-4.

Chu DT, Wong WL, Mavlight GM: Immunotherapy with chinese medicinal herbs: Immune restoration of local xenogeneic graft-versus-host reaction in cancer patients by fractionated astragalus membranaceus in vitro. *Journal of Clinical Laboratory Immunology* 1988b; 25(3):1 19-23.

Clark PI, Slevin ML, Webb JAW, et al: Oral urea in the treatment of secondary tumours in the liver. *Br J Cancer* 1988; 57:317-18.

Clark W, Brater D, Johnson A, eds. *Goth's Medical Pharmacology* 13th ed. St. Louis: Mosby Year Book, 1992.

Clemens MR, Ladner C, Schmidt H, Ehninger G, Einsele H, Buehler E, Waller HD, Gey KF: Decreased essential antioxidants and increased lipid hydroperoxides following high-dose radiochemotherapy. *Free Radical Res Commun* 1989; 7(3-6):227-32.

Clifford C, Kramer B: Diet as a risk and therapy for cancer. *Clinical Nutrition* 1993; 77(4):725-40.

Cohen LA, Choi K, Weisburger JH, et al: Effect of varying porportions of dietary fat on the development of N-nitrosomethylurea-induced rat mammary tumors. *Anticancer Res.* 1986b; 6:215.

Cohen LA, Thompson DO, Maeura Y, et al: Dietary fat and mammary cancer. Promoting effects of different dietary fats on N-nitrosomethylurea-induced mammary tumorigenesis. *J Natl Cancer Inst.* 1986a; 77:33.

Collins TM, Denish A, Sheffield J, Mitra A, et al: Nicotinamide enhances skin flap survival. *Scand J Plast Reconstr Surg Hand Surg* 1989; 23(3):177-9.

Colston KW, Berger U, Coombes RC: Possible role for vitamin D in controlling breast cancer cell proliferation. *Lancet* 1989; 1(8631):188-91.

Comroe J Jr: *Proc Natl Acad Sci USA* 1978; 75:4543.

Comstock G, et al: Prediagonostic serum levels of carotenoids and vitamin E as related to subsequent cancer in Washington County, Maryland. *Am J Clin Nutr* 1991; 53:260s-264s.

Comstock GW, Bush TL, Helzlsouer K: Serum retinol, beta-carotene, vitamin E, and selenium as related to subsequent cancer of specific sites. *American Journal of Epidemiology* 1992; 135(2):115-21.

Constantinou A, Kiguchi K, Huberman E: Induction of differentiation and DNA strand breakage in human HL-60 and K-562 leukemia cells by genistein. *Cancer Res* 1990; 50(9):2618-24.

Cooper R, Joffe BI, Lamprey JM, et al: Hormonal and biochemical responses to transcendental meditation. *Postgraduate Med J* 1985; 61:301-4.

Copland SA, McHardy KC, Wahle KW, et al: Altered platelet stearic to oleic acid ratio in malignancy. *Eur J Cancer* 1992; 28A(6-7):1135-7.

Corbe CH, Boissin JP, Siou A. *J Fr Ophatalmol* 1988; 11(5)453-460.

Cos S, Sanchez-Barcelo EJ: Differences between pulsatile or continuous exposure to melatonin on MCF-7 human breast cancer cell proliferation. *Cancer Lett* 1994 Sep 30; 85(1):105-109.

Cotgreave I, Moldeus P, Schuppe I: The metabolism of N-acetylcysteine by human endothelial cells. *Biochem Pharmacol* 1991 Jun 21; 42(1):13-6.

Covington W, Ho DH, Newman RA, et al: Enzyme depletion of plasma l-tryptophan (TRP). *Proc Annu Meet Am Soc Clin Oncol* 1990; 9:A316.

Coward L, Barnes NC, Setchell KDR, et al: Genistein, daidzein, and their B-Glycoside conjugates: antitumor isoflavones in soybean foods from american and asian diets. *J Agric Food Chem* 1993; 41:1961-67.

Creagan, et al: *N Engl J Med* 1979; 301:687-90.

Creasey W: *Diet and Cancer.* Philadelphia: Lea & Febiger; 1985.

Crespo D, Fernandez-Viadero C, Verduga R, et al: Interaction between melatonin and estradiol on morphological and morphometric features of MCF-7 human breast cancer cells. *J Pineal Res* 1994 May; 16(4):215-222.

Crommelin DJA, Midha KK: *Topics in Pharmaceutical Sciences 1991.* Stuttgart: Medpharm Scientific Publishers, 1992.

Crowell PL, Lin S, Vedejs E, et al: Identification of metabolites of the antitumor agent d-limonene capable of inhibiting protein isoprenylation and cell growth. *Cancer Chemother Pharmacol* 1992; 31(3):205-212.

Cullis P, Hope MJ: "Physical properties and functional roles of lipids in membranes." *Biochemistry of Lipids, Lipoproteins and Membranes.* DE Vance and JE Vance editors. Amsterdam: Elsevier, 1991.

Czernicki Z: Effects of agents which increase the resistance of the vascular wall and the proteinase inhibitor trasylol on experimental brain edema. *Neurol Neurochir Pol* 1977; 11(4):457-60.

Dai Y, Hang BQ, Mong QY, et al: Anti-inflammatory effect of fructus Ligustri Lucidi. *Chung Kuo Chung Hsi I Chieh Ho Tsa Chih* 1989; 14(7):431-3.

Daly L: The first international urokinase/warfarin trial in colorectal cancer. *Clin Exp Metastasis* 1991; 9(1):3-11.

Daniel PT, Holzschuh J, Berg PA: The pathogenesis of cianidanol-induced fever. *Eur J Clin Pharmacol* 1988; 34:241-47.

Danopoulos ED, Danopoulou, IE: Urea treatment of liver metastases. Correspondence. *Clin Oncol* 1981; 7:385-91.

Danopoulos ED, Danopoulou IE: Correspondence. *Clin Oncol* 1983; 9:89-91.

Danopoulos ED, Danopoulou IE: Effects of urea treatment in combination with curettage in extensive periophthalmic malignancies. *Ophthalmogica* 1979; 179:52.

Danopoulos ED, Danopoulou IE: Regression of liver cancer with oral urea. Letter. *Lancet* 1974a Jan 26; 1(848):132.

Danopoulos ED, Danopoulou IE: The results of urea treatment in liver malignancies. *Clin Oncol* 1975; 1:341.

Danopoulos ED, Danopoulou IE: Urea treatment of skin malignancies. *Lancet* 1974b; 1:132.

Danopoulos ED, Danopoulou IE, Besbeas S, et al: The effects of urea treatment in combination with curettage in extensive lip cancers. *J Surg Oncol* 1982 Mar; 19(3):127-31.

Das UN: Gamma-linolenic acid, aracidonic acid, and eicosapentaenoic acid as potential anticancer drugs. *Nutrition* 1990; 6(6):429-34.

Das UN: Tumoricidial action of cis-unsaturated fatty acids and their relationship to free radicals and lipid peroxidation. *Cancer Lett* 1991; 56(3):235-43.

Das UN, Huang YS, Begin ME, et al: Uptake and distribution of cis-unsaturated fatty acids and their effect on free radical generation in normal and tumor cells in vitro. *Free Radic Biol Med* 1987; 3(1):9-14.

Davis DL, Bradlow HL, Wolff M, et al: Medical hypothesis: xenoestrogens as preventable causes of breast cancer. *Environ Health Perspect* 1993 Oct; 101(5):372-7.

Davis RH, Stewart GJ, Bregman PJ: Aloe vera and the inflamed synovial pouch model. *J Am Podiatr Med Assoc* 1992; 82(3):140-8.

De Bravo MG, De Antueno RJ, Toledo J, et al: Effects of eicosapentaenoic and docosahexaenoic acid concentrate on a human lung carcinoma grown in nude mice. *Lipids* 1991; 26(11):866-70.

De la Torre JC editor. *Biological actions and medical applications of dimethyl sulfoxide.* New York: Annals of the New York Academy of Sciences, 1983.

De Quay B, Malinverni R, Lauterburg BH: Glutathione depletion in HIV-infected patients: role of cysteine deficiency and effect of oral N-acetylcysteine. *AIDS* 1992; 6, 815-19.

De Vries N, De Flora S: N-acetyl-l-cysteine. *J Cell Biochem Suppl* 1993; 17F:270-7.

De Vries TJ, Quax PH, Denijn M, et al: Plasminogen activators, their inhibitors, and urokinase receptor emerge in late stages of melanocytic tumor progression. *Am J Pathol* 1994(1):70-81.

De Witte P: Metabolism and Pharmacokenetics of anthranoids. *Pharmacology* 1993; 47(suppl 1):86-97.

De Witte P, Lemli J: Excretion and distribution of [14C] rhein [14C] rhein anthrone in rats. *J Pharm. Pharmacol* 1988a; 40(1):652-655.

De Witte P, Lemli J: Metabolism of [14C] rhein [14C] rhein anthrone in rats. *Pharmacology* 1988b; 36(suppl 1):152-57.

Del Giacco GS, Mantovani G, Cengiarotti L, et al: Secondary immunodeficiency in advanced lung cancer. *Tissue React* 1984; 6(6):499-504.

Delos S, Iehle C, Martin PM, Raynaud JP: Inhibition of the activity of 'basic' 5 alpha-reductase (type 1) detected in DU 145 cells and expressed in insect cells. *J Steroid Biochem Col Biol* 1994; 48(4):347-52.

Delpino A, Paggi M, et al: Protien synthetic activity and andenylate energy charge in rhein-treated cultured human glioma cells. *Cancer Biochem Biophys* 1992; 12(4):241-52.

Demetrakopoulos GE, Brennan MF: Tumoricidal potential of nutritional manipulations. *Cancer Res (Suppl)* 1982; 42:756s-65s.

Denekamp J: Review article: Angiogenesis, neovascular proliferation and vascular pathophysiology as targets for cancer therapy. *The British Journal of Radiology* 1993; 66:181-96.

Derogatis LR, Morrow GR, Fetting J, et al: The prevalence of psychiatric disorders among cancer patients. *JAMA* 1983 Feb 11; 249(6):751-7.

Deschner EE, Cohen BI, Raicht RF: The kinetics of the protective effect of beta-sitosterol against MNU-induced colonic neoplasia. *J Cancer Res Clin Oncol* 1982; 103(1):49-54.

Desoize B, Sen S: Apoptosis or programmed cell death: concepts, mechanisms and contribution in oncology. *Bull Cancer* (Paris) 1992; 79(5):413-25.

Desser L, Rehberger A: Induction of tumor necrosis factor in human peripheral-blood monnuclear cells by proteolytic enzymes. *Oncology* 1990; 47:475-77.

Desser L, Rehberger A, Kokron E, et al: Cytokine synthesis in human peripheral blood mononuclear cells after oral administration of polyenzyme preparations. *Oncology* 1993; 50:403-7.

Deutsch E, Dragosics B, Kopsa H, et al: Prekallikrein, HMW-kininogen and factor XII in various disease states. *Thromb Res* 1983; 31(2):351-64.

Dev SB, Hoffman GA: Electrochemotherapy—a novel method of cancer treatment. *Cancer Treat Rev* 1994; 20(1):105-15.

DeVita VT, Hellman S, Rosenberg SA, (eds): *Cancer Principles & Practice of Oncology. Vol. 1.* 2nd edition. Philadelphia: JB Lippincott Co, 1985.

Deyo RA, Inui TS, Leininger J, Overman S: Measuring functional status in chronic disease: a comparison of traditional scales and a self administered health status questionnaire in patients with rheumatoid arthritis. *Med Care* 1983; 21:180-92.

Deyo RA, Inui TS, Leininger J, Overman S: Physical and psychosocial function in rheumatoid arthritis. Clinical use of a self administered instrument. *Arch Internal Med* 1982; 142:879-82.

Di Sorbo DM, Wagner R Jr, Nathanson L: In vivo and in vitro inhibition of B16 melanoma growth by vitamin B6. *Nutr Cancer* 1985; 7(1-2):43-52.

Dietzel F: Basic principles in hyperthermic tumor therapy. Recent results. *Cancer Res* 1983; 86:177-90.

Dobrowsky E, Newell K, Tannock IF: The potential of lactate and succinate to kill nutrient deprived tumor cells by intracellular acidification. *Int J Radiat Oncol Biol Phys* 1991; 20(2):275-9.

Doll R, Peto R: The causes of cancer: quantitative estimates of avoidable risks of cancer in the United States today. *J Natl Cancer Inst* 1981; 66:1 191-1308.

Dombradi CA, Foldeak S: Screening report on the antitumor activity of purified arctium lappa extracts. *Tumori* 1966; 52(3):173-175.

Donden Y: *Health Through Balance. An Introduction to Tibetan Medicine.* Trans., ed. by Jeffrey Hopkins. Ithaca: Snow Lion Publications, 1986.

Douros J, Suffness M: New natural products under development at the national cancer institute. *Recent Results in Cancer Research, Vol. 76.* SK Carter, Y Sakurai, H Umezawa editors. Berlin: Springer-Verlag, 1981.

Downer SM, Cody MM, McCluskey P, Wilson PD, et al: Pursuit and practice of complementary therapies by cancer patients receiving conventional treatment. *BMJ* 1994; 9309(6947):86-9.

Droge W, Wolf M, Mihm S: The effect of prostaglandins on the intracellular signal transmission and regulation of T-cell functions. *Prostaglandins in Cancer Research* E. Garaci, R Paoletti, MG Santoro eds. New York: Springer-Verlag, 1987.

Drozdova TS, Makhonova LA, Maiakova SA, et al: Immunologic correction using thymus gland preparation (T-activin) in the programmed treatment of patients with non-lymphoid leukemia. *Gematol Transfuziol* 1990; 35(1):14-6.

Duke JA. *Handbook of Biochemically Active Phytochemicals and Their Activities* Boca Raton, FL: CRC Press; 1992.

Duke JA: Weeds? or wonder drugs? *Organic Gardening* 1994; 41(6):38-40.

Dundee JW, Ghaly RG, Fitzpatrick KT, Abram WP, Lynch GA: Acupuncture prophylaxis of cancer chemotherapy-induced sickness. *JR Soc Med* 1989; 82(5):268-71.

Dunnick JK, Hailey JR: Toxicity and carcinogenicity studies of quercetin, a natural component of foods. *Fundam Appl Toxicol* 1992; 19(3):423-31.

Durie BG, Soehnlen B, Prudden JF: Antitumor activity of bovine cartilage extract (Catrix-S) in the human tumor stem cell assay. *J Biol Response Mod* 1985; 4(6):590-5.

Dvorak HF, Harvey VS, Estrella P, et al: Fibrin containing gels induce angiogensis. *Lab Invest* 1987; 57 (6):673-86.

Dwyer JT: "Dietary fat and breast cancer: testing interventions to reduce risks." *Exercise, Calories, Fat and Cancer* MM Jacobs editor, New York: Plenum Press, 1992.

Dyerberg J: "Conference summary and future directions." *Health effects of w-3 polyunsaturated fatty acids in seafoods. World Rev Nutr Diet* Simopoulos AP et al., editors. Basel, Karger, 1991, 66:16-9.

Ebisuno S, Hirano A, Kyoku I, et al: Basal studies on combination of Chinese medicine in cancer chemotherapy: protective effects on the toxic side effects of CDDP and antitumor effects with CDDP on murine bladder tumor (MBT-2). *Nippon Gan Chiryo Gakkai Shi* 1989 20; 24(6):1305-12.

Edward MS, Levin VA, Wilson CB: Brain tumor chemotherapy: an evaluation of agents in current use for phase II and phase III trials. *Cancer Treat Rep* 1980; 64(12):1179-205.

Egorin MJ, Kaplan RS, Salcman M, Aisner J, Colvin M, Wiernik PH: Cyclophosphamide plasms and cerebrospinal fluid kinetics with and without dimethyl sulfoxide. *Clin Pharmacol Ther* 1982; 32:122-128.

El-Domeiri AA, Messiha FS, Hsia WC: Effect of alkali salts on sarcoma I in A/J mice. *J Surg Oncol* 1981; 18:423-429.

El-Sheikh MM, Dakkak MR, Saddique A: The effect of Permixon on androgen receptors. *Acta Obstet Gynecol Scand* 1988; 67(5):397-9.

Eldridge AC, Kwolek WF: Soybean isoflavones; Effect of environment and variety on composition. *J Agri Food Chem* 1983; 31:394-96.

Elegbede JA: Prospective roles of plant secondary metabolites in the treatment of mammary cancer. *Diss Abstr Int* 1985; 46(6):1874.

Elia G, Santoro MG: Regulation of heat shock protein synthesis by quercetin in human erythroleukaemia cells. *Biochem J* 1994; 15; 300(Pt 1):201-9.

Ernst E: Garlic therapy? Theories of a folk remedy (author's translation). *MMW Munch Med Wochenschr* 1981; 123(41):1537-8.

Etienne A, Hecquet F, Soulard C, Spinnewyn B, et al: In vivo inhibition of plasma protein leakage and Salmonella enteritidis-induced mortality in the rat by a specific paf-acether antagonist: BN 52021. *Agents Actions* 1986 Jan; 17(3-4):368-70.

Evans SM, Van Winkle T, Szuhaj B, et al: Protection against metastasis of radiation-induced thymic lymphosarcoma an weight loss in C57B1/6NCr1BR mice by an autoclave-resistant factor present in soybeans. *Radiat Res* 1992; 132(2):259-62.

Fahim MS, Fahim Z, Harman JM, Clevenger TE, et al: Effect of Panax ginseng on testosterone level and prostate in male rats. *Arch Androl* 1982 Jun; 8(4):261-3.

Fan TP, Hu DE, Guard S, et al: Stimulation of angiogenesis by substance P and interleukin-1 in the rat and its inhibition by NK1 or interleukin-1 receptor antagonists. *Br J Pharmacol* 1993; 110(1):43-9.

Fan YP: Enhancing effect of jian pi jin dan on immune functions of normal and cyclophosphamide induced immunosuppressed mice. *Chung Kuo Chung Hsi I Chieh Ho Tsa Chih* 1993; 13(4):223-5.

Farnsworth N: Relative safety of herbal medicines. *Herbalgram.* Summer/Spring 1993; 29:36A-36H.

Favalli C, Mastino A, Garaci E: "Prostaglandins in immunotherapy of cancer." *Prostaglandins in Cancer Research.* E Garaci, R Paoletti, MG Santoro editors. Berlin: Springer-Verlag; 1987.

Fazioli F, Blasi F: Urokinase-type plasminogen activator and its receptor: new targets for anti-metastatic therapy? *Trend Pharmacol Sci* 1994; 15(1):25-9.

Felton GE: Does kinin released by pineapple stem bromelain stimulate production of prostaglandin E1-like compounds. *Hawaii Medical Journal* 1977; 36(2):39-47.

Felton GE: Fibrinolytic and antithrombotic action of bromelain may eliminate thrombosis in heart patients. *Med Hypothesis* 1980; 6:1123-33.

Fernandes G, Venkatraman JT: "Possible mechanisms through which dietary lipids, calorie restriction and exercise modulate breast cancer." *Exercise, Calories, Fat and Cancer.* MM Jacobs editor. New York: Plenum Press; 1992.

Ferraroni M, LaVecchia C, et al: Selected micronutrient intake and the risk of colorectal cancer. *Br J Cancer* 1994 Dec; 70(6):1150-5.

Fibach E, Treves A, Kidron M, Mayer M: Induction of differentiation in human myeloid leukemic cells by proteolytic enzymes. *J Cell Physiol* 1985; 123:228-34.

Ficarra P, Ficarra R, Villari A, et al: High-performance liquid chromatography and diffuse reflectance spectroscopy of flavonoids in Crataegus oxyacantha L. III—analysis of 2-phenyl-chroman derivitaves and caffeic acid. *Farmaco* 1990; 45(2):237-45.

Finnegan MCM, Goepel JR, Royds J, et al: Elevated levels of MDM-2 and p53 expressions are associated with high grade non-Hodgkin's lymphoma's. *Cancer Letters* 1994; 86:215-21.

Fischer M, Levine PH, Weiner B, et al: The effect of vegetarian diets on plasma lipid and platelet levels. *Arch Intern Med* 1986; 146:1 193-97.

Fischer S, Slaga T: *Arachidonic Acid Metabolism and Tumor Promotion.* Boston: Martinus Nijhoff Publishing; 1985.

Fitzgerald DE, Frisch P, Milliken JC: Relief of chronic arterial obstruction using intravenous brinase. *Scand J Thor Cardiovasc Surg* 1979; 13:327-32.

Flagg EW, Coates RJ, Jones DP, et al: Dietary glutathione intake and the risk of oral and pharyngeal cancer. *Am J Epidemiol* 1994 Mar 1; 139(5):453-465.

Flamm WG, Lehman-Mckeeman LD: The human relevance of the renal tumor-inducing potential of d-limnene in male rats; Implications for risk assessment. *Regul Toxicol Pharmacol* 1991; 13(1):70-86.

Flanagan RJ, Meredith TJ: Use of N-acetylcysteine in clinical toxicology. *Am J Med* 1991 Sep 30; 91(3C):131S-139S.

Fletcher RH, Fletcher SW: Glutathione and ageing: ideas and evidence. *Lancet* 1994 Nov 19; 344(8934):1379-80.

Floridi A, Castiglione S, Bianchi C, et al: Effect of rhein on the glucose metabolism of ehrlich ascites tumor cells. *Biochem Pharmacol* 1990a; 40(2):217-22.

Floridi A, Gentile FP, Bruno T, et al: Growth inhibition by rhein and lonidamine of human glioma cells in vitro. *Anticancer Res* 1990b; 10(6):1633-6.

Folkman J: The vascularization of tumors. *Sci Amer* 1976; 234(5):58-64, 70-3.

Folkman J: Tumor angiogenesis. *Cancer Medicine* Third edition, JF Holland, E Frei III, RG Bast, et al. editors. Philadelphia: Lea & Febiger, 1993a. pp. 153-170.

Folkman J: Tumor angiogenesis: diagnostic and therapeutic clinical applications. *Proceedings of The American Association for Cancer Research* 1993b; 34.

Folkman J, Hochberg M. *J Exp Med* 1972; 138:745.

Folkman J, Klagsburn M: Angiogenic factors. *Science* 1987; 235:442-7.

Fortmeyer HP, Timm C, Blum U, et al: Vitamin B6 responsive growth of human tumors. *Anticancer Res* 1988; 8(4):813-8.

Foster S, Yue C: *Herbal Emissaries.* Rochester, VT: Healing Arts Press, 1992.

Foster WG, Pentick JA, McMahon A, Lecavalier PR: Body distribution and endocrine toxicity of hexachlorobenzene (HCB) in the female rat. *J Applied Toxicol* 1993; 13(2):79-83.

Fotsis T, Pepper M, Adlercreutz H, Fleischmann G, et al: Genistein, a dietary-derived inhibitor of in vitro angiogenesis. *Proc Natl Acad Sci USA* 1993; 90(7):2690-4.

Frawley D: *Ayurvedic Healing. A Comprehensive Guide.* Salt Lake City: Passage Press, 1989.

Fredrikson M, Furst CJ, Lekander M, et al: Trait anxiety and anticipatory immune reactions in women receiving adjuvant chemotherapy for breast cancer. *Cancer Invest* 1993; 11(4):440-50.

Freedman LS, Clifford C, Messina M: Analysis of dietary fat, calories, body weight, and the development of mammary tumors in rats and mice: a review. *Cancer Rev* 1990; 50(18):5710-9.

Friedmann CA: Structure-activity relationships of anthraquinones in some pathological conditions. *Pharmacology* 1980; 20(suppl 1):113-22.

Fuchs AG, DeLustig ES: Localization of tissue copper in mouse mammary tumors. *Oncology* 1989; 46(3):183-7.

Fujiki H, Takahiko H, Yamashita K, et al: "Inhibition of tumor promotion by flavonoids." *Plant Flavonoids in Biology and Medicine II* Alan R. Liss, Inc., 1986; 429-40.

Fujimoto GI, Morrill GA, O'Connell ME, Kostellow AB: Effects of cannabinoids given orally and reduced appetite on the male rat reproductive system. *Pharmagology* 1982; 24(5):303-13.

Fujita Y, Yamane T, Tanaka M, et al: Inhibitory effect of (-)-epigallocatechin gallate on carcinogenesis with N-ethyl-N'-nitro-N-nitroguanidine in moude duodenum. *Jpn J Cancer Res* 1989; 80(6):503-5.

Fujiyoshi T, Hayashi I, Oh-ishi S: Kaolin-induced writhing response in mice: activation of the plasma killikrein-kinin system by kaolin. *J Pharmamacobiodyn* 1989; 12(8):483-7.

Fuks JZ, Egorin MJ, Aisner J, Ostrow SS, et al: Cyclophosphamide and dimethylsulfoxide in the treatment of squamous carcinoma of the lung. Therapeutic efficacy, toxicity, and pharmacokinetics. *Cancer Chemother Pharmacol* 1981; 6(2):117-20.

Furman MI, Grigoryev, D, Bray PF, Dise KR, Goldschmidt-Clermont PJ: Platelet tyrosine kinases and fibrinogen receptor activation. *Circ Res* 1994 Jul; 75(1):172-80.

Furukawa F, Takigawa M, Matsuyoshi N, Shirahama S, et al: Cadherins in cutaneous biology. *J Dermatol* 1994; 21(11):802-13.

Furusawa E, Chou SC, Furusawa S et al: Antitumor activity of ganoderma lucidium, an edible mushroom, on intraperitoneally implanted lewis lung carcinoma in synergenic mice *Phytotherapy Research* 1992; 6:300-304.

Furuya Y, Yamamoto K, Kohno N, et al: 5-fluorouracil attenuates an oncostatatic effect of melatonin on estrogen-sensitive human breast cancer cells (MCF7). *Cancer Lett* 1994 June 15; 81(1):95-8.

Gabrijelcic D, Svetic B, Spaic D, et al: Determination of cathespins B, H, L and kininogen in breast cancer patients. *Agents Actions Suppl* 1992; 38 (Pt 2):350-7.

Gali HU, Perchellet EM, Gao XM, et al: Antitumor-promoting effects of gallotannins extracted from various sources in mouse skin in vivo. *Anticancer Res* 1993; 13(4):915-22.

Gan W, Cheng, B, Li Z, et al: Studies on the [antitumor] mechanism of indirubin by treatment of chronic myelocytic leukemia (CML). *Shengwu Huaxue Zazhi* 1987; 3(3):225-230.

Gandolfo GM, Girelli G, Conti L, et al: Hemolyitc anemia and thrombocytopenia induced by cianidanol. *Acta Haematol* 1992; 88:96-99.

Gardner MLG: Gastrointesinal absorption of intact proteins. *Ann Rev Nutr* 1988; 8:329-50.

Gardner MLG: Intestinal assimilation of intact peptides and proteins from the diet—a neglected field? *Biol Rev* 1984; 59:289-331.

Garland CF, Comstock GW, Garland FC, et al: Serum 25-hydroxyvitamin D and colon cancer: eight-year prospective study. *Lancet* 1989; 2(8673):1176-8.

Ge JY, Zhang ZL: [Progress in pharmacology and clinical application of Ligusticum wallichii.] *Chi Chung Kuo Chung Hsi I Chieh Ho Tsa Chih* 1994; 14(10):638-40.

Gebbia V, Valenza R, Testa A, et al: Weekly 5-fluorouracil and folinic acid plus escalating doses of cisplatin with glutathione protection in patients with advanced head and neck cancer. *Med Oncol Tumor Pharmacother* 1992; 9(4):165-8.

Gebhard KJ, Gridley DS, Stickney DR, et al: Enhancement of immune status by high levels of dietary vitamin B-6 without growth inhibition of human malignant melanoma in athymic nude mice. *Nutr Cancer* 1990; 14(1):15-26.

Geboes K, Spiessens C, Nijs G, et al: Anthranoids and the mucosal immune system of the colon. *Pharmacology* 1993; 47(suppl 1):49-57.

Geder L, Metz KR, Towfighi J, Mikus JL, et al: Effect of dimethylsulfoxide on human gliomas: correlations between the nuclear magnetic resonance spectra and the transformed phenotypes of the tumor cells. *Neurofibromatosis* 1989; 2(1):23-34.

Geng CS, Xing ST, Zhou JH, et al: Enhancing effect of Lycium barbarum polysaccharides in the interleukin-2 activity in mice. *Chinese J of Pharmac and Toxicology* 1989; 3(3):175-9.

Gerard G: Therapeutique anti-cancreuse et bromelaines. *Agressologie* 1972; 3:261-74.

Gey, KF: Prospects for the prevention of free radical disease, regarding cancer and cardiovascular disease. *Brit Med Bulletin* 1993; 49(3):679-99.

Gibaldi M: *Biopharmaceutics and clincial pharmacokinetics.* Philadelphia: Lea & Febiger, 1991.

Giedanowski J, Lemmel EM, Baszczyk B: The influence of thymus hormones on the NK cells activity. *Arch Immunol Ther Exp* (Warsz) 1987; 35(5):657-61.

Ginsburg J: Environmental oestrogens. *Lancet* 1994; 343:284-285.

Glaser JL, Brind JL, Vogelman JH, et al: Elevated serum dehydroepiandrosterone sulfate levels in practitioners of the transecendental meditation (TM) and TM-sidhi programs. *J Behav Med* 1992; 15(4):327-41.

Glaves D, Huben RP, Weiss L: Haematogenous dissemination of cells from human renal adenocarcinomas. *Br J Cancer* 1988:57:32-35.

Goel RK, Das Gupta G, Ram SN, et al: Antiulcerogenic and anti-inflammatory effects of emodin, isolated from rhamnus triquerta wall. *J Exp Biol* 1991; 29(3):230-2.

Goel RK, et al: Anti-ulcerogenic effect of banana powder (Musa sapientum var. paradisiaca) and its effect on mucosal resistance. *Journal of Ethno-Pharmacology* 1986; 18:33-44.

Gong P, Xie SS, Qin FH: Enhancing effect of kang shuai sen fang on immune functions of mice. *Chung Hsi I Chieh Ho Tsa Chih* 1991 Apr; 11(4):223-4, 197-8.

Gonzalez R, Sanchez A, Ferguson JA, et al: Melatonin therapy of advanced human malignant melanoma. *Melanoma Res* 1991 Nov-Dec; 1(4):237-43.

Goodman LS, Gilman A: *The Pharmacological Basis of Therapeutics.* 7th ed. New York: Macmillan Publish Co, 1985.

Gotze H, Rothman SS: Enteropancreatic circulation of digestive enzyme as a conservation mechanism. *Nature* 1975 Oct 16; 257(5527):607-9.

Gould MN: Chemoprevention of mammary cancer by monterpenes. *Proceedings of the Am Assoc for Can Res* 1993; 34:572.

Grauffel V, Kloareg B, Mabeau S, et al: New natural polysaccharides with potent antithrombic activity; fucans from brown algae. *Biomaterials* 1989; 10(6):363-8.

Graziani Y, Winikoff J, Chayoth R: Regulation of cyclic amp level and lactic-acid production in ehrlich ascites tumor cells. *So Biochim Biophys ACTA* 1977; 497(2):499-506.

Greenwald HP. *Who survives Cancer?* Los Angeles: University of California Press, Ltd.; 1992.

Greenwald P, Kelloff G, Burch-Whitman C, et al: Chemoprevention. *CA Cancer J Clin* 1995 45:31-49.

Greer S, Morris T, Pettigale KW: Psychological response to breast cancer: effects on outcome. *Lancet* 1979; 2:785-7.

Grekin DA, Epstein JH: Psoralens, UVA (PUVA) and photcarcinogenesis. *Photochmeistry and Photobiology* 1981; 33(Yearly Review):957-60.

Gribel NV, Pashinskii VG: Antimetastatic properties of aloe juice. *Vopr Onkol* 1986; 32(12):38-40.

Gridley DS, Kettering JD, Slater JM, Nutter RL: Modification of spontaneous mammary tumors in mice fed different sources of protein, fat and carbohydrate. *Cancer Lett* 1983; 19(2):133-46.

Griffin DT, Dodd NJ, Moore JV, Pullan BR, Taylor TV: The effects of low-level direct current on a preclinical mammary carcinoma: tumour regression and systemic biochemical sequelae. *Br J Cancer* 1994; 69(5):875-8.

Grimminger W, Witthohn K: Analytics of senna drugs with regard to the toxicological discussion of anthranoids. *Pharmacology* 1993; 47(suppl 1):98-109.

Grinnell F, Fukamizu H, Pawelek P, et al: Collagen processing, crosslinking, and fibril bundle assembly in matrix produced by fibroblasts in long-term cultures supplemented with ascorbic acid. *Exp Cell Res* 1989; 181(2):483-91.

Gruber BL, Hersh SP, Hall NR, Walezky LR, et al: Immunological responses of breast cancer patients to behavioral interventions. *Biofeedback Self Regul* 1993; 18(1):1-22.

Grunt TW, Somay C, Oeller H, Dittrich C: Comparative analysis of the effects of dimethyl sulfoxide and retinoic acid on the antigenic pattern of human ovarian adenocarcinoma cells. *J Cell Sci* 1992 Oct; 103(Pt2):501-9.

Grunwald J: The European phytomedicines market figures, trends, analyses. *Herbalgram* Summer 1995; 34:60-5.

Gugler R, Leschik M, Dengler HJ: Disposition of quercetin in man after single oral and intravenous doses. *Europ J Clin Pharacol* 1975; 9:229-34.

Guillaume M, Padioleau F: Veinotonic effect, vascular protection, antiinflammatory and free radical scavengering properties of horse chestnut extract. *Arzneim-Forsch* 1994; 44(1):25-35.

Guo CY, Zhao SY, Lin CR: Effects of rhubarb on aracidonic acid metabolism of the renal medulla in the rabbit. *Chung Hsi I Chieh Ho Tsa Chih* 1989; 9(3):161-3.

Guzley GJ: Alternative cancer treatments: impact of unorthodox therapy on the patient with cancer. *South Med J* 1992; 85(5):5 19-23.

Haag JD, Gould MN: Mammary carcinoma regression induced by perillyl alcohol, a hydroxylated analog of limonene. *Cancer Chemotherapy and Pharmacology* 1994; 34:477-483.

Haag JD, Lindstrom MJ, Gould MN: Limonene-induced regression of mammary carcinomas. *Cancer Research* 1992 Jul 15; 52:4021-6.

Haak-Frendscho M, Kino K, Sone T, et al: Ling Zhi-8: a novel T cell mitogen induces cytokine production and upregulation of ICAM-1 expression. *Cell Immunol* 1993; 150(1):101-13.

Hagen TM, Grazyna T, et al: Bioavailability of dietary glutathione: effect on plasma concentration. *Am Physiol Soc* 1990:G524-G529.

Hagmann W: Cell proliferation status, cytokine action and protein tyrosine phosphorylation modulate leukotriene biosynthesis in a basophil leukaemia and a mastocytoma cell line. *Biochem J* 1994 Apr 15; 299(pt2):467-72.

Hague A, Manning AM, van der Stappen JW, et al: Escape from negative regulation growth by transforming growth factor beta from the induction of apoptosis by the dietary agent sodium butyrate may be important in colorectal carcinogensis. *Cancer Metastasis Rev* 1993; 12(3-4):227-37.

Hamada H, Hiramatsu M, Edamatsu R, Mori A: Free radical scavenging action of baicalein. *Japan Arch Biochem Biophys* 1993; 306(1):261-6.

Hamanaka T, Ohgoshi M, Kawahara K, et al: A novel antitumor cyclic hexapeptide (RA-700) obtained from rubiae radix. *J Pharmacobiodyn* 1987 Nov; 10(11):616-623.

Hamilos DL, Mascali JJ, Wedner HJ: The role of glutathione in lymphocyte activation--II. Effects of buthionine sulfoximine and 2-cyclohexene -1-one on early and late activation events. *Int J Immunopharmacol* 1991; 13(1):75-90.

Hampel H, Hofrichter G, Liehn H, et al: Pharmacology of escin isomers, especially alpha-escin. *Arzneim-Forsch* 1970; 20(2):209-15.

Han GQ, Wei LH, Li CL, et al: The isolation and identification of PAF inhibitors from Piper wallichii (Miq.) Hand-Mazz and P. hancei Maxim. *Yao Hsueh Hsueh Pao* 1989; 24(6):438-43.

Han R: Highlight on the studies of anticancer drugs derived from plants in China. *Stem Cells (Dayt)* 1994; 12(1):53-63.

Hanna MG Jr, Peters LC, Hoover H Jr: "Immunotherapy by active specific immunization: basic principles and preclinical studies." *Biologic Therapy of Cancer*. VT DeVita, S Hellman, SA Rosenberg editors. Philadelphia: JB Lippincott, 1991.

Hannan GN, McAuslan BR: Modulation of synthesis of specific proteins in endothelial cells by copper, cadmium, and disulfiram: an early response to an angiogenic inducer of cell migration. *J Cell Physiol* 1982; 111(2):207-12.

Haranaka K, Satomi N, Sakurai A, et al: Antitumor activities and tumor necrosis factor producibility of traditional Chinese medicines and crude drugs. *J Tradit Chin Med* 1985a; 5(4):271-8.

Haranaka K, Satomi N, Sakurai A, et al: Antitumor activities and tumor necrosis factor producibility of traditional Chinese medicines and crude drugs. *Cancer Immunol Immunother* 1985b; 20(1):1-5.

Harborne JB, Baxter H, editors: *Phytochemical Dictionary: A Handbook of Bioactive Compounds from Plants*. Bristol: Taylor & Frances, Inc, 1991.

Hardell L, Danell M, Angqvist CA, et al: Levels of selenium in plasma and glutathione peroxidase in erythrocytes and the risk of breast cancer. A case-control study. *Biol Trace Res* 1993 Feb; 36(2):99-108.

Harguindey S: Hydrogen ion and dynamics cancer: an appraisal. *Medical and Pediatric Oncology* 1982; 10:217-36.

Harmening DM, editor. *Clinical hematology and fundamentals of hemostasis*. Philadelphia: FA Davis Co, 1992.

Harper JM, Levine AJ, Rosenthal DL, et al: Erythrocyte folate levels, oral contraceptive use and abnormal cervical cytology. *Acta Cytol* 1994 May-Jun; 38(3):324-30.

Harris C, Pierce K, King G, et al: Efficacy of acemannan in treatment of canine and feline spontaneous neoplasms. *Mol Biother* 1991; 3(4):207-13.

Hartwell JL: Plants used against cancer. A survey. *Lloydia* 1970 Sep; 33(3):288-392.

Hartwell JL: Plants used against cancer. A survey. *Lloydia* 1971a Dec; 34(4):386-425.

Hartwell JL: Plants used against cancer. A survey. *Lloydia* 1971b Mar; 34(1):103-160.

Hasui Y, Nishi S, Kitada S, et al: Urokinase-type plasminogen activator antigen as prognostic factor in bladder cancer. *Nippon Hinyokika Gakki Zasshi* 1993; 84(9):1624-8.

Hau DM, You ZS: Therapeutic effects of ginseng and mitomycin C on experimental liver tumors. *Int J of Oriental Med* 1990; 15(1):10-14.

Hauser SP: Unproven methods in cancer treatment. *Curr Opin Oncol* 1993; 5(4):646-54.

Hayes, WA. *Principles and Methods of Toxicology.* New York: Raven Press 1984.

Hayes NA, Foreman JC: The activity of compounds extracted from feverfew on histamine release from rat mast cells. *J Pharm Pharmacol* 1987; 39(6):466-70.

He J, Li Y, Wei S et al: Effects of mixture of astragalus membranaceus, fructus ligustri and eclipta prostrata on immune function in mice. *Hua Hsi I Ko Ta Hsueh Pao* 1992; 23(4):408-11.

Heber D, Ashley JM, Leaf DA, et al: Reduction of serum estradiol in postmenopausal women given free access to low-fat high carbohydrate diet. *Nutrition* 1991; 7:137.

Hedley DW: Na+/H+ antiport blockers as possible inhibitors of in vivo tumor growth (meeting abstract). *Cancer Chemother Pharmacol* 1989; 24(suppl 2):s86.

Hei TK, Sudilovsky O: Effects of a high-sucrose diet on the development of enzyme-altered foci in chemical hepatocarcinogenesis in rats. *Cancer Res* 1985; 45(6):2700-5.

Heiberg E, Nalesnik WJ, Janney C: Effects of varying potential and electrolytic dosage in direct current treatment of tumors. *Acta Radiol* 1991; 32(2):174-7.

Heidemann A, Miltenburger HG, Mengs U: The genotoxicity status of senna. *Pharmacology* 1993; 47(suppl 1):178-86.

Heino J, Kahari VM, Jaakkola S, et al: Collagen in the intracellular matrix of cultured scleroderma skin fibroblasts: changes related to ascorbic acid-treatment. *Matrix* 1989; 9(1):34-9.

Hennekens CH, Buring JE: Antioxidant vitamins—benefits not yet proved. *The New England Journal of Medicine* 1994; 330(15):1080-1.

Henson DE, Block G, Levine M: Ascorbic acid: biologic functions and relation to cancer. *Journal of the National Cancer Institute* 1991; 83(8):547-50.

Herberman R, Santoni A: "Regulation of NK-cell activity." *Biological Responses in Cancer: Progress Toward Potential Applications* Vol 1. E Mihich editor. New York: Plenum Press, 1982.

Hersh EM, Taylor CW: "Immunotherapy by active immunization of the host using nonspecific stimulants and immunomodulators." *Biologic Therapy of Cancer.* VT DeVita Jr., S Hellman, SA Rosenberg editors. Philadelphia: JB Lippincott, 1991.

Heur YH, Zeng W, Stoner GD, et al: Synthesis of ellagic acid O-alkyl derivatives and isolation of ellagic acid as a tetrahexanoyl derivative from Fragaria ananassa. *J Nat Prod* 1992; 55(10):1402-7.

Hiai, S: "Chinese medicinal medicine material and the secretion of ACTH and corticosteroid." *Advances in Chinese Medicinal Materials Research.* HM Chang, HW Yeung, WW Tso, A Koo editors. Singapore: World Scientific, 1985, 49-60.

Hietanen E, Bartsch H, Bereziat JC, et al: Diet and oxidative stress in breast, colon and prostate cancer patients: a case-control study. *Eur J Clin Nutr* 1994 Aug; 48(8):575-586.

Hildenbrand G: Nutritionally superiority of organically grown foods. *Healing Newsltr* 1989; 5(2).

Hill RP, Young SD, Cillo C, Ling V: Metastatic cell phenotypes: Quantitative studies using the experimental metastasis assay. *Cancer Rev* 1986; 5:118-151.

Hill SM, Spriggs LL, Simon MA: The growth inhibitory action of melatonin on human breast cancer cells is linked to the estrogen response system. *Cancer Lett* 1992 Jul 10; 64(3):249-56.

Hirano T, Gotoh M, Oka K: Natural flavanoids and lignans are potent cytostatic agents against human leukemic HL60 cells. *Life Sciences* 1994; 55(13):1061-9.

Hirono I, Ueno I, Hosaka S, et al: Carcinogenicity examination of quercitin and rutin in ACI rats. *Cancer Letters* 1981; 13:15-21.

Hitzenberger G: The therapuetic effectiveness of chestnut extract. *Wein Med Wochenschr* (Austria) 1989; 139:385-9.

Hjortso E, Fomsgaard JS, Fogh-Andersen N: Does N-acetylcysteine increase the excretion of trace metals (calcium, magnesium, iron, zinc and copper) when given orally? *Eur J Clin Pharmacol* 1990; 39(1):29-31.

Hladon B, Kowalewski Z, Bobkiewicz T, et al: Cytotoxic activity of some chelidonium maius alkaloids on human and animal tumor cell cultures in vitro. *Ann Pharm* 1978; 13:61-8.

Hocman G: Chemoprevention of cancer: selenium. *Int J Biochem* 1988; 20(2):123-32.

Hofsli E, Waage A: Effect of pyridoxine on tumor necrosis factor activities in vitro. *Biotherapy* 1992; 5(4):285-90.

Hojima Y, Pierce JV, Pisano JJ: Pumpkin seed inhibitor of human factor XIIa (activated Hageman factor) and bovine trypsin. *Biochem* 1982 Aug 3; 21(16):3741-6.

Holcenberg JC, Kien CL: The effects of protein or amino acid intake on the nitrogen balance and antitumor activity of glutaminase treatment. *Current Topics in Cellular Regulation* 1985; 26:395-402.

Holdiness MR: Clinical pharmacokinetics of N-acetylcysteine. *Clin Pharmacokinet* 1991 Feb; 20(2):123-34.

Holland JF, Frei E, Bast R, et al: *Cancer Medicine* Third Edition. Philadelphia: Lea & Febiger; 1993.

Holleb AI, Fink DJ, Murphy GP: *American Cancer Society Textbook of Clinical Onocology* Atlanta: American Cancer Society, 1991.

Holmes TH, Masuda M: Life changes and illness susceptibility. *Stressful Life Events: Their Nature and Effects.* BS Dohrenwend, BP Dohrenwend (eds). New York: Wiley, 1974.

Homma M, Oka K, Kobayashi H, et al: Impact of free magnolol excretions in asthmatic patients who responded well to saiboku-to, a chinese herbal medicine. *J Pharm Pharmacol* 1993; 45(9):844-6.

Honn KV: Tumor cell-platelet aggregation: Induced by cathepsin B-like proteinase and inhibited by prostacyclin. *Science* 1982; 217:540-42.

Honn KV, Menter DG, Steinert BW, et al: Analysis of platelet, tumor cell, and endothelial cell interactions in vivo and in vitro. *Prostaglandins in Cancer Research* E. Garaci, R. Paoletti, MG Santoro eds. New York: Springer-Verlag, 1987a.

Honn KV, Steinert BW, Onoda JM, et al: The role of platelets in metastasis. *Biorheology* 1987b; 24(2):127-137.

Hooper TL, Rahman M, Magell J: Oral urea in the treatment of colo-rectal liver metastases. *Clin Oncol* 1984; 10:341-4.

Hoover HC, Hanna, MG: "Immunotherapy by active specific immunization: clinical applications.". *Biologic Therapy of Cancer.* VT DeVita, . Hellman, S Rosenberg, editors. Philadelphia: JB Lippincott, Co, 1991.

Horii A, Kyo M, Asakawa M, et al: Multidisciplinary treatment for bladder carcinoma—biological response modifiers and kampo medicines. *Urol Int* 1991; 47 Suppl 1:108-12.

Hornick SB: Factors affecting the nutritional quality of crops. *Am J Alter Agri* 1992; 7(1-2).

Hossain MZ, Shibib BA, Rahman R: Hypoglycemic effects of Coccinia indica: inhibition of key gluconeogenic enzyme, glucose-6-phosphatase. *Indian J Exp Biol* 1992; 30(5):418-20.

Hou J, Liu S, Ma Z, et al: Effects of Gynostemma pentaphyllum makino on the immunological function of cancer patients. *J Tradit Chin Med* 1991; 11(1):47-52.

Hou Y, Ma GL, Wu SH, et al: Effect of radix Astralagi seu hedysari on the interferon system. *Chinese Medical Journal (Engl)* 1981; 94(1):35-40.

Hsu HY. *Treating Cancer With Chinese Herbs* Long Beach, CA: OHAI Press; 1990.

Hsu HY, Chen, YP, Hong, M: *The Chemical Constituents of Chinese Herbs* Vol 1. Long Beach, CA: Oriental Healing Arts Institute; 1982.

Hsu HY, Chen, YP, Hong, M: *The Chemical Constituents of Chinese Herbs* Vol 2. Long Beach, CA.: Oriental Healing Arts Institute; 1985.

Hsu HY, Chen YP, Shen SJ, et al. *Oriental Materia Medica* Long Beach, CA: Ohai Press; 1986.

Hu DE, Fan TP: [Leu8] des-Arg9-bradykinin inhibits the angiogenic effect of bradykinin and interleukin-1 in rats. *Br J Pharmacol* 1993; 109(1):14-7.

Hu H, Hang B, Wang P: Anti-inflammatory effect of radix Angelicae chinensis. *Chung Kuo Chung Hsi I Chieh Ho Tsa Chih* 1991; 16(11):684-6.

Hu WL, Ma YJ: Effect of glycerol-induced acute renal failure in rabbit with Ligusticum wallichii on thromboxane B2, 6-ket-prostaglandin F1 alpha/thromboxane B2. *Chung Kuo Chung Hsi I Chieh Ho Tsa Chi* 1993; 13(9):549-50.

Huang B, Wang Y: *Thousand Formulas and Thousand Herbs of Traditional Chinese Medicine. Volume Two: Formulas.* China: Heilongjiang Education Press; 1993.

Huang BS. *Syndromes of Traditional Chinese Medicine* Harbin, P. R. China: Heilnogjiang Education Press; 1993.

Huang HC, Chang JH, Tung SF, et al: Immunosuppressive effect of emodin, a free radical generator. *Eur J Pharmacol* 1992a; 211(3):359-64.

Huang HC, Chu SH, Lee Chao PD: Vasorelaxants from chinese herbs, emodin and scoparone, possess immunosuppressive properties. *European Jouranl of Pharmacology* 1991; 198:211-13.

Huang HC, Lee CR, Weng YI, et al: Vasodilator effect of scoparone (6,7-dimethoxycoumarin) from a Chinese herb. *Eur J Pharmacol* 1992b; 281(1):123-8.

Huang KC. *The Pharmacology of Chinese Herbs* Boca Raton, FL: CRC Press; 1993.

Huang YS, Zhang JT: [Antioxidative effect of three water-soluble components isolated from Salvia miltiorrhiza in vitro.] *Yao Hsueh Hsueh Pao* 1992; 27(2):96-100.

Hudson EA, Beck SA, Tisdale MJ: Kinetics of the inhibition of tumour growth in mice by eicosapentaenoic acid—reversal by linoleic acid. *UK Biochem Pharmacol* 1993; 45(11):2189-94.

Hunnisett AG, Kars A, Howard JMH, Davis S: Changes in plasma amino acids during conditioning therapy prior to bone marrow transplantation: their relevance to antioxidant status. *Amino Acids* 1993; 4(1-2):177-85.

Iaffaioli RV, Frasci G, Tortora G, et al: Effects of thymic extract 'thymostimulin' on the incidence of infection and myelotoxicity during adjuvant chemotherapy for breast cancer. *Thymus* 1988-89; 12(2):69-75.

Iishi H, Tatsuta M, Baba M, et al: Protection by oral Phenylalanine against gastric carcinogenesis induced by N-methyl-N'-nitro-N-nitrosoguanidine in Wistar rats. *Cancer* 1990; 62(2):173-6.

Ikeda I, Imasato Y, Sasaki E, et al: Tea catechins decrease micellar solubility and intestinal absorption of cholesterol in rats. *Biochem Biophys Acta* 1992; 1127(2):141-6.

Imanishi N, Kawai H, Hayashi Y, Yatsunami K, Ichikawa A: Effects of glycyrrhizin and glycyrrhetinic acid on dexamethasone-induced changes in histamine synthesis of mouse mastocytoma P-185 cells and in histamine release from rat peritoneal mast cells. *Biochem Pharmacol* 1989; 38(15):2521-6.

Imaoka K, Inouye S, Takahashi T, et al: Effects of Perilla frutescens extract on anti-DNP IgE anti-body production in mice. *Arerugi* 1993; 42(1):74-80.

Imbasciati E, DeCristofaro V, Scherini A, et al: Acute renal failure due to (+)-cyanidanol-3-induced hemolytic anemia. *Nephron* 1987; Letter to the Editor 46:323.

Infante M, Pastorino U, Chiesa G, et al: Laboratory evaluation during high-dose vitamin A administration: a randomized study on lung cancer patients after surgical resection. *J Cancer Res Oncol* 1991; 117:156-62.

275

Ingber D, Folkman J: Inhibition of angiogenesis through modulation of collagen metabolism. *Lab Invest* 1988 Jul; 59(1):44-51.

Ingram DM, Roberts A, Nottage EM: Host factors and breast cancer growth chracteristics. *Eur J Cancer* 1992; 28A(6-7):1153-61.

Iosi F, Santini MT, Malorni W: Membrane and cytoskeleton are intracellular targets of rhein in A431 cells. *Anticancer Res* 1993; 13(2):545-54.

Isaacs WB, Bova GS, Morton RA, Bussemakers MJ, et al: Molecular biology of prostate cancer. *Semin Oncol* 1994; 21(5):514-21.

Isemura M, Suzuki Y, Satoh K, et al: Effects of catechins on the mouse lung carcinoma cell adhesion to the endothelial cells. *Cell Biol Int* 1993; 17(6):559-64.

Ishikawa M, Oikawa T, Hosokawa M, Hamada J, et al: Enhancing effect of quercetin on 3-methylcholanthrene carcinogenesis in C57B1/6 mice. *Neoplasma* 1985; 32(4):435-41.

Ishiwara F: Ueber den einfluss 58 verschiedener chemischer verbindungen auf den tierkrebs. *Gann* 1927; 21:1-5.

Israel L, Hajji O, Grefft-Alami A, et al: Vitamin A augmentation of the effects of chemotherapy in metastatic breast cancers after menopause. *Ann Med Interne* (Paris) 1985; 136(7):551-4.

Istfan N, Wan J, Bistrian B: Nutrition and tumor promotion: in vitro methods for measurement of cellular proliferation and protein metabolism. *J of Parenteral and Enteral Nutrition* 1992; 6(6) supp:76s-81s.

Ito H, Shimura K: Effects of a blended Chinese medicine, xiao-chai-hu-tang, on Lewis lung carcinoma growth and inhibition of lung metastasis, with special reference to macrophage activation. *Jpn J Pharmacol* 1986; 41(3):307-14.

Ito H, Shimura K: Studies on the antitumor activity of traditional Chinese medicines. (I) *Gan To Kagaku Ryoho* 1985b; 12(11):2145-8.

Ito H, Shimura K: Studies on the antitumor activity of traditional Chinese medicines. (II). The antitumor mechanism of traditional Chinese medicines. *Gan To Kagaku Ryoho* 1985a; 12(11):2149-54.

Ito N: Is quercetin carcinogenic? *Jpn J Cancer Res*; Letter to the editor 1992; 83:312-14.

Ito N, Hagiwara A, Tamano S, Kagawa M, et al: Lack of carcinogenicity of quercetin in F344/DuCrj rats. *Jpn J Cancer Res* 1989; 80(4):317-25.

Jaeger A, Walti M, Neftel K: "Side effects of flavonoids in medical practice." *Plant Flavonoids in Biology and Medicine II* Alan R. Liss, Inc, 1988; 379-94.

Jaffe BM, Santoro MG: Prostaglandin production by tumors. *Prostaglandins in Cnacer Research.* E Garaci, R Paoletti, MG Santoro editors. Berlin: Springer-Verlag, 1987.

Jain RK: Determinants of tumor blood flow: a review. *Cancer Res* 1988 May 15; 48(10):2641-58.

Jain RK: Vascular and interstitial barriers to delivery of therapeutic agents in tumors. *Cancer Metastasis Rev* 1990 Nov; 9(3):253-66.

Jakobson AM, Hahnenberger R: Antiangiogenic effect of heparin and other sulphaed glycosaminoglycans in the chick embryo chorioallantoic membrane. *Pharmacol Toxicol* 1991 Aug; 69(2):122-6.

Jalink K, Moolenaar WH: Thrombin receptor activation causes rapid neural cell rounding and neurite retraction independent of classic second messengers. *J Cell Biol* 1992; 118(2):411-9.

Janicke F, Pache L, Schmitt M, et al: Both the cytols and detergent extracts of breast cancer tissues are suited to evaluate the prognostic impact of the urikinase-type plasminogen activator and its inhibitor, plasminogen activator inhibitor type 1. *Cancer Res* 1994; 54(10):2527-30.

Jankun J, Merrick HW, Goldblatt PJ: Expression and localization of elements of the plasminogen activation system in benign breast disease and breast cancers. *J Cell Biochem* 1993; 53(2):135-44.

Jansen MA, Muenz LR: A retrospective study of personality variables associated with fibrocystic disease and breast cancer. *J Psychosom Res* 1984; 28:35.

Jansson B: Dietary, total body, and intracellular potassium-to-sodium ratios and their influence on cancer. *Cancer Detection and Prevention* 1990; 14(5):563-5.

Jansson B: Intercellular electrolytes and their role in cancer etiology. *Stat Textbooks Monogr* 1987; 83:1-59.

Jayasuriya H, Koonchanok NM, Geahlen RL, et al: Emodin, a protein tyrosine kinase inhibitor from polygonum cuspidatum. *J Nat Prod* 1992; 55(5):696-8.

Ji XJ, Liu XM, Kun L, et al: Pharmacological studies of meisoindigo; Absorption and mechanism of action. *Biomedical and Environmental Sciences* 1991; 4:332-37.

Jiang SZ, Yu G, Cao JN, et al: Advers effect of indirubin on cardiovascular system. *Chinese Journal Of Hematology* 1986; 7(1):30.

Jiang T, Yan S, Wang S, et al: Effect of "Liuwei Dihuang decoction" on prevention and treatment of tumor. *J of Trad Chinese Med* 1984; 4(1):59-68.

Jing Y, Nakaya K, Han R: Differentiation of promyeloctic leukemia cells HL-60 induced by daidzen in vitro and in vivo. *Anticancer Res* 1993; 13(4):1049-54.

Jing Yk, Han R: Differentiation of B16 melanoma cells induced by daidzein. *Chinese Journal of Pharmacology and Toxicology* 1992; 6(4):278-80.

Jirtle RL, Haag JD, Gould MN: Increased levels of TGF-B1 and mannose-6-phosphate/insulin-like growth factor-II (M6P/IGH-II) receptor in limonen-induced mammary tumor regression. *Proceedings of the American Association for Cancer Research #3266* 1993; 34:548.

Johri RK, Zutshi U, Kameshwaran L, Atal CK: Effect of quercetin and albizzia saponins on rat mast cell. *J Physiol Pharmacol* 1985; 29(1):43-6.

Jones DP, Coates RJ, Flagg EW, et al: Glutathione in Foods Listed in the National Cancer Institute's Health Habits and History Food Frequency Questionnaire. *Nutr Cancer* 1992; 17:57-75.

Jones DP, Hagen TM, Weber R: Oral administration of glutathione (GSH) increases plasma GSH concentration in humans. *FASEBJ* 1989; 3:1250A.

Juliano R: Signal transduction by integrins and its role in the regulation of tumor growth. *Cancer Metastasis Rev* 1994; 13(1):25-30.

Juliano RL, Varner JA: Adhesion molecules in cancer: the role of integrins. *Curr Opin Cell Biol* 1993; 5(5):812-8.

Kabuki T, Noma T, Kawano Y, et al: Suppressive effect of Saibokuto on dermatophagoides farinae (Df) antigen-induced IL2 responsiveness of lymphocytes from asthmatic children. *Arerugi* 1990; 39(7):610-4.

Kaji T, Kaga K, Miezi N, et al: A stimulatory effect of artemesia leaf extract on the proliferation of cultured endothelial cells. *Chem Pharm Bull (Tokyo)* 1990a; 38(2):538-40.

Kaji T, Kaga K, Miezi N, et al: Possible mechanism of stimulatory effect of artemesia leaf extract on the proliferation of cultured endothelial cells. *Chem Pharm Bull* 1990b; 38(9):2494-7.

Kanatani Y, Kasukabe T, Hozumi M, Motoyoshi K, et al: Genistein exhibits preferential cytotoxity to a leukemogenic variant but induces differentiation of a non-leukemogenic variant of the mouse monocytic leukemia Mm cell line. *Leuk Res* 1993; 17(10):847-53.

Kandaswami C, Perkins E, Soloniuk DS, et al: Ascorbic acid-enhanced antiproliferative effect of flavinoids on squamous cell carnimoa in vitro. *Anti-Cancer Drugs* 1993; 4:91-96.

Kane MA, Johnson A, Nash AE, et al: Serum melatonin levels in melanoma patients after repeated oral administration. *Melanoma Res* 1994 Feb; 4(1):59-65.

Karakiulakis G, Missirlis E, Maragoudakis ME: Mode of action of razoxane: inhibition of basement membrane collagen-degradation by a malignant tumor enzyme. *Methods Find Exp Clin Pharmacol* 1989 Apr; 11(4):255-61.

Karlsrud TS, Buo L, Aasen AO, et al: Characterization of kininogens in human malignant ascites. *Thromb Res* 1991; 63(6):641-50.

Karmali RA: "Lipid nutrition, prostaglandins and cancer." *Biochemistry of Arachidonic Acid Metabolism*, W Lands editor, Boston: Martinus Nijhoff Publishing, 1985.

Karmali RA, Marsh J, Fuchs C: Effect of omega-3 fatty acids on growth of a rat mammary tumor. *JNCL* 1984; 73(2):457.

Karmali RA, Reichel P, Cohen LA, et al: The effects of dietary omega-3 fatty acids on the DU-145 transplantable human prostatic tumor. *Anticancer Res* 1987; 7(6):1173-9.

Kashiwada Y, Nonaka G, Nishioka I: Studies on rhubarb (rhei rhizoma) XV; Simultaneous determination of phenolic constituents by high-performance liquid chromatography. *Chem Bull* 1989; 37(4):999-1004.

Kataoka T, Akagawa KS, Tokunaga T, et al: Activation of macrophages with Hochu-ekkito. *Gan To Kagaku Rhoyo* 1989; 16(4Pt 2-2):1490-3.

Katiyar SK, Agarwal R, Mukhtar H: Inhibition of both stage I and stage II skin tumor promotion in SENCAR mice by a polyphenolic fraction isolated from green tea: inhibition depends on the duration of polyphenol treatment. *Carcinogenesis* 1993b; 14(12):2641-3.

Katiyar SK, Agarwal R, Mukhtar H: Inhibition of spontaneous and photo-enhanced lipid peroxidation in mouse epidermal microsomes by epicatechin derivatives from green tea. *Cancer Lett* 1994 Apr 29; 79(1):61-6.

Katiyar SK, Agarwal R, Mukhtar H: Protection against malignant conversion of chemically induced benign skin papillomas to squamous cell carcinomas in SENCAR mice by a polyphenolic fraction isolated from green tea. *Cancer Res* 1993c; 53(22):5409-12.

Katiyar SK, Agarwal R, Mukhtar H: Protective effects of green tea polyphenols administered by oral intubation against chemical carcinogen-induced forestomach and pulmonary neoplasia in A/J mice. *Cancer Lett* 1993a; 73(2-3):167-72.

Katiyar SK, Agarwal R, Wang ZY, et al: (-)-Epigallocatechin-3-gallate in camellia sinensis leaves from himalayan region of sikkim: inhibitory effects against biochemical events and tumor initiation in sencar mouse skin. *Nutr Cancer* 1992; 18(1):73-83.

Kato T, Okamoto R: Effect of shakuyaku-kanzo-to on serum estrogen levels and adrenal gland cells in ovariectomized rats. *Nippon Sanka Fujinka Gakkai Zasshi* 1992; 44(4):433-9.

Kaufman PB, Thompson A, Melia J (University of Michigan-Ann Arbor); Duke JA, (USDA, Maryland): *Untitled, work in progress.*

Kawakita T, Nakai S, Kumazawa Y, et al: Induction of interferon after administration of a traditional Chinese medicine, xiao-chai-hu-tang (shosaiko-to). *Int J Immunopharmacol* 1990; 12(5):515-21.

Kelley WD: *One answer to cancer*. USA: Wedgestone Press, 1972.

Kelly SB, Miller J, Wood CB, et al: Erythrocyte acid desaturation in patients with colorectal carcinoma. *Dis. Colon Rectum* 1990; 33(12):1026-30.

Kennedy AR, Szuhaj BF, Newberne PM, et al: Preparation and production of a cancer chemopreventive agent, Bowman-Birk inhibitor concentrate. *Nutr Cancer* 1993; 19(3):281-302.

Kennedy BJ: Use of questionable methods and physician education. *J Cancer Educ* 1993; 8(2):129-31.

Kennedy KA, Rockwell S: Microenvironmental variability and heterogeneity in transplanted and spontaneous mouse tumors (meeting abstract). *Proc Annu Meet Assoc Cancer Res* 1990; 31:A351.

Key T, Reeves G: Organochlorines in the environment and breast cancer. [editorial] *BMJ* 1994 Jun11; 308(6943):1520-1.

Kiecolt-Glaser JK, Stephens R, Lipetz P, et al: Distress and DNA repair in human lymphocytes. *J Behav Med* 1985; 8:311.

Kiesewetter H, Jung F, Pindur G, et al: Effect of garlic on thrombocyte aggregation, microcirculation, and other risk factors. *Int J Clin Pharmacol Ther Toxicol* 1991; 29(4):151-5.

Kiguchi K, Constantinou AI, Huberman E: Genistein-induced cell differentiation and protein-linked DNA strand breakage in human melanoma cells. *Cancer Commin* 1990; 2(8):271-7.

Kim H, Chen X, Gillis CN: Ginsenosides protect pulmonary vascular endothelium against free radical-induced injury. *Biochem Biophys Res Commun* 1992; 189(2):670-6.

Kim JH, Kim SH, Alfieri A, et al: Quercetin an inhibitor of lactate transport and hyperthermic sensitizer of hela cells. *Cancer Res* 1984; 44(1):102-6.

Kim KJ, Li B, Winer J, et al: Inhibition of vascular endothelial growth factor-induced angiogenesis suppresses tumour growth in vivo. *Nature* 1993; 362:841-4.

Kimura I, Nagaura T, Kobayashi S, et al: Inhibitory effects of magnoshinin and magnosalin, compound from Shin-i (Flos magnoliae), on the competence and progression phases in prolifereation of subcultured rat aortic endothelial cells. *Jpn J Pharmacol* 1992; 60(1):59-62.

Kimura M, Amemiya K, Suzuki J: Insulin-induced granuloma tissue formation and angiogenesis in alloxan-treated diabetic mice. *Endocrinol Jpn* 1987 Feb; 34(1):55-63.

Kimura M, Kobayashi S, Luo B, Kimura I: Selective inhibition by magnosalin and magnoshinin, compounds from 'shin-i' (Flos magnoliae), of adjuvant-induced angiogenesis and granuloma formation in the mouse pouch. *Int Arch Allergy Appl Immunol* 1990; 93(4):365-70.

Kimura M, Kobayashi S, Luo B, Kimura I: Selective inhibition by magnosalin and magnoshininin, compounds from Shin-i (Flos magnoliae), of adjuvant-induced angiogenesis and granuloma formation in the mouse pouch. *Agents Actions Suppl* 1991; 32:197-201.

Kingston RD, Fielding JW, Palmer MK: Peri-operative heparin: a possible adjuvant to surgery in colorectal cancer? *Int J Colorectal Dis* 1993 Jul; 8(2):111-5.

Kinscherf R, Fischbach T, Mihm S, et al: Effect of glutathione depletion and oral N-acetyl-cysteine treatment on CD4[+] and CD8[+] cells. *FASEB Journal* 1994 Apr; 8:448-51.

Kioka N, Hosokawa N, Komano T, et al: Quercetin, a biflavonoid, inhibits the increase of human multi-drug resistance gene (MDR1) expression caused arsenite. *Federation of European Biochemical Societies* 1992; 301(3):307-9.

Kiremidjian-Schumacher L, Roy M, et al: Regulation of cellular immune responses by selenium. *Biol Trace Elem Res* 1992 Apr-Jun; 33:23-35.

Klein AD, Penneys NS: Aloe vera. *Journal of the American Academy of Dermatology* 1988; 18(4):714-20.

Kliachkin BM, Basargin ST, Glushkov AN, et al: Mechanism of formation of blocking factors and method antiblocking immunotherapy in malignant tumors. *Vopr Onkol* 1985; 31(2):78-84.

Knighton DR, Hunt TK, Scheuenstuhl H, et al: Oxygen tension regulates the expression of Angiogenesis factor by macrophges. *Science* 1983; 221:1283-5.

Kobayashi H, Fujie M, Shinohara H, et al: Effects of urinary trypsin inhibitor on the invasion of reconstituted basement membranes by ovarian cancer cells. *Int J Cancer* 1994a; 57(3):378-84.

Kobayashi H, Shinohara H, Takeuchi K, et al: Inhibition of the soluble and the tumor cell receptor-bound plasmin by urinary trypsin inhibitor and subsequent effects on tumor cell invasion and metastasis. *Cancer Res* 1994b; 54(3):844-9.

Koch AE, Burrows JC, Polverini PJ, Cho M, Leibovich SJ: Thiol-containing compounds inhibit the production of monocyte/macrophage-derived angiogenic activity. *Agents Actions* 1991 Nov; 34(3-4):350-7.

Koch AE, Cho M, Burrows JC, et al: Inhibition of production of monocyte/macrophage-derived angiogenic activity by oxygen free-radical scavengers. *Cell Biology Int Reports* 1992; 16(5):415-25.

Kohda H, Tokumoto W, Sakamoto K, et al: The biologically active constituents of ganoderma lucidum. *Chem Pharm Bull* 1985; 33(4):1367-74.

Koizumi A: On the mechanisms of retardation of aging and inhibition of mammary tumorigenesis by energy restriction in SNH/C3H F1 female mice. *Nippon Eiseigaku Zasshi* 1991; 46(4):855-66.

Kojima R, Fukushima S, Ueno A, et al: Anti tumor activity of leguminosae plants constituents. I. Antitumor activity of constituents of sophora subprostrata. *Chem Pharm Bull* 1970; 18(12):2555-63.

Kolonel LN, Nomura AM, Hirohata T, et al: Association of diet and place of birth with stomach cancer incidence in Hawaii Japanese and Caucasians. *Am J Clin Nutr* 1981 Nov; 34(11):2478-85.

Koman A, Cazaubon S, Adem A, Couraud PO, Strosberg AD: Different regulatory patterns of M1 and M2 muscarinic receptor subtype RNA in SH-SY5Y human neuroblastoma induced by phorbolester or DMSO. *Neurosci Lett* 1993 Jan 4; 149(1):79-82.

Komori A, Yatsunami J, Okabe S, et al: Anticarcinogenic activity of green tea polyphenols. *Jpn J Clin Oncol* 1993; 23(3):186-90.

Kondo K, Tsuneizumi K, Watanabe T, Oishi M: Induction of in vitro differentiation of mouse embryonal carcinoma F9 cells. *Cancer Res* 1991; 51(19):5398-404.

Koretz MJ, Lawson DH, York RM, Graham SD, et al. *Arch Surg* 1991; 126(7):898-903.

Koshiura R, Miyamoto K, Ikeya Y, et al: Antitumor activity of methanol extract from roots of Agrimonia pilosa Ledeb. *Jpn J Pharmacol* 1985; 38(1):9-16.

Kotsy MP, Fleishman SB, Herndon JE, et al: Cisplatin, vinblastine, and hydrazine sulfate in advanced, non-small-cell lung cancer: a randomized placebo-controlled, double-blind phase III study of the cancer leukemia group B. *J Clin Oncol* 1994; 12:1113-20.

Krahenbuhl S, Hasler F, Krapf R: Analysis and pharmacokinetics of glycyrrhizic acid and glycyrrhetinic acid in humans and experimental animals. *Steroids* 1994; (59):121-26.

Kronfol Z, Silva J Jr, Greden J: Impaired lymphocyte function in depressive illness. *Life Sciences* 1983; 33:241-7.

Krumbiegel G, Schulz HU: Rhein and aloe-emodin kinetics from senna laxatives in man. *Pharmacology* 1993; 47(suppl 1):120-24.

Kuang AK, Chen JL, Chen MD: Effects of yang-restoring herb medicines on the levels of plasma corticosterone, testoterone and triiodothyronine. *Chung Hsi I Chieh Ho Tsa Chih* 1989 Dec; 9(12):737-8, 710.

Kubo M, Matsuda H, Tokuoka K, et al: Anti-inflammatory activities of methanolic extract and alkaloidal components from Corydalis tuber. *Biol Pharm Bull* 1994 Feb; 17(2):262-5.

Kubo M, Tong CN, Matsuda H: Influence of the 70% methanolic extract from red ginseng on the lysosome of tumor cells and on the cytocidal effect of mitomycin C. *Planta Med* 1992; 58(5):424-8.

Kuhnau J: The flavonoids: a class of semi-essential food components: their role in human nutrition. *Wld Rev Nutr Diet* 1976; 24:117-91.

Kull FC Jr, Brent DA, Parikh I, Cuatrecasas P: Chemical identification of a tumor-derived angiogenic factor. *Science* 1987 May 15; 236(4803):843-5.

Kumakura S, Yamashita M, Tsurufuji S: Effect of bromelain on kaolin-induced inflammation in rats. *European Journal of Pharmacology* 1988; 150:295-301.

Kumazawa Y, Itagaki A, Fukumoto M, et al: Activation of peritoneal macrophages by berberine-type alkaloids in terms of induction of cytostatic activity. *Priority Journals* 1984; 6(6):587-92.

Kun J. *Prevention and Treatment of Carcinoma in Traditional Chinese Medicine* Hong Kong: The Commercial Press; 1985.

Kuna P, Petyrek P, Dostal M: Modification of toxic and radioprotective effects of cystamine by glutathione in mice. *Radiobio Radiother* 1978 May; 599-601.

Kuprina NI, Savushkina NK, Andreev AV, Gleiberman AS: The modulation of the phenotype of the human hepatoblastoma cell line HepG2 under the action of dimethyl sulfoxide. *Ontogenez* 1993 Jul-Aug; 24(4):57-67.

Kuroda M, Imura T, Morikawa K, et al: Decreased serum levels of selenium and glutathione peroxidase activity associated with aging, malignancy and chronic hemodialysis. *Trace Elements in Medicine* 1988; 5(3):97-103.

Kusen SI, Gurskaia NI, Pashkovskaia IS, et al: Insulin-degrading neutral proteinases of the plasma membrane of loach liver and embroyo cells. *Ukr Biokhim Zh* 1989 Jan-Feb; 61(1):23-7.

Kuttan G: Tumoricidal activity of mouse peritoneal macrophages treated with Viscum album extract. *Immunol Invest* 1993; 22(6-7):431-40.

Kuttan R, Bhanumathy P, Nirmala K, et al: Potential anticancer activity of turmeric (Curcuma longa). *Cancer Lett* 1985; 29(2):197-202.

Kuttan R, Sudheeran PC, Josph CD: Tumeric and curcumin as topical agents in cancer therapy. *Tumori* 1987; 73:29-31.

Kuzmina EG, Degtiareva AA: Restoration of immunologic indices following reflexotherapy in the combination treatment of radiation-induced edema of the upper limbs. *Med Radiol* 1987a; 32(7):42-6.

Kuzmina EG, Degtiareva AA, Zubova ND, Guseva LI, Klimanov ME: Effectiveness of various therapeutic schemes for patients with radiation edema of the extremeties. *Med Radiol* 1987b; 32(3):18-22.

La Vecchia C, Franceschi S, Dolara P, Bidoli E, Barbone F: Refined-sugar intake and the risk of colorectal cancer in humans. *Int J Cancer* 1993; 55(3):386-9.

Lagrua G, Olivier-Martin F, Grillot A: A study of the effects of procyanidololigomers on capillary resistance in hypertension and in certain nephropathies. *Sem Hop* 1981; 57:1399-1401.

Lagrue G, Behar A, Kazandjian M, Rahbar K: Idiopathic cyclic edema. The role of capillary hyperpermeability and its correction by ginkgo biloba extract. *Presse Med* 1986 Sep 25; 15(31):1550-3.

Landau BJ, Kwaan HC, Varrusio EN, et al: Elevated levels or urokinase-type plasminogen activator and plasminogen activator inhibitor type-1 malignant human brain tumors. *Cancer Res* 1994; 54(4):1105-8.

Lang, W: Pharmacokinetics of ^{14}C-labelled rhein in rats. *Pharmocology* 1988; 36(1):158-171.

Langer R, Brem H, Falterman K, et al: Isolation of cartilage factor that inhibits tumor neovascularization. *Science* 1976; 193:70-2.

Langer R, Conn H, Vacanti J, et al: Control of tumor growth in animals by infusion of angiogenesis inhibitor. *Proc Natl Acad Sci* 1980; 77(7):4331-5.

Larocca LM, Giustacchini M, Maggiano N, Ranelletti FO, et al: Growth-inhibitory effect of quercetin and presence of type II estrogen binding sites in primary human transitional cell carcinomas. *J Urol* 1994; 152(3):1029-33.

Larocca LM, Teofili L, Leone G, Sica S, et al: Antiproliferative activity of quercetin on normal bone marrow and leukaemic progenitors. *Br J Haematol* 1991; 79(4):562-6.

Lasekan JB, Clayton MK, Gendron-Fitzpatrick A: Dietary olive and safflower oils in the promotion of DMBA-induced mammary tumorgenesis in rats. *Nutr Cancer* 1990; 13:153-63.

Lashner BA: Red blood cell folate is associated with the development of dysplasia and cancer in ulcerative colitis. *J Cancer Res Clin Oncol* 1993; 119(9):549-54.

Lau BH, Qian XJ, Wong BY, et al: Chinese medicinal herbs restore tumor-associated immunosuppression (Meeting abstract). *FASEB J* 1992; 6(5):A1930.

Lawson DH, Stockton LH, Bleier JC, et al: The effect of phenylalanine and tyrosine restricted diet on elemental balance studies and plasma aminograms of patients with disseminated malignant melanoma. *Am J of Clin Nutr* 1985; 41:73-84.

Lea MA, Xiao Q, Sadhukhan AK, Cottle S, et al: Inhibitory effects of tea extracts and (-)-epigallocatechin gallate on DNA synthesis and proliferation of hepatoma and erythrleukemia cells. *Cancer Letters* 1993a; 68:231-36.

Lea MA, Xiao Q, Sadhukan AK, et al: Inhibitory action of tea extracts and (-)-epigallocatechin gallate on cell proliferation. *Proc Annual Meeting American Cancer Assoc Cancer Res* 1993b; Meeting Abstract:34.

Lee A, Langer R: Shark cartilage contains inhibitors of tumor angiogenesis. *Science* 1983; 221:1185-7.

Lee CM, Jiang LM, Shang HS, et al: Prehispanalone, a novel platelet activating factor receptor antagonist from leonurus heterophyllus. *Br J Pharmacol* 1991; 103(3):17 19-24.

Lee ES, Steiner M, Lin R: Thioallyl compounds: potent inhibitors of cell proliferation. *Biochim Biophys Acta* 1994; 1221(1):73-7.

Lee I, Boucher Y, Jain RK: Nicotinamide can lower tumor interstitial fluid pressure: mechanistic and therapeutic implications. *Cancer Res* 1992 Jun 1; 52(11):3237-40.

Leeper DB, Wang GH, Li DJ: Effect of 100g oral glucose on tumor pH in Chinese patients (meeting abstract). Thrityeight Annual Meeting of the Radiation Research Society and Tenth Annual Meeting of the North American Hyperthermia Group. April 7-12, 1990, New Orleans, LA, p.11, 1990.

Legnani C, Frascaro M, Guazzaloca G, et al: Effects of dried garlic preparation on fibrolysis and platelet aggregation in healthy subjects. *Arzneimittelforschung* 1993; 43(2):1 19-22.

Leibovitz BE: Polyphenols & Bioflavonoids the Medicines of Tomorrow -Pts 1 & 2. *Townsend Letters for Doctors* April-May 1994

Leibow C, Rothman SS: Enteropancreatic circulation of digestive enzymes. *Science* 1975 Aug 8; 189(4201):472-4.

Lemli J, Lemmens L: Metabolism of sennosides and rhein in the rat. *Pharmacology* 1980; 20(1):50-57.

Leung A: *Encyclopedia of Common Natural Ingredients Used in Foods, Drugs, and Cosmetics.* New York: J Wiley & Sons, 1980.

Levin L, Kocha W, Driedger A: Oral urea in treatment of liver metastases from colorectal adenocarcinoma. *Cancer Treatment Reports* 1987 Nov; 71(11):1119.

Levine L: "Tumor promoters, growth factors and arachidonic acid." *Prostaglandins in Cancer Research.* E Garaci, R Paoletti, MG Santoro editors. Berlin: Springer-Verlag, 1987.

Levine M, Hirsh J, Gent M, Arnold A, et al: Double-blind randomised trial of a very-low-dose warfarin for the prevention of thromboebolism in stage IV breast cancer. *Lancet* 1994; 343(8902):867-8.

Levy S, Heberman R, Maluish A, et al: Prognostic risk assessment in primary breast cancer by behavioral and immunological parameters. *Health Psychol* 1985; 4:99.

Levy S, Lee J, Bagley C, et al: Survival hazards analysis in first recurrent breast cancer patients: seven-year follow-up. *Psychosom Med* 1988; 50:520-8.

Levy SA. *Behavior and Cancer* San Francisco: Jossey-Bass Publishers; 1985.

Lewis PJ: Risk factors for breast cancer. Pollutants and pesticides may be important. [letter] *BMJ* 1994 Dec 17; 309(6969):1662.

Lewith GT and Aldridge D, editors. *Clinical research methodology for complementary therapies.* London: Hodder & Stoughton, 1993.

Li GH, Wang QL, Liu FQ: Experimental study of warming and recuperating kidney yang by you-gui-yin. *Chung Hsi I Cheih Ho Tsa Chih* 1990; 10(9):547-8.

Li L, Chen X, Li J: Observations on the long-term effects of "yi qi yang yin decoction" combined with radiotherapy in the treatment of nasopharyngeal carcinoma. *J Tradit Chin Med* 1992a; 12(4):263-6.

Li L, Jiao L, Lau BH: Protective effect of gypenosides against oxidative stress in phagocyctes, vascular endothelial cells and liver microsomes. *Cancer Biother* 1993 Fall; 8(3):263-72.

Li L, Jin YY: The influence of Gynostemma pentaphyllum extract on platelet aggregation and arachidonate metabolism in rabbits. *Chin Pharmacol Bull* 1989; 5:213-17.

Li L, Lau BHS: Protection of vascular endothelial cells from hydrogen peroxide-induced oxidant injury by gypenosides, saponins of Gynostemma pentaphyllum. *Phytotherapy Research* 1993; 7:299-304.

Li NQ: Clinical and experimental study on shen-qi injection with chemotherapy in the treatment of malignant tumor of digestive tract. *Chung Kuo Chung Hsi I Chieh Ho Tsa Chih* 1992; 12(10):588-92, 579.

Li PP: Treatment of tumors and their progress by improving blood circulation to remove stasis.*Chung Kuo Chung Hsi I Chieh Ho Tsa Chih* 1992; 12(10):634-6, 623.

Li SH, Fei X, Wu ZL, et al: Effect of an extract from cauline of Piper kadsura ohwi on endotoxin-induced hypotension and lung injury in rats. *Chung Kuo Chung Yao Tsa Chih* 1989; 14(11):683-5, 704.

Li W, et al: Effects of Codonopsis pilosula-astralagus injection on platelet aggregation and activity of PGI2-like substance. *J of Tradit Chinese Med* 1986; 6(1):9-12.

Li W, Zhou CH, Lu QL: Effects of Chinese materia medica in activating blood stimulating menstrual flow on the endocrine function of ovary-uterus and its mechanisms. *Chung Kuo Chung Hsi I Chieh Ho Tsa Chih* 1992b; 12(3):165-8.

Li X, Wu XG: Effects of ginseng on hepatocellular carcinoma in rats induced by diethylnitrosamine—a further study. *J Tongji Med Univ* 1991; 11(2):73-80.

Li XL: Blood platelets, neoplasm metastasis and anti-metastatic effect of huoxue-huayu drugs. *Chung Hsi I Chieh Ho Tsa Chih* 1989; 9(10):637-40.

Li XM: The general situation of treating leukemia with traditional Chinese medicine. *Chung Hsi I Chieh Ho Tsa Chih* 1989; 9(6):378-9.

Li Y, Yu G: A comparative clinical study on prevention and treatment with selected chronomedication of leukopenia induced by chemotherapy. *J of Trad Chin Med* 1993; 13(4):257-261.

Liao J, et al: Clinical and experimental studies of coronary heart disease treated with Yi-Qi Huo-Xue injection. *J Trad Chin Med* 1989; 9(3):193-8.

Liburdy RP, Sloma TR, Sokolic R, et al: ELF magnetic fields, breast cancer, and melatonin: 60 Hz fields block melatonin's oncostatic action on ER + breast cancer cell proliferation. *J Pineal Res* 1993 Mar; 14(2):89-97.

Lien EJ, Li WY: *Structure Activity Relationship Analysis of Anticancer Chinese Drugs and Related Plants*. University of Southern California: The Oriental Healing Arts Institute of the United States; 1985.

Lieu CW, Lee SS, Wang SY: The effect of Ganoderma lucidum on induction of differentiation in leukemic U937 cells. *Anticancer Res* 1992; 12(4):1211-5.

Lin L, Wu S, Tang J: Clinical observation and experimental study of the treatment of aplastic anemia by warming and tonifying the spleen and kidney. *Chung Hsi I Cheih Ho Tsa Chih* 1990; 10(5):272-4.

Lin PF: Antitumor effect of actinidia chinensis polysaccharide on murine tumor. *Chung Hua Chung Liu Tsa Chih* 1988; 10(6):441-4.

Linder J: The thymus gland in secondary immunodeficiency. *Arch Pathol Lab Med* 1987; 111(12):1118-22.

Linder MC, editor. *Nutritional Biochemistry and Metabolism* 2nd edition. New York: Elsevier Science Publishing Co. Inc.; 1991.

Lipkin M, Newmark H: Effect of added dietary calcium on colonic epithelial-cell proliferation in subjects at high risk for familial colonic cancer. *N Engl J Med* 1985; 313:1381-4.

Lissoni P, Barni S, Ardizzoia A, et al: A randomized study with the pineal hormone melatonin versus supportive care alone in patients with brain metastases due to solid neoplasms. *Cancer* 1994c Feb 1; 73(3):699-701.

Lissoni P, Barni S, Ardizzoia A, et al: Randomized study with the pineal hormone melatonin versus supportive care alone in advanced nonsmall cell lung cancer resistant to a first-line chemotherapy containing cisplatin. *Oncology* 1992a; 49(5):336-9.

Lissoni P, Barni S, Cattaneo G, et al: Clinical results with the pineal hormone melatonin in advanced cancer resistant to standard antitumor therapies. *Oncology* 1991b; 48(6):448-50.

Lissoni P, Barni S, Cazzaniga M, et al: Efficacy of the concomitant administration of the pineal hormone melatonin in cancer immunotherapy with low-dose IL-2 in patients with advanced solid tumors who had progressed on IL-2 alone. *Oncology* 1994b Jul-Aug; 51(4):344-7.

Lissoni P, Barni S, Rovelli F, et al: Neuroimmunotherapy of advanced solid neoplasms with single evening subcutaneous injection of low-dose interleukin-2 and melatonin: preliminary results. *Eur J Cancer* 1993b; 29A(2):185-9.

Lissoni P, Barni S, Tancini G, et al: Pineal-opioid system interactions in the control of immunioinflammatory responses. *Ann NY Acad Sci* 1994a Nov 25; 741:191-196.

Lissoni P, Barni S, Tancini G, Rovelli F, et al: A study of the mechanisms involved in the immunostimulatory action of the pineal hormone in cancer patients. *Oncology*. 1993c; 50(6):399-402.

Lissoni P, Brivio F, Ardizzoia A, et al: Subcutaneous therapy with low-dise interleukin-2 plus the neurohormone melatonin in metastatic gastric cancer patients with low performance status. *Tumori* 1993a Dec 31; 79(6):401-4.

Lissoni P, Tisi E, Barni S, et al: Biological and clinical results of a neurimmunotherapy with interleukin-2 and the pineal hormone melatonin as a first line threatment in advanced non-small cell lung cancer. *Br J Cancer* 1992b Jul; 66(1):155-8.

Lissoni P, Tisi E, Brivio F, et al: Modulation of interleukin-2 induced macrophage activation in cancer patients by the pineal hormone melatonin. *J biol Regul Homeost Agents* 1991a Oct-Dec; 5(4):154-6.

Liu C, Lu S, Ji MR: Effects of Cordyceps sinensis (CS) on in vitro natural killer cells. *Chung Kuo Chung Hsi I Chieh Ho Tsa Chih* 1992a; 12(5):267-9, 259.

Liu CX, He WG: Leukogenic effect of complex indigo powder. *J Ethnopharmacol* 1991; 34(1):83-6.

Liu HM: Wound chamber study of nerve and blood vessel growth. *Proc Natl Sci Counc Repub China* 1992; 16(1):65-9.

Liu HM, Wang DL, Liu CY: Interactions between fibrin, collagen and endothelial cells in angiogenesis. *Adv Exp Med Biol* 1990; 281:3 19-31.

Liu J, Hua G, Liu W, Cui Y, et al: The effect of IH764-3 on fibroblast proliferation and function. *Chin Med Sci J* 1992b Sep; 7(3):142-7.

Liu P, Mizoguchi Y, Morisawa S: Effects of magnesium lithospermate B on D-glalctosamide induced rat liver injury. *Chung Kuo Chung Hsi I Chieh Ho Tsa Chih* 1993a; 13(6):352-3.

Liu T, Soong SJ, Wilson NP: A case control study of nutritional cators and cervical dysplasia. 1993b Nov-Dec; 2(6):525-30.

Liu XH, Bravo-Cuellar A, Florentin I, et al: In vivo immuno-pharmacological properties of the traditional Chinese medicine kang fu-xin. *Int J Immunotherapy* 1989; 5(1):25-33.

Liu XY, Ang NQ: Effect of liu wei di huang or jin gui shen qi decoction on adjuvant treatment in small cell lung cancer. *Chung Hsi I Chieh Ho Tsa Chih* 1990; 10(12):720-2, 708.

Liu Z: Effects of Ligusticum wallichii on the plasma levels of beta-thromboglobulin, platelet factor 4, thromboxane B2 and 6-keto-PGF1 alpha in patients with acute cerebral infarction. *Chung Hsi I Chieh Ho Tsa Chih* 1991; 11(12):711-3.

Liu Z: Effects of Ligusticum wallichii on the plasma levels of beta-thromboglobulin, platelet factor 4, thromboxane B2 and 6-keto-PGF1 alpha in rabbits under acute experimental cerebral ischemia. *Chung Hsi I Chieh Ho Tsa Chih* 1990; 10(9):543-4.

Loesche W, Mazurov AV, Voyno-Yasenetskaya TA, et al: Feverfew—an antithrombotic drug? *Folia Haematol Int Mag Klin Morphol Blutforsch* 1988; 115(1-2):181-4.

Longiave D, Omini C, Nicosia S, et al: The mode of action aescin on isolated veins: relationship with PGF2.alpha. *Pharmacol Res Commun* 1978; 10(2):145-52.

Lonnbro P, Wadso I: Effect of dimethyl sulphoxide and some antibiotics on cultured human T-lymphoma cells as measured by microcalorimetry. *J Biochem Biophys Methods* 1991 May-June; 22(4):331-6.

Loprinizi CL, Kuross SA, O'Fallon JR, et al: Randomized placebo-controlled evaluation of hydrazine sulfate in patients with advanced colorectal cancer. *J Clin Oncol* 1994a; 12:1121-5.

Loprinzi CL, Goldberg RM, Su JQ, et al: Placebo-controlled trial of hydrazine sulfate in patients with newly diagnosed non-small-cell lung cancer. *J Clin Oncol* 1994b; 12:1126-9.

Loscher W, Wahnschaffe U, Mevissen M, et al: Effects of weak alternating magnetic fields on nocturnal melatonin production and mammary carcinogenesis in rats. *Oncology* 1994 May-Jun; 51(3):288-95.

Lotz-Winter H: On the pharmacology of bromelain: an update with special regard to animal studies on dose-dependent effects. *Planta Med* 1990; 56:249-53.

Lotze MT, Rosenberg SA: "Interleukin-2: clinical applications." *Biologic Therapy of Cancer*. Philadelphia: JB Lippincott, 1991.

Lu CY, Dustin LB, Vazquez MA: "Macrophage tumoricidal activity is inhibited by docosahexaenoic acid (DHA), an omega-3 fatty acid." *Exercise, Calories, Fat, and Cancer.* MM Jacobs, editor. New York: Plenum Press, 1992.

Lu M, Chen Q: Biochemical study of chinese rhubarb; Inhibitory effects of antraquinone derivatives on P388 lekemia in mice. *Zhongguo Yaoke Daxue Xuebao* 1989; 20(3):155-7.

Lu XF: Experimental study on the immunosuppressive effects of gui zhi tang. *Chung Hsi I Chieh Ho Tsa Chih* 1989; 9(5):283-5.

Lu ZH, Yang YC, Shen SY, et al: The inhibitory effects of psoralen plus ultraviolet irradiation on human leukemic cell lines. *Zhongguo Yaoli Xuebao* 1993; 14(Zengkan):28-30.

Lukacs GL, Nagy I, Lustyik G, et al: Microfluorimetric and X-ray microanalytic studies on the DNA content and Na+:K+ ratios of the cell nuclei in various types of thyroid tumors. *J Cancer Res Clin Oncol* 1983; 105(3):280-4.

Luo D, Li Y: Preventive effect of green tea on MNNG-induced lung cancers and precancerous lesions in LACA mice. *Hua Hsi I Ko Ta Hsueh Hsueh Pao* 1992; 23(4):433-7.

Ma L: Experimental study on the immunomodulatory effects of rhubarb. *Chung Hsi I Chieh Ho Tsa Chih* 1991; 11(7):418-9, 390.

Ma M, Yao B: Progress in indirubin treatment of chronic myelocytic leukemia. *Journal of Traditional Chinese Medicine* 1983; 3(3):245-248

Ma Y, Han GQ, Liu ZJ: Studies on PAF antagonistic bicyclo(3,2,1) octanoid neolignans from Piper kadsura. *Yao Hsueh Hsueh Pao* 1993a; 28(3):207-11.

Ma Y, Han GQ, Wang YY: PAF antagonistic benzofuran neolignans from Piper kadsura. *Yao Hsueh Hsueh Pao* 1993b; 28(5):370-3.

Macchiarini P, Danesi R, Del Tacca M, et al: Effects of thymostimulin on chemotherapy-induced toxicity and long-term survival in small cell lung cancer patients. *Anticancer Res* 1989; 9(1):193-6.

MacGregor JT: "Mutagenic and carcinogenic effects of flavonoids." *Plant Flavonoids in Biology and Medicine II* Alan R. Liss, Inc., 1986; 411-424.

Maciocia G. *The Foundations of Chinese Medicine* New York: Churchill Livingstone; 1989.

Mahadevan V, Hart IR: Divergent effects of flavone acetic acid on established versus developing tumour blood flow. *Br J Cancer* 1991 Jun; 63(6):889-92.

Mahajani SS, Kulkarni RD: Effect of disodium cromoglycate and picrorrhiza kurroa root powder on sensitivity of guinea pigs to histamine and sympathomimetic amines. *Allergy Appl Immunol* 1977; 53:137-44.

Mahnensmith RL, Aronson PS: The plasma membrane sodium-hydrogen exchanger and its role in physiological and pathophysiological processes. *Circ Res* 1985; 56(6):773-88.

Majewski S, Szmurlo A, Marczak M, Jablonska S, Bollag W: Inhibition of tumor cell-induced angiogenesis by retinoids, 1,25-dihydroxyvitamins D3 and their combination. *Cancer Lett* 1993 Nov 30; 75(1):35-9.

Maki PA, Kennedy AR: Humoral and cellular immune functions are not compromised by the anticarcinogenic bowman-birk inhibitor. *Nutr Cancer* 1992; 18:165-73.

Makimura M, Hirasawa M, Kobayashi K, et al: Inhibitory effect of tea catechins on collagenase activity. *J Periodontal* 1993; 64(7):630-6

Malaker K, Anderson BJ, Beecroft WA, et al: Management of oral mucosal dysplasia with beta-carotene retinoic acid: a pilot cross-over study. *Cancer Detect Prev* 1991; 15(5):335-40.

Malter M, Schriever G, Eilber U: Natural killer cells, vitamins, and other blood components of vegetarian and omnivorous men. *Nutr Cancer* 1989; 12:271-78.

Malterud KE, Farbrot TL, Huse AE, Sund RB: Antioxidant and radical scavenging effects of anthraquinones and anthrones. *Pharmacology* 1993; 47(suppl 1):77-85.

Mantovani G, Proto E, Lai P, et al: Controlled trial of thymostimulin treatment of patients with primary carcinoma of the larynx resected surgically. *Recenti Prog Med* 1992; 83(5):303-6.

Marathe GK, Krishnakantha TP, D'Souza CJ: PAF-acether in AK-5 tumour cells. *Cell Biol Int Rep* 1991; 15(1):85-90.

Mareel MM, De Mets M: Anti-invasive activities of experimental chemotherapeutic agents. *Crit Rev Oncol Hematol* 1989; 9(3):263-303.

Marks PA, Rifkind RA: "Differentiating Factors." *Biologic Therapy of Cancer* VT DeVita Jr., S Hellman, SA Rosenberg editors. Philadelphia: JB Lippincott, 1991.

Maruyama H, Yamazaki K, Murofushi S, et al: Antitumor activity of Sarcodon aspratus (Berk.) S. Ito and Ganoderma lucidum (Fr.) Karst. *J Pharmacobiodyn* 1989; 12(2):118-23.

Masquelier J: Natural products as medicinal agents. *Planta Med* 1980; 242S-256S.

Mathews J: Media feeds frenzy over shark cartilage as cancer treatment. *J NCI* 1993 Aug 3; 85(15):1190-1.

Matin A, Hung MC: Repression of neu-induced clonogenicity by dimethylsulfoxide correlates with decreased levels of neu-encoded cell-surface p185 and changes in phosphotyrosine content of endogenous proteins. *Cancer Lett* 1993 Jan 15; 68(1):55-60.

Matsubara T, Saura R, Hirohata K, Ziff M: Inhibition of human endothelial cell proliferation in vitro and neovascularization in vivo by D-penicillamine. *J Clin Invest* 1989; 83(1):158-67.

Matsuda H, Yano M, Kubo M, et al: Pharmacological study on citrus fruits. II.; Anti-allergic effect of fruit of citrus unshiu markovich (2). *Yakugaku Zasshi* 1991; 111(3):193-8.

Matsukawa Y, Marui N, Sakai T, Satomi Y, et al: Genistein arrests cell cycle progression at G2-M. *Cancer Res* 1993; 53(6):1328-31.

Matsukawa Y, Yoshida M, Sakai T, et al: The effect of quercetin and other flavonoids on cell cycle progression growth of human gastric cancer cells. *Planta Med* 1990; 56:677-78.

Matsumoto M: Inhibitors for protein tyrosine kinases, erbstatin, genistein and herbimycin A, induce differentiation of human neural tumor cell lines. *Jpn Nippon Geka Hokan* 1991; 60(2):113-21.

Matsumura Y, Maruo K, Kimura M, et al: Kinin-generating cascade in advanced cancer patients and in vitro study. *Jpn J Cancer Res* 1991; 82 (6):732-41.

Matsura K, Kawakita T, Nakai S, et al: Role of B-lymphocytes in the immunopharmacological effects of a traditional Chinese medicine, xiao-chai-hu-tang (shosaiko-to). *Int J Immunopharmacol* 1993; 15(2):237-43.

Maurer HR, Hozumi M, Honma Y, et al: Bromelain induces the differentiation of leukemic cells in vitro: an explanation for its cytostatic effects? *Planta Med* 1988:377-81.

Mayne ST, Graham S, Zheng TZ: Dietary retinol: prevention or promotion of carcinogenesis in humans? *Cancer Causes Control* 1991; 2(6):443-50.

McAuslan BR, Gole GA: Cellular and molecular mechanisms in angiogenesis. *Trans Ophthalmol Soc UK* 1980; 100(3):354-8.

McDevitt CA, Lipman JM, Ruemer RJ, et al: Stimulation of matrix formation in rabbit chondrocyte cultures by ascorbate. *J Orthop Res* 1988; 6(4):518-24.

McDonald S, Meyerowitz C, Smudzin T, Rubin P: Preliminary results of a pilot study using WR-2721 before fractionated irradiation of the head and neck to reduce salivary gland dysfunction. *Int J Radiat Oncol Biol Phys* 1994; 29(4):747-54

McGinnis LS: Alternative therapies, 1990. An Overview. *Cancer* 1991; 67(6 Suppl):1788-92.

McNamee D: Limonene trial in cancer. *The Lancet* 1993; 342:801.

McNicol A: The effects of genistein on platelet function are due to thromboxane receptor antagonism rather than inhibition of tyrosine kinase. *Prostaglandins Leukot Essent Fatty Acids* 1993; 48(5):379-84.

Meares A: A form of intensive meditation associated with the regression of cancer. *Amer J of Clinical Hypothesis* 1983a; 25(2-3):114-21.

Meares A: Psychological mechanisms on the regression of cancer. *The Med J of Australia* June 11, 1983b:58-59.

Meares A: Regression of cancer of the rectum after intensive meditation? *Med J Aust* 1979; 2(10):539-40.

Meares A: Stress, meditation and the regression of cancer. *The Practioner* 1982; 226:1607-9.

Meares A: What can the cancer patient expect from intensive meditation? *Aust Fam Physician* 1980; 9(5):322-5.

Mengeaud V, Nano JL, Fournel S, et al: Effects of eicosapentaenoic acid, gamma-linolenic acid and prostaglandin E1 on three human colon carcinoma cell lines. *Prostaglandins Leukot Essent Fatty Acids* 1992; 47(4):313-9.

Mengs U, Klein M: Genotoxic effects of aristolochic acid in the mouse micronucleus test. *Plant Medica* 1988:502.

Messiha FS: Biochemical aspects of cesium administration in tumor-bearing mice. *Phar Biochem & Behavior* 1984b; 21(1):27-30.

Messiha FS: Effect of cesium and ethanol on tumor bearing rats. *Phar Biochem & Behavior.* 1984a; 21(1):35-40.

Messiha FS, El-Domeiri A, Sproat HF: Effects of lithium and cesium salts on sarcoma-I implants in the mouse. *Neurobehav Toxicol* 1979; 1:27-31.

Messiha FS, Stocco DM: Effect of cesium and potassium salts on survival rats bearing novikoff hepatoma. *Phar Biochem & Behavior* 1984; 21(1):31-34.

Messina M, Barnes S: The role of soy products in reducing risk of cancer. *Journal of the National Cancer Institute* 1991; 83(8):541-6.

Metcalf D, Morstyn G: Colony-stimulating factors: general biology. *Biologic Therapy of Cancer*. VT DeVita, S Hellman, SA Rosenberg editors. Philadephia: JB Lippincott Co, 1991.

Mettlin C, Graham S, et al: Diet and cancer of the esophagus. *Nutr Cancer* 1981; 2(2):143-147.

Meyn RE, Stephens LC, Hunter NR, et al: Induction of apoptosis in murine tumors by cyclophosphamide. *Cancer Chemother Pharmacol* 1994; 33(5):410-4.

Miller BA, Reis LAG, Hankey BF, et al, editors. *Cancer Statistics Review 1973-1989*. National Cancer Institute. NIH Pub. No. 92-2789. 1992.

Milner JA: Effect of selenium on virally induced and transplanted tumor models. *Fed Proc* 1985; 44(9):2568-72.

Milner JA, Stepanovich LV: Inhibitory effect of dietary arginine on growth of Ehrlich ascites tumor cells in mice. *J Nutr* 1979; 109:489-93.

Mir LM, Orlowski S, Poddevin B, Belehradek J Jr: Electrochemotherapy tumor treatment is improved by interleukin-2 stimulation of the host's defenses. *Eur Cytokine Netw* 1992; 3(3):331-4.

Mitter CG, Zielinski CC: Plasma levels of d-dimer: a crosslinked fibrin-degradation product in female breast cancer. *J Cancer Res Clin Oncol* 1991; 117(3):259-62.

Moertel CG, Fleming TR, Creagan ET, et al: High-dose vitamin C versus placebo in the treatment of patients with advanced cancer who have had no prior chemotherapy. *N Eng J Med* 1985; 312:137-41.

Molto LM, Carballido JA, Manzano L, et al: Thymostimulin enhances the natural cytotoxic activity of patients with transitional cell carcinoma of the bladder. *Int J Immunopharmacol* 1993; 15(3):335-41.

Monboisse JC, Braquet P, Randoux A, et al: Non-enzymatic degradation of acid-soluble calf skin collagen by superoxide ion: protective effect of flavonoids. *Biochem Pharmacol* 1983; 32(1):53-8.

Monjan AA, Collector MI: Stress-induced modulation of the immune response. *Science* 1977; 196:307-8.

Moongkardni P, Srivattana A, Bunyaprpphatsara N, et al: Cytotoxicity assay of hispidulin and quercetin using colorimetric technique. *Warasan Phesetchasat* 1991; 18(2):25-31.

Morant R, Jungi WF, Koehli C, Senn HJ: Why do cancer patients use alternative medicine? *Schweiz Med Wochenschr* 1991; 121(27-28):1029-34.

Mori H, Xu Q, Sakamoto O, et al: Mechanisms of antitumor activity of aqueous extracts from Chinese herbs: their immunopharmacological properties. *Jpn J Pharmacol* 1989; 49(3):423-31.

Morino K, Matsukara N, Kawachi T, Ohgaki H, et al: Carcinogenicity test of quercetin and rutin in golden hamsters by oral administration. *Carcinogenesis* 1982; 3(1):93-7.

Morita H, Umeda M, Masuda T, et al: Cytotoxic and mutagenic effects of emodin on cultured mouse carcinoma FM3A cells. *Mutat Res* 1988; 204(2):329-32.

Morrell EM, Hollandsworth JG Jr.: Noreepinephrine alterations under stress conditions following the regular practice of meditation. *Psychosom Med* 1986; 48(3-4):270-7.

Morris DM, Marino AA, Gonzalez E: Electrochemical modification of tumor growth in mice. *J Surg Res* 1992; 53(3):306-9.

Morris T, Greer S, Pettingale KW, et al: Patterns of expression of anger and their psychological correlations in women with breast cancer. *J Psychosom Res* 1981; 25:111-17.

Moses MA, Sudhalter J, langer R: Identification of an inhibitor of neovascularization from cartilage. *Science* 1990; 248:1408-10.

Motoo Y, Sawabu N: Antitumor effects of saikosaponins, baicalin and baicalein on human hepatoma cell lines. *Cancer Letters* 1994; 86:91-95.

Mousavi Y, Adlercreutz H: Genistein is an effective stimulator of sex hormone-binding globulin production in hepatocarcinoma human liver cancer cells and suppresses proliferation of those cells in culture. *Steroids* 1993; 58(7):301-4.

MUCOS Pharma GmbH & Co.: *Wobe-mugos*. Alpentrabe, West Germany, undated.

Murakami S, Muramatsu M, Otomo S: Gastric H+, K(+)-At pase inhibition by catechins. *J Pharm Pharmacol* 1992; 44(11):926-8.

Murata A, Morishige F, Yamaguchi H: Prolongation of survival times of terminal cancer patients by administration of large doses of ascorbate. *Int J Vitam Nutr Res Suppl* 1982; 23:103-13.

Murray M, Pizzorno J: *Encyclopedia of Natural Medicine*. Rocklin, CA: Prima Publishing, 1991.

Murray MT: *The Healing Power of Herbs*. Rocklin: Prima Publishing, 1992.

Nagatsu Y, Inoue M, Ogihara Y: Modification of macrophage functions by shosaikoto (kampo medicine) leads to enhancement of immune response. *Chem Pharm Bulletin* 1989; 37(6):1540-2.

Nagy I, Lustyik G, Lukacs G, et al: Correlation of malignancy with the intracelluar NA+:K+ ratio in human thyroid tumors. *Cancer Res* 1983; 43(11):5395-402.

Nagy I, Toth L, Szallasi Z, Lampe I: Energy-dispersive, bulk specimen X-ray microanalytical measurement of the intracellular Na+/K+ ratio in human laryngeal tumors. *J Cancer Res Clin Oncol* 1987; 113(2):197-202.

Nagy IZ, Lustyik G, Nagy VZ, et al: Intracellular Na+:K+ ratios in human cancer cells as revelaed by energy dispersive x-ray microanalysis. *J Cell Biol* 1981; 90(3):769-77.

Nagy JA, Brown LF, Senger DR, et al: Pathogenesis of tumor stroma generation: a critical role for leaky blood vessels and fibrin deposition. *Biochim Biophys Acta* 1989; 948(3):305-26.

Nair PP, Turjman N, Kessie G, et al: Diet, nutrition intake, and metabolism in populations at high and low risk for colon cancer. *Am J Clin Nutr* 1984; 40(4 Suppl):927-30.

Nair SC, Pannikar B, Panikkar KR: Antitumour activity of saffron (Crocus sativus). *Cancer Lett* 1991; 57(2):109-14.

Nair SC, Salomi MJ, Varghese CD, et al: Effect of saffron on thymocyte proliferation, intracellular glutathione levels and its antitumor activity. *Biofactors* 1992; 4(1):51-4.

Nakajima S, Tohda Y, Ohkawa K, et al: Effect of saiboku-to (TJ-96) on bronchial asthma. Induction of glucocorticoid receptor, beta-adrenaline receptor, IgE-Fc epsilon receptor expression and its effect on experimental immediate and late asthmatic reaction. *Ann N Y Acad Sci* 1993; 685:549-60.

Nakamura T, Kuriyama M, Kosuge E, et al: Effects of saiboku-to (TJ-96) on the production of platelet-activating factor in human neutrophils. *Ann N Y Acad Sci* 1993; 685:572-9.

Nakane H, Ono K: Differential inhibitory effects of some catechin derivatives on the activities of human immunodeficiency virus reverse transcriptase and cellular deoxyribonucleic and ribonucleic acid polymerases. *Biochemistry* 1990; 29:2841-45.

Nakashima S, Koike T, Nozawa Y: Genistein, a protein tyrosine kinase inhibitor, inhibits thromboxane A2-mediated human platelet responses. *Mol Pharmacol* 1991; 39(4):475-80.

Nathan CF, Cohn ZA: Antitumor effects of hydrogen peroxide in vivo. *J Exp Med* 1981; 154:1539-53.

Natori S, Ikekawa N, Suzuki M, editors. *Advances in natural products chemistry; Extraction and isolation of active compounds.* New York: John Wiley & Sons, 1981.

NCI. *Investigators Handbook; A Manual for Participants in Clinical Trials of Investigative Agents* Sponsored by the Division of Cancer Treatment, National Cancer Institute. Bethesda.: US Department of Health and Human Services, 1993.

Negri E, La Vecchia C, Franceschi S, et al: Attributable risk for oral cancer in northern Italy. *Cancer Epidemiol Biomarkers Prev* 1993 May-Jun; 2(3):189-93.

Neri B, Fiorelli C, Moroni F, Nicita G, et al: Modulation of human lymphoblastoid interferon activity by melatonin in metastic renal cell carcinoma. A phase II study. *Cancer* 1994 Jun 15; 73(12):3015-9.

Neve J, Vertongen F, Molle L: Selenium deficiency. *Clin Endocrinol Metab* 1985; 14(3):629-56.

Neves PC, Neves MC, Cruz AB, et al: Differential effects on mandevilla velutina compounds on paw oedema induced by phospholipase A2 and phospholipase C. *Eur J Pharmacol* 1993; 243(3):213-9.

Newberne PM, Voranunt S, Locniskar M, et al: Inhibition of hepatocarcinogenesis in mice by dietary methyl donors methionine and choline. *Nutr Cancer* 1990; 14:175-81.

Newell K, Franchi A, Pouyssegur J, et al: Studies with glycolysis-deficienct cells suggest the production of lactic acid is not the only cause of tumor acidity. *Proc Natl Acad Sci* 1993; 90:1127-31.

Nicosia RF, Belser P, Bonanno E, Diven J: Regulation of angiogenesis in vitro by collagen metabolism. *In Vitro Cell Dev Biol* 1991 Dec; 27 A(12):961-6.

Nieper HA: Bromelain in der kontrolle malignen washstums. *Krebsgeschehen* 1976; 1:9-15.

Nigam S, Muller S, Benedetto C: Elevated plasma levels of platelet-activating factor (PAF) in breast cancer patients with hypercalcemia. *J Lipid Mediat* 1989; 1(6):323-8.

Ning CH, Wang GM, Zhao TY, et al: Therapeutical effects of jian pi yi shen prescription on the toxicity reactions of postoperative chemotherapy in patients with advanced gastric carcinoma. *J Tradit Chin Med* 1988; 8(2):113-6.

Nishiyori T, Tsuchiya H, Inagaki N, et al: Effect of saiboku-to, a blended Chinese traditional medicine, on Type I hypersensitivity reactions, particularly on experimentally-caused asthma. *Nippon Yakurigaku Zasshi* 1985; 85(1):7-16.

Niwa M, Yuasa K, Kondo S, et al: Studies of Wakan-Yakus (traditional herbal drugs): especially on the effects of Gaiyoh (Artemisiae folium) on blood coagulation. *Thromb Res* 1985; 38(6):671-9.

Norman A, Bennett LR, Mead JF, et al: Antitumor activity of sodium linoleate. *Nutrition and Cancer* 1988; 11:107-15.

Novi AM: Regression of aflatoxin B$_1$-induced hepatocellular carcinomas by reduced gluthione. *Science* 1981; 212(1):541-2.

O'Dwyer ST, Michie HR, Ziegler TR, Revhaug M, Smith RJ, Wilmore DW: A single dose of endotoxin increases intestinal permeability in healthy humans. *Arch Surg* 1988; 123:1459-64.

O'Leary A: Stress, emotion, and human immune function. *Psychological Bulletin* 1990; 108(3):363-77.

OAM. *Office of alternative medicine workshop on the collection of clinical research data relevant to alternative medicine and cancer.* Bethesda: Office of Alternative Medicine, 1994.

Oates KK, Goldstein AL: "Thymosin." *Biologic Therapy in Cancer* VT DeVita Jr, S Hellman, SA Rosenberg editors. Philadelphia: JB Lippincott, 1991.

Obolentseva GV, Khadzhai Ya I: Effect of escin and a flavonoid complex prepared from horse chestnut on inflammatory edema. *Farmakol Toksikol* 1969; 32(2):174-7.

Ogura M, Suzuki K, Terumi T, et al: Antiinflammatory action of the horse chestnut saponin (amorphous aescin). *Oyo Yakuri* 1975; 9(6):883-94.

Ohta T, Tawara M, Tatsuka M, et al: An approach to prolongation of survival rate in tumor bearing mice using 5-fluorouracil in combination with various kinds of herb medicine. *Gan To Kagaku Ryoho* 1983; 10(8):1858-65.

Oikawa T, Ashino-Fuse H, Shimamura M, et al: A novel angiogenic inhibitor derived from Japanese shark cartilage (I). Extraction and estimation of inhibitory activities toward tumor and embryonic angiogenesis. *Cancer Letters* 1990a; 51:181-6.

Oikawa T, Hirotani K, Nakamura O, Shudo K, et al: A highly potent antiangiogenic activity of retinoids. *Cancer Lett* 1989 Nov 30; 48(2):157-62.

Oikawa T, Hirotani K, Ogasawara H, Katayama T, et al: Inhibition of angiogenesis by vitamin D3 analogues. *Eur J Pharmacol* 1990b Mar 20; 178(2):247-50.

Okamoto R, Kumai A: Antigonadotropic activity of hop extract. *Acta Endocrinol (Copenh)* 1992 Oct; 127(4):371-7.

Okamoto T, Motohasi H, Takemiya S, et al: Clinical effects of Juzendaiho-to on immunologic and fatty metabolic states in postoperative patients with gastrointestinal cancer. *Gan To Kagaku Ryoho* 1989; 16(4 Pt 2-2):1533-7.

Okamura S, Shimoda K, Yu LX, et al: A traditional Chinese herbal medicine, ren-shen-yang-rong-tang (Japanese name: ninjin-yoei-to) augments the production of granulocyte-macrophage colony-stimulating factor from human peripheral blood mononuclear cells in vitro. *Int J Immunopharmacol* 1991; 13(5):595-8.

Okino M, Tomie H, Kanesada H, Marumoto M, et al: Optimal electric conditions in electrical impulse chemotherapy. *Jpn J Cancer Res* 1992; 83(10):1095-101.

Okita K, Murakamio T, Takahashi M: Anti-growth effects with components of Sho-saiko-to (TJ-9) on cultured human hepatoma cells. *European Journal of Cancer Prevention* 1993; 2:169-76.

Okunieff P: Interactions between ascorbicacid and the radiation of bone marrow, skin, and tumor. *Am J Clin Nutr* 1991; 54:1281S-3S.

Oleinik AN, Ovsiannikova LM: [Mechanism of the pro-oxidant activity of tetracycline.] *Antibiotiki* 1983; 28(11):845-8.

Olin BR, Hebel S, Dombeke et al. editors. *Drug Facts and Comparisons.* St. Louis: Facts and Comparisons; 1993.

Orme-Johnson D: Medical care utilization and the transcendental meditation program. *Psychosom Med* 1987; 49(6):637.

Osawa K, Matsumoto T, Yasuda H, et al: The inhibitory effect of plant extracts on the collagenolytic activity and cytotoxicity of human gingival fibroblasts by Porphyromonas gingivalis crude enzyme. *Bull Tokyo Dent Coll* 1991; 32(1):1-7.

Oshio H, Kawamura N: Quantative analysis of the laxative components in rhubarb by high performance liquid chromatography. *Shoyakugaku Zasshi* 1985; 39(2):131-38.

Ota H, Fukushima M, Maki M: Stimulatory action of shakuyaku on aromatase activity in culuted rat follicles. *Nippon Sanka Fujinka Gakkai Zasshi* 1989 May; 41(5):525-9.

Paige K, Palomares M, D'Amore PA, et al: Retinol-induced modification of the extracellular matrix of endothelial cells: its role in growth control. *In Vitro Cell Dev Biol* 1991; 27A(2):151-7.

Pan M: *Cancer Treatment with Fu Zheng Pei Ben Principle.* Fuijian: Fujian Science and Technology Publishing House, 1992.

Pan MJ, Li YH, Chen LF: Treatment of 320 cases of gastric cancer with liwei huajie decoction combined with surgery and chemotherapy. *Chinese Journal of Combined Traditional and Western Medicine* 1986; 6(5):268-70.

Panday BL, Das PK: Immunopharmacological studies on picrorrhiza kurroa royle ex benth part II: antiallergic activity. *Ind J Allergy Applied Immunol* 1988; 21-34.

Park KG, Heys SD, Blessing K, et al: Stimulation of human breast cancers by dietary L-arginine. *Clin Sci (Colch)* 1992 Apr; 82(4):413-417.

Parke A, Bhattacherjee P, Palmer RM, Lazarus NR: Characterization and quantification of copper sulfate-induced vascularization of the rabbit cornea. *Am J Pathol* 1988; 130(1):173-8.

Pastorino U, Infante M, Maioli M, et al: Adjuvant treatment of stage I lung cancer with high-dose vitamin A. *J Clin Oncol* 1993; 11(7):1216-22.

Pastorino U, Soresi M, Clerci G, et al: Lung cancer chemoprevention with retinol palimate: preliminary data from a randomized trial on stage Ia non small-cell lung cancer. *Acta Oncology* 1988; 27:773-80.

Pauling L, Moertel C: A proposition: megadoese of vitamin C are valuable in the treatment of cancer. *Nutr Rev* 1986 Jan; 44(1):28-32.

Pawlicki M, Rachtan J, Rolski J, Sliz E: Results of delayed treatment of patients with malignant tumors of the lymphatic system. *Pol Tyg Lek* 1991; 46(48-49):922-3.

Payton O D. *Research: the validation of clinical practice,* 2nd edition. Philadelphia: F.A. Davis Co, 1988.

Pedersen H, Grondahl-Hansen J, Francis D, et al: Urokinase and plasminogen activator inhibitor type I in pulmonary adenocarcinoma. *Cancer Res* 1994; 54(1):120-3.

Peng SY, Norman J, Curtin G, et al: Decresed mortality of Norman murine sarcoma in mice treated with immunomodulator, acemannan. *Mol Biother* 1991; 3(2):79-87.

Penn I: "Principles of tumor immunity: immunocompetence and cancer." *Biologic Therapy of Cancer* V DeVita, S Hellman, S Rosenberg editors. Philadelphia: JB Lippincott, 1991.

Pepper MS, Montesano R, Vassalli JD, et al: Chondrocytes inhibit enothelial sprout formation in vitro: evidence for involvement of a transforming growth factor-beta. *J Cell Physiol* 1991; 146(1):170-9.

Persad RA, Gillat DA, Heinemann D, et al: Erythrocyte stearic to oleic acid ratio in prostatic carcinoma. *J Urol* 1990; 65(3):268-70.

Peterson G, Barnes S: Genistein and biochanin A inhibit the growth of human prostate cancer cells but not epidermal growth factor receptor tyrosine autophosphylation. *Prostate* 1993; 22(4):335-45.

Peterson G, Barnes S: Genistein inhibition of the growth of human breast cancer cells: independence from estrogen receptors and the multi-drug resistance gene. *Biochem Biophys Res Commun* 1991; 179(1):661-7.

Piantelli M, Rinelli A, Macri E, Maggiano N, et al: Type II estrogen binding sites and antiproliferative activity of quercetin in human meningiomas. *Cancer* 1993; 71(1):193-8.

Piccoli B, Parazzoli S, Zaniboni A, et al: Non-visual effects of light mediated via the optical route: review of the literature and implications for occupational medicine. *Med Lav* 1991 May-Jun; 82(3):213-32.

Pieri C, Marra M, Moroni F, Recchioni R, Marcheselli F: Melatonin: a peroxyl radical scavenger more effective than vitamin E. *Life Sci* 1994; 55(15):PL271-6.

Pignatelli M, Vessey CJ: Adhesion molecules: novel molecular tools in tumor pathology. *Hum Pathol* 1994; 25(9):849-56.

Pignol B, Etienne A, Crastes de Paulet A, et al: "Role of flavonoids in the oxygen-free radical modulation of the immune response." *Plant flavonoids in Biology and Medicine II* Alan R. Liss, Inc. 1988; 173-82.

Pinsky C, Bose R: Pharmacological and toxicological investigations of cesium. *Phar Biochem & Behavior* 1984; 21(1):17-23.

Piontek, M, Hengels, KJ, Porschen R, Strohmeyer G: Antiproliferative effect of tyrosine kinase inhibitors in epidermal growth factor-stimulated growth of human gastric cancer cells. *Anticancer Res* 1993 Nov-Dec; 13(6A):21 19-23.

Pitton C, Lanson M, Besson P, et al: Presence of PAF-acether in human breast carcinoma: relation to axillary lymph node metastasis. *J Natl Cancer Inst* 1989; 81(17):1298-302.

Pizzorno J, Murray M: Vaccinium Myrtillus. *A Textbook of Natural Medicine* Seattle, John Bastyr College Publications, 1987.

Plotnikof M, Faith W. *Stress and Immunity* Boca Raton, FL: CRC Press; 1991.

Pommier RF, Woltering EA, Milo G, et al: Synergistic cytotoxicity between dimethyl sulfoxide and antineoplastic agents against ovarian cancer in vitro. *Am J Obstet Gynecol* 1988 Oct; 159(4):848-52.

Pommier RF, Woltering EA, Milo G, Fletcher WS: Synergistic cytotoxicity of combinations of dimethyl sulfoxide and antineoplastic agents against P388 leukemia in CD-F1 mice. *Anticancer Drugs* 1992 Dec; 3(6):635-9.

Popowicz, P, Engel G, Marshall H, Linder S: Repression of stromelysin metalloprotease expression in rat fibrosarcoma cells by dimethylsulfoxide. *Clin Exp Metastasis* 1993 Jan; 11(1):77-82.

Potapenko AY, Kyagova AA, Bezdetnaya LN, et al: Products of psoralen photooxidation posess immunomodulative and antileukemic effects. *Photochem Photobiol* 1994; 60(2):171-4.

Powles TJ, Coombes RC, Smith IE, et al: Failure of chemotherapy to prolong survival in a group of paitents with metastic breast cancer. *The Lancet* 1980; March 15:580-2.

Powles TR: "Prostaglandins and cancer: clinical approaches." *Prostaglandins in Cancer Research*. E Garaci, R Paoletti, MG Santoro editors. Berlin: Springer-Verlag; 1987.

Prados J, Melguizo C, Fernandez JE, Aranega AE, et al: Actin, tropomyosin and alpha-actinin as markers of differentiation in human rhabdomyosarcoma cell lines induced with dimethyl sulfoxide. *Cell Mol Biol* 1993 Jul; 39(5):525-36.

Pritchard GA, Jones DL, Mansel RE: Lipids in breast carcinogenesis. *Br J Surg* 1989; 76:1069-73.

Prudden JF: The treatment of human cancer with agents prepared from bovine cartilage. *J Biol Response Mod* 1985; 4(6):551-84.

Prudden JF, Allen J: The clincal acceleration of wound healing with a cartilage preparation. *J Am Med Assoc* 1965; 192:352.

Prudden JF, Balassa LL: The biological activity of bovine cartilage preparations. *Semin Arthritis Rheum* 1974; 3(4):287-321.

Prudden JF, Migel P, Hanson P, et al: The discovery of potent pure chemical wound-healing accelerator. *Am J Surg* 1970; 1 19(5):560-4.

Prudden JF, Wolarsky E: The reversal by cartilage of steroid-induced inhibition of wound healing. *Surg Gynecol Obstet* 1967; 125(1):109-13.

Prudden JF, Wolarsky ER, Balassa LL: The acceleration of healing. *Surg Gynecol Obstet* 1969; 128(6):1321-6.

Purohit V, Ahluwahlia BS, Vigersky RA: Marihuana inhibits dihydrotestoterone binding to the androgen receptor. *Endrocrinology* 1980 Sep; 107(3):848-50.

Qi XG: Protective mechanism of Slavia miltiorrhiza and Paeonia lactiflora for experimental liver damage. *Chung Hsi I Chieh Ho Tsa Chih* 1991 Feb; 11(2):102-4.

Qin LP, Wu H, Zhou QH: Effects of total coumarins, essential oil and water extracts of Cnidium monnieri on plasma prostaglandin and cyclic nucleotide in the rats of kidney yang insufficiency. *Chung Kuo Chung Hsi I Chieh Ho Tsa Chih* 1993; 13(2):100-1.

Qin Z, Den H, Zhuang H: Effect of oxymatrine on prolonging the survival time of the cardiac tissue allograft in mice and its immunologic mechanisms. *Chung Hsi I Chieh Ho Tsa Chih* 1990; 10(2):99-100.

Ralamboranto L, Rakotovao LH, Le Deaut JY, et al: Immunomodulating properties of an extract isolated and partially purified from Aloe vahombe. Study of antitumoral properties and contribution to the chemical nature and active principle. *Arch Inst Pasteur Madagascar* 1982; 50(1):227-56.

Ramanathan R, Das NP, Tan CH: Effects of gamma-linolenic acid, flavonoids, and vitamins on cytotoxicity and lipid peroxidation. *Free Radic Biol Med* 1994a; 16(1):43-8.

Ramnathan R, Das NP, Tan CH: Inhibition of tumor promotion and cell proliferation by plant polyphenols. *Phytother Res* 1994b; 8(5):293-6.

Ranelletti FO, Ricci R, Larocca LM, Maggiano N, et al: Growth-inhibitory effect of quercetin and presence of type-II estrogen-binding sites in human colon-cancer cell lines and primary colorectal tumors. *Int J Cancer* 1992; 50(3):486-92.

Ransberger, K: Use of bromelain in cancer and metasasis treatment. Patent Identification DE 4302060 A1 940728, abstract undated.

Rao CN, Rao VH, Steinmann B: Bioflavonoid-mediated stabalization of collagen in adjuvant-induced arthritis. *Scand J Rheumatol* 1983; 12(1):39-42.

Rao XQ: Clinical and experimental studies of shengxue tang combined with chemotherapy in the treatment of late-stage gastric cancer. *Chung Hsi I Chieh Ho Tsa Chih* 1987; 7(12):715-7, 707.

Rao XQ, Yu RC, Zhang JH: Sheng xue tang on immunological functions of cancer patients with spleen deficiency syndrome. *Chung Hsi I Chieh Ho Tsa Chih* 1991; 11(4):218-9, 197.

Razina TG, Udintsev SN, Prishchep TP, et al: Enhancement of the selectivity of the action of the cytostatics cyclophosphane and 5-fluorouracil by using an extract of the Baikal skullcap in an experiment. *Vopr Onkol* 1987; 33(2):80-4.

Razina TG, Udintsev SN, Tiutrin II, et al: The role of thrombocyte aggregation function in the mechanism of the antimetastatic action of an extract of Baikal skullcap. *Vopr Onkol* 1989; 35(3):331-5.

Reich R, Royce L, Martin GR: Eicosapentaenoic acid reduces the invasive and metastic activities of malignant tumor cells. *Biochem Biophys Res Commun* 1989; 160(2):559-64.

Reichel H, Norman AW: Systemic effects of vitamin D. *Annu Rev Med* 1989; 40:71-8.

Reiter RJ: Interactions of the pineal hormone melatonin with oxygen-centered free radicals: a brief review. *Braz J Med Biol Res* 1993; 26(11):1141-55.

Reiter RJ, Melchiorri D, Sewerynek E, Poeggeler B, et al: A review of the evidence supporting melatonin's role as an antioxidant. *J Pineal Res* 1995; 18(1):1-11.

Rhee YH, Ahn JH, Choe J, et al: Inhibition of mutagenesis and transformation by root extracts of Panax ginseng in vitro. *Planta Medica* 1991; 57:125-28.

Rhodes L, Primka RL, Berman C, Vergult G, et al: Comparison of finasteride (Proscar), a 5 alpha reductase inhibition. *Prostate* 1993; 22(1):43-51.

Richards BA: The enzyme knife—a renewed direction for cancer therapy? *J of the Royal Society of Medicine* 1988; 81:284-5.

Richie JP Jr, Leutzinger Y, Parthasarathy S, et al: Methionine restriction increases blood glutathione and longevity in F344 rats. *FASEB J* 1994 Dec; 8(15):1302-7.

Ring K, Ehle H, Schwarz M: Influence of the flavonoid (+)-catechin on the permeability of ehrlich mouse ascites tumor cell membranes. *Arch Pharmacol* 1976; 294(3):217-24.

Rittenhouse JR, Lui PD, Lau BH: Chinese medicinal herbs reverse macrophage suppression induced by urological tumors. *J Urol* 1991; 146(2):486-90.

Robert L, et al: The effect of procyanidolic oligomers on vascular permeability. A study using quantitative morphology. *Pathol Biol* 1990; 38:608-16.

Rockwell S, Hughes CS, Kennedy KA: Effect of host age on microenvironomental heterogeneity and efficacy of combined modality therapy in solid tumors. *Int J Radiat Biol Phys* 1991; 20(2):259-63.

Roeise O, Sivertsen S, Ruud TE, et al: Studies on components of the contact phase system in patients with advanced gastrointestinal cancer. *Cancer* 1990; 65(6):1355-9.

Rogentine GN, Vankammen DP, Fox BH, et al: Psychological factors in the prognosis of malignant melanoma: a prospective study. *Psychosom Med* 1979; 41:647-55.

Rogers AE, Nields HM, Newberne PM: Nutritional and dietary influences on liver tumorigenesis in mice and rats. *Arch Toxicol Suppl* 1987; 10:231-43.

Rohan TE, Howe GR, Friedenreich GM, et al: Dietary fiber, vitamins A, C, and E, and the risk of breast cancer: a cohort study. *Cancer Causes Control* 1993 Jan; 4(1):29-37.

Romano CF, Lipton A, Harvey HA, et al: A phase II study of Catrix-S in solid tumors. *J Biol Response Mod* 1985 Dec; 4(6):585-9.

Roschlau WHE, Fisher AM: Thrombolytic therapy with local perfusions of CA-7 (fibrinolytic enzyme from aspergillus oryzae) in the dog. *Angiology* 1966; 17:670.

Rose D: Diet hormones, and cancer. *Annu Rev Publ Health* 1993; 14:1-17.

Rosen J, Sherman WT, Prudden JF, et al: Immunoregulatory effects of catrix. *J Biol Response Mod* 1988; 7(5):498-512.

Rosenberg SA: "Adoptive cellular therapy: Graft-versus-tumor responses after bone-marrow transplantation." *Biologic Therapy of Cancer.* VT DeVita, S Hellman, SA Rosenberg editors. Philadelphia: JB Lippincott, 1991.

Rossi-Fanelli F, Cascino A, Muscaritoli M: Abnormal substrate metabolism and nutritional strategies in cancer management. *Journal of Parenteral and Enteral Nutrition* 1991; 15(6):680-3.

Roth J: Tumors—disorders of cell adhesion. *Verh Dtsch Ges Pathol* 1994; 78:22-5.

Rubin D, Laposata M: Cellular interactions between n-6 and n-3 fatty acids; a mass analysis of fatty acid elongation/desturation, distribution among complex lipids, and conversion to eicosanoids. *Journal of Lipid Research* 1992; 33:1431-40.

Rucker G, Mayer R, Shin-Kim JS: Triterpene saponins from the Chinese drug Daxueteng (Caulis sargentodoxae). *Planta Med* 1991; 57(5):468-70.

Rudofsky G: Improving venous tone and capillary sealing. Effect of a combination of Ruscus extract and hesperidine methyl chalcone in healthy probands in heat stress. *Fortschr Med* 1989 Jun 30; 107(19):52, 55-8.

Ryan JJ, Clarke MF: Alteration of p53 conformation and induction of apoptosis in a murine erythroleukemia cell line by dimethylsulfoxide. *Leuk Res* 1994 Aug; 18(8):617-21.

Sadove AM, Keuttner KE: Inhibition of mammary carcinoma invasiveness with cartilage-derived inhibitors. *Surg Forum Orthopaed* 1977; 28:499-501.

Sagesaka-Mitane Y, Miwa M, Okada S: Platelet aggregation inhibitors in hot water extract of green tea. *Chem Pharm Bull* 1990; 38:790-3.

Saito H, Kagawa T, Tada S, Tsunematsu S, et al: Effect of dexamethasone, dimethylsulfoxide and sodium butyrate on a human hepatoma cell line PLC/PRF/5. *Cancer Biochem Biophys* 1992 Nov; 13(2):75-84.

Sakagami H, Asano K, Hara Y, et al: Stimulation of human monocyte and polymorphonuclear cell iodination and interleukin-1 production by epigallocatechin gallate. *J Leukoc Biol* 1992; 51(5):478-83.

Sakaguchi S, Tutumi E, Yokota K, et al: Preventive effects of a Chinese herb medicine (sho-saiko-to) against lethality after recombinant human tumor necrosis factor administration in mice. *Mirobiol Immunol* 1991; 35(5):389-94.

Sakalova A, Mikulecky M, Holomanova D, Langer D, et al: The favorable effect of hydrolytic enzymes in the treatment of immunocytomas and plasmacytomas. *Vnitr Lek* 1992; 38(9):921-9.

Sakamoto S, Kudo H, Kawasaki T, Kuwa K, et al: Effects of a Chinese herbal medicine, keishi-bukuryo-gan, on the gonadal system of rats. *J Ethnopharmacol* 1988 Jul-Aug; 23(2-3):151-8.

Sakamoto S, Mori T, Sawaki K, et al: Effects of Kampo (Japanese herbal) medicine "sho-saiko-to" on DNA-synthesizing enzyme activity in 1,2-dimethylhydrazine-induced colonic carcinomas in rats. *Planta Med* 1993; 59:152-54.

Sakamoto S, Yoshino H, Shirahata Y, Shimodairo K, Okamoto R: Pharmacotherapeutic effects of kuei-chih-fu-ling-wan (keishu-bukuryo-gan) on human uterine myomas. *Amer J Chin Med* 1992; 20(3-4):313-7.

Salama A, Meuller-Eckhardt: Cianidanol and its metabolites bind tightly to red cells and are resposible for the production of auto- and drug-dependent antibodies against these cells. *British Journal of Hematology* 1987; 66:263-66.

Salim AS: Oxygen-derived free-radical scavengers prolong survival in colonic cancer. *Chemotherapy* 1992a; 38(2):127-34.

Salim AS: Oxygen-derived free-radical scavengers prolong survival in gastric cancer. *Chemotherapy* 1992b; 38(2):135-44.

Sanchez-Crespo M, Fernandez-Gallardo S, Nieto ML, et al: Inhibition of the vascular actions of IgG aggregates by BN 52021, a highly specific antagonist of paf-acether. *Immunopharmacology* 1985 Oct; 10(2):69-75.

Sanders TAB, Roshanai F: The influence of different types of w-3 polyunsaturated fatty acids on blood lipids and platelet function in healthy volunteers. *Clinical Science* 1983; 64:91-99.

Sandyk R, Anastasiadis PG, Anninos PA, et al: Is the pineal gland involved in the pathogenesis of endometrial carcinoma. *Int J Neurosci* 1992 Jan; 62(1-2):89-96.

Sankawa U, Chun Y: Anti-allergic substances from chinese medicinal plants. *Advances in Chinese Medicinal Materials Research*. Singapore: World Scientific, 1985.

Sartori HE: Cesium therapy in cancer patients. *Phar Biochem & Behavior* 1984; 21(1):11-13.

Sawyer MG, Gannoni AF, Toogood IR, Antoniou G, Ricw M: The use of alternative therapies by children with cancer. *Med J Aust* 1994; 160(6):323-4.

Saynor R: Effects of fatty acids on serum lipids. *The Lancet* 1984; September 14:696-97.

Scambia G, Benedetti Panici P, Ranelletti FO, et al: Quercetin enhances transforming growth factor B_1 secretion by human ovarian cancer cells. *Int J Cancer* 1994a; 57:211-15.

Scambia G, Ranelletti FO, Benedetti PP, Bonanno G, et al: Synergistic antiproliferative activity of quercetin and cisplatin on ovarian cancer cell growth. *Anticancer Drugs* 1990a; 1(1):45-8.

Scambia G, Ranelletti FO, Benedetti PP, et al: Quercetin potentiates the effect of adriamycin in a multidrug-resistant MCF-7 human breast-cancer cell line; P-glycoprotein as a possible target. *Cancer Chemother Pharmacol* 1994b; 34:459-64.

Scambia G, Ranelletti FO, Benedetti PP, Piantelli M, et al: Quercetin inhibits the growth of a multidrug-resistant estrogen-receptor-negative MCF-7 human breast-cancer cell line expressing type II estrogen-binding sites. *Cancer Chemother Pharmacol* 1991; 28(4):255-8.

Scambia G, Ranelletti FO, Panici PB, et al: Inhibitory effect of quercetin on OVCA 433 cells and presence of type II oestrogen binding sites in primary ovarian tumours and cultured cells. *Br J Cancer* 1990b Dec; 62(6):942-946.

Scambia G, Ranelletti FO, Panici PB, Piantelli M, et al: Quercetin induces type-II estrogen-binding sites in estrogen-receptor-negative (MDA-MB231) and estrogen-receptor-positive (MCF-7) human breast-cancer cell lines. *Int J Cancer* 1993; 54(3):462-6.

Schapira DV: Nutrition and cancer prevention. *Prim Care* 1992; 19(3):481-91.

Schlappack OK, Zimmermann A, Hill RP: Microenvironmental influences on metastic ability and drug sensitivity of murine tumor cells (meeting abstract). *Proc Annu Meet Am Assoc Cancer Res* 1990; 31:A406.

Schleifer SJ, et al: Supression of lymphocyte stimulation following bereavement. *JAMA* 1983; 250:374-7.

Scholar EM, Wolterman K, Birt DF, et al: The effect of diets enriched in cabbage and collards on murine pulmonary metastasis. *Nutr Cancer* 1989; 12:121-26.

Schuff-Werner P, Lohr G, Rauschning W, et al: Effect of thymostimulin on chemotherapy-induced changes in lymphocyte subset distribution. A longitudinal study in patients with primary inoperable oropharyngeal cancers. *Onkologie* 1987; 10(3 Suppl):17-21.

Schuschke DA, Reed MW, Saari JT, Olson MD, et al: Short-term dietary copper deficiency does not inhibit angiogenesis in tumours implanted in striated muscle. *Br J Cancer* 1992; 66(6):1059-64.

Schwartz EL, Chamberlin H, Ravichander P, Whitbread JA: Dimethyl sulfoxide inhibits the binding of granulocyte/macrophage colony-stimulating factor and insulin to their receptors on human leukemia cells. *Cancer Res* 1993 Mar 1; 53(5):1142-8.

Schwartz MA, Ingber DE: Integrating with integrins. *Mol Biol Cell* 1994; 5(4):389-93.

Schwartzman RA, Cidlowski JA: Apoptosis: The biochemistry and molecular biology of programmed cell death. *Endocrine Reviews* 1993; 14(2):133-45.

Schweigerer L, Christeleit K, Fleischmann G, Adlercreutz H, et al: Identification in human urine of a natural growth inhibitor for cells derived from solid paediatric tumours. *Eur J Clin Invest* 1992; 22(4):260-4.

Schwitters B, Masquelier J. *OPC in practice; bioflavinoids and their application.* Rome, Italy: Alfa Omega Publishers 1993.

Sciacca FL, Sturzl M, Bussolini F, et al: Expression of adhesion molecules, platelet-activating factor and chemokines by kaposi's sarcoma cells. *J Immunol* 1994; 153(10):4816-25.

Scott PA, Harris A: Current approaches to targeting cancer using antiangiogenesis therapies. *Cancer Treatment Reviews* 1994; 20:393-412.

Scutt A, Meghji S, Canniff JP, et al: Stabalisation of collagen by betel nut polyphenols as a mechanism in oral submucous fibrosis. *Experientia* 1987; 43(4):391-3.

See WA, Xia Q: Regional chemotherapy for bladder neoplasms using continuous intravesical infusion of doxorubicin: impact of concomitant administration of dimethyl sulfoxide on drug absorption and antitumor activity. *J Natl Cancer Inst* 1992 Apr 1; 84(7):510-5.

Seligman M, Beagley G: Learned helplessness in the rat. *J Comp and Physiol Psych* 1975; 88:534-41.

Serraino M, Thompson L: The effect of flaxseed supplementation on the initiation and promotional stages of mammary tumorigenesis. *Nutr Cancer* 1992; 17:153-59.

Sersa G, Miklavcic D, Bastista U, Novakovic S, et al: Antitumor effect of electrotherapy alone or in combination with interleukin-2 in mice with sarcoma and melanoma tumors. *Anticancer Drugs* 1992; 3930; 253-60.

Sersa G, Novakovic S, Miklavcic D: Potentiation of bleomycin antitumor effectiveness by electrotherapy. *Cancer Lett* 1993; 69(2):81-4.

Sessions JL, Walker M. *Coping with Cancer.* Greenwich CT: Devin Adair, 1985.

Setchell KDR, Borriello SP, Hulme P, et al: Nonsteroidal estrogens of dietary origin: possible roles in hormone-dependent disease. *Am J of Clin Nutr* 1984; 40:569-78.

Shen ML, Zhai SK, Chen HL, et al: Immunomopharmacological effects of polysaccharides from Acanthopanax senticosus on experimental animals. *Int J Immunopharmacol* 1991; 13(5):549-54.

Shen TY, Hwang SB, Chang MN, et al: The isolation and characterization of kadsurenone from haifenteng (Piper futokadsura) as an orally active specific receptor antagonist of platelet-activating factor. *Int J Tissue React* 1985; 7(5):339-43.

Shi J: Experimental pharmacological studies on the volatile oil of wen-e-zhu (Curcuma aromatica salisb.): study on the antitumor activity of beta-elemene. *Zhongyao Tongbao* 1981; 6(6):32-3.

Shibata S: "Chemical studies on chinese medicinal materials." *Advances in Chinese Medicinal Materials Research* HM Chang, HW Yeung, WW Tso, A Koo editors. Singapore: World Scientific, 1985.

Shibib BA, Khan LA, Rahman R:Hypoglycemic activity of Coccinia indica and Momordica charantia in diabetic rats: depression of the hepatic gluconeogenic enzymes ... . *Biochem J* 1993; 292 (Pt 1):267-70.

Shikano M, Masuzawa Y, Yazawa K: Effect of docosahexaenoic acid on the generation of platelet-activating factor by eosinophilic leukemia cells, Eol-1. *J Immunol* 1993; 150(8 Pt 1):3525-33.

Shinkai K, Mukai M, Akedo H: Superoxide radical potentiates invasive capacity of rat ascites hapatoma cells in vitro. *Cancer Letters* 1986; 32:7-13.

Shinomiya N, Shinomiya M, Wakiyama H, et al: Enhancement of CDDP cytotoxicity by caffeine is characterized by apoptotic cell death. *Exp Cell Res* 1994; 210(2):236-42.

Shively FL: *Multiple Proteolytic Enzyme Therapy of Cancer.* Dayton: Johnson-Watson Printing & Bookbinding Co, 1969.

Shultz TD, Santamaria AG, Gridley DS, et al: Effect of pyridoxine and pyridoxal on the in vitro growth of human malignant melanoma. *Anticancer Res* 1988 Nov-Dec; 8(6):1313-8.

Shvarev IF, Tsetlin AL: Antiblastic properties of berberine and its derivatives. *Farmakol Tsoikol* 1972; 35(1):73-5.

Siguel EN: Cancerostatic effect of vegetarian diets. *Nutr Cancer* 1983; 4(4):285-291.

Simons LA, Hickie JB, Balasubramaniam S: On the effects of dietary n-3 fatty acids (maxepa) on plasma lipids and lipoproteins in patients with hyper lipidemia. *Atherschlerosis* 1985; 54:75-88.

Simonton OC, Matthews-Simonton S, Sparks TF: Psycological intervention in the treatment of cancer. *Psychosomatic* 1980; 21(3):226-33.

Skotnicki AB: Therapeutic application of calf thymus extract (TFX). *Med Oncol Tumor Pharmacother* 1989; 6(1):31-43.

Sloman R, Brown P, Aldana E, Chee E: The use of relaxation for the promotion of comfort and pain relief in persons with advanced cancer. *Contemp Nurse* 1994; 3(1):6-12.

Smillie MV, Griffiths LA, Male PJ, et al: The disposition and metabolism of (+)-cyanidanol-3 in patients with alcoholic cirrhosis. *Eur J Pharmacol* 1987; 33:255-59.

Smith BL: Organic foods vs. supermarket foods: element levels. *J Appl Nutrition* 1993; 45(1):35-9.

Smith KL, Tisdale MJ: Mechamism of muscle protein degradation in cancer cachexia. *Br J Cancer* 1993; 68(2):314-8.

Solomon GF: Stress and antibody response in rats. *Inter Archives of Allergy* 1969; 35:97-104.

Spiegel D, Bloom JR, Kraemer HC, et al: Effect of psychosocial treatment on survival of patients with metastatic breast cancer. *The Lancet* 1989; Oct 14; 888-91.

Spinks EA, Fenwick GR: The determination of glycyrrhizin in selected UK licorice products. *Food addit Contam* 1990; 7(6):769-78.

Spinozzi F, Pagliacci MC, Migliorati G, et al: The natural tyrosine kinase inhibitor genistein produces cell cycle arrest and apoptosis in Jurkat T-leukemia cells. *Leuk Res* 1994; 18(6):431-9.

Stamp D, Zhang XM, Medline A, Bruce WR, Archer MC: Sucrose enhancement of the early steps of colon carcinogenesis in mice. *Carcinogenesis* 1993; 14(4):777-9.

Stavraky KM: Psychological factors in the outcome of human cancer. *J Psychosom Res* 1968; 12:251-9.

Steinmetz KA, Potter JD: Vegetables, fruit, and cancer. *Cancer Causes Control* 1991; 2(6):427-42.

Stetler-Stevenson WG: The balance of matrix metalloproteinases and their inhibitors: a critical deterent of tumor invasion and angiogensis. *Proc Annu Meet Am Assoc Cancer Res* 1992; 33:A573-4.

Stetler-Stevenson WG, Aznavoorian S, Liotta LA: Tumor cell interactions with the extracellular matrix during invasion and metastasis. *Annu Rev Cell Biol* 1993; 9:541-73.

Stio M, Iantomasi T, Favilli F et al: Glutathione metabolism in heart and liver of the aging rat. *Biochem Cell Biol* 1994 Jan-Feb; 72(1-2):58-61.

Stolk LML, Siddiqui AH: Biopharmaceutics, pharmacokinetics and pharmacology of psoralens. *Gen Pharmac* 1988; 19(5):649-53.

Stone OJ: Pyridoxine deficiency and antagonism produce increased ground substance viscosity with resulting seborrheic dermatitis and increased tumor resistance. *Med Hypothesis* 1989; 30(4):277-80.

Stormer R, Reistad R, Alexander J: Glycyrrhizic acid in licorice-evaluation of health hazard. *Fd Chem Toxic* 1993; 31(4):303-12.

Stryer L: *Biochemistry*. New York: W.H. Freeman and Company; 1988.

Sudsuang R, Chentanez V, Veluvan: Effect of Buddhist meditation on serum cortisol and total protein levels, blood pressure, pulse rate, lung volume and reaction time. *Physiol Behav* 1991; 50(3):543-8.

Suffness M, Douros J: Chapter III: Drugs of plant origin. *Methods in Cancer Research, Vol. XVI*. Academic Press, Inc: 1979.

Suffness M, Newman D, Snader K: Discovery and development of antineoplastic agents from natural sources. *Bioorganic Marine Chemistry, Vol 3*. Berlin: Springer-Verlag, 1989.

Suffness M, Pezzuto JM: Assays related to cancer drug discovery. *Methods in Plant Biochemistry Vol. 6*. Academic Press Limited, 1991.

Suganuma M, Komori A, Okabe S, et al: Mechanisms of anticarcinogenic action of EGCG and tea polyphenols. *13th Internation Symposium on Cancer (Meeting Abstract)* 1993; p. 23.

Sugimura M, Kobayashi H, Terao T: Plasmin modulators, aprotunun and anti-catalytic plasmin antibody, efficiently inhibit destruction of bovine vascular endothelial cells by choriocarcinoma cells. *Gynecol Oncol* 1994; 52(3):337-46.

Sugiura H, Nishida H, Inaba R, Iwata H: [Effects of exercise in the growing stage in mice and of Astragalus membranaceus on immune function.] *Nippon Eiseigaku Zasshi* 1993; 47(6):1021-31.

Sultan C, Terraza A, Devillier C, Carilla E, et al: Inhibition of androgen metabolism and binding by a liposterolic extract of Serenoa repens B in human foreskin fibroblasts. *J Steroid Biochem* 1984 Jan; 20(1):515-9.

Sun WJ, Ma N, Ma LX, Zhang YL, Feng WL: [The effect of ginseng stem, leaf and rhizoma saponins on the formation of lipid peroxides in rats of various ages.] *Chung Kuo Chung Yao Tsa Chih* 1989; 14(5):300-2,319-20.

Sun Y: The role of traditional Chinese medicine in supportive care of cancer patients. *Recent Results in Cancer Research* 1988; 108:327-334.

Sun Y, Hersh EM, Talpaz M, et al: Immune restoration and/or augmentation of local graft versus host reaction by traditional Chinese medicinal herbs. *Cancer* 1983; 52(1):70-3.

Suzuki F, Schmitt A, Utsunomiya T, et al: Stimulation of host resistance against tumors by glycyrrhizin, an active component of licorice roots. *In Vivo* 1992; 6:589-96.

Suzuki M, Nikaido T, Ohmoto T: The study of Chinese herbal medicinal prescription with enzyme inhibitory activity. *Jpn Yakugaku Zasshi* 1991; 111(11):695-701.

Suzuki T, Koayashi Y, Uchida MK, et al: Calcium antagonist-like actions of coumarins isolated from qian-hu on anaphylactic mediator release from mast cell induced by concanavalin. *J Pharmacobiodyn* 1985; 8(4):257-63.

Sweet F, Kao MS, Lee SCD: Ozone selectively inhibits growth of human cancer cells. *Science* 1980; 209(22):931-2.

Takabe H, Yagi T, Satoh Y: Cancer-prone hereditary diseases in relation to DNA repair. *International Cancer Congress, Part B, Biology of Cancer*. EA Mirand, WB Hutchinson, E Mihich, eds. New York: Alan R. Liss, 1983.

Takahashi H, Horikoshi T, Wakamatsu K, Ito S, Parsons PG: Alteration of melanoma melanogenesis by phenotypic modifiers. *J Dermatol* 1992 Nov; 19(11):814-7.

Takahashi K, Kitao M: Effect of TJ-68 (shakuyaku-kanzo-to) on polycystic ovarian disease. *Int J Fertil Menopausal Stud* 1994 Mar-Apr; 39(2):69-76.

Takeda Y, Tominaga T, Tei N, et al: Inhibitory effect of L-arginine on growth of rat mammary tumors induced by 7, 12-dimethylbenz(a)anthracene. *Cancer Res* 1975; 35:2390-3.

Takeuchi T, Nishii O, Okamura T, Yaginuma T: Effect of traditional herbal medicine, shakuyaku-kanzo-to on total and free serum testosterone levels. *Am J Chin Med* 1989; 17(1-2):35-44.

Takeuchi T, Nishii O, Okamura T, Yaginuma T: Effects of paeoniflorin, glycyrrhizin and glycyrrhetic acid on ovarian androgen production. *Am J Chin Med* 1991; 19(1):73-8.

Tamaoki J, Takeyama K, Chiyotani A, et al: Stimulation of Na absorption by the antiasthmatic Kampo drug Saiboku-to in cultured airway epithelium. *Jpn J Pharmacol* 1992; 58(1):47-53.

Tanaka, M: The effect of glycyrrhizin on carcinogenesis in the duodenum of mice given N-ethyl-N'-nitro-N-nitrosoguanidine. *Kyoto-furitsu Ika Daigaku Zasshi* 1991; 100(12):1139-46.

Tanaka T, Kojima T, Kawamori T, et al: Inhibition of 4-nitroquinoline-1-oxide-induced rat tongue carcinogenesis by the naturally occurring plant phenolics caffeic, ellagic, chlorogenic and ferulic acids. *Carcinogenesis* 1993; 14(7):1321-5.

Taniguchi S, Fujiki H, Kobayashi H, et al: Effect of (-)-epigallocatechin gallate, the main constituent of green tea, on lung metastasis with mouse B16 melanoma cell lines. *Cancer Letters* 1992; 65:51-4.

Tannock IF, Hill RP, editors. *The Basic Science of Oncology* 2nd edition. New York: Mc Graw-Hill, Inc.; 1992.

Tapadinhas JM, Rivera IC, Bignamini AA: Oral glucosamine sulphate in the management of arthrosis: report on a multicentre open investigation in Portugal. *Pharmatherapeutica* 1982; 3(3):157.

Tas MP, Simons PJ, Balm FJ, et al: Depressed monocyte polarization and clustering of dendritic cells in patients with head and neck cancer. *Cancer Immunol Immunother* 1993; 36(2):108-14.

Tatarintsev AV, Vrzhets PV, Ersshov DE, Shchegolev AA, et al: The ajoene blockade of integrin-dependent processes in an HIV- infected cell system *Vestn Ross Akad Med Nauk* 1992; (11-12):6-10.

Tatsuta M, Iishi H, Baba M, et al: Inhibition by xiao-chai-hutang (TJ-9) of development of hepatic foci induced by N-nitrosomorpholine in Sprague-Dawley rats. *Jpn J Cancer Res* 1991; 82(9):987-92.

Taubes G: Pesticides and breast cancer: no link? [news] *Science* 1994 Apr 22; 264(5158):499-500.

Taussig SJ: The Mechanism of the psychological action of bromelain. *Med Hypotheses* 1980; 6:99-104.

Taussig SJ, Batkin S: Bromelain, the enzyme complex of pineapple (Ananas comosus) and its clinical application. An update. *J of Ethnopharmacol* 1988; 22:191-203.

Taussig SJ, Szekerczes J, Batkin S: Inhibition of tumour growth in vitro by bromelain, an extract of the pineapple plant (ananas comosus). *Planta Medica* 1985; 538-9.

Teicher BA, Holden SA, Rudolph MB, Sotomayor EA, Herman TS: Effect of environmental conditions (pH, oxygenation and temperature) on the cytotoxicity of flavone acetic acid and its dimethylaminoethyl ester. *Int J Hyperthermia* 1991; 7(6):905-15.

Temoshok L: Biopsychosocial studies on cutaneous malignant melanoma: Psychosocial factors associated with prognostic indicators, progression, psychophysiology, and tumor-host response. *Soc Sci Med* 1985; 20:833-40.

Teofili L, Pierelli L, Iovino MS, Leone G, et al: The combination of quercetin and cytosine arabinoside synergistically inhibits leukemic cell growth. *Leuk Res* 1992; 16(5):497-503.

Thompson WD, Harvey JA, Kazmi MA, et al: Fribrinolysis and angiogensis in wound healing. *UK J Pathol* 1991; 165(4):311-8.

Thompson WD, Smith EB, Stirk CM, et al: Angiogenic activity of fibrin degradation products is located in fibrin fragment E. *UK J Pathol* 1992; 168(1):47-53.

Thompson WD, Smith EB, Stirk CM, et al: Atherosclerotic plaque growth: presence of stimulatory fibrin degradation products. *Blood Caogul Fibrinolysis* 1990a; 1(4-5):489-93.

Thompson WD, Smith EB, Stirk CM, et al: Factors relevant to stimulatory activity of fibrin degradation products in vivo. *Blood Coagul Fibrinolysis* 1990b; 1(4-5):517-20.

Thorgeirsson U, Turpeenniemi-Hujanen T, Liotta L: "Mechanisms of tumor invasion and their potential therapeutic modifications." *Biological Responses in Cancer: Progress Toward Potential Applications* Vol 1. E Mihich editor. New York: Plenum Press, 1985.

Thuning CA, Fanshaw MS, Warren J: Mechanisms of the synergistic effect of oral dimethyl sulfoxide on antineoplastic therapy. *Annals of the New York Academy of Sciences* 1983; 411:150-60.

Tierney LM, Mc Phee SJ, Papadakis MA, et al. editors. *Current Medical Diagnosis and Treatment* Norwalk, CT: Appleton & Lange; 1993.

Tierra M. *Planetary Herbology* Twin Lakes: Lotus Press, 1988.

Tilly JL, Billig H, Kowalski KI, Hsueh AJ: Epidermal growth factor and basic fibroblast growth factor supress the spontaneous onset of apoptosis in cultured rat ovarian granulosa cells and follicles by a tyrosine kinase-dependent mechanism. *Mol Endocrinol* 1992; 6(11):1942-50.

Tisdale MJ: Mechanism of lipid mobilization associated with cancer cachexia: interaction between the polyunsaturated fatty acid, eicosapentaenoic acid, and inhibitory guanine nucleotide-regulatory protein. *Prostaglandins Leukot Essent Fatty Acids* 1993; 48(1):105-9.

Tisdale MJ, Beck SA: Inhibition of tumour-induced lipolysis in vitro and cachexia and tumour growth in vivo by eicosapentaenoic acid. *Biochemical Pharmacology* 1991; 41(1):103-7.

Tixier JM, Godeau G, Robert AM, et al: Evidence by in vivo and in vitro studies that binding of pycnogenols to elastin affects its rate of degradation by elastases. *Biochem Pharmacol* 1984 Dec 15; 33(24):3933-9.

REFERENCES

Toda S, Kimura M, Ohnishi M, et al: Effects of the chinese herbal medicine saiboku-to on histamine release from and the degranulation of mouse peritoneal mast cells induced by compound 48/80. *J Ethnopharmacol* 1988; 24(2-3):303-9.

Toma S, Micheletti A, Giachero A, et al: Selenium therapy in patients with precancerous and malignant oral cavity lesions: preliminary results. *Cancer Detection and Prevention* 1991; 15(6):491-94.

Toren A, Rechavi G: What really cures in autologous bone marrow transplantation? *Med Hypotheses* 1993 Dec; 41(6):495-8.

Traganos F, Ardelt B, Halko N, Bruno S, Darzynkiewicz Z: Effects of genistein on the growth and cell cycle progression of normal human lymphocytes and human leukemic MOLT-4 and HL-60 cells. *Cancer Res* 1992; 52(22):6200-8.

Traganos F, Kapuscinski J, Gong J, et al: Caffeine prevents apoptosis and cell cycle effects induced by camptothecin or topotecan in HL-60 cells. *Cancer Res* 1993; 53(19):4613-8.

Treleaven J, Meller S, Farmer P, et al: Arsenic and ayurveda. *Leuk Lymphoma* 1993; 10(4-5):343-5.

Troll W, Klassen A, Janoff A: Tumorigenesis in mouse skin: inhibition by synthetic inhibitors of proteases. *Science* 1970 Sep 18; 169(451):1211-3.

Tseng J, Chang JG: Suppression of tumor necrosis factor-alpha interleukin-1 beta, interleukin-6 and granulocyte-monocyte stimulating factor secretion from human monocytes by an extract of Poria cocos. *Chung Hua Min Kuo Wei Sheng Wu Chi Mien I Hsueh Tsa Chih* 1992; 25(1):1-11.

Tsopanoglou NE, Pipili-Synetos E, Maragoudakis ME: Thrombin promotes angiogenesis by a mechanism independent of fibrin formation. *Am J Physiol* 1993 May; 264(5 Pt 1):C1302-7.

Tsuraga T, Ebizuka Y, Nakajima J, et al: Biologically active constituents of magnolia salicifolia; inhibitors of induced histamine release from rat mast cells. *Chem Pharm Bull* 1991; 39(12):3265-71.

Tsutani H, Ueda T, Uchida M, et al: Pharmacological studies of the retinol palmitate and its clinical effect in patients with acute non-lymphocytic leukemia. *Leuk Res* 1991; 15(5):335-40.

Tucker EJ, Carrizo A: Haemotoxylon dissolved in dymethylsulfoxide used in recurrent neoplasms. *Internal Surgery* 1968; 49(6):516-27.

Tufte MJ, et al: The response of colon carcinoma in mice to cesium, zinc and vitamin A. *Phar Biochem & Behavior* 1984; 21(1):25-26.

Uchida S, Hisashi O, Edamatsu R, et al: "Active oxygen free radicals are scavenged by condensed tannins." *Plant Flavonoids in Biology and Medicine II* Alan R. Liss, Inc. 1988; 135-38.

Uchida Y, Katori M: Independent consumption of high and low molecular weight kininogens in vivo. *Adv Exp Med Biol* 1986; 198 PtA:113-8.

Ueno I, Nakano N, Hirono I: Metabolic fate of [14C] quercetin in the ACI rat. *Jpn J Exp Med* 1983; 53(1):41-50.

Umehara K, Sugawa A, Kuroyanagi M, et al: Studies on differentiation-inducers from arctium fructus. *Chem Pharm Bull* 1993; 41(10):1774-9.

Umehara K, Takagi R, Kuroyanagi M, et al: Studies on differentiation-inducing activities of triterpenes. *Chem Pharm Bull* 1992; 40(2):401-5.

Umeyana A, Shoji N, Takei M, et al: Ciwujianosides D1 and C1; powerful inhibitors of histamine release induced by anti-immunoglobulin E from rat peritoneal mast cells. *J Pharm Sci* 1992; 81(7):661-2.

Unverferth DV, Mehegan JP, Nelson RW, et al: The efficacy of N-acetyl cysteine in preventing doxorubicin-induced cardiomyopathy in dogs. *Seminars in Oncology* 1983; 10(1) supp 1:2-6.

Ushio Y: Effect of ginsenoside Rgl on the release of enzymes by cultured endothelial cells. *Am J Chin Med* 1992; 20(1):91-101.

Usuki S: Effects of hachimijiogan, tokishakuyakusan, keishibukuryogan, ninjinto and unkeito on estrogen and progesterone secretion in preovulatory follicles incubated in vitro. *Am J Chin Med* 1991; 19(1):65-71.

Usuki S: Hachimijiogan produces testosterone in adult rat testes. *Am J Chin Med* 1988; 16(3-4):93-105.

Van der Merwe SA, Van der Berg AP, Van der Zee et al: Measurement of tumor pH during microwave induced experimental and clinical hyperthermia with fiber optic pH measurement system. *Int J Radiat Oncol Biol Phys* 1990; 18(1):51-7.

Van der Zee J, Van der Berg AP, Broekmeyer-Reurink MP: Temperature and pH during hyperthermic perfusion (meeting abstract). Thirty-seventh Annual Meeting of the Radiation Research Society and Ninth Annual Meeting of the North American Hyperthermia Group. March 18-23, 1989, Seattle, WA, 1989. p. 105.

Van der Zouwe N, Van Dam FS, Aaronson NK, Hanewald GJ: Alternative treatments in cancer; extent and background of utilization. *Ned Tijdschr Geneeskd* 1994; 138(6):300-6.

Van Miert AS: Extrapolation of pharmacological and toxicological data based on metabolic weight. *Arch Exp Veterinar med* 1989; 43(4):481-8.

Van Poppel G: Carotenoids and cancer: an update with emphasis on human intervention studies. *Eur J Cancer* 1993; 29A(9):1335-44.

Vane JR: "Anti-inflammatory drugs and the arachidonic acid cascade." *Prostaglandins in Cancer Research* E Garaci, R Paoletti, MG Santora editors. Berlin: Springer-Verlag, 1987.

Vanhove PH, Donati MB, Claeys R, et al: Action of brinase on human fibrinogen and plasminogen. *Thrombos Haemostas* 1979; 42:571.

Vasterling J, Jenkins RA, Tope DM, Burish TG: Cognitive distraction and relaxation training for the control of side

293

effects due to cancer chemotherapy. *J Behav Med* 1993; 16(1):65-80.

Vaughan-Jones, RD: Regulation of intracellular pH in cardiac muscle. *Proton passage across cell membrane* Ciba Foundation Symposium 139. Sussex: John Wiley & Sons, 1988.

Vaz AL: Double-blind clinical evaluation of the relative efficacy of ibuprofen and glucosamine sulphate in the management of osteoarthritis of the knee in out-patients. *Curr Med Res Opin* 1982; 8:145-9.

Verma AK, Johnson JA, Gould MN, et al: Inhibition of 7,12-dimethylbenz(a)antracene- and n-nitrosommethylurea-induced rat mammary cancer by dietary flavonol quercetin. *Cancer Res* 1988; 48:5754-58.

Vesey DA, Cunningham JM, Selden AC, Woodman AC, Hodgson HJ: Dimethyl sulphoxide induces a reduced growth rate, altered cell morphology and increased epidermal-growth-factor binding in Hep G2 cells. *Biochem J* 1991 Aug 1; 277(Pt 3):773-7.

Vessey SH: Effects of grouping on levels of circulating antibodies in mice. *Proceedings of the Society for Biology* 1964; 115:252-5.

Visudhiphan S, Poolsuppasit S, Piboonnukarintr O, et al: The relationship between high fibrinolytic activity and daily capsicum ingestion in Thais. *Am J Clin Nutr* 1982; 35(6):1452-8.

Vitaliano PP, Lipscomb PA, Carr JE: Letter to the Editor *New Engl J Med* 1985; 313:1355.

Vlietinck AJ, Dommisse RA: *Advances in Medicinal Plant Research: plenary Lectures of the 32nd International Congress on Medicinal Plant Research, Antwerp, July 23-28, 1984.* Stuttgart: Wissenschaftliche Verlagsgesellschaft, 1985.

Vodovnik L, Miklavcic D, Sersa G: Modified cell proliferation due to electrical currents. *Med Biol Eng Comput* 1992; 30(4):CE21-8.

Vogel G, Marek ML, Oertner R: Mechanisms of therapeutic and toxic actions of the horse chestnut saponin escin. *Arzneim-Forsch* 1970; 20(5):699-703.

Vogel G, Stroecker H: Effect of pharmacologically active principles, especially flavonoids and escine, on lymph flow and permeability of the intact plasma-lymph barrier for fluids and defined macromolecules in rats. *Arzneim-Forsch* 1966; 16(12):1630-4.

Vogel R, Assjaig-Machleid I, Ester A, et al: Proteinase-sensitive regions in the heavy chain of low molecular weight kininogen map to the inter-domain junctions. *Journal of Biological Chemistry* 1988; 263(25):12661-8.

Von Ardenne M: Fundamentals of combating cancer metastasis by oxygen multistep immunostimulation processes. *Medical Hypothesis* 1985; 17:47-65.

Von Ardenne M: Selective multiphase cancer therapy: conceptual aspects and experimental basis. *Adv Pharmacol Chemother* 1972; 10:339-380.

Wada H, Kumeda Y, Ogasawara Z, et al: Stimulation of tissue type plasminogen activator by leukaemic cell homogenates. *Blood Coagul Fibrolysis* 1993; 4(4):591-7.

Wagner H: "Immunostimulants from medicinal plants." *Advances in Chinese Medicinal Materials Research* Chang HM, Yeung W, Tso W, Koo A editors. Singapore: World Scientific, 1985.

Walker BR, Edwards CR: Licorice induced hypertension and syndromes apparent mineralocorticoid excess. *Endocrine Metab Clin North Am* 1994; 23(2):359-77.

Walker M. *DMSO Nature's Healer* New York: Avery Publishing, 1993.

Wallerstein R Jr, Davidson W, Dutcher J, et al: Safety, efficacy, and preliminary anticancer activity of blood tryptophan depletion (BTD) therapy using a new extracorporeally placed device. (Meeting abstract). *Proc Annu Meet Am Soc Clin Oncol* 1990; 9:A317.

Walters R: *Options: The Alternative Cancer Therapy Book.* Garden City Park, NY: Avery Publishing Group, Inc; 1993.

Wang B, Cui J, Lui A: The effect of ginseng on immune responses. *Advances in Chinese Medicinal Materials Research.* Singapore: World Scientific, 1985.

Wang DQ, Shen WM, Tian YP, Yun SM, Jiang CG: [The effect of honey-frying on anti-oxidation activity of Astragalus mongholicus Bunge.] *Chung Kuo Chung Yao Tsa Chih* 1994; 19(3):150-2,190.

Wang GT: Treatment of operated late gastric carcinoma with prescription of strengthening the patient's resistance and dispelling the invading evil in combination with chemotherapy: followup study of 158 patients and experimental study in animals. *Chung Hsi I Chieh Ho Tsa Chih* 1990; 10(12):712-6, 707.

Wang GT, Xu JY, Zheng A, et al: Treatment of operated late gastric carcinoma with prescriptions of 'strengthen the patient's resistance and dispel the invading evil' in combination with chemotherapy: follow-up study of 158 patients and experimental study in animals (Meeting Abstract) *First Shanghai International Symposium on Gastrointestinal Cancers.* November 14-16, 1988. p. 244.

Wang JD, Narui T, Kurata H, et al: Hemotological studies on naturally occuring substances. Effects of animal crude drugs on blood coagulation and fibrinolysis systems. *Chem Pharm Bull* (Tokyo) 1989; 37(8):2236-8.

Wang JP, Hsu MF, Teng, CM: Antiplatelet effect of capsaicin. *Thrombosis Research* 1984a; 36:497-507.

Wang JZ, Tsumura H, Ma N, et al: Biochemical and morphological alterations of macrophages and spleen cells produced by antitumor polysaccharide from Acanthopanax obovatus roots. *Planta Med* 1993a; 59(1):54-8.

Wang JZ, Tsumura H, Shimura K, et al: Antitumor activity of polysaccharide from a Chinese medicinal herb, Acanthopanax giraldii Harms. *Cancer Lett* 1992a; 65(1):79-84.

Wang KR, Zhao YL, Wang DS, et al: Effects of traditional Chinese herbs, toad tincture and adenosine 3',5' cAMP on

Ehrlich ascites tumor cells in mice. *Chinese Medical Journal* 1982a; 95(7):527-32.

Wang Q, Chen SQ, Zhang ZH: Determiniation of polysaccharide contents in fructus Lycii. *Chinese Traditional and Herbal Drugs* 1991; 22(2):67-8.

Wang S, Zhu G: Effects of Codonopsis pilosulae on the synthesis of thromboxane A2 and prostacyclin. *Chung Hsi I Chieh Ho Tsa Chih* 1990; 10(7):391-4.

Wang SR, Guo ZQ, Liao JZ: Experimental study on the effects of 18 kinds of Chinese herbal medicine for synthesis of thromboxane A2 and PGI2. *Chung Kuo Chung Hsi I Chieh Ho Tsa Chih* 1993b; 13(3):167-70.

Wang XM, Zie ZF: Effects of wuzi yanzong liquid on hypothalamus, monoamines, sexual hormones and reproductivity in male rats. *Chung Kuo Chung Hsi I Chieh Ho Tsa Chih* 1993 Jun; 13(6):349-51, 325-6.

Wang XQ, Gan WJ, Yang TY, et al: Effect of indirubin on the cell surface of chronic myoelocytic leukemia. *Tianjin Yiyao* 1984b; 12(12):707-10.

Wang Y, Ma R: Effect of an extract of paeonia lactiflora on the blood coagulative and fibrinolytic enzymes. *Chi Chung Hsi I Chieh Ho Tsa Chih* 1990; 10(2):101-2.

Wang Y, Qian XJ, Hadley HR, et al: Phytochemicals potentiate interleukin-2 generated lymphokine activated killer cell cytotoxicity against murine renal cell carcinoma. *Mol Biother* 1992b; 4(3):143-6.

Wang Z, Roberts JM, Grant PG, et al: The effect of a medicinal Chinese herb on platelet function. *Thromb Haemost* 1982b; 48(3):301-6.

Wang ZY, Huang MT, Ho CT, et al: Inhibitory effect of green tea on the growth of established skin papillomas in mice. *Cancer Res* 1992c; 52(23):6657-65.

Wargovich MJ: New dietary anticarcinogens and prevention of gastrointestinal cancer. *Dis Colon Rectum* 1988; 31:72-75.

Wargovich MJ, Lynch PM, Levin B: Modulating effects of calcium in animal models of colon carcinogenesis and short-term studies in subjects at increased risk for colon cancer. *Am J Clin Nutr* 1991; 54:202S-5S.

Watanabe K, Bois FY, Zeise L: Interspecies extrapolation; a reexamination of acute toxicity data. *Risk Analysis* 1992; 12(2):301-10.

Wattenberg L, Leong J: Inhibition of the carcinogenic action of benzopyrene by flavones. *Cancer Research* 1970; 30:1922-5.

Wattenberg LW: Inhibition of carcinogenesis by minor dietary constituents. *Cancer Res* (Supp) 1992; 52:2085s-91s.

Waymack PJ, Chance WT: Effect of prostaglandin E in multiple experimental models; V effect on tumor/host interaction. *Jouranl of Surgical Oncology* 1990; 45:110-16.

Waymack PJ, Klimpel G, Haithcoat J, et al: Effect of prostaglandin E on immune function in normal healthy volunteers. *Surgery, Gynecology & Obstetrics* 1992; 175:329-32.

Wei Y: Effects of fu-zheng jie-du decoction and cyclophosphamidum on the production of tumor necrosis factor in

mice. *Chung Hsi I Chieh Ho Tsa Chih* 1990; 10(6):353-5, 326.

Wei YQ, Zhao X, Kariya Y, Fukata H, et al: Induction of apoptosis by quercetin: involvement of heat shock protein. *Cancer Res* 1994; 54(18):4952-7.

Weidner N, Semple JP, Welch WR, et al: Tumor angiogenesis and metastasis-correlation in invasive breast carcinoma. *New England Journal of Medicine* 1991; 324:1-8.

Weindruch R: Dietary restriction, tumors, and aging in rodents. *J of Gerontology* 1989; 44(6):67-71.

Weindruch R: Effect of caloric restriction on age-associated cancers. *Exp Gerontol* 1992; 27(5-6):575-81.

Weisburger JH: Nutritional approach to cancer prevention with emphasis on vitamins, antioxidants, and carotenoids. *Am J Clin Nutr* 1991; 53:226s-37s.

Weisburger JH, et al: Prevention of arginine glutamate of the carcinogenicity of acetamide in rats. *Appl Pharma Toxicol* 1969; 14:163-75.

Weisman AD, Worden JW: Psychosocial analysis of cancer deaths. *Omega* 1975; 6:61-75.

Weiss GR, Margolin KA, Aronson FR, Sznol M, et al. *J Clin Oncol* 1992; 10(2):275-81.

Weiss RF: *Herbal Medicine*. England: Beaconsfield Publishers, 1991.

Welsch CW: Dietary fat, calories, and mammary gland tumorigenesis. *Adv Exp Med Biol* 1992; 322:203-22.

Welton AF, Hurley J, Will P: "Flavonoids and arachidonic acid metabolism." *Plant Flavonoids in Biology and Medicine II* Alan R. Liss, Inc. 1988; 301-02.

Wendel A, Cikryt P: The level and half-life of gluthione in human plasma. *FEBS Lett* 1980; 120:209-211.

Weng XC, Zhang P, Gong SS, et al: Effect of immunomodulating agents on murine IL-2 production. *Immunol Invest* 1987; 16(2):79-86.

Werner OR, Wallace RK, Charles B, et al: Long-term endocrinologic changes in subjects practicing the transcendental meditation and TM-sidhi program. *Psychosom Med* 1986; 48(1-2):59-66.

Westin JB: Carcinogens in Israeli milk: a study in regulatory failure. *Int J Health Serv* 1993; 23(3):497-517.

Whiteside T, Herberman R: The role of natural killer cells in human disease. *Clinical Immunology and Immunotherapy* 1989; 53:1-23.

Whittemore AS, Wu-Williams AH, Lee M, et al: Diet, physical activity, and colorectal cancer among Chinese in North America and China. *J Natl Cancer Inst* 1990; 82(11):915-26.

Wiernik PH, Yeap B, Vogl SE, et al: Hexamethylmelamine and low or moderate dose cisplatin with or without pyridoxine for treatment of advanced ovarian carcinoma: a study of the Eastern Cooperative Oncology Group. *Cancer Invest* 1992; 10(1):1-9.

Willett WC, Polk BF, Morris JS, et al: Prediagnostic serum selenium and risk of cancer. *Lancet* 1983 Jul 16; 2(8342):130-134.

Willett WC, Stampfer MJ: Selenium and human cancer. *Acta Pharmacol Toxicol* 1986; 59 Suppl 7:240-7.

Williams M: Eleutherococcus senticosus: The use of biological response modifiers in oncology. *British J of Phytotherapy* 1993; 3(1):32-37.

Wilson J, Braunwald E, Isselbacher K, et al. *Harrison's Priciples of Internal Medicine* 12th edition. New York: McGraw-Hill, Inc.; 1991.

Wilson ST, Blask DE, Lemus-Wilson AM: Melatonin augments the sensitivity of MCF-7 human breast cancer cells to tamoxifen in vitro. *J Clin Endrocrinol Metab* 1992 Aug; 75(2):669-70.

Wingo PA, Tong T, Bolden S: Cancer Statistics, 1995. *Ca Cancer J Clin* 1995; 45:8-30.

Wirsching M, Stierlin H, Hoffman F, et al: Psychological identifications of breast cancer patients before biopsy. *J Psychosom Res* 1982; 26:1-10.

Witschi a, Reddy S, Stofer B,et al: The systemic availability of oral glutathione. *Eur J Clin Pharmacol* 1992; 43(6):667-9.

Witte MM, Parker RF, Wang H, Scott RE: Repression of SV40T oncoprotein expression by DMSO. *J Cell Physiol* 1992 Apr; 151(1):50-5.

Wolarsky ER, Finke SR, Prudden JF: Acceleration of wound healing with heterologous cartilage. *Proc Soc Exp Biol Med* 1966; 123(2):556-61.

Wolf M, Ransberger K: *Enzyme Therapy.* New York: Vantage Press; 1972.

Wolfle D, Schmutte, Westendorf J, et al: Hydroxyanthraquinones as tumor promoters: enhancement of malignant transformation of C3H mouse fibroplasts and growth stimulation of primary rat hepatocytes. *Cancer Res* 1990; 50(20):6540-4.

Wong CK, Leung KN, Fung KP, et al: Effects of Pseudostellaria heterophylla on proliferation and differentiation of murine bone marrow cells. *Immunopharmacol Immunotoxicol* 1994; 16(1):71-84.

Wong CK, Leung KN, Fung KP, et al: Mitogenic and tumor necrosis factor producing activities of Pseudostellaria heterophylla. *Int J Immunopharmacol* 1992; 14(8):1315-20.

Wong CK, Lin CS: Remarkable response of lipoid proteinosis to oral dimethyl sulphoxide. *Br J Dermatol* 1988; 119(4):541-4.

Wu JB, Chun YT, Ebizuka Y, et al: Biologically active constituents of centipeda minima; sesquiterpenes of potential anti-allergy activity. *Chem Pharm Bull* 1991; 39(12):3272-5.

Wu JZ, Situ ZQ, Wang W, et al: Antitumor activity of psoralen on the mucoepidermoid carcinoma cell line MEC-1. *Chinese Medical Journal* 1992; 105(11):913-17.

Wynder EL, Taioli E, Rose DP: "Breast cancer — the optimal diet." *Exercise, Calories, Fat and Cancer* MM Jacobs editor. New York: Plenum Press, 1992.

Xiang DB, Li XY: Effects of Achyranthes bidentata polysaccharides on interleukin-1 and tumor necrosis factor-alpha production from mouse peritoneal macrophages. *Chung Kuo Yao Li Hsueh Pao* 1993; 14(4):332-4.

Xiao J, Cui F, Ning T, Zhao W: Effects of alcohol extract from Polygonatum odoratum (Mill.) Druce and Cuscuta australis R. Br. on immunological function of mice injured by burns. *Chung Kuo Chung Yao Chih* 1990 Sep; 15(9):557-9, 578.

Xie SS: Immunoregulatory effect of polysaccharide of Acanthopanax senticosus (PAS). I. Immunological mechanism of PAS against cancer. *Chung Hua Chung Liu Tsa Chih* 1989; 11(5):338-40.

Xie T: Herbal decoction of qingwen baidu yin in treating endotoxic fever in rabbits. *Chung Kuo Chung Hsi I Chieh Ho Tsa Chih* 1993; 13(2):94-7.

Xin YL: Direct current therapy (DCT) for malignant tumors. *Chung Hua Chung Liu Tsa Chih* 1992; 13(6):467-9.

Xin YL: Traditional and western medical treatment of 211 cases of late stage lung cancer. *Chung Kuo Chung Hsi I Chieh Ho Tsa Chih* 1993; 13(3):135-8.

Xu JP: Research on liu wei Rehmannia oral liquid against side effect of drugs of anti-tumor chemotherapy. *Chung Kuo Chung Hsi I Chieh Ho Tsa Chih* 1992; 12(12):734-7, 709-10.

Xu RH, Peng XE, Chen GZ, et al: Effects of cordyceps sinensis on natural killer activity and colony formation of B16 melanoma. *Chin Med J (Engl)* 1992; 105 (2):97-101.

Xu X, Wang HJ, Murphy PA, Cook L, Hendrich, S: Daizein is a more bioavailable soymilk isoflavone than is genistein in adult women. *J Nutr* 1994 Jun; 124(6):825-32.

Yabushita H, Sartorelli AC: Effects of sodium butyrate, dimethylsulfoxide and dibutyryl cAMP on the poorly differentiated ovarian adenocarcinoma cell line AMOC-2. *Oncol Res* 1993; 5(4-5):173-82.

Yagi A, Harada N, Shimomura K, et al: Bradykinin-degrading glycoprotein in Aloe arborescens var. natalensis. *Planta Med* 1987:19-21.

Yagi A, Harada N, Yamada H, et al: Antibradykinin active material in Aloe saponaria. *J Pharm Sci* 1982; 71(10):1172-4.

Yam D: Insulin-Cancer Relationships: Possible Dietary Implication. *Med Hypothesis* 1992; 38:111-17.

Yamada H: Chemical characterization and biological activity of the immunologically active substances in Juzen-taiho-to (Japanese kampo prescription). *Gan To Kagaku Ryoho* 1989 Apr; 16(4 Pt 2-2):1500-5.

Yamada H, Komiyama K, Kiyohara H, et al: Structural characterization and antitumor activity of a pectic polysaccharide from the roots of angelica acutiloba. *Planta Medica* 1990; 56:182-186.

Yamaguchi N, Yoshida J, Ren LJ, et al: Augmentation of various immune reactivities of tumor-bearing hosts with an extract of Cordyceps sinensis. *Biotherapy* 1990; 2(3):199-205.

Yamashiki M, Asakawa M, Kayaba Y, et al: Herbal medicine sho-saiko-to induces in vitro granulocyte colony-stimulating factor production on peripheral blood mononuclear cells. *J Clin Lab Immunol* 1992a; 37(2):83-90.

Yamashiki M, Kosaka Y, Nishimura A, et al: Efficacy of herbal medicine sho-saiko-to on the improvement of impaired cytokine production of peripheral blood mononuclear cells in patients with chronic viral hepatitis. *J Clin Lab Immunol* 1992b; 37(3):111-21.

Yamauchi K, Yagi T, Kuwano S: Suppression of the purgative action of rhein anthrone, the active metabolite of sennosides A and B, by calcium channel blockers, calmodulin antagonists and indometacin. *Pharmacology* 1993; 47(suppl 1):22-31.

Yan L, Boylan LM, Spallholz JE: Effect of dietary selenium and magnesium on human mammary tumor growth in athymic nude mice. *Nutr Cancer* 1991; 16(3-4):239-248.

Yan YS: Effect of Chinese tea extract on the immune function of mice bearing tumor and their antitumor activity. *Chung Hua Yu Fang I Hsueh Tsa Chih* 1992; 26(1):5-7.

Yanagihara K, Ito A, Toge T, Numoto M: Antiproliferative effects isoflavones on human cancer cell lines established from the gastrointestinal tract. *Cancer Res* 1993 Dec 1; 53(23):5815-21.

Yang G, Yu Y: Effects of ginsenoside on the natural killer cell-interferon-interleukin-2 regulatory network and its tumor inhibiting effect. *J of Trad Chin Med* 1988; 8(2):135-140.

Yang YZ, Jin PY, Guo Q, et al: Effect of Astralagus membranaceus on natural killer cell activity and induction of alpha- and gamma-interferon in patients with coxsackie B viral myocarditis. *Chin Med J* (Engl) 1990; 103(4):304-7.

Yano H, Mizoguchi A, Fukuda K, et al: The herbal medicine sho-saiko-to inhibits proliferation of cancer cell lines by inducing apoptosis and arrest at the G0/G1 phase. *Cancer Res* 1994; 54(2):448-54.

Yarbro W, et al eds: N-acetylcysteine: a significant chemoprotective adjunct. *Seminars on Oncology* 1983; (1)(Suppl 1).

Yasukawa K, Takido M, Takeuchi M, et al: "Effect of flavonoids on tumor promoter's activity." *Plant Flavonoids in Biology and Medicine II* Alan R. Liss, Inc., 1988; 247-50.

Yeatman TJ, Risley GL, Brunson ME: Depletion of dietary arginine inhibits growth of metastic tumor. *Arch Surg* 1991; 126:1376-81.

Yeh SF, Chou TC, Liu TS: Effects of anthraquinones of polygonum cuspidatum on hl-60 cells. *Planta Med* 1988; 413-14.

Yeung HW, Cheung K, Leung KN: Immunopharmacology of Chinese medicine I, ginseng induced immunosuppression in virus-infected mice. *Am J Chin Med* 1982; 10(1-4):44-54.

Yeung HW, Poon SP, Li WW, et al: Isolation and characterization of an immunosuppressive protein from Trichosanthes

kirilowii root tubers. *Immunopharmacol Immunotoxicol* 1987; 9(1):25-46.

Yi NY, Feng FP, Yu YM, et al: The action of radix Rehmanniae and Plastrum testudinis on beta-adrenergic receptor-cAMP system. *Chinese Medical Journal* 1987; 100(11):893-8.

Yim CY, Hibbs JB Jr, MeGregor JR, et al: Use of N-acetyl cysteine to increase intracellular glutathione during the induction of antitumor responses by IL-2. *J Immunol* 1994; 152:5796-5805.

Ying SW, Niles LP, Crocker C: Human malignant melanoma cells express high-affinity receptors for melatonin: antiproliferative effects of melatonin and 6-chloromelatonin. *Eur J Pharmacol* 1993 Jul 15; 246(2):89-96.

Yokozaki H, Tottora G, Pepe S, et al: Unhydrolyzable analogues of adenosine 3':5'-monophosphate demonstrating growth inhibition and differentiation in human cancer cells. *Cancer Res* 1992 May 1; 52(9):2504-8.

Yokozawa T, Lee TW, Oura H, et al: Effect of magnesium lithospermate B in rats with sodium induced hypertension and renal failure. *Nephron* 1992; 60(4):460-5.

Yonekura K, Kawakita T, Mitsuyama M, et al: Induction of colony-stiumlating factor(s) after administration of a traditional Chinese medicine, xiao-chai-hu-tang (Japanese name: shosaiko-to). *Immunopharmacol Immunotoxicol* 1990; 12(4):647-67.

Yonekura K, Kawakita T, Saito Y, et al: Augmentation of host resistance to Listeria monocytogenes infection by a traditional Chinese medicine, ren-shen-yang-rong-tang (Japanese name: ninjin-youei-to). *Immunopharmacol Immunotoxicol* 1992; 14(1-2):165-90.

Yoon Sang CC, Huang FL, Kapoor CL: "Role of cyclic AMP in modifying the growth of mammary carcinomas: genomic regulation." *Biological Responses in Cancer* Vol. 4, E Mihich editor. New York: Plenum Press, 1985. pp. 161-79.

Yoshida J, Takamura S, Yamaguchi N, et al: Antitumor activity of an extract of Cordyceps sinensis (Berk.) Sacc. against murine tumor cell lines. *Jpn J Exp Med* 1989; 59(4):157-61.

Yoshida M, Sakai T, Hosokawa N, Marui N, et al: The effect of quercetin on cell cycle progression and growth of human gastric cancer cells. *FEBS Lett* 1990; 260(1):10-3.

Yu G, Ren D, Sun G, et al: Clinical and experimental studies of JPYS in reducing side effects of chemotherapy in late-stage gastric cancer. *J Tradit Chin Med* 1993; 13(1):31-7.

Yu SY, Zhang LA, Yang JX, Qian ZK, Peng YW: Dialectic classification of syndrome diagnosis in traditional Chinese medicine used as new criterion for evaluating prognosis of patients with cervical cancer. *J Tongji Med Univ* 1991a; 11(2):123-5.

Yu SY, Zhu YJ, Li WG, et al: A preliminary report on the intervention trials of primary liver cancer in high-risk populations with nutritional supplementation of selenium in China. *Biol Trace Elem Res* 1991b; 29(3):289-94.

Yuan W: Changes in renal cortical thromboxane A2, prostaglandin F1 alpha and effects of dazoxiben, chuan xiong on in situ immune complex glomerulonephritis in rats. *Chung Hua I Hsueh Tsa Chih* 1993; 73(9):528-31.

Yue Z, et al: Effect of allitridi on platelet aggregation, a preliminary study. *J of Tradit Chinese Med* 1984; 4(1):29-32.

Yung BY, Hsiao TF, Wei LL, et al: Sphinganine potentiation of dimethylsulfoxide-induced granulocyte differentiation, increase of alkaline phosphatase activity and decrease of protein kinase C activity in a human leukemia cell line (HL60). *Biochem Biophys Res Commun* 1994; 199(2):888-96.

Yurkow EJ, Laskin JD: Mechanisim of action of psoralens; Isobologram analysis reveals that ultraviolet light potentiation of psoralen action is not additive but synergistic. *Cancer Chemotherapy Pharmacology* 1991; 27(4):315- 19.

Zacharski LR, Henderson WG, Rickles FR, et al: Effect of warfarin anticoagulation on survival in carcinoma of the lung, colon, head and neck, and prostrate: final report of VA cooperative study #75. *Cancer* 1984; 54:2046-51.

Zaridze D, Evstifeeva T, Boyle P: Chemoprevention of oral leukoplakia and chronic esophagitis in an area of high incidence of oral and esophageal cancer. *Ann Epidemiol* 1993 May; 3(3):225-34.

Zaridze DG, Shevchenko VE, Levchuk AA, et al: Fatty acid composition of phospholipids of erythrocytemembranes and risk of breast cancer. *Vopr Onkol* 1990; 36(12):1442-8.

Zeng XL, Li XA, Zhang BY: Immunological and hematopoietic effect of Codonopsis pilosula on cancer patients during radiotherapy. *Chung Hua Min Kuo Wei Sheng Wu Chi Mien I Hsueh Tsa Chih* 1992:12(10):607-8.

Zhang C, Yang X, Xu L: Immunomodulatory action of the total saponin of gynostemma pentaphylla. *Chung Hsi I Chieh Ho Tsa Chih* 1990d Feb; 10(2):96-98.

Zhang DZ: Effects of traditional Chinese medicine and pharmacology on increasing sensitivity and reducing toxicity in tumor patients undergoing radio-chemical therapy *Chung Kuo Chung Hsi I Chieh Ho Tsa Chih* 1992; 12(3):135-8.

Zhang DZ. *The Treatment of Cancer by Integrated Chinese-Western Medicine* Boulder, Colorado: Blue Poppy Press; 1989.

Zhang DZ: Prevention and cure by traditional Chinese medicine, of the side effects caused by radio-chemotherapy of cancer patients. *Chung Hsi I Chieh Ho Tsa Chih* 1988 Feb; 8(2):114-6.

Zhang E: *Clinic of Traditional Chinese Medicine (II)*. China: Publishing House of Shanghai College of Traditional Chinese Medicine; 1990.

Zhang GL: Treatment of breast proliferation disease with modified xiao yao san and er chen decoction. *Chung Hsi I Chieh Ho Tsa Chih* 1991 Jul; 11(7):400-2, 388.

Zhang H, Xu L, Jin Q, et al: Anti-anaphylactic pharmacological action of water-soluble constituents of gingko biloba L. episperm. *Chi Chung Yao Tsa Chih* 1990a; 15(8):496-7.

Zhang JP, Zhou DJ: Changes in leucocytic estrogen receptor levels in patients with climacteric syndrome and therapeutic effect of luiwei dihuang pills. *Chung Hsi I Chieh Ho Tsa Chih* 1991 Sep; 11(9):521-3, 515.

Zhang L, Nakaya K, Yoshida T, et al: Bufalin as a potent inducer of differentiation of human myeloid leukemia cells. *Biochem Biophys Res Comm* 1991; 178(2):686-693.

Zhang LX, Mong H, Zhou XB: Effect of Japanese Ganoderma lucidum (GL) planted in Japan on the production of interleukin-2 from murine splenocytes. *Chung Kuo Chung Hsi I Chieh Ho Tsa Chih* 1993; 13(10):613-5.

Zhang RJ, Qian JK, Yang GH, et al: Medicinal protection with Chinese herb-compound against radiation damage. *Aviat Space Environ Med* 1990b; 61(8):729-31.

Zhang RX: Laboratory studies of berberine used alone and in combination with 1,3-bis(2-chlorothyl)-1-nitrosourea to treat malignant brain tumors. *Chinese Medical Journal* 1990; 103(8):658-65.

Zhang SL: Changes in cyclic nucleotides and its enzymes in the spleen and plasma of similar spleen deficiency rats induced by rhubarb and the readjusting function of yiqi jianpi decoction. *Chung Hsi I Chieh Ho Tsa Chih* 1990; 10(11):672-4.

Zhang SZ: Treatment of 136 cases of gastrointestinal cancer with chinese medicines. *Shaanxi Traditional Chinese Medicine* 1986; 7(3):111-12.

Zhang TX, Pomerantz DK: Effects of a traditional Chinese herbal medicine (san zhuang wan) on the hypothalamus-pituitary-testis axis of the immature rat. *Am J Chin Med* 1989; 17(3-4):171-7.

Zhang X: [Experiment research on the role of Lycium barbarum polysaccharide in anti-peroxidation.] *Chi Chung Kuo Chung Yao Tsa Chih* 1993; 18(2):110-2,128.

Zhang X, Kuang P, Wu W, Yin X, et al: The effect of radix Slaviae Miltiorrhizae Composita on peroxidation of low density lipoprotein due to copper dichloride. *Beijing J Tradit Chin Med* 1994; 19(3):150-2,190.

Zhang YH, Qi QJ: Anti-tumour study of combined therapy of yi kang ling with chemotherapeutic agents. *Chung Kuo Chung Hsi I Chieh Ho Tsa Chih* 1992 Oct; 12(10):617-9.

Zhang YH, Yoshida K, Isobe SMJ, et al: Modulation by glycyrrhizin of the cell-surface expression of H-2 class I antigens on murine tumour cell lines and normal cell populations. *Immunology* 1990c; 70:405-10.

Zhang Z, Xia SS: Cordyceps sinensis-I as an immunosuppressant in heterotopic heart allograft model in rats. *J Tongji Med Univ* 1990; 10(2):100.

Zhang ZN, Liu EK, Zheng TL, et al: Long term treatment of chronic myeloid leukemia with chinese medicine and busulfan alternately. *Chinese Journal of Integrated Traditional and Western Medicine* 1985b; 5(2):80-82.

Zhang ZN, Liu EK, Zheng TL, et al: Treatment of chronic myelocytic leukemia (CML) by traditional Chinese medicine and Western medicine alternately. *J Tradit Chin Med* 1985a; 5(4):246-8.

Zhao GY: Study on the granule of shencao fuzheng kangai. *Chung Kuo Chung Hsi I Chieh Ho Tsa Chih* 1992; 12(5):292-4, 262.

Zhao HY, Fang WY: Antithrombotic effect of Andrographis paniculata nees in preventing myocardial infarction. *Chin Med J (Engl)* 1991; 104(9):770-5.

Zhao HY, Fang WY: Protective effects of Andrographis paniculata nees on post-infarction myocardium in experimental dogs. *Chin Med J* (Engl) 1990; 10(4):212-7.

Zhao J, Zhang CY, Xu DM, et al: Further study of pollen typhae's effects on the production of tPA and PGI, by cultured endothelial cells. *Thromb Res* 1989; 56(6):677-85.

Zhao J, Zhang CY, Xu DM, et al: The antitherogenic effects of components isolated from pollen typhae. *Thromb Res* 1990; 57(6):957-66.

Zhao KS, Mancini C: Enhancement of the immune response in mice by Astragalus membranaceus extracts *Immunopharmacology* 1990; 20(3):225-33.

Zhao KW, Kong HY: Effect of astragalan on secretion of tumor necrosis factors in human peripheral blood mononuclear cells. *Chung Kuo Chung Hsi I Chieh Ho Tsa Chih* 1993; 13(5):263-5.

Zhao TH: Positive modulating action of shenmaisan with Astralagus membranaceus on anti-tumor activity of LAK cells. *Chung Kuo Chung Hsi Chieh Ho Tsa Chih* 1993; 13(8):471-2.

Zheng W, Blot WJ, Diamond EL, et al: Serum micronutrients and the subsequent risk of oral and pharyngeal cancer. *Cancer Res* 1993 Feb 15; 53(4):795-8.

Zhou QY: "Chinese medicinal herbs in the treatment of viral hepatitis." *Advances in Chinese Medicinal Materials Research.* HM Chang, HW Yeung, WW Tso, A Koo editors. Singapore: Worlld Scientific, 1985.

Zhu XY, HE SZ, Zhong ZH, Zhang FY, et al: Effects of liuwei dihuang granules, pills and decoction on contents of cAMP, E2, T, Zn and Cu in plasma of renal yin deficient patients. *Chung Kuo Chung Yao Tsa Chih* 1993 Aug; 18(8):503-4.

Zhu XY, Yu HY: Immunosupressive effect of cultured Cordyceps sinensis on cellular immune response. *Chung Hsi I Chieh Ho Tsa Chih* 1990; 10(8):485-7.

Ziche M, Morbidelli L, Pacini M, et al: Substance P stimulates neovascularization in vivo and proliferation of cultured endothelial cells. *Microvasc Res* 1990; 40(2):264-78.

Zmewski P, Feit R: *Acumoxa Therapy: A Reference and Study Guide.* Brookline, MA: Paradigm Press; 1989.

Zwi LJ, Baguley BC, Gavin JB, et al: Blood flow failure as a major determinant in the antitumor action of flavone acetic acid. *J Natl Cancer Inst* 1989 Jul 5; 81(13):1005-13.

Addendum

Alessandro R, Kohn EC: Molecular genetics of cancer. *Cancer* 1995; 76(10):1874-1877.

Bagga D, Ashley JM, Geffrey SP, et al: Effects of a very low fat, high fiber diet on serum hormones and menstrual function. *Cancer* 1995; 76:2491-6.

Bussing A, Suzart K, Bergmann J, et al: Induction of apoptosis in human lymphocytes treated with *Viscum album* L. is mediated by the mistletoe lectins. *Cancer Letters* 1996; 99:59-72.

Chihara G: Recent progress in immunopharmacology and therapeutic effects of polysaccharides. *Biol Stand* 1992; 77:191-7.

Chihara G, Hamuro J, Maeda YY et al: Antitumor and metastasis-inhibitory activities of lentinan as an immunomodulator: an overview. *Cancer Detect Prev Supp* 1987; 1:423-43.

Christensen JG, LeBlanc GA: Reversal of multidrug resistance in vivo by dietary administration of the phytochemical indole-3-carbinol. *Cancer Research* 1996; 56:574-581.

Coombe DR, Parish CR, Ramshaw IA, Snowden JM: Analysis of the inhibition of tumor metastasis by sulphated polysaccharides. *Int J Cancer* 1987; 39(1):82-8.

Costelli P, Llovera M, Lopez-Soriano J, et al: Lack of effect of eicosapentaenoic acid in preventing cancer cachexia and inhibiting tumor growth. *Cancer Letters* 1995: 97:25-32.

David G, Van Den Berghe, H: Transformed Mouse Mammary Epithelial Cells Synthesize undersulfated basement membrane proteoglycan. *J Biological Chem* 1983; 258(12):7338-44.

Ebina T, Murata K: Antitumor effect of intratumoral administration of a Coriolus preparation, PSK: inhibition of tumor invasion in vitro. *Gan To Kagaku Ryoho* 1994; 21:2241-3.

Folkers K, Brown R, Judy WV, et al: Survival of cancer patients on therapy with coenzyme Q10. *Biochem Biophys Res Commun* 1993; 192(1):241-5.

Fox AD, DePaula JA, Kripke SA et al: Glutamine-supplemented elemental diets reduce endotoxemia in a lethal model of enterocolitis. *Surg Forum* 1988; 39:46.

Fox AD, Kripke SA, Berman JR et al: Reduction of the severity of enterocolitis by glutamine-supplemented enteral diets. *Surg Forum* 1987; 38:43.

Gogos CA, Ginopoulos P, Zoumbos NC et al: The effect of dietary ω-3 polyunsaturated fatty acids on T-lymphocyte subsets of patients with solid tumors. *Cancer Det and Prev* 1995; 19(5):415-417.

Hardingham TE, Fosang AJ: Proteoglycans: many forms and many functions. *FASEB J* 1992; 6:861-870.

Inohara H, Raz A: Effects of natural complex carbohydrate (citrus pectin) on murine melanoma cell properties related to galectin-3 functions. *Glycoconj J* 1994; 11:527-32.

Jacobs DO, Evans A, O'Dwyer ST, et al: Disparate effects of 5-fluorouracil on the ileum and colon of enterally fed rats with protection by dietary glutamine. *Surg Forum* 1987; 38:45-49.

Jiang WG, Hiscox S, Hallett MB, et al: Regulation of the expression of E-cadherin on human cancer cells by γ-linolenic acid (GLA). *Cancer Res* 1995; 55:5043-48.

Addendum (continued)

Kjellen L, Lindahl U: Proteoglycans: structures and interactions. *Annu Rev Biochem* 1991; 60:443-75.

Klimberg VS, Salloum RM, Kasper M, et al: Oral glutamine accelerates healing of the small intestine and improves outcome after whole abdominal radiation. *Arch Surg* 1990; 125:1040-1045.

Liang JW, Hsiu SL, Wu PP et al: Emodin pharmacokinetics in Rabbits. *Planta Med* 1995 61:406-8.

Lockwood K, Moesgaard S, Folkers K: Partial and complete regression of breast cancer in patients in relation to dosage of coenzyme Q10. *Biochem Biophys Res Commun* 1994a: 199(3):1504-8.

Lockwood K, Moesgaard S, Hanioka T, Folkers K: Apparent partial remission of breast cancer in "high risk" patients supplemented with nutritional antioxidants, essential fatty acids and coenzyme Q10. *Mol Aspects Med* 1994b; 15(suppl):s231-40.

Lockwood K, Moesgaard S, Yamamoto T, Folkers K: Progress on the therapy of breast cancer with vitamin Q10 and the regression of metastasis. *Biochem Biophys Res Commun* 1995: 212(1):172-7.

Naik H, Pilat MJ, Donat T, et al: Inhibition of in vitro tumor cell-endothelial adhesion by modified citrus pectin: a pH modified natural complex carbohydrate. *Proc Am Assoc Cancer Res* 1995; 36:A377.

Nakamura N, Kojima J: Changes in charge density of heparan sulfate isolated from cancerous human liver tissue. *Cancer Research* 1981; 41:278-283.

O'Dwyer ST, Scott T, Smith RJ, et al: 5-Fluorouacil toxicity on small intestinal mucosa but not white blood cells is decreased by glutamine. *Clin Res* 1987; 35:369A.

Okuma K, Furuta I, Ota K: Protective effect of coenzyme Q10 in cardiotoxicity induced by adriamycin. *Gan To kagaku Ryoho* 1984; 11(3):502-8.

Parish CR, Coombe DR, Jakobsen KB et al: Evidence that sulfated polysaccharides inhibit tumor metastasis by blocking tumor-cell-derived heparanases. *Cancer* 1987; 40(4):511-8.

Pienta KJ, Naik H, Akhtar A, et al: Inhibition of spontaneous metastasis in a rat prostate cancer model by oral administration of modified citrus pectin. *J Natl Cancer Inst* 1995; 87:348-353.

Platt D, Raz A: Modulation of the lung colonization of B16-F1 melanoma cells by citrus pectin. *J Natl Cancer Inst* 1992; 84:438-442.

Reichel H, Koeffler HP, Norman AW: The role of the vitamin D endocrine system in health and disease. *NEJM* 1989; 320(15):980-991.

Rita M, Young I, Ihm J, et al: Treating tumor-bearing mice with vitamin D3 diminishes tumor-induced myelopoiesis and associated immunosuppression, and reduces tumor metastasis and recurrence. *Cancer Immunol Immunotherapy* 1995 41:37-45.

Robinson J, Viti M, Hook M: Structure and properties of an under-sulfated heparan sulfate proteoglycan synthesized by a rat hepatoma cell line. *J Cell Biology* 1984; 98:946-953.

Ronca G, Conte A: Metabolic fate of partially depolymerized shark chondroitin sulfate in man. *Int J Clin Pharmacol Res* 1993; 13(suppl):27-34.

Ruoslahti E, Yamaguchi Y: Proteoglycans as modulators of growth factor activities. *Cell* 1991; 64:867-869.

Shi W, Gould MN: Induction of differentiation in neuro-2A cells by the monoterpene perillyl alcohol. *Cancer Letters* 1995; 95:1-6.

Takimoto M, Sakurai T, Kodama K, et al: Protective effect of CoQ10 administration on cardial toxicity in FAC therapy. *Gan To Kagaku Ryoho* 1982; 9(1):116-21.

Tanaka NG, Sakamoto N, Inoue K, et al.: Antitumor effects of an antiangiogenic polysaccharide from an Arthrobacter species with or without a steroid. *Cancer Research* 1989; 49:6727-6730.

Vanderwalle B, Wattez N, Lefebvre J: Effects of vitamin D_3 derivatives on growth, differentiation and apoptosis in tumoral colonic HT 29 cells: possible implication of intracellular calcium. *Cancer Letters* 1995: 97:99-106.

Wang Y, Corr JG, Thaler HY et al: Decreased growth of established human prostate LNCaP tumors in nude mice fed a low-fat diet. *J Natl Cancer Inst* 1995 October 4; 87(19):1456-62.

Yang QY, Kwok CY, editors: *PSP International Symposium 1993*. Shanghai: Fudan University Press, 1993.

Yoon TJ, Yoo YC, Choi OB, et al: Inhibitory effect of Korean mistletoe *(Viscum album coloratum)* extract on tumor angiogenesis and metastasis of haematogenous and non-haematogenous tumor cells in mice. *Cancer Letters* 1995; 97:83-91.

ZhangYW, Zheng QL, Xue Y et al: Treatment of 31 cases of malignant lymphoma with salvia miltiorrhiza. *Journal of Xi'An Medical University* 1989; 10(2):180-83.

ABOUT THE AUTHOR

John Boik is a licensed acupuncturist (LAc.) in Oregon. John received his Masters degree in Acupuncture and Oriental Medicine (MAcOM) from the Oregon College of Oriental Medicine, Portland, and his Bachelors degree in civil engineering from the University of Colorado, Boulder. He is national board certified in both acupuncture and Chinese herbology by the National Commission for the Certification of Acupuncturists (NCCA). He is currently a scientific advisor to the University of Texas Center for Alternative Medicine and serves on the Editorial Review Board for the journal *Alternative Medicine Review*.

INDEX

A

M